Management of Persons with Stroke

MANAGEMENT OF PERSONS WITH STROKE

Editors

MARK N. OZER, M.D.
Medical Director, Stroke Recovery Program
National Rehabilitation Hospital;
Clinical Professor, Department of Neurology
Georgetown University Medical School, Washington, D.C.

with

RICHARD S. MATERSON, M.D.
Senior Vice-President and Medical Director
National Rehabilitation Hospital;
Professor of Physical Medicine and Rehabilitation
Department of Neurology
George Washington University School of Medicine
Washington, D.C.

LOUIS R. CAPLAN, M.D.
Neurologist-in-Chief, New England Medical Center;
Professor and Chairman, Department of Neurology
Tufts University School of Medicine
Boston, Massachusetts

*with **32** illustrations*

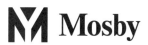 Mosby

St. Louis Baltimore Boston Chicago London Philadelphia Sydney Toronto

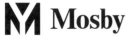 **Mosby**

Dedicated to Publishing Excellence

RC388.5
.M335
1994

Publisher: George Stamathis
Editor: Stephanie Manning
Developmental Editor: Laura DeYoung
Project Manager: Patricia Tannian
Manuscript Editor: Kathy Lumpkin
Designer: Gail Morey Hudson
Manufacturing Supervisor: Kathy Grone
Cover illustration from J Perry: *Clinical Orthopaedics* 63:32-38, 1969.

Printed in the United States of America
Composition by Graphic World, Inc.
Printing/binding by Maple-Vail Book Mfg Group

Mosby–Year Book, Inc.
11830 Westline Industrial Drive, St. Louis, Missouri 63146

Library of Congress Cataloging in Publication Data

Management of persons with stroke / [edited by] Mark N. Ozer.
    p. cm.
    Includes bibliographical references and index.
    ISBN 0-8016-6801-8
    1. Cerebrovascular disease — Treatment. 2. Cerebrovascular
disease — Patients — Rehabilitation. I. Ozer, Mark N.
    [DNLM: 1. Cerebrovascular Disorders — therapy. WL 355 M2655 1994]
RC388.5.M335 1994
616.8'1 — dc20
DNLM/DLC
for Library of Congress   93-7571
                                         CIP

93 94 95 96 97 / 9 8 7 6 5 4 3 2 1

To E.E.

Contributors

T. K. ASADI, M.D.

Consulting Neurologist, Department of Medical Affairs
National Rehabilitation Hospital
Washington, D.C.

CHRISTINE R. BARON, M.A.

Clinical Supervisor, Department of Speech Language Pathology
National Rehabilitation Hospital
Washington, D.C.

CHRISTINE BIRD, M.A., O.T.R./L.

Senior Occupational Therapist
National Rehabilitation Hospital
Washington, D.C.

JOSEPH BLEIBERG, Ph.D.

Director, Department of Psychology
National Rehabilitation Hospital;
Clinical Associate Professor, Department of Neurology
Georgetown University School of Medicine
Washington, D.C.

LOUIS R. CAPLAN, M.D.

Neurologist-in-Chief, New England Medical Center;
Professor and Chairman, Department of Neurology
Tufts University School of Medicine;
Boston, Massachusetts

MAUREEN FREDA, MS, O.T.R./L.

Director, Department of Occupational Therapy
National Rehabilitation Hospital
Washington, D.C.

JAN C. GALVIN

Director, Assistive Technology/Rehabilitation Engineering Program
National Rehabilitation Hospital
Washington, D.C.

WILLIAM GARMOE, Ph.D.

Psychology Service, National Rehabilitation Hospital
Washington, D.C.

THERESE M. GOLDSMITH, M.S., C.C.C.-S.L.P.

Assistant Director, Department of Speech-Language Pathology
National Rehabilitation Hospital
Washington, D.C.;
Adjunct Faculty, Department of Speech-Language Pathology and Audiology
Loyola College
Baltimore, Maryland

JANET M. LIECHTY, M.S.W.

Clinical Social Worker, Social Work Service
National Rehabilitation Hospital
Washington, D.C.

REBECCA C. MAHONEY, B.S., O.T.R./L.

Clinical Specialist, Department of Occupational Therapy
National Rehabilitation Hospital
Washington, D.C.

RICHARD S. MATERSON, M.D.

Senior Vice-President and Medical Director
National Rehabilitation Hospital;
Professor of Physical Medicine and Rehabilitation
Department of Neurology
George Washington University School of Medicine
Washington, D.C.

ANNE C. NEWMAN, Ph.D.

Psychology Service, National Rehabilitation Hospital
Washington, D.C.

LORENZ K.Y. NG, M.D.

Director, Chronic Pain Program
National Rehabilitation Hospital;
Assistant Clinical Professor, Department of Neurology
George Washington University
Washington, D.C.

MARK N. OZER, M.D.

Medical Director, Stroke Recovery Program
National Rehabilitation Hospital;
Clinical Professor, Department of Neurology
Georgetown University Medical School
Washington, D.C.

MICHAEL H. PHILLIPS, M.D.

Consultant Urologist, National Rehabilitation Hospital;
Clinical Assistant Professor, Department of Urology
George Washington University,
Washington, D.C.

PAUL R. RAO, Ph.D.

Co-Director, Stroke Recovery Program
Director, Speech-Language Pathology Service
National Rehabilitation Hospital
Washington, D.C.;
Adjunct Professor, University of Maryland
College Park, Maryland,
Loyola College, Baltimore, Maryland,
Gallaudet University, Washington, D.C.

Acknowledgments

This book represents in large part work done in the Stroke Recovery Program at the National Rehabilitation Hospital. It is appropriate that the book be dedicated to our patients who provided the impetus for this effort; to the professional staff who contributed to the development of the ideas; and most specifically to Edward Eckenhoff, whose vision in the founding of the National Rehabilitation Hospital this book reflects. My special thanks to Paul Rao, Ph.D., who has been my colleague in the development of the care of persons with stroke, and to Sue Hipschen for her extraordinary helpfulness in the production of the book.

Foreword

The ability to define the world and our place in it distinguishes our humanity. Stroke forever alters this world-making capacity. The stroke patient's cosmos, once comprehensible and manageable, is transformed into a confusing, intimidating, and hostile environment. The skills of intellect, sensation, perception, and movement, which are honed over the course of a lifetime and which, when taken together, so characterize our humanity, are the very endowments most compromised by stroke.

Stroke continues to be vastly misunderstood by the public and remains one of the most confounding medical conditions confronting modern health care. To the patient and the family, stroke represents a profound mystery and crisis. The family expects the physician not only to treat the condition, but also to demystify stroke for them and to proclaim a definitive prognosis. To address these concerns responsibly, the clinician assumes the obligations of practitioner and care manager. The mobilization and management of acute care and rehabilitative resources are the essential challenges to the clinician who treats persons with stroke.

Management of Persons with Stroke offers the most comprehensive approach yet taken to stroke treatment and recovery. The text includes a thorough discussion of medical management and offers insights into the broader set of principles that the members of the health delivery team must address in concert with the stroke patient and family. Worthy of particular note is the perspective of stroke survivors themselves. The authors explore the reorganization and reintegration of function and how it is enhanced by contributions the stroke survivor makes at various stages of the recovery process. This book also provides an enlightened perspective on employing an integrated, interdisciplinary team approach for the most effective use of professional resources in achieving optimal patient outcomes.

The National Stroke Association commends the authors of this book for offering the most definitive guidance yet published on stroke care and rehabilitation. We believe health care providers will find this text to be an invaluable new resource as they coordinate their approaches to the management of persons with stroke.

Gary R. Houser
Vice President, National Stroke Association,
Denver, Colorado

Preface

The management of persons with stroke offers an extraordinary opportunity to develop new models for care. Stroke is already the largest single cause of neurologic disability, and the increasingly aging population necessitates greater attention to making care of persons with stroke more effective and less expensive. Because of the enormity of the resources required to deal with this problem and the human costs of inadequate response, innovative approaches are needed.

This book is designed for use by physicians and other health professionals who deal with persons with stroke. Medical specialists such as those in internal medicine, geriatrics, neurology, and physiatry interact with persons with stroke at various stages of the disease. All those specialists must recognize the essential continuity of the disease process and the consequent need for continuity of care. One innovation therefore is to view the management of persons with stroke as a coordinated approach, over time, in which primary prevention and prevention of recurrent stroke are integral parts of care. There is need to prevent impairment as well as alleviate disabilities.

The book emphasizes several other principles by which innovative approaches can be developed to alleviate disabilities once impairments have occurred. Physicians and other health professionals, such as psychologists, social workers, and speech, physical, and occupational therapists, interact with one another and with persons with stroke. All these efforts must be coordinated, with emphasis on areas that help the patient return to and live in the community. There is the need to measure outcomes intrinsic to the process of management, to establish goals, and to revise such goals in light of ongoing experience. Thus undergirding the effective management of persons with stroke is a system in which planning is continuous.

The second principle is that the product of such a planning system is data dealing not only with outcomes but also with techniques for achieving those outcomes. The process is a *problem-solving* planning system. The focus on problem-solving strategies emphasizes the ongoing nature of the problems being faced. The problems and the outcomes vary over time; the strategies for solving them may have more general application. What is to be generated is resourcefulness.

The third principle relates to the development of resources not only in the professionals but also in the persons with the stroke and their families. The resources to be developed are the techniques for solving problems and the ongoing application of these techniques to life problems. Thus one may call the approach a *collaborative* problem-solving planning system.

The major sections of the book deal with the development and implementation of plans during the phases of acute care, rehabilitation, and continuing care. The organization of each section reflects the planning process being described. After the several goals of each phase are identified, the overall problems and the plans for their alleviation are discussed. Thus each phase in the life of a person following a stroke requires the health care professional to develop plans for medical treatment and for prevention of impairments and alleviation of disabilities appropriate to that phase. Within each of the problem areas the organization recapitulates the problem-solving process. For example, the medical plan during the rehabilitation phase deals with the problem of carrying out therapeutic exercise in the context of diabetes and cardiac disease, which are common comorbidities. Identifying the problem and planning to deal with it involve collaboration between health care professionals and the person with stroke in setting goals, finding solutions, and evaluating outcomes. Case reports are used to illustrate application to real-life situations.

The authorship of the various chapters and sections of chapters is indicated, as well as those responsible for editorial direction for the several phases in the life of the person with stroke. When not otherwise stated, the authorship of the several chapters, sections of chapters, and overall editorial responsibility is that of the senior author.

Health care professionals may profit from reading the book sequentially or from focusing on a single phase that is particularly relevant to their concern.

By the end of the book readers should be able to apply the process described to the treatment of persons with stroke. In addition, these self-management principles can be applied more generally to the treatment of the even larger number of persons with other long-term medical problems leading to disabilities.

Mark N. Ozer

Contents

PART I **PRINCIPLES OF MANAGEMENT**

1 **Nature of the Problem,** 2

2 **Natural History of Stroke,** 11

3 **Character of the Solution,** 18

PART II **ACUTE CARE PHASE**
Louis R. Caplan, *editor*
NATURE OF THE PROBLEM, 27

4 **Medical Management Plan,** 30

Nature of the problem, 30
Comorbidity and its effects, 32
Deep vein thrombosis and pulmonary embolus, 34
Bladder management, 43
Michael H. Phillips
Management of seizures, 50
T.K. Asadi

5 **Neurologic Management Plan,** 61
Louis R. Caplan

Nature of the problem, 62
Neurologic assessment of the acute stroke, 63
Treatment, 83
Patterns of neurologic impairment, 92

6 **Rehabilitation Management Plan,** 114

Nature of the problem, 114
Disorders of sensorimotor control, 116
Efficacy of rehabilitation, 131

PART III REHABILITATION CARE PHASE

Richard S. Materson, *editor*

NATURE OF THE PROBLEM, 143

7 Medical Management, 146

Nature of the problem, 146
Diabetes, 147
Cardiac disease, 153

8 Prevention of Recurrent Stroke, 164

Nature of the problem, 164
Management of hypertension, 172
Management of cardiac factors, 180

9 Rehabilitation Management: Principles, 195

Nature of the problem, 196
Management of the interdisciplinary team, 198
Neuropsychologic aspects of normal aging and stroke
rehabilitation, 219
William Garmoe, Anne C. Newman, and Joseph Bleiberg
Preparing the family for discharge: an interdisciplinary approach,
251
Janet M. Liechty

10 Rehabilitation Management: Alleviating Specific Disabilities,
279
Communication disorders, 281
Paul R. Rao
Dysphagia and its management, 310
Therese M. Goldsmith and Christine R. Baron
Enhancing motor function, 332
Training in activities of daily living, 346
Christine Bird and Rebecca C. Mahoney
Training in mobility, 367
Richard S. Materson and Mark N. Ozer

PART IV **CONTINUING CARE PHASE**

Mark N. Ozer, *editor*

NATURE OF THE PROBLEM, 413

11 Enhancing Quality of Life, 416

Nature of the problem, 416
Enhancing family life, 421
Maureen Freda
Enhancing community integration, 433
Jan C. Galvin

12 Ensuring Continuity of Medical Care, 448

Nature of the problem, 448
Stroke prevention, 449
Management of spasticity, 459
Central poststroke pain, 463
Mark N. Ozer and Lorenz K.Y. Ng

APPENDIX **COMMUNITY RESOURCES, 471**

PART I

Principles of Management

1 Nature of the Problem
2 Natural History of Stroke
3 Character of the Solution

CHAPTER 1

Nature of the Problem

Cerebrovascular disease leading to stroke is a principal cause of mortality and morbidity in the United States. Nearly 400,000 Americans suffer a stroke each year, and of these, 150,000 die. The number of stroke survivors in the United States approaches 2 million.[3] Although the incidence is decreasing, stroke still represents the third leading cause of death (after heart disease and malignant neoplasms), and its prevalence in the population appears to be increasing, partially because of increased survival.[12]

The mortality from cerebrovascular disease per se has fallen from 88:100,000 persons in 1950 to 31:100,000 in 1986 — a decrease of about 55%. The incidence of death from cerebrovascular disease fell to 7% of all deaths in 1986 (from almost 11% in 1950). The mortality from cardiovascular disease has remained relatively unchanged; it is still high, comprising nearly 37% of deaths in 1950 and 36% in 1986.[13] The causes of the decline in cerebrovascular deaths remain somewhat unclear; however, improvements in diagnostic accuracy and the widespread treatment of hypertension undoubtedly contributed.[11]

In 1986, 150,000 persons with an underlying diagnosis of stroke died in the United States. One measure used to calculate the effects of such loss is that of years of potential life lost before 65 years of age. This figure is the number of deaths in each age group weighted by 65 minus the midpoint of that age group; for cerebrovascular disease, the loss is in the range of 250,000 years.[5] Age-adjusted mortality rates were 1.2 times higher for males than for females and 1.8 times higher for blacks than for whites. In addition, age-adjusted rates were generally highest in the southeastern states. The management of persons with stroke must be responsive to these statistics.

Mortality is but one of the important measures of the severity of the problem. Another measure is the likelihood of stroke recurrence with a consequent greater degree of significant impairment. Studies on the incidence of stroke and the burden of its recurrence are derived from the National Survey of Stroke carried out in the mid-1970s.[8] During the period of this survey, approximately 400,000 persons with stroke were discharged from short-term-care general hospitals. Of these, approximately 75% were treated for an initial stroke. Approximately one fourth were treated for a recurrent stroke. The overall incidence rate for initial stroke used the total population as a base; the rate for stroke recurrence is based on those at-risk patients having had a previous stroke. In the 45- to 64-year-old age group, the attack rate for initial strokes was about 180:100,000, compared with a 1800 to 3700:100,000 subsequent attack rate in the same age group. In this age group the average rate of recurrence was 15 times the incidence rate for an initial stroke. (The incidence of recurrence figures reflect the various estimates of stroke survivorship, ranging from 1.7 to 2.9 million during the years 1976 to 1977.) The relative incidence rate among persons 65 years of age or older was about 1000:100,000 for initial strokes and about seven times that in those who had had a previous stroke. Thus it appears that the likelihood of stroke recurrence is generally high although greater for those in the younger age group.

The Framingham Heart Disease Epidemiology Study offers a more specific prospective sample of the age-adjusted incidence of stroke and recurrence.[9] In this study, "strokes" included both transient ischemic attacks (TIAs) and completed strokes. The latter included atherothrombotic infarction (ABI), cerebral embolism (CE), and intracerebral hemorrhage (ICH). Subarachnoid hemorrhage was also included. Survival rates were calculated for the ABI group alone and for all strokes combined.

The fatality rate during the first 30 days following a vascular event varied with the type of stroke. Fig. 1-1 describes the 30-day case fatality rate (CFR). The CFR was 46% for subarachnoid hemorrhage and 67% for ICH. The overall CFR for CE and ABI was approximately the same — about 15% — although there was an inexplicable marked difference in early death between males and females with CE.

Long-term survival was reported only for the ABI group (Fig. 1-2). After surviving the original vascular event, those patients with ABI who were free of hypertension and cardiac comorbidity survived nearly as well at the end of the first 5 years as did the general population in the same age group. For men with both cardiac comorbidity and hypertension, the cumulative 5-year survival rate was reduced from 85% to 35%. Cardiac comorbidity alone reduced the ABI 5-year survival rate in men substantially — from 69% to 41%. Hypertension alone reduced the male survival rate to 51%. For women, there was somewhat less effect; however, in the presence of both risk factors, a substantial reduction (from 70% to 55%) was seen in the 5-year survival rates. For a second stroke after ABI, men experienced a 42% 5-year cumulative recurrence rate and women a 24% rate, despite a similarity in age in the two groups. This high rate in males was reduced to 28% by excluding those with cardiac comorbidity and a history of hypertension before the initial vascular episode. A similar exclusion in females reduced the rate of recurrence only slightly (to 19%).

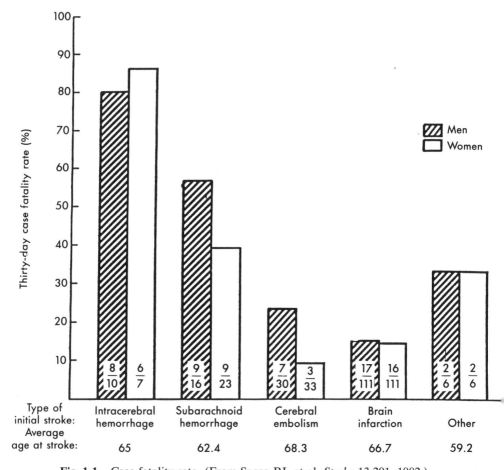

Fig. 1-1 Case fatality rate. (From Sacco RL et al: *Stroke* 13:291, 1982.)

Thus, among long-term survivors, cardiovascular disease is a leading contributor to death. Cardiovascular disease and hypertension are also important factors causing stroke recurrence, particularly in men. These findings have provided the basis for intervention that attempts to reduce the effects of these risk factors and to prevent initial stroke, its recurrence, and mortality. The management of specific risk factors is discussed throughout this book; it forms an important part of management during the several life phases of the person with stroke.

The extent to which the treatment of risk factors contributes to a reduction in stroke mortality has been calculated for many disorders. Hypertension is just one example. Based on data from 1986 it is estimated that almost one third of the 150,000 deaths from stroke might be eliminated by maintaining systolic blood

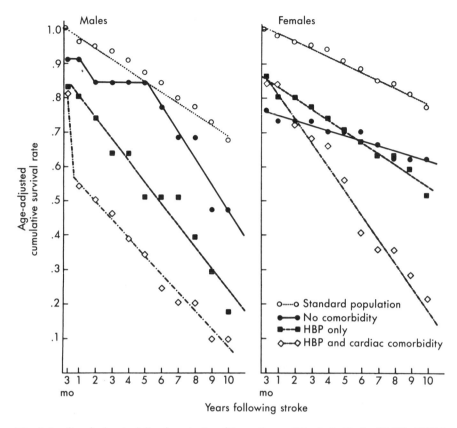

Fig. 1-2 Survival rate following stroke. (From Sacco RL et al: *Stroke* 13:291, 1982.)

pressure below 140 mm Hg. The overwhelming proportion of that reduction could be achieved by maintaining systolic blood pressure below 160 mm Hg. Table 1-1 illustrates this finding along with other risk factors, such as smoking and diabetes.[6] Deaths caused by coronary artery disease would be substantially reduced by lowering cholesterol levels, another potentially treatable risk factor; the reduction is projected to be approximately 40%.[6] Similarly, in a clinical follow-up, survival during the postacute period of a stroke was reviewed in patients who underwent rehabilitation.[14] The absence of a history of myocardial disease was particularly relevant to 2-year survival rates.

Studies of mortality and the incidence of stroke occurrence reflect the extent of the problem only in its broadest outlines. The associated morbidity is more difficult to delineate, particularly in respect to the disabilities resulting from brain injury. The burden of care that falls on the population as a result of stroke is difficult to estimate. Levels of disability and the care involved vary with the

TABLE 1-1   Effects of Risk Factors

RISK FACTOR	PREVALENCE (%)	RELATIVE RISK	POPULATION-ATTRIBUTABLE RISK (%)	ESTIMATED DEATHS
Hypertension				
Systolic pressure:				
140-159 mm Hg	12.0	1.56	4.6	6,863
>159 mm Hg	17.7	3.25	27.2	40,583
TOTAL			31.8	47,446
Smoking among males				
Former	28.9	1.29	5.7	3,363
Current	31.2	2.24	26.3	15,518
Smoking among females				
Former	17.4	1.06	0.8	722
Current	26.5	1.84	18.1	16,326
TOTAL			24.1	35,929
Diabetes				
Male	5.7	1.60	3.3	1,947
Female	7.4	1.80	5.6	5,051
TOTAL			4.7	6,998

From Hahn RA, Teutsch SM, Rothenberg RB: *Chronic disease reports from the MMWR*, Atlanta, 1990, US Department of Health and Human Services.

severity of the injury and the specific character of the impairments. Care also varies with the availability of family and community resources that can help supplant or at least mitigate the need for institutional care.

The percentage of patients requiring institutional care is a useful gross estimate of the burden of care needed as a result of stroke. This figure ranges from 10% to 30%.[12] Based on one recent estimate of the number of patients with initial strokes who were discharged from short-term-care hospitals — 300,000[8] — those requiring institutional care (about 20%) are approximately 50,000 to 60,000 persons. At a cost of approximately $36,000 per year for "intermediate care,"[4] the projected costs are in the range of $1 billion per year. For those patients with recurrent stroke, the requirement for institutional care increases. If, of the 100,000 persons suffering a recurrent stroke, 30% require institutional care, the cost would be an additional $500 million, for a total minimal cost of $1.5 billion for the first year after stroke. A more accurate estimate of the cost for those institutionalized with stroke uses the prevalence figure of 2.5 million.[7] If the lowest figure for the incidence of institutionalization is used (10% rather than

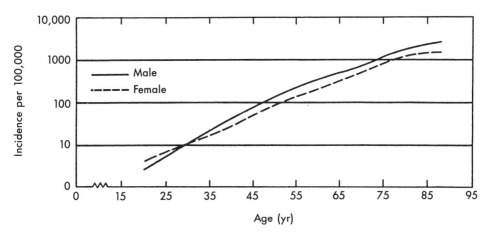

Fig. 1-3 Initial attacks of strokes. Age-specific incidence rates of persons hospitalized for initial strokes per 100,000 population by sex, 1975-1976. (From Robins M, Baum HM: *Stroke* I [suppl 12]:I45, 1981.)

20% or 30%), 250,000 patients require such care at a total cost of $9 billion each year for care in long-term facilities. These costs reflect charges only for basic care in intermediate-term-care facilities.

Costs include not only financial expenditures but the price paid in human terms if treatment is less effective. The costs for those requiring institutionalized care include the loss of independence; for society and the family, the burden of providing care must be met. For many the specter of being severely impaired and unable to live independently is so devastating that they would prefer not to live at all. Additional costs accrued in caring for the remaining 90% of those patients with stroke living in community settings are undoubtedly high, although they cannot be estimated as readily as for those in institutions. The effects of stroke are clearly devastating to the individual, the family, and society.

Despite the decrease in incidence, the severity of the problem is likely to increase because the incidence of initial stroke is related to age and the age distribution of the population shows a steadily increasing elderly fraction. Fig. 1-3 illustrates the usual pattern of rise in incidence with increased age.[8] For example, the incidence of "stroke admissions" in 1975 to 1976 in Table 1-2 shows the relationship between the various decades. The average rate of increase in age-specific rates doubles each decade in those between the ages of 45 and 85 years. The average risk for stroke is particularly high for men, reflecting a 60% higher age-adjusted incidence for the more common nonhemorrhagic strokes. More recent data continue to show that the median incidence of stroke (excluding subarachnoid hemorrhage) is in the decade of 60 to 70 years of age.[1] In the age distribution for thrombotic stroke, somewhat greater than two thirds of patients are in the age group 61 years old and older.

TABLE 1-2 Incidence Rates of Initial Strokes per 100,000 Population, 1975-1976*

AGE (YR)	TOTAL	MALE	FEMALE
Under 35	3.3	2.5	4.1
35-44	31.3	41.5	25.7
45-54	106.2	123.3	90.3
55-64	262.2	341.6	191.1
65-74	582.5	658.4	524.2
75-84	1382.6	1713.6	1180.2
85 and older	1824.8	2504.0	1501.1

Modified from Robins M, Baum HM: *Stroke* I(suppl 12):I45, 1981.
*Data from short-term general hospitals in conterminous United States.

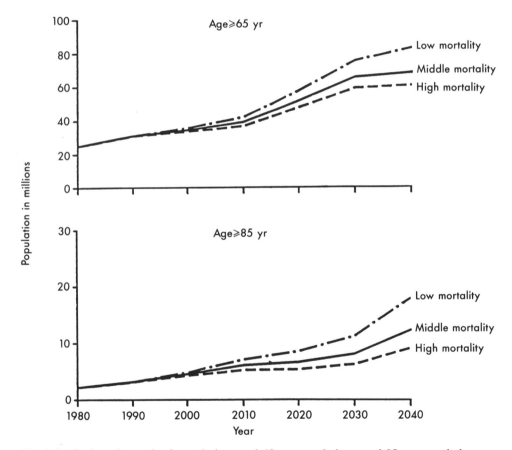

Fig. 1-4 Projected growth of population aged 65 years and above and 85 years and above. Projections are based on low (series 9), middle (series 14), and high (series 19) mortality assumptions from the U.S. Bureau of Census. (From Schneider EL, Guralnick JM: *JAMA* 263:1335, 1990.)

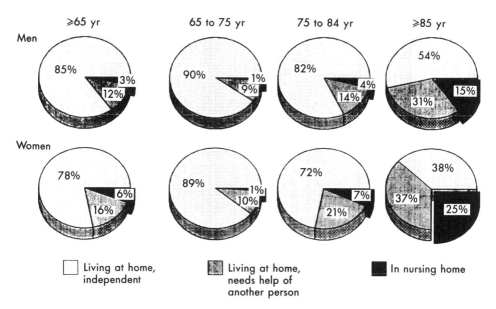

Fig. 1-5　Percentage of the population by age group and sex who (1) live at home independently, (2) live at home but require the help of another person, or (3) reside in a nursing home. The percentages of older persons in nursing homes by age group are from the 1985 National Nursing Home Survey. The percentages of persons living at home and needing assistance are from analyses of data from The Supplement on Aging to the 1984 National Health Interview Survey, applied to the total population. Assistance is defined as needing help with one or more of the following activities: eating, dressing, bathing, transferring from bed to chair, using the toilet, walking, cooking, shopping, managing money, using the telephone, and performing light housekeeping. (From Schneider EL, Guralnick JM: *JAMA* 263:2335, 1990.)

The present and projected rapid growth in the oldest age groups is illustrated in Fig. 1-4.[10] The projected population of persons over 65 years of age (using the current Census Bureau middle mortality series) will rise to 52 million by the year 2020. If low mortality occurs, the projection will increase to 57 million. An examination of the projected increase in the group over 85 years of age is even more impressive; the middle mortality projection forecasts 6.7 million by the year 2020.

The dramatic impact of these figures becomes clear when one considers the likelihood of the increase in disability and institutionalization. The burden of care resulting from disability in 1985 was based on data about those requiring nursing homes and those needing help from another person although living at home. Fig. 1-5 describes these data.[10] The percentage of persons in the 65- to 74-year-old age group residing in nursing homes is only 1%, with an additional 10% requiring help at home. These figures increase substantially in the next decade, 75 to 84 years of age. For those over 85 years of age, a majority of women (62%) and a substantial proportion of men (46%) either reside in nursing homes or need assistance to live at home.

The specific contribution of stroke to this pattern of disability in the elderly is substantial although difficult to evaluate. There is no doubt that the incidence of morbidity and the burden of care will increase as the population ages and that at least some part of these effects will be due to stroke. The prevention of stroke, the reduction of the burden of care, and most particularly the reduction in the number of those requiring institutionalization must be seen as a high priority and an increasing problem. The goal must be to postpone disability until later in life, if at all, and to minimize the degree of such disability, particularly the loss of independence.[2]

Thus it is particularly incumbent on health care workers to develop new models that might be responsive to these important needs. The price of failure is high. The severity of the problem is clear. What is necessary is an exploration of the opportunities for affecting these issues.

REFERENCES

1. Foulkes MA et al: The stroke data bank: design, methods and baseline characteristics, *Stroke* 19:547, 1988.
2. Fries JF: The sunny side of aging, *JAMA* 263:2354, 1990.
3. Goldstein M: The decade of the brain: challenge and opportunities in stroke research, *Stroke* 21:373, 1990.
4. *Guide to retirement living in metropolitan Washington,* McLean, Va, 1991, Douglas Publishing.
5. Hahn RA, Teutsch SM, Rothenberg RB: *Chronic disease reports from the MMWR,* Atlanta, 1990, US Department of Health and Human Services.
6. Hahn RA et al: Excess deaths from nine chronic diseases in the United States, *JAMA* 264:2654, 1990.
7. National Institute of Disability Related Research: *National health interview survey, 1983–1985: data on disability,* Washington, DC, 1988, The Institute.
8. Robins M, Baum HM: Incidence, *Stroke* 1(suppl 12):145, 1981.
9. Sacco RL et al: Survival and recurrence following stroke: the Framingham study, *Stroke* 13:291, 1982.
10. Schneider EL, Guralnik JM: The aging of America and impact on health care costs, *JAMA* 263:2335, 1990.
11. Sheinberg P: Controversies in the management of cerebral vascular disease, *Neurology* 38:1609, 1988.
12. Stineman MG, Granger CV: Epidemiology of stroke related disability and rehabilitation outcome, *Phys Med Rehabil Clin North Am* 2:457, 1991.
13. Sutherland JE, Persky VW, Brody JA: Proportionate mortality trends: 1950 through 1986, *JAMA* 264:3178, 1990.
14. Wade DT et al: Long-term survival after stroke, *Age Aging* 13:76, 1984.

CHAPTER 2

Natural History of Stroke

The early mortality and age incidence for persons with subarachnoid hemorrhage differ markedly from other stroke patient subgroups. The etiologic factors of their strokes, such as congenital aneurysm, may also differ. This group of patients are thus not dealt with in the text. The demographics of the incidence of intracerebral hemorrhage (ICH) may also be different, with an etiology presumably related in part to cerebral angiomata. However, the availability of computed tomography (CT) has changed the management and prognosis of persons with ICH, and the improvement in the early survival of those with ICH has been marked.[7] A large percentage of ICH can be attributed to hypertension.[8] Thus the medical histories of patients with ICH now approximate those whose pattern has been thrombotic or embolic disease leading to cerebral infarction. The etiology and prognosis for nonhemorrhagic stroke somewhat resemble ICH: there is a concomitant history of hypertension, more widespread cardiovascular disease, and the possibility of recurrence. Thus patients with ICH are considered here along with those who have nonhemorrhagic stroke.

The relative incidence of the various disease entities is described in Table 2-1, derived from the Stroke Data Bank.[6] Excluding those with primary subarachnoid hemorrhage, the subject of this book is the management of "stroke" in persons with vascular disease. Included are hemorrhagic intracerebral stroke and infarction. Thus this text pertains to the health care of 85% of those who experience stroke and 95% of those who live beyond the first 30 days after a vascular event.

At this point, it is useful to consider the well-established distinction between "impairment" and "disability."[10] "Impairment" refers to the loss of sensation and coordination of motor actions or language that may occur with injury to the brain. "Disability" refers to the functional consequences of such impairments—that is, the life actions of the person affected. For example, the impairments in motor coordination called "hemiparesis" frequently lead to a disability in mobility. The disturbances found on visual field examination are impairments that can lead to a disability in propelling a wheelchair around obstacles. Impairments in cognition may lead to disabilities in learning the

TABLE 2-1 Distribution of Diagnosis by Subtype of Stroke

SUBTYPE	PERCENT
Cerebral infarctions	
Infarct, unknown cause	32
Embolic	14
Atherosclerotic	6
Lacune	19
Hemorrhage	
Intracerebral	13
Subarachnoid	13
Other	3

Modified from Foulkes MA et al: *Stroke* 19:547, 1988.

compensatory strategies helpful in overcoming problems such as safely propelling a wheelchair.

The management of persons with stroke requires recognition of the several phases at which an opportunity exists to affect the medical course. The life of the person with stroke has been divided into three phases: acute, rehabilitation, and continuing care. Each of these phases is defined by criteria and expected outcomes. For example, in the acute care phase a major effort is devoted to minimizing the degree of impairment. Fig. 2-1 describes the development of impairment from brain injury and some of the actions that can be taken.

It is first necessary to recognize that, at any stage, the effects of stroke result from the interaction of multiple factors, which are subject (at least in part) to modification. The first stage involves the underlying disease process leading to cerebrovascular disease; the occurrence of a stroke is a sudden expression of a disease process involving the distribution of nutrients to the brain via the vascular system. The suddenness of the episode belies the long-standing chronicity of the underlying vascular disease and its high likelihood of further progression over time. The disturbance in blood supply to the brain is also an expression (within a limited, although crucial, area of the body) of a more diffuse process involving the vascular system, with particular effects on the heart. As mentioned earlier, one of the major opportunities in the management of stroke patients is that of lessening the effects of those ongoing risk factors that contribute to both the initial appearance of stroke and its subsequent recurrence.

Vascular insufficiency can appear in the anterior (carotid) or posterior (vertebral and basilar) circulation and in any one of the arteries in either of those systems. Occlusion within one portion of the vascular tree is but one factor affecting the distribution or extent of injury. Vascular insufficiency in any portion

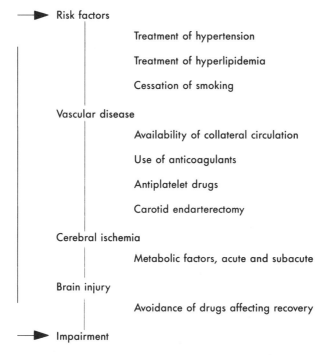

Fig. 2-1 Cascade leading to impairment.

of the vascular tree results from more than merely the vessel occluded. The effects also result from the degree to which the vascular system can respond to that occlusion by providing nutrients to the brain via alternative collateral routes. The diffuse nature of atherosclerotic disease affects the degree of responsiveness. The rate at which the obstruction occurs can further modify the degree to which collateral circulation can respond; for instance, a slower onset can mitigate the degree of insufficiency through the development of collateral circulation.

The degree to which the anterior or posterior circulation is affected and the extent to which the disease process is intracranial or extracranial and implicates the heart and the vascular system is important. Some of the opportunities of management are to improve heart function and lessen the likelihood of arrhythmia; to lessen the likelihood of blood clots from the heart by treatment with anticoagulant medication, and to diminish obstruction within the major extracranial arteries via surgery or antiplatelet drugs.[2] Although generally initiated during the acute phase, there is a need for ongoing management of these treatments during the subsequent phases.

The degree to which infarction occurs with consequent impairment in neurologic function is affected by more than just the metabolic supply provided by the vascular system. A sequence of initiating events occurs, particularly concerning the continued breakdown of glucose in the absence of oxygen. Th process of nonaerobic glycolysis leading to relative lactic acidosis can increase the severity and extent of the neuronal damage. Further metabolic derangements occur, the early mitigation of which can limit the extent and severity of injury. This provides another opportunity to affect the cascade of events that appears at first to be inexorable.[9]

Another opportunity to affect the course of the patient's condition lies in the relationship between the degree of neuronal injury and its consequent disturbance in neurologic function. These disturbances are considered "impairments," with the signs and symptoms affecting the motor, sensory, and other systems of the body. The extent and duration of such impairments are explained only in part by the site and extent of the neural injury, which are usually evident on an examination of the nervous system using single photon emission computed tomography or another imaging technique. It is well established that early recovery of neurologic function does occur, although the mechanism is unclear. For example, *diaschisis* is the term given to relatively temporary distant effects of the neural injury that appear initially. Such disruptions in function reflect a physiologic change but not necessarily permanent destruction of tissue.[4]

One of the tasks of management in the acute phase is to minimize such impairments by protecting the integrity of brain tissue that is metabolically deranged but not yet destroyed. It is necessary to recognize the development of edema and other factors leading to further neural injury and to minimize their extent; this is the major task of management in the acute phase. During the acute and subsequent phases, avoiding the administration of drugs that could disrupt function is another means of mitigating the effects of injury to the brain.

Even with a constant degree of injury, restoration can occur. Reorganization takes place, with a subsequent return of function. Presumably, such recovery occurs through the development of new connections between the existing neural elements. One of the management tasks initiated during the acute phase and continued during the rehabilitation phase is to enhance such recovery to the fullest extent possible. At a minimum, an effort must be made to prevent secondary impairments such as pain and limitation in motion caused by soft tissue derangements.

In addition, it is important to determine the nature of impairments that remain — that is, whether their distribution is mainly within the brainstem, in the portion above the tentorium, or both and whether they are located on the right or left sides and more anterior or posterior. One of the management tasks during the acute phase is to consider the implications of a particular set of impairments to formulate a prognosis and to plan the long-term rehabilitation program. For example, a person with marked motor impairment and impairment in position sense may have difficulty in learning to transfer safely from a bed to a chair. Particularly relevant to rehabilitation planning is the degree to which communication and learning abilities are impaired because the patient frequently needs to acquire new modes of carrying out activities of daily living. For example, the

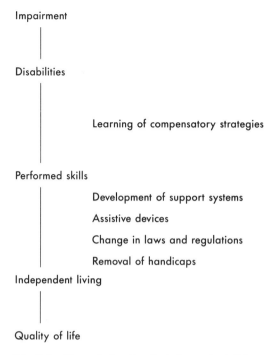

Fig. 2-2 Cascade leading to independent living.

ability to compensate for impairment in motor skills is influenced by the extent to which there is intact comprehension of instructions. Rehabilitation is primarily a learning opportunity.

The next level of analysis is also of primary importance in the rehabilitation phase. Fig. 2-2 describes the interaction of the several elements contributing to the amelioration of the functional disabilities arising from impairment in the brain. The character of the impairments determines to a significant degree, but not completely, the severity and quality of the problems faced by the patient in accomplishing activities of daily living. Achieving mobility, caring for oneself and others, communicating thoughts and feelings, and organizing and performing other more complex activities of daily living are affected by disturbances in previously established modes of function. However, the development of compensatory strategies can significantly contribute to overcoming disabilities despite continued impairment. The context in which those compensatory strategies are most effectively acquired is the major management opportunity described in this book. Rehabilitation is primarily a learning opportunity, and the environment for such learning must be adjusted so that disabilities can be alleviated by learning to perform new skills.

The patient's eventual living arrangements depend on still another level of analysis. Functional problems or disabilities vary, not only with the impaired person and the ability to learn compensatory strategies, but also with the availability of support systems within the family and the community. The presence or absence of such support systems often determines whether the patient lives in an institutional or noninstitutional setting. An ongoing goal of management is to develop within such support systems the requisite degree of confidence and competence to care for the person with stroke.

The patient's eventual outcome is also a result of the interaction between the patient and the environment. Major criticism about outcome measurement has come about from the independent living (IL) movement. "Quality of life" is the degree to which the person with disabilities is able to function in the full range of social roles — that is, to work (including employment) and to participate in other social and leisure activities (including family life). Measures have been developed that reflect the basic premise of the IL movement, which maintains that self-determination rather than institutional life and supervision by others is necessary for the optimum quality of life. These measures include an evaluation not only of the restrictiveness of living arrangements but also of the patient's productivity (both inside and outside the home) and (on an even broader level) of his or her contribution to community and family life.

A number of environmental variables should be considered in light of the IL thesis that these factors contribute more heavily to the results achieved than do the classic measures that focus on the individual's level of impairment and disability. When the IL version of patient outcome is considered, the ability to get into a vehicle is particularly important. Access to transportation is an example of a significant determinant in achieving the optimum quality of life. Awareness of these issues must be integral to the planning and training of patient management during the rehabilitation phase and should be implemented during the continuing care phase. Individual limitations, such as functional deficits as measured by the Barthel Index, interact significantly with environmental factors to affect ultimate results. The dynamic nature of the interactions between the individual and environmental factors must be considered.[3]

Handicaps is the term that refers to the deleterious effects of the physical and social environment on the patient's outcome.[5] For example, a person with hemiparesis may have learned to become mobile by using a wheelchair. However, this disability cannot be alleviated if doorways are too narrow and stairs block entrances. Becoming employed once again may be enhanced by the ability to commute to work via accessible transportation. Enhancing the availability and access to resources can improve the patient's outcome, despite the severity of disability. The removal of physical handicaps, such as stairs that block entrances, can aid the patient's integration into the community. Other assistive devices can provide a more effective interface between the person with disabilities and a relatively unchanged environment. The wheelchair is a prime example. Even more important are changes in social attitudes and in laws concerning income maintenance that discourage employment.[1]

The sequence of events in the process of vascular disease (Figs. 2-1 and

2-2) is not as a sudden inexorable unidirectional process; rather, at multiple stages, interventions can occur that can change the direction of events. The problem can be seen in terms of its potential for solution and amelioration.

From the perspectives of the health care system and the person who has experienced stroke, the focus of intervention traditionally has been the sudden loss of function — hence the term *stroke*. However, it is necessary to view this episode in the context of time, both before and after. The person who has had a stroke can live for many years and, in most instances, can live an active and independent life with a disease process that can be ameliorated considerably. Thus life after a stroke should be viewed both with greater hope and with a greater sense of possibility.

Opportunities for modifying the sequence of events leading to and following stroke exist throughout the various phases. However, at present, the major opportunities exist in the modification of those risk factors amenable to change, preventing primary stroke or reducing the likelihood of recurrence. These risk factors include hypertension and cardiac disease. Major opportunities also exist to learn new compensatory strategies that enable the person with stroke to regain independent function. In the near future, it is anticipated that further opportunities to mitigate the degree of neural injury caused by vascular insufficiency will exist in treatment during the acute phase — primarily by early recognition of stroke warning signs and prompt treatment.

The commonality in all these opportunities lies in the degree to which one may enhance the results by involving the person with stroke. Given the magnitude of the problem and the need for cost-effective solutions, the goal is to solve problems by creating resourcefulness and by considering the person with stroke and family members as valuable sources for doing so.

REFERENCES

1. Bowe F: *Handicapping America: barriers to disabled people,* New York, 1978, Harper & Row.
2. Caplan LR: *Stroke: a clinical approach,* Boston, 1991, Butterworth.
3. De Jong G, Branch LG: Predicting the stroke patient's ability to live independently, *Stroke* 12:648, 1982.
4. Feeney DM, Baron JC: Diaschisis, *Stroke* 17:817, 1986.
5. Finkelstein V: Attitudes and disabled people: issues for discussion, *World Rehabilitation Fund Monographs*, No. 5, 1980.
6. Foulkes MA et al: The stroke data bank: design, methods and baseline characteristics, *Stroke* 19:547, 1988.
7. Garraway WM, Whisnant JP, Drury I: The changing pattern of survival following stroke, *Stroke* 14:699, 1983.
8. Helweg-Larsen S et al: Prognosis for patients treated conservatively for spontaneous intracerebral hematomas, *Stroke* 15:1045, 1984.
9. Plum F: What causes infarction in ischemic brain, *Neurology* 33:222, 1983.
10. Wood PH, Barley EM: *People with disabilities,* New York, 1980, World Rehabilitation Fund.

CHAPTER 3

Character of the Solution

In the management of the person who has experienced stroke, the goals are to enable the person to function free of illness, to prevent recurrent stroke, to minimize impairments arising from resulting brain injury, and to ameliorate the functional disabilities of persons who experience impairment. The purpose of this text is to provide methods to deal with these major goals at the different phases of the patient's life. The enormity of the problem requires the effective use of all resources.

Each of these overall goals includes the development of a series of plans. Supporting these plans is the process by which the plans are generated. To maximize the contribution of resources by all participants in implementing the plan, these same participants must contribute to the process by which the plan is generated. Particularly important is the contribution by the primary participants — that is, the person with stroke and his or her family. Therefore it is necessary for such persons to contribute to the planning process to the maximal extent possible.

Fig. 3-1 describes the basic cyclical structure of the planning process. Plans must incorporate the goals, the means, and time for evaluation. At the appointed time, the plans are reviewed and revised. The degree to which an individual goal or several goals have been achieved can aid in setting new goals. The methods that were helpful in reaching the initial goals also must be reviewed and revised in light of experience. Not only can one define new goals at this time, one must also revise and make more appropriate the means of achieving them. The time when evaluation takes place can also be revised in light of the rate with which one anticipates results. Although the cyclical structure implies a time interval between the plan, its implementation, and its review, it is valuable to carry out this process in an ongoing way. At any point in the implementation, one can choose to review the techniques or methods in use, the outcomes being achieved, and the rate with which reassessment and review are carried out.

The planning process can be defined as a set of questions to be answered. The box on p. 19 lists those questions. Ordinarily the question about a problem or concern precedes the question about goals during the delineation of the initial plan. A review of the outcomes, methods, or both is appropriate some time after

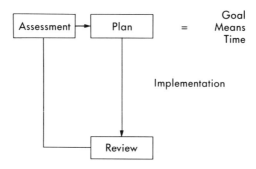

Fig. 3-1 The planning cycle.

Planning Questions

1. What are the concerns? What problems exist?
2. What are the goals?
3. What outcomes have been achieved?
4. What has succeeded in producing such outcomes?

---

the plan has been made and implemented. One may choose to emphasize another question at any time. One may choose to address the question about outcome alone on a daily basis and to revise one's means less frequently. One may address the question about concerns and goals more or less frequently.

The initial question addressed in all basic medical interviews is the one dealing with problems or concerns. A working alliance must be established between the physician (or other health professional) and the patient. The interview is the most powerful and sensitive instrument by which to achieve this alliance. Prerequisite to that alliance is the patient's feeling that he or she is being understood, based on that individual's interaction with the physician (or other health professional). If the patient senses that his or her experiences are understood, trust is enhanced. It is essential that the patient's main concerns and fears be uncovered rather than hasty reassurances being given. Reassurance should be used only after the complaint has been clarified and empathy with the concerns has been conveyed. As Peabody stated, "The secret of the care of the patient is in caring for the patient."[4]

Cassell makes an important distinction between "disease" and "illness." The latter is the subjective source of the suffering for which the person seeks relief; the relief of suffering becomes even more imperative if there is chronicity of disease. For suffering to be effectively treated, its presence must be recognized. Yet the difficulty of such recognition is inherent in the subjectivity of the data.[5] For instance, a threat of, or injury caused by, a stroke may be so overwhelming that any individual may be expected to suffer because of it. Nevertheless, the suffering of each patient is individual and particular despite the common characteristics that make suffering possible.

The recognition of an individual's suffering by others is enhanced if the individual can describe it. One way to get such a description is to ask for it. This may not suffice, but it is at least worth trying. Total knowledge of another person is impossible. Yet the patient must have evidence that someone cares. Thus the successful interview must meet the characteristics of a "dialogue."[9]

The expression of concerns by the patient is an important part of the healing interaction. The physician can then recognize the existence of such concerns. The actions of the interviewer can help the patient develop statements about concerns. Frequently and perhaps unwittingly, the patient's expression of concerns is inhibited or interrupted.[3] In one study it was reported that control of the interaction by the physician generally occurred after only 18 seconds; at that time the physician asked direct questions that could be answered with a yes or no. The physician's use of open-ended questions elicited a more complete range of patient concerns. When dealing with concerns other than physical complaints, there is a particular requirement for open-ended interaction. The patient's initial statement of concern ("chief complaint") determines the patient's primary problem in as much as 76% of somatic, but only 6% of psychosocial, problems. It is necessary to solicit additional concerns periodically throughout the visit to overcome (at least partially) this loss of potentially relevant information from the patient.

In answering questions about concerns, the person with stroke can begin to identify the effects of the impairments in terms of his or her individual needs. For example, when several persons with weakness on the left side of the body were asked about their concerns, the answers varied in a way that the questioner could not foresee. When one woman was asked, her eventual answer was, "I'm afraid that I will lose my balance on my steep front steps." Another described her concern about no longer being able to carry out her gardening or care for her granddaughter. One man described his concern about no longer being able to care for his wife, who was disabled. These patients each defined their disabilities in terms of their individual lives, despite similar degrees of impairment.

Therefore it is important to adequately explore all the questions in the planning process. It is helpful to permit at least threefold exploration of the initial question about concerns to identify what are indeed the major concerns. The threefold exploration of answers to this question helps to establish the issue most important for that particular person. For instance, the woman first described above came to her eventual answer after a series of statements. The first answer was general: "My left side is weak." When asked, "What problems does the weakness of your left side cause you?" she replied, "I have trouble going up and down steps." When asked again, she made her own problem even more explicit, as defined by her setting. This threefold process of exploration helped to transform the focus from a discussion of impairments ("My left side is weak") to the functional consequences of disabilities in the life of the specific person. In dealing with chronic illness, one needs to define the problem in such functional terms that one can design ways of alleviating the problem, even if the impairments remain.

The process of defining a problem is ongoing. The answers will, of course, vary with the individual's degree and type of impairment and the idiosyncratic setting in which he or she is required to function. The answers will also change over time as thoughts become clearer, as old problems are solved and new ones appear, and as the patient feels more trust in the person asking the questions. Ultimately, the question about concerns is one the person with disabilities must recurrently ask himself or herself. This cyclical process also is applicable to other questions in the planning process.

When addressing the question about goals, the threefold exploration of possible goals generally permits the development of a series of objectives, with the last more likely to be a short-term rather than a global initial response to goals. This same threefold exploration also is useful when dealing with the question about outcomes. A sense of positive accomplishment will more likely be engendered if several outcomes, rather than just one, have been achieved. This same principle is even more relevant when answering the question "What works?" to define the means by which outcomes are achieved.

One of the major problems in the management of persons with impairments is the loss of methods previously used to accomplish important life activities. For example, weakness of the leg may deprive the person of walking as a means of getting around. It is important to recognize that what has been lost is a means and not the ultimate goal. "Getting around" – that is, mobility – is the aim. Doing so by means of walking has obviously been important. It is not, however, the only way by which one got around in the past, nor will its unavailability preclude getting around in the future.[7] However, the patient must overcome the sense of loss and the despair that occur after losing such a normal ability. The patient is being asked to consider what is essentially an abnormal method – one that is unusual for that person and one that may be abnormal in the view of the patient's overall culture.

It is particularly helpful to question what works in the context of actual outcomes. In the context of having achieved a goal, one can consider what may have contributed to such an achievement. It is necessary to evoke the setting so that the search for what works can be made appropriate to the individual. Therefore, although this question may be addressed when making the initial plan, its particular value for the person with stroke is to address it in the context of that person's own experience of success.[6]

In answering this crucial question about what worked, it is useful to explore at least several different instances of successful outcome or several aspects that could describe that result. For example, a man with long-standing, severe poststroke central pain identified some of the strategies he found helpful in managing his pain. He described several positive experiences in relation to his overall goal of "carrying on my life despite the pain." Some of them included "traveling to my son's house," "taking a graduation trip," and "going out to dinner." It is in the context of describing at least several such experiences that the person can begin to consider that such events do occur. One such experience may be of interest, but it is helpful to understand that such events can come on a more frequent level. At least three experiences can help to establish a sense that they do occur.

In the context of these episodes, the previously mentioned patient was better able to generate some of the strategies he found useful. Some of those strategies were recurrent, but others became clearer or arose anew when the question was explored on several occasions. Some of the strategies were quite specific to a situation; others had general applicability. Not only were the specific strategies important, but the realization that there were a number of them was significant. The message learned is that there are a number of ways to accomplish the goal; if one way does not work, one can seek another, with some likelihood of success in finding a method that helps. Even more important is the knowledge that these compensatory strategies can be defined by the patient out of the patient's own experiences. It is the role of the professional to aid the patient in achieving this sense of empowerment.

In considering the overall cyclical structure of the planning system and some of its components, it becomes clear that the products of such a planning system are data that deal not only with outcomes but also with techniques useful in achieving those outcomes. What is designed is a *planning system* devoted to *problem solving.*

The focus on problem-solving strategies emphasizes the ongoing nature of the problems being faced. The problems and outcomes vary over time, and the strategies for solving problems may have more general application. The first major goal is to generate resourcefulness or to unleash resourcefulness already present, not to make the patient's situation worse by stifling resourcefulness that already exists. The second major goal is to develop the resources not only of professionals but of the patient with the stroke and the family. The resources to be developed, the techniques for solving problems, and their ongoing generation must ultimately be those of the primary participants—that is, the patient and family. Thus one may call the approach a *collaborative* problem-solving planning system. During the life of the person who has experienced a stroke, the development of these problem-solving planning skills is a major task of the rehabilitation phase and is implemented later during the continuing care phase.

TABLE 3-1 Degrees of Patient Participation in the Planning Process

	PROFESSIONAL	PERSON WITH STROKE	PERCENTAGE CONTRIBUTION
Independence	–	Asks self; answers for self	100
Free choice	Asks open-ended questions without providing answers	Answers for self; explores and selects	80
Multiple choice	Asks by providing several (three) answers; suggests	Selects answer(s) for self	60
Forced choice	Asks by recommending (one) answer before action	Agrees (or disagrees)– "yes" or "no"	40
No choice	Does not ask; prescribes; action predetermined	Compliant (or noncompliant)	20

The management of persons with stroke is considered as a set of plans dealing with each of the major problem areas. The first of these is the development of a medical treatment plan to prevent medical illness relating to stroke. In both the acute and the rehabilitation phases, prevention of illness is of the highest priority. Prevention may also be an ongoing concern during the continuing care phase in light of the frequent comorbidities associated with stroke. The second set of plans relates to the treatment of risk factors to prevent further impairments caused by recurrent stroke. The implementation of this plan takes place in the acute and rehabilitation phases, but it also extends into the future life of the person with stroke. The third set of plans deals with the alleviation of disabilities relating to impairments. The management of disabilities with patient and family participation is an ongoing problem-solving process. The ability of the primary participants to take part in a problem-solving planning process initiated during the rehabilitation phase extends into the ongoing continuing care phase in all three problem areas.

Table 3-1 describes the level of participation achieved in relation to the questions addressed in generating such plans. We focus particularly on increased participation in answering the questions about outcome and means. Participation can vary, not only with the questions, but also with the degree to which the patient has been accustomed to dealing with his or her problems in the past. For some, even "multiple choice" questions are difficult to answer; for others, the levels of participation in answering planning questions may be much greater.

The degree of participation by the person with stroke in answering the question about "what works" can also vary depending on the area being addressed. The treatment procedures in the prevention of illness are frequently technical. They include the use of medication and other modalities less likely to be initiated by the person with stroke. The level of participation may be that of "agreement" to recommendations made by professional staff ("forced choice"). Even in this area, however, the potential exists for the person to be involved to a somewhat greater degree in the setting of goals and the evaluation of outcome.

The prevention of further impairment caused by recurrent stroke requires more participation in management from the person with stroke. A given level of participation in the setting of goals and the evaluation of outcome can also elicit a higher degree of participation in the development and implementation of problem-solving strategies. Participation in managing risk factors can perhaps be achieved at a level of selection from suggestions made by professional staff ("multiple choice").

The alleviation of disabilities and their ongoing management during the rehabilitation and continuing care phases offer an even greater opportunity for participation in all aspects of planning, in particular, for higher levels of participation in the exploration of problem-solving strategies and for independent use of the entire process. The aim is for the person with stroke to contribute ideas about techniques freely in answer to open-ended questions ("free choice").

The focus is on the person learning about himself or herself, discovering what works, and finding new ways to achieve goals. Learning that one's answers to a question have validity can lead to asking the question independently. Learning takes place when the patient recognizes that alternatives do exist; understands that solutions are not worse because they are "different"; identifies what some solutions are; and knows how to generate others. The degree to which compensatory strategies become part of the repertoire of the person with stroke varies with each person. Not only does fitting those strategies to the person make the strategies more appropriate, but also the very process of involvement ensures commitment along with the modifications.

Thus, during the various phases described, the overall degree of participation by the person with stroke and the family varies. (See Table 3-2 to illustrate the defining of problems.) In the acute phase and in the medical setting, the level of participation may be at the level of forced choice or even lower; during the rehabilitation phase, there is both an opportunity and a need for the relationship to move toward greater degrees of freedom in decision making. During this phase, *collaboration* can be used in the rehabilitation plan and in the plan for the management of risk factors and medical issues.

For example, during the rehabilitation phase, a joint search by the professional staff and primary participants is made for compensatory strategies dealing with disabilities. By the end of that phase, relatively independent use of the compensatory strategies has been generated. During the continuing care phase an even greater degree of independence is encouraged: the primary participants may generate new plans on their own to deal with unforeseen

TABLE 3-2   Information Gathering Process to Define Problem

STAGE	PROFESSIONAL	PATIENT	GOAL
Acute phase	Asks the question via neurologic assessment; focuses on signs	Relatively passive	To determine impairment
Rehabilitation	Asks the question via an interview; focuses on symptoms	Collaborative	To determine disabilities
Continuing care		Independent; asks questions of self	To determine need for professional care

problems involving disabilities. This same developmental process can be employed in controlling risk factors for stroke, such as hypertension. In the acute phase the medication or other means for controlling blood pressure may be prescribed; during the rehabilitation phase the person is made more aware of medication and agrees to its use; during the continuing care phase the person or caregiver is responsible for seeing that the medication is taken.

The exploration of answers to the various questions used in the planning process generally requires suggestions or recommendations initiated by the professional staff. At the minimum the professional staff provides the structure for planning, including the principle of ongoing review and adaptation. The professional staff functions as a planning consultant to the primary participants, enabling them to express their thoughts on concerns, goals, outcomes, and strategies for problem solving.

In most settings, carrying out this principle of collaboration requires a group of professionals who function as a team. Coordination within an interdisciplinary team is particularly important during the rehabilitation phase. Recognizing the needs of the person with stroke is necessary in making interdisciplinary plans and in evaluating the outcomes of those plans and the strategies effective in bringing them about before any revisions. In this text, examples illustrate this ongoing *coordinated* problem-solving planning process in various problem areas, such as mobility and communication.

The aim of the healing relationship, in Pellegrino's words,[8] is to "restore wholeness or, if this is not possible, to assist in striking some new balance between what the body imposes and the self aspires to." If full restoration is not possible, amelioration, adaptation, or coping becomes the goal of the healing relationship.[9] It is essential that the actions taken not only be technically correct, but also ultimately be "good" for that patient. Good healing actions refer to those that the individual patient perceives as worthwhile and that are personally derived from and incorporated into the patient's own life. Thus there is a shift in emphasis from what may be merely technically correct to what is worthwhile. Pellegrino goes on to emphasize that the "unequivocal criterion of a good decision is the enhancement of the patient's moral agency," even if this is contrary to the physician's opinion.

This principle of the patient's empowerment must underlie the entire process of rehabilitation.[2] The goal is to energize and catalyze the rehabilitation patient's capacity for life and to enable the patient to ambulate, communicate, and perform other activities of daily living to the best of his or her abilities. The entire process must be directed toward this overall goal. The process of engendering and channeling active participation can enhance the sense of empowerment. It has been suggested that a high degree of active and interested participation can enhance the meeting of the more classic goals, such as ambulation and communication.[1] This book is designed to illustrate both care continuity over time and coordination within the team of professionals devoted to a goal of problem-solving in collaboration with the person with stroke or the caregiver.

REFERENCES

1. Bach-y-Rita P, Bach-y-Rita E: Hope and active patient participation in the rehabilitation environment, *Arch Phys Med Rehabil* 71:1084, 1990.
2. Banja JD: Rehabilitation and empowerment, *Arch Phys Med Rehabil* 71:614, 1990.
3. Bechman HB, Frankel RM: The effect of physician behavior on the collection of data, *Ann Intern Med* 101:692, 1984.
4. Bellet PS, Maloney MJ: The importance of empathy as an interviewing skill in medicine, *JAMA* 266:1831, 1991.
5. Cassell EJ: Recognizing suffering, *Hastings Center Rep* 21:24, 1991.
6. Ozer MN: *The management of persons with spinal cord injury,* New York, 1988, Demos.
7. Payton OD, Nelson CE, Ozer MN: *Patient participation in program planning: a manual for therapists,* Philadelphia, 1990, FA Davis.
8. Pellegrino ED: The healing relationship: the architectonics of clinical medicine. In Shelp EA, editor: *The clinical fabric of the physician-patient relationship,* Boston, 1983, D Reidel.
9. Zaner RM: Medicine and dialogue, *J Med Philos* 15:303, 1990.

PART II

Acute Care Phase

Edited by
Louis R. Caplan

NATURE OF THE PROBLEM
4 **Medical Management Plan**
5 **Neurologic Management Plan**
6 **Rehabilitation Management Plan**

NATURE OF THE PROBLEM

The acute care phase is initiated by the relatively sudden appearance of symptoms of focal neurologic impairments in sensory, or motor function, as well as cognitive and behavioral abnormalities. The overall goal of the acute phase is the establishment of medical and neurologic stability with a minimization of brain injury and subsequent impairment. The immediate short-term plan is to determine the pathophysiology of the stroke and to minimize the impairment resulting from the present episode of vascular insufficiency. This can involve alleviating the metabolic consequences of the ischemia. Focal ischemia leads to injury to the entire neuropil in that area, and the goal is to minimize the spatial extent of such injury. The effects of more diffuse vascular ischemia caused by hypotension are on those areas that are particularly vulnerable, such as the hippocampus and sensitive cellular elements. In this situation the goal is to minimize the severity, degree, and type of cellular injury of such diffuse effects. These activities must take place within minutes to hours of the onset of the stroke.

A slightly longer time frame (in the range of hours to days) exists when dealing with the medical complications. These include both the underlying disease processes associated with stroke, such as diabetes and cardiac disease, and those aspects that arise in the aftermath of the stroke. Problems occur in bladder management and in swallowing that can lead to infection and illness. Seizures may appear. Particularly problematic is the development of venous thrombosis with the subsequent pulmonary embolus. The goal is to minimize illness and mortality in the acute phase.

In addition, another plan is necessary for the prevention of recurrent stroke. It is important to recognize the frequently cyclic nature of the history of the person with stroke. There may be a subsequent stroke early in the course of the initial stroke, or one may occur later, the likelihood of which must be minimized and for which the patient must be prepared to seek care. Assessment during this initial phase must explore the appropriateness of surgical versus medical management, such as the use of anticoagulant or antiplatelet medication. The implementation of the stroke prevention plan is ongoing. Prevention involves recognition of risk factors and the initiation of educative and other strategies as early as possible, even while managing the acute stroke. Management of risk factors is continued during the following rehabilitation phase and is implemented by the person with stroke more independently during the ongoing continuing care phase.

The acute phase also sees the initiation of the rehabilitation plan for minimizing the disabilities (i.e., the effects of the impairments caused by brain injury on the life of the person with stroke). The type and severity of the impairment are of major importance in determining the prognosis for independence (i.e., in the patient caring for his or her own needs). This plan is developed in greater detail during the subsequent rehabilitation phase. During the initial acute phase, there is ongoing assessment of the degree of injury. The severity and type of neurologic impairment are major determinants of the extent of rehabilitation activities to be provided during the subsequent phase.

The rehabilitation program can be initiated during the acute phase to optimize later retraining outcomes. Safeguards need to be instituted so that subsequent retraining can take place. For example, a goal during the acute phase is to guard against changes, such as those in the soft tissues of the hemiplegic arm, that could interfere with later function.

At the outset, the physician must consider the appropriate setting for carrying out retraining—at the patient's home or in an outpatient or inpatient setting. The patient's alternatives are returning home (with no formal care but often family burdens); ambulatory care; home care; skilled nursing care; or a rehabilitation unit care. Recent focus on the costs of health care requires a determination of the cost effectiveness of the various alternatives.

Each of the following sections deals with problems encountered in each of the preceding areas and the activities and treatments designed to alleviate them. Thus a "plan" is generated in each area to achieve the goals of medical stabilization and of minimization of neurologic impairment while laying the basis for a more long-term plan to alleviate resultant disabilities and to prevent future impairment caused by stroke recurrence.

CHAPTER 4

Medical Management Plan

Nature of the problem
Comorbidity and its effects
Deep vein thrombosis and pulmonary embolus
  Nature of the problem
  Identification of deep vein thrombosis
  Prevention of deep vein thrombosis
  Identification of pulmonary embolism
Bladder management
  MICHAEL H. PHILLIPS
  Nature of the problem
  Pathophysiology
  Evaluation and treatment
Management of seizures
  T.K. ASADI
  Nature of the problem
  Temporal relation of stroke and seizure
  Management of seizure disorder

NATURE OF THE PROBLEM

The achievement of medical stability is affected by the medical problems associated with stroke. These include problems related to the disease processes, of which stroke is but a reflection. The major comorbidities include diabetes and cardiac disease. In addition, medical problems arise in the wake of the stroke itself. The hypercoagulability and immobilization can lead to a higher incidence of deep vein thrombosis with embolization to the lungs. Dysfunction of the swallowing mechanism can lead to both nutritional deficiencies and aspiration pneumonia. Disturbances in bladder function can lead to incontinence with skin breakdown and a higher likelihood of urinary tract infection. During the acute phase, a decision must generally be made about appropriate ongoing seizure management. These medical issues impinge on the mortality and morbidity of the person with stroke during the acute phase. They also affect the readiness with which the person with stroke is available for rehabilitation training. Medical stability and the ability to maintain activity for approximately 3 hours are requirements for entry into more intensive rehabilitation.

Case mortality and morbidity during the 30 days immediately after the onset of stroke generally reflects the duration of the acute phase. Medical stability usually is achieved far sooner in many instances. Referral to a more intensive rehabilitation phase can be made at any time depending on the degree of neurologic impairment and medical illness. Nevertheless, much of the statistical data reflects this 30-day time frame.

The actual incidence of mortality varies with several factors. The person's age at the onset of stroke, the severity of the concomitant cardiac disease and other associated factors, the character of the stroke, and the severity of impairment can all affect mortality and morbidity. Still another factor in the analysis of data is the years during which the data were collected. Some evidence exists that the changes in diagnosis and management over the years may have an effect.

Of particular significance is the contribution of the character of the stroke to the results. As one would expect, death early in the period after onset is associated particularly with hemorrhagic stroke. In one study reflecting experience over the decades 1950 to 1980, mortality resulting from intracerebral hemorrhage (ICH) was about 80%.[3] Another study contrasts the experience during 1945 to 1949 and 1975 to 1979.[1] Mortality caused by ICH was 100% at 21 days in the early era and was reduced to 58% at 30 days during the late era. During the period 1975 to 1980 (with the availability of the computed tomography [CT] scan since 1978), mortality remains at 60% in those with supratentorial hemorrhage.[4]

An even more recent study carried out in Sweden examined two cohorts.[5] The first cohort was treated during the period 1975 to 1978; the second, 1983 to 1986. The first period was before the widespread use of CT, and the presence of hemorrhage was determined by use of spinal taps. The chance of surviving 1 month after stroke did not change between these two periods despite the development of a separate hospital stroke unit that had a significant effect in reducing mortality *after* the first 30 days. The primary mechanism of death in the cases occurring during the first week was transtentorial herniation, the pathophysiology of which was either edema or extension of hemorrhage.[4] In almost all cases the functional status of those patients who were dying was that of coma. These data suggest that, despite some reduction in mortality, the effect of more severe intracerebral hemorrhage remains insoluble even with recent advances.

Mortality for the larger number of persons with nonhemorrhagic stroke over the long time period of 1950 to 1980 was 14%.[3] In those with infarction (either supratentorial or infratentorial) during the more recent period of 1975 to 1980, mortality remained about 15%.[4] In this latter study, deaths in the first week occurred mainly as a result of transtentorial herniation. However, unlike the cases of hemorrhagic stroke, a substantial number of deaths occurred later in the first month after stroke. In those who died of "noncerebral" causes, the largest number had pneumonia; the next largest number of deaths were due to cardiac failure, with another group of deaths characterized as sudden or from unknown causes. Particularly noteworthy was the high incidence of death from cardiac causes in those who were relatively less impaired by the stroke and who were described as "requiring only assistance or supervision" or as "independent."

Particularly hopeful are the findings of a study conducted in Norway during the period 1986 to 1987.[2] A comparison was made between patients hospitalized in a general medical unit and those in a more specialized stroke unit. Mortality did not vary between the two groups during the first 5 days, when death was related to the severity of the brain injury. However, the subsequent mortality incidence did vary during the 6 weeks after stroke, with a death rate of 17% in the general unit and 7% in the specialized one.

The higher mortality in the general medical unit was attributed to pneumonia, pulmonary embolism, and recurrent stroke. Treatment in the more specialized stroke unit included intensive and early mobilization; a protocol that precluded glucose infusion during the first 48 hours; no antiedema agents; no treatment for blood pressure lower than 250/130 mm Hg; anticoagulation medication in those less than 75 years of age with embolic infarction; and subcutaneous administration of 5000 U bid of heparin. Thus it appears that the medical management leading to an improvement in mortality is a regimen that mobilizes patients early to help prevent pneumonia and deep vein thrombosis. Functional outcome is also improved. At the end of the 6-week treatment period the mean scores both on the Barthel Index and from a neurologic examination were significantly higher in the specialized treatment group.

COMORBIDITY AND ITS EFFECTS

The medical comorbidities contributing to the mortality during this initial phase are associated cardiovascular disease and hyperglycemia with or without diabetes. These same factors militate against neural recovery and can worsen impairment.

One study[8] identified deterioration on the basis of change on the Canadian Neurological Scale[7] during the first 48 hours. The glycemia level 24 hours after onset of the infarct was related to the progression of the clinical picture and to other factors, including elevated systolic blood pressure at admission and involvement of the carotid vascular territory. This group of factors was associated with particular mortality during the first week after onset. In those who survived, the degree of impairment in function was also more severe. Still another study identified a serum glucose level of 155 mg/dl as the mean at the time of admission.[11] Those below the mean had a significantly greater likelihood of "complete" or "good" recovery than those with the higher level. The group with high glucose values was also far more likely to be diabetic. Effects were documented by positron emission tomography (PET) scan and CT. The glucose level was highly correlated with the extent of metabolic brain abnormalities seen on the PET scan.

Data derived from the Stroke Data Bank also confirm these findings.[16] Early recurrent stroke was defined as a noniatrogenic recurrence within 30 days of the index stroke, with clear evidence of a new deficit in a different anatomic or vascular territory or of a different subtype. This group had increased morbidity with doubling of the length of their hospital stay, a tripling of mortality, and a major worsening of the degree of motor impairment. The risk of occurrence was significantly affected by a history of hypertension, diastolic pressure greater than 100 mm Hg, history of diabetes, and blood sugar concentration greater than 140 mg/dl. The estimated risk of early recurrence rose from 0.77% in the absence of both hypertension and hyperglycemia to 8.56% in those with coexisting hypertension and an initial blood sugar concentration of 300 mg/dl. The cumulative overall 30-day recurrence risk was 3.3%. Particularly susceptible were those individuals with a pathogenetic process of hemodynamic insufficiency. Embolic disease had a somewhat lower recurrence rate, perhaps reflecting the use of anticoagulant medication in those with a clear diagnosis of emboli. A relatively low level of recurrence was found in patients with documented lacunar infarct.

In one study it was posited that the presumed relationship between poor outcome and hyperglycemia may relate not to the presence of underlying diabetes but rather to the effects of the stroke per se.[19] These authors used as their criteria for underlying diabetes the levels of glycosylated hemoglobin, fructosamine, and glucose. Thus "diabetics" were those with an elevation of all these factors. Those with hyperglycemia alone ("nondiabetics") had increased mortality, reflecting mainly a higher incidence of concomitant intracerebral hemorrhage. Diabetics and nondiabetics with comparable sugar levels had similar outcomes. The authors postulate that hemorrhage may induce hyperglycemia secondary to stress. The association of glucose concentration and eventual outcome was a reflection of the severity of the stroke rather than a direct harmful effect of glucose per se. This issue is discussed again in the section dealing with the metabolic changes leading to neural injury during the acute phase.

Still another study that followed patients closely during the early period after stroke found a mortality of 25% in those with thromboembolic disease. Death resulted mainly because of cerebral complications, but a substantial percentage of deaths occurred because of cardiac pathologic conditions (35%) and pulmonary embolism (20%) documented at autopsy.[9]

It is not surprising that mortality and possibly increases in the severity of neurologic impairment are associated with the coexistence of cardiac disease. A strong association exists between carotid artery disease and coronary artery disease (CAD). Over the long term, CAD is the major cause of death among patients with different manifestations of cerebrovascular atherosclerosis.[15] It has been suggested that the finding of cerebrovascular disease should occasion a search for the corresponding myocardial disease.[17] The search is relevant not only to the proper treatment for prevention of emboli of cardiac origin but as an important determinant of longevity. One prospective study included persons with transient ischemic attacks (TIAs) or stroke mild enough to enable participation in cardiac exercise testing. The incidence of CAD as evidenced by radionucleotide cardiac tests was confirmed by coronary angiography. The incidence of CAD was quite high (58%), with a 42% incidence in those with no history suggestive of CAD.[14] Even more recently, studies in those with TIAs or asymptomatic carotid stenosis confirm a high incidence of abnormality on thallium-201 scan, with the additional finding of a high likelihood of subsequent myocardial events on follow-up.[12]

The problem with diagnosing significant CAD is complicated by the degree to which persons with stroke are asymptomatic. Therefore screening has been advocated. One report describes the value of Holter monitoring when documenting ST segment depression.[10] Particularly relevant is the identification of persons with asymptomatic three-vessel or left main CAD because of the associated worsened prognosis. Criteria for the selection of patients for screening are not yet in place.[6] It has been suggested that those with carotid artery disease who are younger than 65 years of age be screened. The particular screening method used varies. Stress thallium-201 imaging is recommended for those able to exercise and dipyridamole thallium-201 imaging in those unable to do so. The sensitivity of the thallium studies as measured by follow-up coronary angiography was 93% in a recent study.[12]

Not only does the presence of cardiac disease contribute to death and morbidity in those with cerebrovascular disease, but also the effects of acute stroke may contribute to the cardiac arrhythmias by increased sympathetic tone.[13] Electrocardiographic (ECG) changes suggestive of myocardial ischemia occur particularly in those with hemorrhage (either intracerebral or subarachnoid). Changes include peaked P waves, short PR intervals, long QT intervals, pathologic Q waves, abnormal ST segments, and peaked T waves. The incidence in persons with nonhemorrhagic ischemic stroke ranges from 15% to 40%. Such findings can account for episodes of sudden death. The pathophysiology of these effects has been attributed to epinephrine release causing hypercontracted muscle fibers that become necrotic—so-called myocytolysis.[18]

DEEP VEIN THROMBOSIS AND PULMONARY EMBOLUS
Nature of the Problem

The incidence of pulmonary embolism [PE] as the proximate cause of death in persons with supratentorial infarction has been estimated to range from 2% to 13%.[21,50] The incidence varies with the population surveyed and the degree to which autopsy findings are used. For example, one autopsy study found a 3% incidence of PE in those dying with stroke who were below 45 years of age and a 16% incidence in those 60 to 74 years of age.[47] Mortality tends to occur 2 to 4 weeks after the onset of stroke when the patient has survived possible neurologic death caused by transtentorial herniation.

The pathophysiology of the relatively high incidence of deep vein thrombosis (DVT) as a source of potential PE in persons with stroke is not entirely clear. Immobility leading to stasis amplified by paresis has been the usual explanation. That the incidence is particularly high in the paretic leg and in the presence of edema supports this.[52] DVT was not found in those who were ambulant or who had minor deficits.[20] Immobilization appears to be the common element. Additional factors such as hypercoagulability may also contribute. There has been evidence of enhanced thrombin activity in the month after the onset of stroke.[37] Other studies have shown a hyperactivity of platelets and of the coagulation system with signs of increased thrombin formation in the circulation as a consequence of the cerebral insult. The occurrence of DVT early after stroke supports some factor other than immobilization alone. The findings of both early occurrence and a far higher incidence in the paretic (53%) than the nonparetic (7%) leg also suggest the possible combined causes of hypercoagulability and immobilization.[57]

The ongoing occurrence of DVT in the postacute period was demonstrated in several studies. One study found an incidence of between 30% and 40% among persons admitted to a rehabilitation center with an average poststroke interval of 45 days.[52] The time at which the DVT first appeared was unknown. The coincidence of DVT and other parameters of hypercoagulability was noted in a population entering a rehabilitation center even earlier, with a mean interval of 16 days after the stroke.[44] The determination of the presence of DVT was based on clinical grounds and confirmed by phlebography. (One should note that such a protocol based on clinician presentation may obscure the true incidence.) The incidence of DVT was 12%. Particularly noteworthy was the increased incidence of DVT and PE in those with associated atrial fibrillation; the incidence was 25 times that of those without atrial fibrillation. It is postulated that impaired venous return is the additional factor contributing to the increased risk in these persons. In our experience the positive incidence was about 2% in persons screened at an average of 10 days after onset.

The significance of PE has generally been measured by mortality. The effects of this problem can also be measured by other criteria. The following case report illustrates the disruptive nature of DVT with PE in the course of rehabilitation, even when mortality does not occur.

CASE REPORT

L.R. is a 76-year-old woman with a history of hypertension and type II diabetes who had been in good health and living alone independently. She had an acute onset of left-sided weakness. A head CT scan showed a low-density lesion in the right internal capsule and parietal cortex. No evidence of arrhythmia was seen. The ECG showed evidence of an old myocardial infarct. L.R. was described as obese with poor peripheral pulses in her legs. No leg edema was present. Left lower extremity weakness was found throughout, with less than antigravity strength. She required substantial physical assistance for transfers and marked assistance for ambulation. Discharge to her home would require her to be independent in carrying out positional transfers. There was no family member available to help at home. It was initially projected that L.R. would meet the goal of independent movement by the time of discharge which was 6 weeks after the onset of stroke.

L.R. developed superficial phlebitis in the right thigh which was treated with warm compresses, leg elevation, and thromboembolytic disease (TED) hose. At 30 days after the onset of stroke and while walking in physical therapy, L.R. experienced an acute onset of chest tightness with shortness of breath. An arterial blood gas (ABG) analysis showed a PCO_2 of 40.9, a PO_2 of 67.2 with room air, and a PO_2 of 133.9 with 4 L of oxygen. An ECG showed no significant changes. Venous Doppler ultrasound demonstrated DVT in both femoral and popliteal veins. L.R. began heparin and later coumadin therapies for presumed PE. She returned to the rehabilitation program after 1 week of bed rest. (It was now 5 weeks after the onset of stroke.)

At this point there was a change in projected discharge plan. The goals initially set had not been met. When, at 6 weeks after onset, she still required physical assistance in ambulation and transfers, her discharge was delayed and projected to be 2 weeks later (for a total of 8 weeks after onset). The goal remained eventual independent ambulation with use of a walker, but L.R. would require some physical assistance on discharge. The original plan for her to return to her home had to be changed. Instead, she would live with her daughter who would take a leave of absence from her job until an improvement in L.R.'s ability to ambulate enabled her to be at home alone.

This case illustrates the relationship of DVT and subsequent PE despite the use of graded compression hose in a person who is ambulating 30 days after the onset of stroke. The cost of such an episode was high. Despite prompt treatment and prevention of mortality, the patient's rehabilitation program was interrupted and her return home prolonged for an additional 3 weeks. The level of independence originally projected was also reduced. The patient was no longer able to return to her previous home but required alternative housing.

Identification of Deep Vein Thrombosis

The goal is to prevent PE, which can lead to significant morbidity and mortality. The first level of prevention is to identify DVT when it exists as the precursor of PE. DVT is an important indicator of PE risks. Defects seen on CT lung-series scan and suggestive of PE could be found far more frequently (10 times) in those with evidence of DVT.[28] However, many episodes of PE are silent. Thus the problem lies in identifying the existence of DVT before embolization to the lungs.

The most reliable clinical finding is unilateral swelling. It is suggested that the area of minimal circumference of the ankles be monitored rather than the more commonly used maximum circumference of the calves. In persons with PE documented by angiography, 58% had no symptoms referable to the leg. Thus there is a low level of sensitivity. Specificity is also low with venography, which identifies fresh proximal thrombosis in only 29% of those in whom DVT is suspected clinically.[58] It is clear that the clinical presentation is neither sensitive nor specific.

Screening tests are superior to clinical signs alone and yield both an earlier identification and greater sensitivity.[20] For instance, one third of the cases demonstrable on screening tests (and confirmed on venography) were not identified based on clinical grounds. Venography has been the "gold standard," yet its accuracy is less than 90% because of both failure to visualize some aspect of the venous system and false-positive findings based on clinical evidence. Its invasive nature has led to the development of alternative methods.

Fibrinogen tagged with radioactive iodine has been used to identify DVT in the calf, whereas impedance plethysmography (IP) has been useful for identifying DVT in the proximal leg. The use of IP has been particularly advocated as the appropriate screening test because DVT in the thigh is particularly likely to lead to PE, as was seen in the positive findings from CT lung series scans in one study.[42] In that report all patients with proximal thigh vein thrombosis also had calf vein thrombosis; none of the patients with calf vein thrombosis alone showed evidence of PE; and over half the patients with thigh vein thrombosis revealed evidence of PE. Another study using both screening methods found a combined incidence of 22%, with DVT occurring mainly in the deep calf without apparent overlap between the two sites. Two cases of PE were cited; however, one was in a person with calf DVT.[20] In still another study the use of IP alone gave an incidence of 34%, with clinical evidence of DVT in only 6% of those.[52] There was no mention of PE in this group.

The relative likelihood of DVT occurring in the proximal veins and leading to embolization of the lungs was confirmed once again.[28] Ongoing screening by IP (and confirmation by venography) demonstrated proximal vein thrombosis in 88% of those who were positive on screening. The remainder had isolated calf vein thrombosis. The incidence of an abnormal finding on CT lung scan was 27% in those with calf vein thrombosis alone, whereas 78% with proximal vein thrombosis had an abnormal finding on CT lung scan (heavily weighted toward a high probability on CT lung scan). The value of IP as a single screening measure was demonstrated in another group of patients with clinical evidence of DVT.

Adding iodinated fibrinogen studies to the screening regimen added no new cases of DVT or PE beyond those already demonstrated on venography and angiography.[33] In general, the reported sensitivity of IP alone was considered to be greater than 90%.[32]

More recently the use of Doppler ultrasound has been advocated as an alternative noninvasive test. In a study of those with clinical DVT (and in whom venography was done) Doppler flow in the common femoral vein was considered normal when it was detectable and when there was an increase during expiration and decrease during inspiration. Less than a 10% increase in the anteroposterior diameter of the common femoral vein during the Valsalva maneuver was considered diagnostic of thrombus. Ultrasound was used to image the deep veins in order to detect the presence or absence of visible thrombus. Real-time Doppler ultrasound studies were found to be 100% sensitive in detecting thrombus involving the common femoral vein. It is recommended that ultrasound be used as a screen before venography.[56] The additional use of Doppler did not add to specificity or sensitivity, confirming the value of ultrasound alone without the need for venography based on clinical follow-up.[25] In another large study series of outpatients, those with signs of DVT were studied with ultrasound.[38] The single criterion of "compressibility of the vein" was used as a sign of abnormality. Venography was also done. Ultrasound revealed noncompressibility in all patients in whom venography showed proximal vein thrombosis affecting the popliteal or femoral veins. Abnormal ultrasound findings in proximal veins were also found in approximately one third of those with calf vein thrombosis. The overall sensitivity was 91%. It is important to establish both the specificity and the sensitivity of all tests used. In the outpatient study described previously, all those without DVT on venography also had negative findings on the compressibility measure; thus ultrasound achieved a specificity of 100%. Other criteria useful in other studies, such as the response to the Valsalva maneuver, were less specific.

In summary, the radioiodine-labeled fibrinogen uptake test (RFUT) is highly sensitive for small calf vein thrombi but insensitive above the midthigh. IP has been shown to be effective in identifying particularly significant, more proximal thrombi. Ultrasound studies approach the accuracy of venography for both calf veins and thigh veins. Scanning involving ultrasonic imaging has been recently shown to be highly sensitive and specific and can serve as an alternative to IP. One recent review once again confirms the value of laboratory evaluation over clinical examination in establishing the existence of DVT.[22]

Prevention of Deep Vein Thrombosis

The high incidence of DVT and resultant PE, along with the relative poor predictive value of risk factors,[57] has led to the development of treatment protocols to prevent DVT. These treatment protocols include both anticoagulant medication and techniques to increase muscle action or other methods to reduce stasis. The cost effectiveness and clinical value of prophylaxis in persons after surgery has been established.[31]

In persons with stroke the use of low-dose heparin (5000 U q8h) is associated with a significant reduction in the incidence of DVT as measured by leg CT scans with fibrinogen [131]I.[40] More recent studies confirmed the value of fixed-dose low-molecular-weight heparin in the prevention of DVT in acute stroke.[55] Treatment was started within 7 days and continued for 14 days or until discharge. Both fibrinogen ^{131}I and IP were used for surveillance, and venography was carried out if the results were positive. All thrombi occurred in patients with severe paresis (i.e., those in whom movements of the distal part of the leg occurred only with gravity eliminated if at all) and almost always (8:9) in the paretic limb. DVT occurred in 28% of the placebo group and 4% of the treated group, with no DVT in the crucial proximal thigh in the treated group.

In another study with an equivalent observation period of up to 14 days and postmortem examination of those patients who did die, tagged fibrinogen surveillance was also used.[40] The incidence of DVT peaked at the fifth day and diminished thereafter. The incidence of DVT was reduced from 73% in the control group to 22% in those treated with 5000 U of heparin subcutaneously q8h, with significant reductions in those with PE present at death (fivefold reduction) and in the death rate. The mortality resulting from PE was particularly affected by treatment in those with less severe stroke, as measured by both the degree of hemiplegia and the level of consciousness.

Still another randomized double-blind study[49] used a dose of low-molecular-weight heparin adjusted for body weight (3000 to 5000 U qd). Again, treatment was started early in acute stroke and continued for up to 14 days. Surveillance was by venography of the paretic limb, clinical examination, and IP. Contrary to the other studies, no evidence of a positive effect was found with this regimen.

The effect of TED hose in persons with stroke is unclear. The studies available for review include the effects of TED after general surgical procedures rather than after stroke. After general surgery the usefulness of graded compression stockings was found to be equivalent to that of fixed low-dose heparin (5000 U q12h).[26] The presence of DVT was assessed by technetium-plasmin uptake. In still another study of persons undergoing general surgery, the incidence of DVT was assessed by tagged fibrinogen with low fixed doses of heparin (5000 U q12h) and graded compression hose applied to one leg. The frequency of DVT in the legs of control patients (i.e., those who received no stockings but low-dose heparin) was 12%; in patients who received low-dose heparin and whose legs were encased in stockings, the incidence was 4%.[54] Therefore graded compression stockings contribute some degree of protection, and their low cost makes them a useful adjunct.

Several methodologic issues should be raised when considering the studies described previously. Tagged fibrinogen or technetium-enhanced scans image the calf rather than thigh. Although one may be preventing DVT in the calf, it is unclear whether one is preventing DVT in the thigh. It is DVT in this area that is most likely to give rise to PE, and ultimately any efforts are directed toward the prevention of PE.

The form, amount, and dosage frequency of heparin and the duration of treatment have not been adequately assessed for persons with stroke. Nevertheless, it is recommended that persons with nonhemorrhagic stroke receive low-dose heparin for prevention of DVT.[45] For all other stroke patients, external pneumatic compression is recommended. In general, it is advised that heparin therapy cease with ambulation. The risk of venous thromboembolic events is reduced if independent ambulation is greater than 50 feet. In those without known hemorrhagic risk and who are not yet walking with a quadruped cane, even with bracing and physical assistance, the use of subcutaneous heparin is indicated.[23] Thus the management of DVT and PE ultimately lies in the prompt and active mobilization of persons with stroke; with prophylactic low-dose anticoagulation therapy and graded compression hose, mobilization aids in the prevention of DVT and PE. Data from a recent study suggest that subcutaneous heparin improves the incidence of PE-contributory mortality.[35]

Once DVT is diagnosed, treatment with anticoagulant therapy is justified to prevent PE. Although it is generally agreed that proximal vein thrombosis should be treated, treatment of calf vein thrombosis is of questionable value. Heparin is given intravenously to maintain a partial thromboplastin time of $1.5 \times$ control, after which warfarin is administered for 3 to 6 months.[27] Use of a vena cava filter is indicated in patients for whom anticoagulant therapy has failed or is contraindicated.

Identification of Pulmonary Embolism

PE may occur despite use of the prophylactic regimen outlined previously. The clinical presentation of PE is well established and classically includes tachycardia, low-grade fever, and less specific symptoms, such as anxiety. A high index of suspicion and the finding of arterial saturation below that normally found is useful. The increased likelihood of communication difficulties in persons with stroke makes it even more necessary to maintain a high index of suspicion.[24]

Pulmonary angiography is the accepted method for establishing the presence or absence of pulmonary embolism.[34] However, despite the technique of selective angiography, the invasiveness and side effects of pulmonary angiography have fueled a search for alternatives. The perfusion scan with technetium-labeled albumin has gained widespread acceptance but lacks specificity. It fails to correctly identify the absence of disease, yielding a relatively high incidence of false-positive findings. Pulmonary angiography revealed PE in only about 40% of patients with abnormal technetium-labeled albumin scan findings.[34]

In a prospective study,[34] patients with an abnormal perfusion lung scan finding underwent a ventilation-perfusion lung scan followed by pulmonary angiography. The two diagnostic studies were evaluated separately and independently. Ventilation-perfusion mismatch occurs when ventilation is preserved in areas of reduced perfusion caused by PE. Ventilation and perfusion are both thought to be affected in the presence of parenchymal disease, and thus a "match" is said to exist.

The basic premise has been found to be incorrect. Those with large perfusion defects and mismatches do have a high probability of PE, as defined by angiography (86%). However, the mismatch principle was not helpful in those with smaller defects. In those with small perfusion defects (one or more subsegments), angiography confirmed PE in 40% with mismatch and 25% with match. Thus the finding of a match does *not* rule out PE in those with small defects. The strategy of using a "low-probability" lung scan pattern to rule out PE is incorrect. The frequency of positive findings of thromboembolism in such cases ranged from 29% to 46%.

Recognizing the association of DVT and PE, proximal venous thrombosis also indicates the presence of PE. Although proximal venous thrombi are mainly clinically silent, almost 90% were detected by IP; such positive results are highly predictive of venous thromboembolism. Using pulmonary angiography as the reference standard, negative venogram findings can occur in 30% of cases. Thus, although a positive result with IP or venography can be used as a basis for starting therapy, a negative result cannot be used to exclude venous thromboembolism.

The following diagnostic algorithm is recommended: after a history, physical examination, ECG, and chest x-ray examination, a perfusion lung scan is done.[31] A negative perfusion lung scan finding rules out significant PE. A study to rule out DVT may be used. Anticoagulant therapy is withheld unless venous thrombosis is suspected clinically and is demonstrable by studies on the leg, as outlined previously.

A positive perfusion scan finding leads to several alternatives. If the defect is large, a ventilation lung scan is performed. If a mismatch is present, one can assume the presence of PE (positive predictive value of 86%). If a match exists, one cannot rule out PE. In those with small perfusion defects, the ventilation scan does not add information. The alternative to pulmonary angiography in these patients is a study of the leg with venography, IP, or Doppler ultrasound. If DVT is present, anticoagulant therapy should be instituted without confirming the presence of PE. Only if the results are negative for DVT is angiography indicated. In PE, the therapeutic levels of anticoagulant medication are essentially the same as for DVT.

In summary, DVT prophylaxis is useful in preventing PE in persons with stroke. The selection of patients for prophylaxis is based on the degree of hemiplegia and a general reduction in activity. The concomitant finding of atrial fibrillation also may help in selection. Prophylaxis should be instituted early in the patient's course and should continue until the patient achieves mobility. There is a continued likelihood of DVT and possibly PE occurring, even in the rehabilitation phase. The first 30 days after onset, in particular, are associated with a hypercoagulable state, but the relevance of this to DVT has not been clearly demonstrated. Anticoagulation with subcutaneously administered heparin is the basis for achieving prophylaxis. The use of low-molecular-weight heparin appears to be particularly useful.

Despite ongoing prophylaxis, monitoring the patient for the development of DVT with noninvasive techniques appears to be useful. Such monitoring should be done on a routine basis rather than in response to clinical findings alone. Based on the literature, IP appears to be a useful and cost-effective monitoring technique. However, more recently the availability of ultrasound has made it the test of choice for monitoring. Certainly, if clinical findings such as swelling exist, sonography can also be used for noninvasive confirmation before therapeutic anticoagulant therapy is begun.

Thus the management of venous thromboembolic disease can be seen as operating on three levels. The first is prophylaxis of DVT with low-dose anticoagulant medication and other measures. If prophylaxis of DVT fails, a therapeutic level of anticoagulant medication is indicated for treating DVT. It is necessary to monitor the patient for DVT to avoid PE. The measure of success of a prophylaxis program is the reduced necessity to evaluate and treat patients for PE. Other measures of success include a reduction in the number of days a patient must be hospitalized. This clinical problem provides an opportunity to apply cost-effectiveness analysis (CEA) to health care.[33]

The following case report illustrates the need for ongoing vigilance and the value of assessing for DVT whenever possible.

CASE REPORT

B.K., a 69-year-old, left-handed, white male with a history of obesity and hypertension, had a sudden onset of left-sided weakness and dysarthria. His blood pressure was 190/110 mm Hg. A head CT scan performed on the day of onset yielded negative results for hemorrhage, but it demonstrated multiple lucencies consistent with small vessel disease. A repeat CT scan several days later showed an evolving nonhemorrhagic right middle cerebral artery territory infarct with moderate edema of the right parietal lobe. An ECG showed normal sinus rhythm with a first-degree atrioventricular node block and occasional supraventricular tachycardia. When examined 15 days after the onset, the patient used mouth breathing and was experiencing Cheyne-Stokes respirations. He was alert and able to understand spoken language and to answer by nodding yes or no appropriately. His left-sided weakness was greater in the arm than the leg; strength against resistance was present throughout the leg. The patient's position sense was affected up to his wrist and ankle on the left. Venous Doppler ultrasound studies showed no evidence of DVT. He required maximal assistance (75%) with ambulation and minimal physical assistance (25%) with transfer. He received TED hose and heparin, 5000 U subcutaneously bid.

B.K. ambulated 50 feet with a large-based quadruple leg cane by 31 days after the onset of stroke, and heparin was discontinued. Two days later (33 days after onset), he complained of difficulty in breathing and showed evidence of atrial fibrillation. His complaints improved when he converted once again to normal sinus rhythm. After converting to atrial fibrillation a second time, he was given quinidine. The patient's ABG analysis revealed a Po_2 of 70, a Pco_2 of 35.5, an O_2 saturation level of 94%, and a pH of 7.41.

On the following day the patient once again complained of shortness of breath, and his blood pressure fell to 90 mm Hg systolic. There was no evidence of cardiac arrythmia on the ECG. The ABG analysis showed a pH of 7.44, a Po_2 of 68, a Pco_2 of 29, and an O_2 saturation level of 94%. There was no evidence of DVT on clinical examination. A repeat venous Doppler ultrasound study showed incomplete compressibility of the left popliteal vein, which was consistent with intraluminal clots. The ventilation-perfusion CT scan showed pulmonary embolus, and the patient was started on an anticoagulant medication regimen.

This case illustrates the need to consider that a hypercoagulable state is present, even in the context of adequate ambulation approximately 30 days after the onset of stroke. A history of paroxysmal atrial fibrillation may be relevant to the later development of DVT. Approximately 1 week after cessation of heparin prophylaxis, the patient presented with PE in the absence of clinical signs of DVT. The presence of a new clot in the left popliteal vein was demonstrated. Thus treatment with anticoagulant therapy was justified on the basis of the finding of DVT. However, it was elected to perform a lung CT scan before starting anticoagulant therapy.

BLADDER MANAGEMENT

Michael H. Phillips

Nature of the Problem

Urinary bladder dysfunction arising from stroke can be one of the greatest problems facing patients and their families. The symptoms may vary from simple urgency to incontinence or retention. Although urgency is the most common symptom encountered in this group of patients, it has been estimated that 50% or more of patients will be incontinent at some point during the first year following their stroke.[59,62,65]

The cost attributed to incontinence underscores the importance of addressing potential urinary tract problems in this patient population. The costs of managing incontinence resulting from all causes range from $2.50 per day for outpatients to $6.00 per day for inpatients.[66] Inclusive in these figures are the costs of direct medical care and evaluation and of treatment for the potential consequences of the incontinence, such as skin breakdown and urinary tract infection. In 1987 overall cost exceeded $10 billion.[66] As a major cause of disability in the United States, stroke contributes significantly to this total expense.

Although placement of an indwelling Foley catheter may result in a "quick fix" of most bladder problems associated with stroke, it often creates new problems. For monitoring purposes, short-term use of a catheter may be unavoidable, but it may also result in infection or even urosepsis. Hematuria from local irritation is also common. With long-term use of a Foley catheter, traumatic injury such as bladder neck erosion in females and urethral stricture or fistulae in men has been seen. Bladder stones and squamous cell carcinoma have been reported in both sexes with long-term indwelling Foley catheters. All of these factors must be weighed against the convenience.

In the urologic evaluation of the stroke patient, an assement of the individual's underlying medical problems and how they might contribute to bladder infection should be included. The presence of metabolic disorders, such as diabetes mellitus, or anatomic problems, including benign prostatic hypertrophy (BPH), prostate cancer, or cystocele, can have a significant impact on the patient's urinary rehabilitation potential.

CASE REPORT

A 67-year-old man with right hemiparesis and aphasia following a stroke was examined. He was febrile, had a urinary tract infection and urinary retention, and required the insertion of a Foley catheter because intermittent catheterization proved to be too painful. Despite adequate antibiotic treatment, he failed to empty his bladder completely. Residual urine volume determinations were in excess of 120 ml. For 1 year before the stroke the patient complained of progressive hesitancy, urgency, and frequency, and benign prostatic hyperplasia was diagnosed.

After multiple failed voiding trials, a urodynamic evaluation demonstrated elevated intravesical voiding pressures in the presence of an abnormally slow urine flow. Treatment consisted of a transurethral prostatectomy performed with the patient under spinal anesthesia. Shortly after surgery the patient's residual urine volume fell to normal. Although he persisted in having irritation and was treated with imipramine (25 mg at bedtime), the medication was subsequently discontinued with complete resolution of his symptoms.

This case illustrates the superimposition of stroke on a previously diagnosed anatomic problem of the urinary tract seen commonly in elderly men. The urodynamic evaluation gave objective evidence of an outflow obstruction and was instrumental in planning therapy. The persistence of irritative voiding symptoms after surgery was thought to be related to the surgical procedure because the preoperative urodynamic study did not reveal the presence of uninhibited bladder contractions. This was borne out in the relatively rapid resolution of the symptoms.

Also important to bladder function are the changes in cognition and mobility that frequently accompany stroke. An evaluation of all these factors, taking into account the individual's social and environmental situation, may make the difference between dryness and incontinence or the need for institutional versus home care.[74]

CASE REPORT

An elderly woman with a past history of hypertension, mild congestive heart failure, and osteoarthritis became hemiplegic following a stroke. Before the stroke she complained of both urinary frequency during the day and nocturia. However, she was independently living at home and was continent of both bowel and bladder. Following the stroke she was incontinent of both.

On the woman's admission to the hospital the urologic examination findings were consistent with atrophic vaginitis and the presence of a small cystocele. Her perineal sensation was intact and rectal tone normal. The patient's postvoid residual urine volumes were between 50 and 75 ml.

The mobility problems present before the stroke were worsened by the hemiplegia, making it impossible for the patient, who was cognizant of her problem, to reach even a bedside commode. When she became recumbent, peripheral edema was mobilized, resulting in an increase in nocturia and ultimate worsening of incontinence. Because she was unable to ambulate, absorptive pads were used as a temporary measure. A caregiver was obtained, and a timed voiding program was initiated. The presence of a caregiver enabled the patient to execute transfers to a bedside commode, ultimately resulting in a resumption of both bowel and bladder continence. Institutionalization was not required.

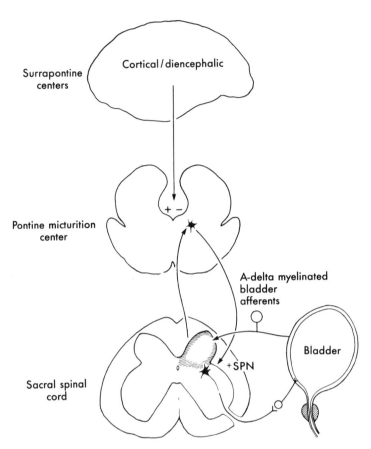

Fig. 4-1 Schematic of supraspinal micturition reflex pathway. Bladder distention activates unmyelinated A-delta fiber afferents. Ascending input is relayed to a region of the pons termed the pontine micturition center. Depending on cortical input, excitatory descending input activates neurons in the sacral parasympathetic nucleus *(SPN)* that cause bladder contraction. (From Walsh PC: *Campbell's urology,* ed 6, Philadelphia, 1992, WB Saunders.)

In the preceding instance the use of anticholinergic medication was contraindicated because of coexisting medical problems. The use of absorptive pads was also avoided to preserve a measure of the patient's self-esteem and control of her bodily functions.

Pathophysiology

Many theories on the neurologic pathways involved in voiding have been proposed. Based on neurophysiologic studies in animals and on clinical studies in humans, it was concluded that normal micturition is a brainstem reflex rather than a simple sacral reflex.[60] Afferent discharges resulting from a full bladder

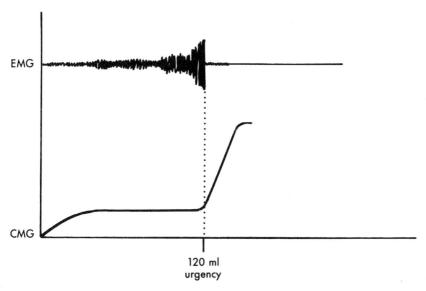

EMG

CMG

120 ml
urgency

Fig. 4-2 Schematic representation of a urodynamic study exhibiting "first sensation" and the urgent need to void at 120 ml. This is associated with a sudden elevation in detrusor pressure, an involuntary cessation of striated sphincter electromyographic (EMG) activity, and incontinence. *CMG,* Cystometrogram. (From Walsh PC: *Campbell's urology,* ed 6, Philadelphia, 1992, WB Saunders.)

travel through the pelvic nerve and pathways within the spinal cord to synapse in a supravesical micturition center thought to be in the rostral pons. It is at this level that the coordination between bladder contraction and sphincter relaxation is accomplished. Furthermore, it is thought that volitional control of voiding depends on communication between the frontal cortex and the micturition center (Fig. 4-1).[60,63] When these lines of communication are disturbed, as is often seen in stroke, the most common occurrence is loss of cortical inhibition, resulting in detrusor hyperreflexia.

Attempts at relating the location of the brain injury following stroke to the pattern of voiding dysfunction have not been entirely conclusive.[67,68,71] Detrusor areflexia is common immediately following stroke. This has often been attributed to "cerebral shock" for which the physiologic mechanism is unknown.[70] Detrusor decompensation resulting from urinary retention has been implicated as a possible contributing source. Frequency and urgency, with or without incontinence, are the most common findings during the recovery phase. Urodynamic findings are most often consistent with detrusor hyperreflexia. This is often associated with the inability to volitionally contract the striated sphincter (Fig. 4-2). Although occasionally detrusor sphincter dyssynergy may appear to be demonstrated electromyographically, this is actually thought to be a volitional attempt to abort voiding brought on by an involuntary detrusor contraction (pseudodyssynergia). Pseudodyssynergia is in direct contrast to the true dyssynergy observed in suprasacral and subpontine spinal cord injuries. In this instance there is involuntary opposition of the detrusor contraction by a spastic contraction of the striated sphincter.[61]

Evaluation and Treatment

During the immediate poststroke period an indwelling Foley catheter may be required to monitor the patient's urine output. Once overall stability has been achieved, the patient can be monitored for spontaneous voiding, keeping in mind any underlying metabolic or anatomic problems.

Intermittent catheterization may be instituted for persistent urinary retention, beginning on a schedule of every 4 to 6 hours. The frequency of the catheterization should attempt to recapitulate normal voiding, with the goal being volumes of 350 to 450 ml. During this period, attempts at eliminating any medication with anticholinergic or sympathomimetic side effects should be made. Patients should be allowed to attempt voiding on a commode as often as possible. If spontaneous voiding begins, catheterization for postvoid residual urine should continue until the catheterization volumes are consistently less than 100 ml. A sterile urine stream should be ensured before the discontinuation of catheterization. If retention persists, referring the patient for urodynamic analysis and endoscopy is appropriate to help differentiate detrusor failure from bladder outlet obstruction.

In instances in which detrusor failure is noted in men, continuation of intermittent catheterization is preferred if tolerated by the patient. Surgery to decrease an outlet obstruction in this instance is likely to fail in promoting complete evacuation of the bladder. Periodic reevaluation of the patient is appropriate to assess for recovery of detrusor tone, which subsequently may allow a successful surgical remedy.

The diagnosis of bladder outlet obstruction is made urodynamically through the demonstration of high voiding pressures in the presence of low flow. The postvoid residual urine volume may or may not be elevated. The source of the obstruction is nearly always prostatic, but it may also be located primarily at the level of the bladder neck or in the form of a urethral stricture. Removal of the obstruction through surgical or medical means may alleviate the problem of a large postvoid residual urine volume, but it may also result in incontinence from the now unopposed uninhibited detrusor contractions. It is at this point, however, that pharmacologic intervention may be successful in alleviating the irritative symptoms with less risk for urinary retention. Bladder outlet obstruction in women has rarely been described.

Urgency and frequency, with or without incontinence, should first be evaluated through a simple urinalysis and urine culture. If no infection is present, the presence of overflow incontinence can be ruled out through the measurement of the postvoid residual urine volume. In the presence of a large residual urine volume, referral for urodynamic study should be considered. In patients with small postvoid residual urine volumes, an evaluation of the overall "environment" should be made before attempts at pharmacologic manipulation. In some instances the problem is lack of access to the facilities rather than a urodynamic finding of detrusor hyperreflexia. In these instances and in others in which pharmacologic or surgical intervention is impossible, treatment by prompted or timed voiding has been shown to reduce incontinent episodes.[69]

Medical management for those individuals with negative urine culture results, small residual urine volumes, and persistent irritative symptoms is accomplished using a variety of pharmacologic agents. Musculotropic relaxants (oxybutynin chloride, dicyclomine hydrochloride, flavoxate hydrochloride) and anticholinergic agents (propantheline bromide) may be effective alone or in combination in abolishing symptoms. Tricyclic antidepressants (imipramine) and newer calcium antagonists have also been used effectively.[73] All of those medications can have significant side effects, which may hinder their usefulness in older patients.

CASE REPORT

A 60-year-old man with a history of hypertension became hemiplegic on the left side of his body. The CT scan findings were consistent with a right frontotemporoparietal stroke. The patient's primary urologic complaints were urgency, frequency, and nocturia. Before the stroke he voided normally. He had only moderate prostatic enlargement on examination. His postvoid residual volumes varied between 10 and 50 ml. Urinalysis revealed a 20 to 50 white blood count per high-power field (WBC/hpf). The urine culture grew *Enterococcus* sp. The patient was treated with appropriate antibiotic therapy for the infection. Despite the clearing of the pyuria and negative culture results, the irritative symptoms persisted. The patient was ultimately treated with oxybutynin (5 mg po bid) and became continent without urgency and frequency.

In elderly men the risk for urinary retention from the use of anticholinergic agents is great, regardless of the prostatic size. The doses should be low at first and then titrated as the symptoms improve. Postvoid residual urine volumes must be monitored to ensure that persistent urgency and frequency are not due to pharmacologically induced retention and overflow incontinence.

In situations in which there is no indication for surgery and in which pharmacologic and behavioral therapy produced less than optimal results, external collecting devices, pads, or both are an alternative.[64,72]

MANAGEMENT OF SEIZURES

T.K. Asadi

Nature of the Problem

Patients with stroke frequently have seizures; stroke is a common cause of recurrent seizures in the elderly.[84,85] The decision to treat these patients is a significant one and should be based on many factors, including the time of onset and etiologic factors of the stroke; the patient's metabolic status; and the effects of possible antiepileptic medication use on the patient's general condition.

The purpose of this section is to familiarize the reader with the common factors affecting the decision to use antiepileptic drugs (AEDs). The decision is made most frequently during the acute stage following a stroke, although there is ongoing need for monitoring when AEDs are used. The issues of when to use AEDs, which ones to use, and when to discontinue their use are considered. The many side effects of these drugs, particularly in elderly stroke patients, are also discussed.

Temporal Relation of Stroke and Seizure

A seizure may occur before, at the onset of, or weeks to months after a stroke. In one study 4.5% of patients who were admitted to a hospital with acute stroke had a previous history of epilepsy.[85] The matched control group had a 0.6% epilepsy history rate. The increased incidence of epilepsy in stroke patients was attributed to subclinical cerebral vascular disease. These seizures may have occurred weeks or even years before the presenting stroke. Primarily focal motor in character, the seizures can foreshadow the impending motor deficit and are attributed to poor blood flow.[82] Less often they are generalized and, even more rarely, complex partial defects.[85] Thus the onset of seizures in middle age or older can be a warning sign for further strokes and warrants a study of the patient's cerebral circulation, especially in the absence of other obvious etiologic factors.

Seizures at the onset of stroke are those that occur during the first 2 weeks. The frequency depends on the causes of the stroke and on its location.[78] In one study 4.4% of patients with lobar infarct or extensive hemorrhages developed seizure. Seizure occurred in 6% to 20% of patients at the onset or immediately following the subarachnoid hemorrhage.[86] Of patients with cortical infarcts, 6.5% developed seizure during the acute stage. Of patients with hemispheric transient ischemic attacks, 3.7% had seizures. Lacunar infarcts, infarcts in the posterior fossa, and small deep hemorrhages are not associated with an increased risk for seizures. Patients with cerebral embolism experience more seizures than patients with thrombotic infarcts.[83] The presence of arteriovenous malformation increases the chance of seizures occurring before, during the acute stage of, and after the stroke. Thus seizures are more frequent in patients with hemorrhage and those whose injury is lobar.

In the acute stage almost 60% of seizures are partial. Forty percent are a generalized tonic-clonic type of seizure. Of partial seizures, 75% are simple partial motor; the remaining 25% become generalized.[78] The presence of metabolic abnormalities — including hyperglycemia, hypoglycemia, hypernatremia, hyponatremia, hypocalcemia, hypomagnesemia, renal failure, and infections — increases the chance of seizures.

In one study, at the time of discharge the functional outcome of the stroke patient with early seizures was not significantly different than that of the stroke patient without seizures.[81] However, the prognosis during the first few days was worse for patients with seizures than for those without; after the first few days the outlook was similar to those without seizures. The major exceptions to this include patients with watershed infarcts and paroxysmal lateralized epileptiform discharges on electroencephalogram (EEG). A prolonged focal motor seizure can develop in these patients. This clinical entity is difficult to treat and has a poor prognosis.[82]

Seizures may begin months to a year after a stroke.[81] The reported incidence varies between 12.5% and 20%.[75,84] Generally, 50% of patients who develop late onset seizures have had seizures at the onset of stroke. Almost all stroke-related late onset seizures occur in the first year. In one study, most patients in the late onset group had cerebral embolism and many had cortical involvement. There was no relationship between the size of the nonembolic infarct and the incidence of seizures.[79] The existence of significant neurologic deficits did not predict late onset seizures. Subarachnoid hemorrhage, intracerebral hematoma, and arteriovenous malformations are associated with more frequent seizures. Cortical venous thrombosis is accompanied by a high frequency of recurrent seizures. In the late onset group of stroke-related seizure patients, most seizures are focal, but generalized seizures are also common.

Management of Seizure Disorder

The drug treatment both for recurrent seizures before the stroke and for late onset recurrent seizures is similar to that for patients with epilepsy resulting from other causes. If the patient has previously received AEDs, the serum level should be checked and adjusted to more therapeutic levels. Almost all patients who develop single or recurrent seizures in the first 2 weeks after a stroke receive AEDs. However, 7 months after a stroke, only 37% of surviving patients take these medications.[78]

The size of the stroke should not be considered a factor in making the decision to maintain AED treatment. Even an extremely large lesion may be less epileptogenic. The infarcted tissues are not epileptogenic per se. It is the surrounding damaged or dysfunctioning neurons that are the source of the epileptic discharge. If there is no cortical involvement caused by infarct or lobar hemorrhage, there seems to be no need for long-term AED therapy. In one study, recurrent seizures after a stroke were not seen in patients who had early onset seizures associated with pure subarachnoid hemorrhage.[77]

One of the problems in treating recurrent seizures of any cause is determining whether to stop the treatment and, if so, when termination should take place. In one study, late seizures were significantly more frequent in patients who had experienced early seizures (32%) than in the control group (10%), which was matched for age, sex, and type of stroke (i.e., cortical infarction, lobar or extensive hemorrhage, or subarachnoid hemorrhage).[77] The presence of side effects of AEDs was the most frequent reason for discontinuing the administration of these medications.

Stroke-related epilepsy belongs to a symptomatic group of seizures, and this group has a poor prognosis for spontaneous recovery or permanent remission after successful initial control. Most stroke-related seizures are partial, and partial seizures generally have a poorer prognosis. The presence of major neuropsychiatric handicaps also augurs a poor prognosis, dictating long-term anticonvulsant treatment. Other important factors that have an adverse effect on the long-term prognosis are the presence of cortical lesions; the severity of the seizures; short periods between seizures; the risk of future stroke; and the presence of other factors that may increase the chance of seizures, such as toxic metabolic disorders. Arteriovenous malformations, vasculitis, and possible embolic causes of stroke also tend to result in more persistent seizures. Using the findings from an EEG in making the decision to discontinue AED use is controversial. The presence of epileptic discharges may be indicative of seizure activities, but the lack of them is not a definite indication to discontinue medication therapy.

A major determining factor in the treatment of seizure disorder in the stroke patient (who is usually elderly) is the side effects of these medications. Most of these patients have many other medical problems and are receiving multiple medications. It is likely that AEDs may interact adversely with these medications. The effect of AEDs on the patient's cognitive function during the acute or rehabilitation phases of stroke management is also a limiting factor.

The following case illustrates the possible effect of AEDs on cognitive function and the effect of an interaction of drugs.

CASE REPORT

E.C., an 85-year-old, right-handed retired schoolteacher, was found lying on her floor by a neighbor. She had last been spoken to 48 hours earlier. On admission to an acute care setting, E.C. displayed left facial focal seizures. A head CT scan yielded no evidence of a hemorrhage. Magnetic resonance imaging (MRI) showed multiple ischemic infarcts throughout both hemispheres, the basal ganglia, and the pons. No further seizures occurred when the patient received phenytoin, 300 mg qd. Two weeks after the onset the phenytoin level was 4.8 ng/dl. The patient was fully oriented. On a short-term memory test she recalled two out of three objects at 5 minutes. She began carbamazepine therapy for more appropriate treatment of her focal seizures. The plan was to discontinue the phenytoin when the carbamazepine level reached a therapeutic range. After several days the patient complained of slurred speech and clouding of consciousness. The phenytoin level at that time was 8.3 ng/dl and the carbamazepine was 5.2 ng/dl. The phenytoin was discontinued and a clearing of consciousness resulted. An EEG several days later showed diffuse slowing with right temporal slow wave focus. The patient has remained seizure free while taking carbamazepine, 200 mg bid.

Table 4-1 is a list of the side effects of the most commonly used medications. The side effects may be dose dependent, idiosyncratic, or long term.[80] Physicians should try to control seizures at the lowest dose of medications. The goal is to treat the patient, not the medication's blood level. Often symptoms can be controlled well despite blood levels of medication that are called "subtherapeutic" or "low" by the clinical laboratory. The following case illustrates one of the more common idiosyncratic reactions to phenytoin.

CASE REPORT

C.B. was a 60-year-old woman who, after a sudden onset of severe headache, was found to have a ruptured aneurysm of the right pericallosal artery. She underwent craniotomy with clipping of the aneurysm. Subsequent left hemiparesis and a mild cognitive deficit were present. No seizure was reported. She was administered 500 mg of phenytoin per day for prophylactic purposes and transferred to the rehabilitation unit. Her phenytoin level on admission was 17.2 ng/dl, and she had a mild cognitive impairment with problems of memory and in performing calculations. Three weeks later her cognitive functions remained unchanged, but she had developed a generalized rash and periorbital swelling. Her WBC was 20,500 with 25% eosinophils. Phenytoin therapy was stopped, and steroid treatment was instituted, lasting for several weeks. Her cognitive difficulties improved, and she eventually returned to work.

Stroke patients usually have other medical problems, for which they receive a variety of medications. It is not unusual to see a patient who is taking more than five medications and who needs to begin AED therapy. The possible

TABLE 4-1 Antiepileptic Drugs

	ACUTE, DOSE-RELATED SIDE EFFECTS	EFFECT ON COGNITIVE FUNCTIONS	LONG-TERM EFFECT OR NON-DOSE RELATED
Phenytoin	Usually but not always with serum levels above therapeutic amount—vertigo; ataxia tremor; nystagmus and dysarthria	Both in acute and chronic use; more in elderly; rarely causes encephalopathy	Cognitive disturbances; depression; psychosis; delirium, cerebellar atrophy (?), movement disorder; peripheral neuropathy; hepatic toxicity; folic acid deficiency; aplastic anemia; leukopenia, lymphadenopathy; disturbed vitamin D, calcium metabolism, and osteomalacia; skin rash
Carbamazepine	Very common if initial doses are high—change in mental function; poor coordination; ataxia; blurred vision; dizziness; dyskinesia; asterixis	Mild effect on cognitive function; rare cases of psychosis	Bone marrow depression (0.5/million), eosinophilia, leukocytosis; nausea and vomiting; anorexia; rare but serious hepatic dysfunction; nonsignificant increase in liver enzyme level; skin rash; alopecia; hyponatremia
Phenobarbital	Change in affect and behavior; drug dependency; hallucinations; withdrawal syndrome; sedation; nystagmus; dysarthria; ataxia	Major on initial doses and with higher dosage	Megaloblastic with and without folic acid deficiency; effect on metabolism of calcium with chemical osteomalacia; skin rash; hepatic toxicity
Sodium valproate	Gastrointestinal disturbance (anorexia, nausea, vomiting, diarrhea and constipation); essential type of tremor	Not well known	Pancreatitis (may be fatal); weight gain; skin rash; hair loss; thrombocytopenia; severe hepatotoxicity; hyperammonemia with encephalopathy

interactions between all of these medications is a major medical problem. Some AEDs induce liver enzymes and change the metabolism of other AEDs or other medications. Most AEDs are bound to plasma proteins. This is true for other medications. Competition to bind with the protein has an effect on the serum concentration of many medications. Many drugs interfere with the absorption of other drugs. Table 4-2 describes some of the major known effects of commonly used AEDs with other medications.

In patients with focal motor or generalized seizures as the result of a stroke, carbamazepine and phenytoin have the highest treatment success. Phenobarbital, primidone, and valproic acid are second-line treatments. Most patients in the acute stage following stroke receive phenytoin because of the availability of its parenteral form. However, evidence exists that phenytoin can interfere with the recovery of motor functions. If possible the patient should be maintained on monotherapy. All of the side effects mentioned previously are seen more commonly with polytherapy.

The range of relationships between seizures and stroke are illustrated in the following case report.

CASE REPORT

R.D. was a 77-year-old man with a history of chronic obstructive pulmonary disease (COPD) who had a right cerebrovascular accident (CVA). Several days later, he had left-sided motor seizures, which were treated with phenytoin. The patient's condition was controlled with 400 mg of phenytoin. He also required continuous supplemental oxygen to maintain an adequate arterial oxygen saturation. The only other drugs administered were theophylline and aspirin (325 mg qd). Several months later the patient developed generalized weakness and slurred speech. His serum phenytoin level at that time was 26 ng/dl. The phenytoin dosage was reduced to 200 mg/day, and he improved. Several months later the patient developed transient slurred speech, followed within an hour by generalized seizure and status epilepticus lasting 18 hours. The patient's phenytoin level on admission to the hospital was 9.6 ng/dl. He developed a marked deterioration of his residual left hemiparesis. A head CT scan revealed extension of his previous encephalomalacia. He was treated with more phenytoin and continued to have many generalized and focal motor seizures with increased postictal weakness on the hemiplegic side. He was then placed on carbamazepine therapy. The patient remained seizure free while receiving both phenytoin and carbamazepine. His left-sided hemiplegia progressively improved with intensive rehabilitation.

This case illustrates the association of seizures with the acute onset of stroke. The history of the second episode suggests that the onset of the status

TABLE 4-2   Drug Interactions

	INCREASE THE METABOLISM AND REDUCES THE BLOOD LEVEL OF:	DRUGS THAT INCREASE THE LEVEL OF ANTIEPILEPTIC DRUGS	DRUGS THAT DECREASE THE LEVEL OF ANTIEPILEPTIC DRUGS	DRUG INTERACTIONS WITH NO FIXED END RESULT
Phenytoin	Warfarin, corticosteroids, oral contraceptives, quinidine, digitoxin, vitamin D, rifampin, doxycycline, estrogens, furosemide, carbamazepine, benzodiazepine	Chloramphenicol, dicumarol, isoniazid, phenylbutazone, alcohol, salicylates, chlordiazepoxide, phenothiazines, diazepam, estrogen, cimetidine, and others	Antiacid preparations containing calcium	Phenobarbital, valproic acid and sodium valproate
Carbamazepine	Sodium valproate, ethosuximide, clonazepam, warfarin, oral contraceptives, doxycycline, theophylline, haloperidol	Cimetidine, propoxyphene, erythromycin, isoniazid, calcium channel blocking agents (e.g., verapamil)	Phenobarbital, phenytoin, primidone	Phenobarbital
Sodium valproate				Phenytoin, antiplatelet and anticoagulant agents

epilepticus was preceded by transient cerebral ischemia. This onset of status epilepticus, associated with the second stroke, undoubtedly contributed to the severity of the increased neural injury. It is unclear whether maintenance of the patient's phenytoin level at a somewhat higher level could have protected him from the serious effects of this second stroke. The presence of ongoing COPD with problems in maintaining adequate oxygen saturation was a complicating factor.

REFERENCES

Nature of the Problem

1. Garroway WM, Whisnant MD, Drury I: The changing pattern of survival following stroke, *Stroke* 14:699, 1983.
2. Indredarik B et al: Benefit of a stroke unit: a randomized controlled trial, *Stroke* 22:1026, 1991.
3. Sacco RL et al: Survival and recurrence following stroke: Framingham Study, *Stroke* 13:290, 1982.
4. Silver FL et al: Early mortality following stroke: a prospective review, *Stroke* 15(3):492, 1984.
5. Terent A: Survival after stroke and transient ischemic attacks during the 1970s and 1980s, *Stroke* 20(10):1320, 1989.

Comorbidity and Its Effects

6. Chimowitz MI, Mancini GBJ: Asymptomatic coronary artery disease in patients with stroke, *Stroke* 26:23, 1992.
7. Cote R et al: The Canadian Neurological Scale: a preliminary study in acute stroke, *Stroke* 17:731, 1986.
8. Davalos A et al: Deteriorating ischemic stroke: risk factors and prognosis, *Neurology* 40:1865-1869, 1990.
9. Fieschi C et al: Clinical and instrumental evaluation of patients with ischemic stroke within the first 6 hours, *J Neurol Sci* 91:311, 1989.
10. Kaplan MS, Pratley R, Hawkins WJ: Silent myocardial ischemia during rehabilitation for cerebrovascular disease, *Arch Phys Med Rehabil* 72:59, 1991.
11. Kushner M et al: Relation of hyperglycemia early in ischemic brain infarction to cerebral anatomy, metabolism and clinical outcome, *Ann Neurol* 28:129, 1990.
12. Love BB et al: Coronary artery disease and cardiac events with asymptomatic and symptomatic cerebrovascular disease, *Stroke* 23:939, 1992.
13. Myers MG et al: Cardiac sequelae of a acute stroke, *Stroke* 13:838, 1982.
14. Rokey R et al: Coronary artery disease in patients with cerebrovascular disease: a prospective study, *Ann Neurol* 16:50, 1984.
15. Sacco RL et al: Survival and recurrence following stroke: the Framingham Study, *Stroke* 13:291, 1982.
16. Sacco RL et al: Determinants of the early recurrence of cerebral infarction: the Stroke Data Bank, *Stroke* 20:983, 1989.
17. Sirna S et al: Cardiac evaluation of the patient with stroke, *Stroke* 21:14, 1990.
18. Talman WJ: Cardiovascular regulation and lesions of the central nervous system, *Ann Neurol* 18:1, 1985.
19. Woo J et al: The influence of hyperglycemia and diabetes mellitus on immediate and 3 months morbidity and mortality after acute stroke, *Arch Neurol* 47:1174, 1990.

Deep Vein Thrombosis

20. Bornstein NM, Norris JW: Deep vein thrombosis after ischemic stroke: rationale for a therapeutic trial, *Arch Phys Med Rehabil* 69:955, 1988.
21. Bounds JV et al: Mechanisms and timing of deaths from cerebral infarction, *Stroke* 12:474, 1981.
22. Brandstater ME, Roth EJ, Siebeus HC: Venous thromboembolism in stroke: literature review and implications for clinical practice, *Arch Phys Med Rehabil* 73:S379, 1992.
23. Bromfield EB, Reding MJ: Relative risk of deep venous thrombosis or pulmonary embolism post-stroke based on ambulatory status, *J Neurol Rehabil* 2:51, 1988.
24. Chaudhuri GX, Costa JR: Clinical findings associated with pulmonary embolism in a rehabilitation setting, *Arch Phys Med Rehabil* 72:671, 1991.
25. Cronan JJ, Dorfman GS, Grusmark J: Lower-extremity deep venous thrombosis: further experience with and refinements of US assessment, *Radiology* 168:101, 1988.
26. Fasting H et al: Prevention of postoperative deep venous thrombosis, *Acta Chir Scand* 151:245, 1985.
27. Hirsh J, Hull RD: Treatment of venous thromboembolism, *Chest* 89(suppl):5, 1986.
28. Huisman MV et al: Unexpected high prevalence of silent pulmonary embolism in patients with deep venous thrombosis, *Chest* 95:498, 1989.
29. Huisman MV et al: Serial impedance plethysmography for suspected deep vein thrombosis in outpatients: the Amsterdam Practitioner Study, *N Engl J Med* 314:823, 1986.
30. Hull RD, Raskob GE, Hirsh J: Diagnosis of clinically suspected pulmonary embolism: practical approaches, *Chest* 89(suppl):5, 1986.
31. Hull RD, Raskob GE, Hirsh J: Prophylaxis of venous thromboembolism: an overview, *Chest* 89(suppl):5, 1986.
32. Hull RD et al: Impedance plethysmography using the occlusive cuff technique in the diagnosis of venous thrombosis, *Circulation* 53:4, 1976.
33. Hull LL et al: Cost effectiveness of clinical diagnosis, venography, and noninvasive testing in patients with symptomatic deep-vein thrombosis, *N Engl J Med* 304:1561, 1981.
34. Hull RD et al: Pulmonary angiography, ventilation lung scanning and venography for clinically suspected pulmonary embolism with abnormal perfusion lung scan, *Ann Intern Med* 98:891, 1983.
35. Indredarik B et al: Benefit of a stroke unit: a randomized controlled trial, *Stroke* 22:1026, 1991.
36. Landi G et al: Hypercoagulability in acute stroke: prognostic significance, *Neurology* 37:1667, 1987.
37. Lane DA et al: Activation of coagulation and fibrinolytic systems following stroke, *Br J Hematol* 53:655, 1983.
38. Lensing AWA et al: Detection of deep vein thrombosis by real-time B-mode ultrasonography, *N Engl J Med* 320:342, 1989.
39. Leyvraz PF et al: Adjusted versus fixed-dose subcutaneous heparin in the prevention of deep-vein thrombosis after total hip replacement, *N Engl J Med* 309:954, 1983.
40. McCarthy ST, Turner J: Low-dose subcutaneous heparin in the prevention of deep-vein thrombosis and pulmonary emboli following acute stroke, *Age Aging* 15:84, 1986.
41. McCarthy ST et al: Low-dose heparin as a prophylaxis against deep-vein thrombosis after acute stroke, *Lancet* 2(8042):800-1, 1977.
42. Moser KM, Lemoine JR: Embolic risk conditioned by location of deep venous thrombosis, *Ann Intern Med* 94:439, 1981.
43. Myers MG et al: Cardiac sequelae of acute stroke, *Stroke* 13:838, 1982.

44. Noel P et al: Atrial fibrillation as a risk factor for deep vein thrombosis and pulmonary emboli in stroke patients, *Stroke* 22:760, 1991.
45. Office of Medical Applications of Research, National Institutes of Health: Consensus conference: prevention of venous thrombosis and pulmonary embolism, *JAMA* 256:744, 1986.
46. Reference deleted.
47. Peramas OW et al: Clinicopathologic comparative analysis of pulmonary embolism developed in young and elderly stroke patients, *Neurology* 41(suppl):367, 1991.
48. Russell D et al: Diagnostic efficacy of impedance plethysmography for clinically suspected deep-vein thrombosis: a randomized trial, *Ann Intern Med* 102:21, 1985.
49. Sandset M et al: A double-blind and randomized placebo-controlled trial of low molecular weight heparin once daily to prevent deep-vein thrombosis in acute ischemic stroke, *Semin Thromb Hemost* 16(suppl):25, 1990.
50. Silver FL et al: Early mortality following stroke: a prospective review, *Stroke* 15:492, 1984.
51. Sioson ER: Deep vein thrombosis in stroke patients: an overview, *J Stroke Cerebrovasc Dis* 2:74, 1992.
52. Sioson ER, Crowe WE, Dawson NV: Occult proxima deep vein thrombosis: its prevalence among patients admitted to rehabilitation hospital, *Arch Phys Med Rehabil* 69:183, 1988.
53. Todd JW et al: Deep venous thrombosis in acute spinal cord injury: a comparison of ^{125}I fibrinogen leg scanning impedance plethysmography and venography, *Paraplegia* 14:50, 1976.
54. Torngren S: Low dose heparin and compression stockings in the prevention of postoperative deep venous thrombosis, *Br J Surg* 67:482, 1980.
55. Turpie AGG et al: Double-blind randomized trial of org 10172 low-molecular-weight heparinoid in prevention of deep-vein thrombosis in thrombotic stroke, *Lancet* 1:523, 1987.
56. Vogel P et al: Deep venous thrombosis of the lower extremity: US evaluation, *Radiology* 163:747, 1987.
57. Warlow C, Ogston D, Douglas AS: Deep venous thrombosis of the legs after strokes, *Br Med J* 1:1178, 1976.
58. Wheeler HB, Anderson FA: Diagnostic approaches for deep vein thrombosis, *Chest* 89 (suppl):5, 1986.

Bladder Management

59. Barer DH: Continence after stroke: useful predictor of goal of therapy? *Age Aging* 18(3):183, 1989.
60. Blaivas JG: The neurophysiology of micturition: a clinical study of 550 patients, *J Urol* 127:958, 1982.
61. Blaivas JG et al: Detrusor-external sphincter dyssynergy, *J Urol* 125:542, 1981.
62. Borrie MJ et al: Urinary incontinence after stroke: a perspective study, *Age Aging* 15(3):177, 1986.
63. Bradley WE, Timm GW, Scott FB: Innervation of the detrusor muscle and urethra, *Urol Clin North Am* 1:3, 1974.
64. Brink CA: Absorbent pads, garments, and management strategist, *J Am Geriatr Soc* 38:368, 1990.
65. Brocklehurst JC et al: Incidence and correlates of incontinence in stroke patients, *J Am Geriatr Soc* 33(8):540, 1985.
66. Hu T: Impact of urinary incontinence on health-care costs, *J Am Geriatr Soc* 38:292, 1990.

67. Khan Z et al: Predictive correlation of urodynamic dysfunction and brain injury after cerebrovascular accident, *J Urol* 126:86, 1981.
68. Khan Z et al: Analysis of voiding disorders in patients with cerebrovascular accidents, *Urology* 35:265, 1990.
69. Schnelle JF: Treatment of urinary incontinence in nursing home patients by prompted voiding, *J Am Geriatr Soc* 38:356, 1990.
70. Staskin DR: Intracranial lesions that affect lower urinary tract function. In Krane RJ, Siroky MB, editors: *Clinical neurology*, Boston, 1991, Little, Brown.
71. Tsuchida S et al: Urodynamic studies on hemiplegic patients after cerebrovascular accident, *Urology* 21:315, 1983.
72. Warren JW: Urine-collection devices for use in adults with urinary incontinence, *J Am Geriatr Soc* 38:364, 1990.
73. Wein AJ, Barret DM: *Voiding function and dysfunction: a logical and practical approach*, Chicago, 1988, Year Book.
74. Williams ME, Gaylord SA: Role of functional assessment in the evaluation of urinary incontinence, *J Am Geriatr Soc* 38:296, 1990.

Management of Seizures

75. Adams RD, Victor M: *Principles of neurology*, ed 4, New York, 1989, McGraw Information Services.
76. Dietz MA, McDowell FH: Potentiation of rehabilitation: medication effects on recovery of function after brain injury and stroke, *J Stroke Cerebrovasc Dis* 1:37, 1991.
77. Kilpatrick CJ, Davis SM, Hopper JL: Early seizures after acute stroke: risk of late seizures, *Arch Neurol* 49:509, 1992.
78. Kilpatrick CJ et al: Epileptic seizures in acute stroke, *Arch Neurol* 47:157, 1990.
79. Louis S, McDowell FM: Epileptic seizures in nonembolic cerebral infarction, *Arch Neurol* 17:414, 1967.
80. Laidlaw J, Richens A, Oxley J: *A textbook of epilepsy*, New York, 1988, Churchill Livingstone.
81. Millikan CH, McDowell FM, Easton JD: *Stroke*, Philadelphia, 1987, Lea & Febiger.
82. Niedermeyer E, de Silva FL: *Electroencephalography: basic principles, clinical application and related fields*, Baltimore, 1982, Urban & Schwarzenberg.
83. Patrick J, Whitty CW: Recurrent cerebral emboli and diagnosis of focal epilepsy, *Lancet* 1:1291, 1965.
84. Richardson EP, Dodge PR: Epilepsy in cerebrovascular disease, *Epilepsy* 3:49, 1954.
85. Shinton RA et al: The frequency of epilepsy preceding stroke: case control study in 230 patients, *Lancet* 1:11, 1987.
86. Walton JN: *Subarachnoid hemorrhage*, New York, 1956, Churchill Livingstone.

CHAPTER 5

Neurologic Management Plan

Louis R. Caplan

Nature of the problem
Neurologic assessment of the acute stroke
  Review of the various stroke mechanisms
  Identifying the stroke mechanism
  Localizing the lesion
  Laboratory evaluation
  Review
    If the lesion is hemorrhage
    If the lesion is ischemia
Treatment
  Subarachnoid hemorrhage
  Intracerebral hemorrhage
  Ischemia
Patterns of neurologic impairment
  Left cerebral hemispheric deficits
    Aphasia
    Acquired disorders of written language
    Apraxia
  Right cerebral hemisphere abnormalities
    Neglect
    Anosognosia
    Dysprosodia
    Motor impersistence
    Constructional apraxia
  Abnormalities of the temporooccipital lobes
    Visual symptoms
    Amnesia
    Behavior
  Frontal lobe lesions
  Elementary dysfunctions
    Paresis
    Sensory symptoms

Hemianopia
Nonpyramidal hemimotor syndromes
Diplopia, dizziness, and ophthalmoplegia

NATURE OF THE PROBLEM

Before becoming immersed in the details of diagnosing and selecting treatment for the patient with acute stroke, the physician should step back from the bedside for a moment and broaden his or her perspective. Stroke is nearly always a manifestation of a systemic degenerative vascular disease, most often hypertension, atherosclerosis, or both. The long-range plan for the care of the patient should include the following:

1. Immediate short-term strategies to *diagnose* the cause and pathophysiologic factors of the stroke and to *initiate treatment* to minimize acute brain damage
2. Slightly longer range goals of anticipating and *preventing medical complications* of the stroke and choosing and pursuing *rehabilitation strategies* aimed at overcoming handicaps created by the neurologic deficits
3. *Prevention* of future strokes and other cardiovascular events, involving the recognition of *stroke risk factors* and the institution of educative and other strategies as early as possible, even while managing the acute stroke

Risk factor modification should begin early, be continued throughout the patient's hospitalization, and be emphasized after hospital discharge. Rehabilitative strategies and patient education also must be started early to be effective. The box below enumerates the four key interrelated aspects of the evaluation of every stroke patient.

Key Elements of the Evaluation of Stroke Patients

1. Recognize *stroke risk factors* and begin modification. Knowledge of the risk factors also helps predict stroke mechanism.
2. Identify *medical conditions;* these help predict — and thus prevent — complications. Knowledge of medical illnesses also helps predict stroke mechanism.
3. Determine the *cause of the stroke (stroke mechanism).* The etiologic factors guide treatment.
4. Localize the *brain lesion.* The location of the lesion determines the nature of the neurologic deficits. Localization is essential to plan investigations. Characterization of the deficit is important for planning and facilitating rehabilitation.

NEUROLOGIC ASSESSMENT OF THE ACUTE STROKE
Review of the Various Stroke Mechanisms

Stroke is a very broad term used to characterize any acute central nervous system damage that occurs as a result of blood vessel abnormalities. Under the broad umbrella of stroke are many diverse conditions. Their treatments are specific and depend on identifying the cause and pathophysiology of the stroke in the individual patient. The major stroke categories are reviewed in Fig. 5-1. Before sending in the troops, it is important to know what the enemy looks like and how it behaves. The better stroke mechanisms are known and understood, the more easily they are recognized in patients.

The first key distinction is made between *hemorrhage* and *ischemia*. These are two diametrically opposite conditions. Hemorrhage is bleeding that involves *too much blood* within the cranium in and around the brain, whereas ischemia means that *too little blood* is getting to vital brain regions. In patients with hemorrhage one seeks to limit blood extravasation, whereas in ischemia one tries to augment the supply of blood. Strategies that limit bleeding, such as decreasing blood pressure, might worsen ischemia; treatments to prevent recurrent ischemia caused by vascular occlusion, such as anticoagulation, may promote or worsen hemorrhage.

Within these two broad categories of hemorrhage and ischemia are important subdivisions. Hemorrhage can be divided into *subarachnoid hemorrhage (SAH),* indicating blood localization around the brain within the cerebrospinal fluid pathways, and *intracerebral hemorrhage (ICH)*, indicating bleeding directly into the brain substance. SAH is usually caused by an aneurysm or vascular malformation that abuts the surface of the brain or the ventricular ependymal surface. Rupture of an aneurysm results in the release of blood under high pressure (i.e., systemic arterial pressure) into the cerebrospinal fluid. This causes an abrupt increase in intracranial pressure and headache, sudden cessation of activity, and often vomiting. The blood rapidly disseminates within the subarachnoid space but usually not into the brain substance. The bleeding is usually brief and stops before the patient arrives at the hospital. Treatment is aimed mostly at *preventing the next bleed.* The initial rupture of the aneurysm or malformation makes it more vulnerable to rebleeding, often within the next few hours, days, or weeks. Definitive treatment usually involves surgical or endovascular control of the responsible aneurysm or vascular malformation. Head trauma, bleeding diatheses, amyloid angiopathy, drugs, and hypertension are much less common causes of SAH.

In ICH the bleeding is into the brain parenchyma, and the causes and treatment strategies are different from those in SAH. ICH is most often caused by acute or chronic hypertension.[8] Small penetrating arteries deep within the brain break, causing blood to issue into the local brain tissue at arteriolar or capillary pressure. The earliest symptoms are due to dysfunction of the focal region of the brain that contains the blood.[12] If bleeding is into the left putamen,

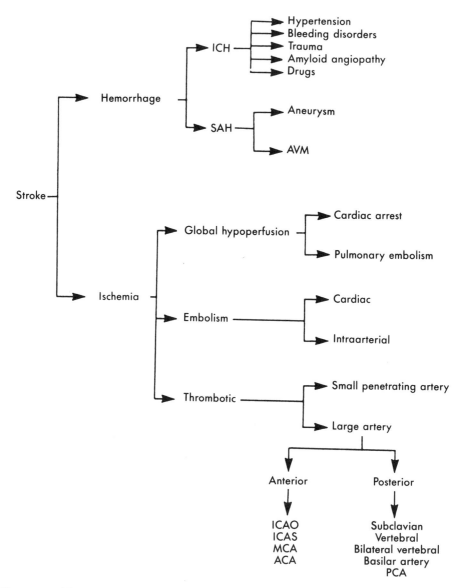

Fig. 5-1 Differential diagnosis of stroke. (From Caplan LR, Kelly JJ: *Consultation in neurology,* Philadelphia, 1988, BC Decker.)

weakness of the right limbs is the first symptom noted. If bleeding is into the right cerebellum, veering to the right and ataxia are usually the first symptoms. Once the bleeding begins, it gradually increases and forms a local collection of blood called a hematoma (Fig. 5-2). The initial bleeding causes an abrupt increase in local tissue pressure. This results in breakage of adjacent capillaries, with

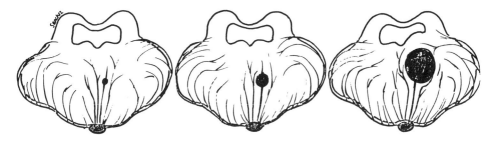

Fig. 5-2 Enlarging pontine hematoma. (From Caplan LR, Stein RW: *Stroke: a clinical approach,* Boston, 1986, Butterworth.)

bleeding developing along the circumference of the initial hemorrhage. Additional pressure develops on the periphery of the hematoma, and more capillaries are compressed and break. The hematoma grows on its periphery much like a snowball rolling downhill in the snow. As the hematoma grows in size, the focal neurologic signs increase. The patient with a left putaminal hemorrhage has increased right limb weakness and might develop numbness of the right limbs, aphasia, and deviation of the head and eyes to the left. If the hematoma becomes moderate sized or large, the surrounding structures are displaced and intracranial pressure rises. The increased pressure causes headache, vomiting, and a reduced level of alertness. The enlarging hematoma may decompress itself by discharging some of its contents into the cerebrospinal fluid on the surface of the brain or into the ventricular system. The increase in tissue pressure around the hematoma helps to contain it and to limit the bleeding. The treating physician's goal is to *limit the size of the hematoma* and prevent a fatal outcome that may ensue from the pressure shifts within the skull. Acute rebleeding is not especially common. Elevated blood pressure, related to acute or chronic hypertension, is by far the most common cause of ICH. Vascular malformations within the brain also cause ICH, and these may rebleed, although usually this does not occur until months or years later. Head trauma, drug use, bleeding disorders, and amyloid angiopathy are less frequent causes of ICH as compared with hypertension and vascular malformations.[8,12]

In patients with brain ischemia the lack of blood flow can be global (*systemic hypoperfusion*) or focal. Focal brain ischemia is almost always due to a focal abnormality affecting the blood vessels that supply the ischemic zone. When the focal vascular abnormality originates and evolves in situ at the site of the occlusive process, the process is termed thrombosis. When the material blocking the vessel originated downstream away from the occlusion, the process is termed embolism. The practical reason for distinguishing between these two processes should be obvious. If the occlusive process developed locally, "fixing" the local abnormality might cure the situation. On the other hand, if the pathologic condition is elsewhere, correcting the local area of blockage will not prevent further obstruction from emboli.

Four rather different pathologic conditions most often cause localized vascular occlusive lesions. They are the following:

1. *Atheromatous plaques* develop along the arterial intimal surface and subintima. These plaques grow and gradually encroach on the arterial lumen. When they reach a critical size, they crack and ulcerate, promoting superimposed thrombus formation.[21]

2. *Thrombi* are formed within the lumen. *White thrombi*, composed of platelets mixed with fibrin, tend to form on irregular surfaces such as craggy atheromatous plaques. Platelets are activated and adhere to one another and to the vascular endothelium. *Red thrombi* tend to form in regions of stagnation and reduced blood flow such as severely stenotic arteries. They are composed of red blood cells mixed with fibrin. In some patients with hypercoagulability, red thrombi form without major vascular lesions.

3. *Thickening of the walls of arteries* occurs when the constituents of the arterial media hypertrophy, and fibrous tissue, collagen, and smooth muscle proliferate. At times, foreign substances such as amyloid and inflammatory tissue are deposited within the arteries. Hypertensive arteriopathies, amyloid angiopathy, and fibromuscular dysplasia are all examples of disorders affecting the arterial wall locally and leading to encroachment on the lumen and altered vascular contractility. Dissection of the arterial wall can result from trauma or abnormal wall composition and leads to an acute intramural hematoma, which compromises the lumen.

4. Altered vascular contractility (*vasoconstriction* and *vasodilation*) lead (1) to vasospasm with constriction and, at times, occlusion of the vascular lumen or (2) to abnormal dilation of arteries with altered blood flow and turbulence. Recent studies have shown that an increased rigidity of the arteries and atherosclerosis may increase the tendency of arteries to vasoconstrict. Strategies to treat these various types of vascular pathologic and pathophysiologic states clearly differ.

Emboli originate from the heart, venous system, and proximal arterial bed.[6] The box on p. 67 lists the most frequent sources and embolic materials from each donor site. Thrombi originating in the venous system must of course traverse the heart or the pulmonary vascular bed to reach the brain (so-called paradoxic embolism). Prevention of further embolization involves the use of systemic anticoagulant agents or control of the local donor site (e.g., repair of an abnormal heart valve, septal defect, or an aortic, carotid, or vertebral artery plaque).

When *systemic hypoperfusion* is responsible for ischemia, the process does not affect a local vessel but instead involves the pump system. The most common

---

Common Embolic Sources and Materials

Cardiac
    Valvular disease (calcium, bacteria, fibrin-platelet white thrombi):
        rheumatic; calcific; bacterial endocarditis; thrombotic marantic
        endocarditis; mitral annulus calcification; mitral valve myxomatous
        change with prolapse
    Coronary artery, disease related (red thrombi): myocardial infarcts; ventric-
        ular aneurysms; mural thrombi; hypokinetic zones
    Lesions within the cardiac chambers (tumor tissues, red thrombi): atrial
        myxomas; other intracardiac tumors, thrombi
    Septal defects (red thrombi): atrial and ventricular septal defects; atrial
        septal aneurysms; patent foramen ovale
    Arrhythmias (red thrombi): atrial fibrillation; sick sinus syndrome
Paradoxical emboli (red thrombi): cardiac septal defects; pulmonary arterio-
    venous fistulae
Aorta (cholesterol particles, calcium, white and red thrombi): plaques with
    superimposed thrombi
Proximal arteries (cholesterol plaques, white and red thrombi): arterial
    plaques and thrombi
Systemic (fat, air, oral pills injected intravenously containing talc and micro-
    crystalline cellulose)

---

cause of systemic hypoperfusion is acute circulatory failure caused by cardiac pump failure (e.g., arrhythmia, acute myocardial ischemia), hypotension, shock, or hypovolemia. The end result is an insufficient amount of blood reaching the brain. The symptoms and signs are those of global brain hypoperfusion. Patients feel light headed and faint. Their vision dims; sounds appear distant and indistinct; thinking becomes less clear; and patients feel as if they will pass out. Usually accompanying the brain ischemia are signs of general circulatory compromise, that is, pallor, tachycardia, sweating, and low blood pressure. The patient's symptoms are improved by lying down. Usually there are no focal unilateral signs of brain dysfunction (e.g., hemiparesis, hemianopia, hemisensory loss), in contrast to thrombotic and embolic strokes in which focal signs predominate. The evaluation of patients with systemic hypoperfusion is aimed at identifying the cause of the circulatory failure. An acute cardiac event, systemic bleeding, hypovolemia, and pulmonary embolism are frequent mechanisms. Time should not be spent studying the brain or extracranial and intracranial arteries because the problem is in the "pump" and "water tank," not in the "pipes." Recovery depends on the rapid correction of the circulatory problem and restoration of adequate blood flow to the brain.

Data Needed to Identify the Stroke Mechanism

1. Demography: age, race, sex
2. Risk factors: patient and family history of hypertension, coronary artery disease, vascular disease, hypercholesterolemia, smoking
3. Presence of transient ischemic attacks or other warning signs before the stroke
4. Time of onset and activity at onset
5. Course of the deficit
6. Accompanying symptoms: headache, vomiting, loss of consciousness, seizures
7. Physical examination findings: blood pressure, pulse, cardiac examination
8. Vascular examination findings: absent pulses, bruits, collateral channels
9. Neuroimaging findings: computed tomography, magnetic resonance imaging, or both, showing infarct or hemorrhage
10. Vascular imaging findings: ultrasound, magnetic resonance angiography, catheter angiography
11. Lumbar puncture results

Identifying the Stroke Mechanism

The enemies have been met; how does one next go about recognizing them? The identification of the stroke mechanism depends primarily on the patient's history, the general physical examination, and the investigations (see the box above). The physician should begin considering the cause of the stroke when first told about a patient. For example, during the initial phone call about a patient, the caller usually transmits demographic data and some medical background. Perhaps the caller relates that a 70-year-old man with a past history of angina, myocardial infarctions, and leg claudication developed paralysis of his left arm and leg that day. The information reveals that this patient has systemic atherosclerosis and cardiac disease. The likelihood is that his stroke is due to associated atherosclerosis of the brain's major supply arteries or to embolism arising from the patient's heart disease. In another example the caller tells the physician about a 35-year-old man with severe hypertension who has developed left limb weakness that day and who has a bad headache and reduced alertness. The patient has no history of other vascular disease. In this patient the history of severe hypertension suggests the strong probability of a hemorrhage. Because the patient is paralyzed on one side of the body, a parenchymatous hemorrhage (an ICH) is much more likely than an SAH. If, instead, the physician was told by the caller that the patient was a 34-year-old normotensive woman with rheumatic mitral stenosis and atrial fibrillation who had suddenly developed a left hemiparesis, embolism from her rheumatic valvular disease or bacterial endocarditis would head the list of probable causes. Knowledge of the *risk factors*

TABLE 5-1   Weighing Pathophysiologic Factors

	THROMBOSIS	LACUNE	EMBOLUS	INTRACEREBRAL HEMORRHAGE	SUBARACHNOID HEMORRHAGE
Hypertension	+ +	+ + +		+ + +	+
Severe hypertension		+		+ + + +	+ +
Coronary artery disease	+ + +		+ +		
Leg claudication	+ + +		+		
Atrial fibrillation			+ + + +		
Sick sinus syndrome			+ +		
Valvular heart disease			+ + +		
Diabetes	+ + +	+	+		
Bleeding diathesis				+ + + +	+ +
Cancer	+ +		+ +	+	+
Old age	+ +	+ +	+ +	+ +	+
Black or Asian descent	+	+ +		+ +	

From Caplan LR, Stein RW: *Stroke: a clinical approach*, Boston, 1986, Butterworth.

and present *medical conditions* helps to rate the probability of various stroke mechanisms. In Table 5-1 are listed some factors that influence the likelihood of the presence of various stroke mechanisms. These factors are identified from the patient's history and the general physical examination (e.g., of blood pressure, pulse, and cardiac status). Data from stroke registries were used to assign these factors' loading weights.[14,23,27]

Demographic factors, including age, race, and sex, are important in estimating the probability of a given stroke mechanism and vascular lesion. Men, especially white men, have a high incidence of atherosclerosis affecting the extracranial arteries at the internal carotid and vertebral artery origins in the neck.[13] They often have accompanying coronary artery and peripheral artery occlusive disease, hypercholesterolemia, and hypertension.[13,27] Women during the childbearing years are less prone to extracranial atherosclerosis and coronary artery disease. Blacks and persons of Japanese, Chinese, and Thai descent are more prone to hypertension, ICH, and vascular occlusive lesions affecting the intracranial arteries.[13] Women of childbearing age are also prone to intracranial occlusive disease. Pregnancy, the puerperium, and high-estrogen-content birth control pills make this group also susceptible to intracranial venous sinus thrombosis. Knowing these predilections helps in emphasizing parts of the general examination and, later, in planning investigations.

After the physician meets the patient and becomes aware of his or her past medical history, information about the period before the stroke should be elicited. Any *warnings* or *transient episodes* that may have occurred before the stroke should be noted.[5] The presence of warning events may provide a crucial clue to the stroke mechanism. For example, if a man who presented with an acute onset of a left hemiparesis had experienced a transient episode of obscured vision in the right eye for 5 minutes the week before, the probability of an occlusive lesion affecting the right internal carotid artery at a position before the ophthalmic artery branch would be quite high. *Transient ischemic attacks (TIAs)* in the same vascular territory as the stroke usually mean the process is "thrombotic." If there were multiple episodes of transient or persisting dysfunction in different vascular territories than the stroke, the stroke mechanism would be more likely to be embolic.

Unfortunately, most patients are ill informed about the functions of the nervous system. Stroke patients with a hemiparesis often attribute the problem to a malfunction of the limbs, and hemianopic patients are certain that the problem is in their eyes. Many people relate brain dysfunction to "crazy" or "dumb" behavior, coma, and epileptic fits but do not think of the brain as controlling the movement of the limbs or as the repository of incoming sensations—they usually do not conceive of the brain as controlling the "puppet strings" going to and from all parts of the body. Patients relay information they believe to be relevant to the current problem. If they have weakness of the left arm, they may not tell the physician about transient weakness of the left leg that occurred 1 week before because the events seem unrelated to them. Certainly they will not mention preceding attacks involving the right eye because they do not understand the relationship. To obtain a history of TIAs, physicians must inquire very specifically, asking questions such as, "Have you had transient leg weakness, periods of loss of speech, double vision, or temporary numbness?" During the initial period of the hospitalization, patients are often ill, worried, tired, and preoccupied. They may not accurately recall preceding transient events. The history must often be retaken later to ensure that all prodromal attacks and symptoms are recognized. A particularly important type of warning has been called "sentinel bleeds." Patients with SAH often have had minor bleeding causing sudden-onset severe headache, frequently accompanied by cessation of activity and vomiting. Inquiry about this type of attack is important in patients whose clinical and laboratory findings are compatible with intracranial hemorrhage.

The *time of onset* and the patient's *activity at onset* of ischemic symptoms may also yield clues to the stroke mechanism. Most ischemic strokes begin between 8 and 12 AM.[26] Physical activity such as lifting or coitus can precipitate SAH and ICH and is unusual at the onset of ischemic stroke. Sudden or severe emotional duress and stress can also precipitate ICH. A sudden cough or sneeze can precipitate a brain embolus.

Most important is the analysis of the *course of development of neurologic signs.*[5,16] Each subtype of stroke has characteristic tempos and time signatures. In patients with thrombotic stroke, premonitory TIAs often precede the onset of stroke caused by transient hypoperfusion resulting from the occlusive vascular lesion and embolization from the arteriosclerotic plaque. When an occlusive thrombus develops, the brain supplied by that artery is hypoperfused. Focal ischemia causes local pressure and chemical and metabolic changes, which promote an increase in collateral circulation to the ischemic zone. At first, collateral circulation is not well established and is vulnerable to systemic factors, especially minor changes in blood volume, blood pressure, and even position in bed.[15] At first the occlusive thrombus is not well organized or adherent to the vascular wall. Embolization from the acute thrombus may occur, leading to temporary or persistent increases in neurologic signs. The clinical consequence of this train of pathophysiologic events is a fluctuation in clinical signs. The stepwise progression, fluctuations between normal and abnormal, and gradual progression of deficits are due to the effects of varying hypoperfusion, collateral circulation, and embolization and propagation of a clot.

In embolism the deficit usually begins suddenly when the embolus arrives at and blocks a recipient artery. Sometimes the embolus passes distally, causing a stepwise increase in neurologic signs, usually within 48 hours of onset.[22] In SAH the signs also begin abruptly and consist of severe headache, cessation of activity, and vomiting, usually without paralysis or other focal neurologic signs. In ICH the symptoms and signs develop over minutes or a few hours. The gradually progressive course is explained by the steady enlargement of the hematoma (Fig. 5-2). Improvement is not expected, even transiently, because the hematoma cannot be absorbed quickly. In contrast, patients with ischemic stroke, either thrombotic or embolic, often recover quickly if blood flow to the ischemic zone is restored.

The course of illness can be plotted on graphs that depict the chain of events (Fig. 5-3). An experienced clinician can usually predict the responsible stroke mechanism simply by reviewing the course of illness graph. However, patients often cannot describe the development of the deficit in detail because they are unaccustomed to and unschooled in how to do this. A technique called "walking through" the early stroke period can be used to construct a course of illness graph.[5,16] This technique involves retracing, with the patient, the steps and activities that occurred during and shortly after the onset of stroke. The following is an example of a patient's reconstruction of the course of illness:

While eating breakfast, Ms. Smith noticed that the spoon fell from her left hand. She tried to use the hand but felt it was weak. She walked upstairs, not noting any difficulty with gait or any limp. After lying down for a few moments, she was reassured to find that she now

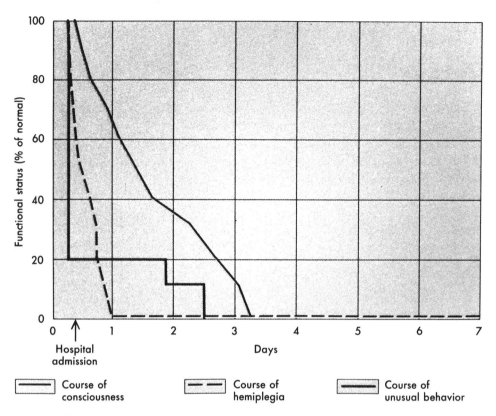

Fig. 5-3 Course of illness in a stroke patient. (From Caplan LR: *Hosp Pract* 20:125, 1985.)

could use the left hand normally. When she awakened from a brief nap she felt normal and walked down the stairs normally. She began to dust the living room and found that her left hand and arm had become weak. When she climbed the stairs to phone her physician, she noted that her left leg was now heavy and weak.

In this patient the deficit fluctuated, which is a typical course for thrombotic occlusion of a large or small penetrating artery. Another example of a patient's reconstruction of events leading to illness is given in the following:

While arguing vigorously with his mother-in-law, Mr. Kelly noted a tingling sensation in his left hand. Moments later he realized his left hand and arm were weak, and when he rose to walk, he had a noticeable limp of his left leg. By the time he walked to his room, he was weak on the left side of his body. He then began to feel a dull headache. When the ambulance arrived 15 minutes later, he could not move his left arm or leg.

This gradual progression of focal neurologic signs is most consistent with an evolving ICH.

Nonneurologic symptoms that accompany the neurologic symptoms and signs are often clues to the stroke mechanisms. By "neurologic symptoms" are meant such conditions as numbness, visual loss, and weakness — that is, symptoms that reflect an abnormality of nervous system function. *Headache at onset* is invariably present in patients with SAH. The absence of headache excludes SAH unless the patient is stuporous, aphasic, or otherwise unable to relate a medical history.[25] Headache preceding the stroke suggests a thrombotic mechanism.[25] As a large artery occludes, collateral circulation develops, and the increased collateral flow causes dilation of the arteries. Vasodilation probably is responsible for the headache that antedates neurologic symptoms. *Seizures* at or shortly after the onset of stroke suggest that ICH or embolism is the cause of stroke. *Vomiting* is common in patients with SAH and ICH but is rarely present in patients with ischemic stroke unless the lesion affects the brainstem or cerebellum.

The general physical examination may also yield clues about the cause of stroke. The presence of such findings as a heart murmur, arrhythmia, purpuric lesions on the skin, and occluded lower extremity arteries can all alter the physician's estimate of the probability of a given stroke mechanism.

Notice that thus far neurologic symptoms or signs have not been described. The diagnosis of the stroke mechanism (i.e., what caused the stroke) does not rely heavily on the neurologic findings. Many general physicians and nonneurologists are daunted by the neurologic examination. Up to this point, little if any knowledge of neurology has been needed to estimate the likelihood of the various stroke mechanisms. The determination of the mechanism of stroke relies heavily on information from the past and present history, on demographic information, and on general physical examination findings.

Localizing the Lesion

Where the lesion is located does give clues about the stroke mechanism. If a plumber knows that a certain sink on the third floor is leaking, he can explore the pipes that he knows lead to that sink. In the same way, if the location of the brain lesion is known and the vascular supply of that region is also known, brain and vascular imaging can be targeted to the region affected. The data needed to identify the location of the lesion are quite different from those needed to determine the type of lesion. Localizing a lesion depends on an analysis of the following:

1. Neurologic symptoms
2. Neurologic signs found on neurologic examination
3. Pattern matching the neurologic symptoms and signs with those of patients with brain lesions at known sites
4. Brain imaging with CT or MRI

Although in this chapter the type of lesion and its location are discussed separately, in practice both questions are pursued concomitantly during the history and general and neurologic examinations.

Hypotheses about the possible and probable stroke mechanisms and locations are actively pursued during the clinical encounter.[9] The probabilities are rarely 100% certain. Usually a number of possibilities concerning the stroke mechanism and location can be roughly ranked by likelihood for the individual patient. For example, in the case of Mr. Kelly, whose history was previously presented, an ICH was the most likely cause of his gradual-onset left hemiparesis. This diagnosis was supported by the history of hypertension and the gradually progressive course. The probability that ICH was the cause was 80%. Thrombosis was also possible, especially with gradual worsening; the probability was 15%. While embolism was unlikely because of the clinical course and the absence of a previously identified source of embolism, it remained within the realm of reasonable possibility (perhaps a 5% probability). Similarly, when localization is considered, the lesion most likely affected the right cerebral hemisphere (a 90% probability), but a right brainstem localization is also possible (10%) from the limited data from the history. The neurologic examination, if properly targeted, should further define the location. The general examination, especially the present blood pressure, and the results of the funduscopic examination of the eyes and the examination of the heart and neck vessels will help refine the probabilities of the various stroke mechanisms.

Clues to location come from the patient's reports about the type of neurologic symptoms, such as language, motor, visual, and somatosensory. The distribution of symptoms in the body is also important. For example, a sensation of numbness in the left hand and left side of the face suggests a superficial right postcentral gyrus perisylvian location. Left hemicorporeal numbness that affects the ear, neck, trunk, back, genitalia, and limbs suggests a lesion of the deep right sensory tract in the internal capsule, thalamus, or brainstem. (There is little cortical representation of the ears and trunk, and a cortical lesion would have to be widespread to include all these areas.) Combinations of symptoms (e.g., a left visual field defect and left hemisensory loss or a right arm and right side of the face weakness along with aphasia) are also helpful in localization.

The process of localization can be compared with trying to find a car on a known route. Crossroads and fellow travelers along segments of the journey help pinpoint the whereabouts of the car on the route. The brain pathways are often long so that a pure motor hemiparesis, reflecting a pyramidal tract lesion on one side, could affect the corticospinal pathway anywhere from the precentral gyrus to the upper spinal cord. Particular attention must be given to the patient's account of the deficit because patients are often aware of dysfunction and abnormalities before physicians detect abnormalities on examination. Once hypotheses of various possible locations are generated from the historical account, these can be tested during the examination, which is focused to separate the various possibilities.

During the examination the clinician should try to define objectively the nature of the neurologic deficits and their distribution in the body. A left upper quadrant visual field deficit identifies either (1) a lesion of the geniculocalcarine visual tract in the temporal or occipital lobe or (2) a lesion of the visual cortex along the inferior bank of the right calcarine fissure. As the examination is performed, the clinician should devise ways to separate and distinguish the various possible locations. For example, in a patient with a right hemiparesis affecting the face, arm, and leg, if the lesion is in the left cerebral hemisphere, aphasia, right visual field loss or visual neglect, or right hemisensory abnormalities might be present. This patient might also have defective right conjugate gaze because of dysfunction of the frontal eye field in the left frontal lobe. If, however, the causative lesion is in the pons, the patient might have defective conjugate gaze to the left because of dysfunction of the left pontine gaze center or might have difficulty in moving the left eye only to the left (sixth cranial nerve palsy) or the left eye to the right on right conjugate gaze (left intranuclear ophthalmoplegia). Nystagmus, bilaterality of weakness, and slight ataxia of the left leg also point to a pontine location. To be effective, the neurologic examination must be targeted and hypothesis driven.

In stroke patients, localizing the stroke depends on *pattern matching*. If the common patterns found in patients with stroke of various kinds at various sites are known, the findings from the history and examination can be readily matched with these known patterns. The box on pp. 76 and 77 lists common stroke localization patterns. The nature and meaning of these neurologic deficits are elaborated later. The key to accurate neurologic localization is a careful assessment of cognitive, behavioral, and neuroophthalmologic abnormalities. The majority of the primate brain is involved in looking, seeing, and visual perceptual analysis. Yet most examiners spend the majority of time during the examination on motor, reflex, and sensory assessment. Abnormalities in these elementary functions are not difficult to evaluate and are often obvious after the history taking or even a brief cursory examination. Neurologic deficits are discussed in more detail later. One cannot overemphasize that *history taking and the general and neurologic examinations must be hypothesis driven.* As Goethe said, "Man sees what he looks for."

In practice, determining the stroke mechanism and locating the brain and vascular lesions should be pursued together. At the conclusion of taking the history, physicians should be prepared to list the most likely stroke mechanisms and most likely brain and vessel sites in the order of probability. During the examination, findings are sought that further confirm, deny, or refine these hypotheses. For example, if the patient gives a history of a sudden, maximal at onset neurologic deficit, the cause of highest probability is embolism. During the examination the physician should carefully examine the patient's pulse for irregularities suggestive of arrhythmia and the heart for a potential embolic source. The major blood vessels that supply the symptomatic region should also be carefully examined as potential sources of intraarterial emboli. If intracranial

Common Stroke Localization Patterns

1. Large hemisphere lesions (full middle cerebral artery territory infarcts, large putaminal ICH)
   Contralateral hemiparesis, hemisensory loss, hemianopsia, neglect
   Decreased alertness, eyes deviated ipsilaterally, and contralateral gaze paresis
   Left lesion: global aphasia
   Right lesion: left neglect, anosognosia, motor impersistence
2. Frontal lobe dorsolateral suprasylvian lesions (upper division middle cerebral artery, frontal lobe hematomas)
   Contralateral hemiparesis and hemisensory loss (mostly arm, hand, face); eyes conjugately deviated ipsilaterally with contralateral gaze palsy
   Left lesion: Broca's aphasia
   Right lesion: left neglect, motor impersistence
3. Temporal lobe and inferior parietal lobe lesions (inferior division middle cerebral artery infarcts, temporal lobe hematomas)
   Contralateral hemianopia or upper quadrantanopia
   Left lesion: Wernicke type of aphasia
   Right lesion: poor drawing and copying ability; agitated delirium
4. Medial frontal lesions (anterior cerebral artery territory infarcts)
   Contralateral lower extremity and shoulder weakness; cortical-type sensory loss in the foot; abulia; left arm apraxia
5. Occipital lobe lesions, unilateral (posterior cerebral artery territory infarcts, occipital lobe hematomas)
   Contralateral hemianopia or upper or lower quadrantanopia
   Left lesion: alexia without agraphia
   Right lesion: disorientation to place
6. Bilateral occipital lobe and temporal lobe lesions (top of basilar embolism)
   Cortical blindness; Balint's syndrome features; prosopagnosia; achromatopsia; amnesia; agitated delirium
7. Cerebellar lesions (cerebellar infarcts and hemorrhages)
   Gait ataxia; dysarthria; veering and leaning to ipsilateral side; ipsilateral CN VI or conjugate gaze paresis
8. Brainstem lesions, bilateral (basilar artery occlusion, pontine hematomas)
   Diplopia; internuclear ophthalmoplegia; nystagmus; crossed motor or sensory signs (ipsilateral cranial nerve to contralateral limbs); bilateral motor, sensory, or cerebellar signs
9. Small, deep white matter or unilateral brainstem lesions (lacunes or atheromatous branch occlusions, small hematomas)
   Pure motor hemiparesis: weakness of contralateral face, arm, and leg with no cognitive, behavioral, sensory, or visual signs (lesion in internal capsule or pons)
   Pure sensory stroke: paresthesia or numbness of contralateral face, arm, leg, and trunk with no cognitive, behavioral, motor, or visual signs (lesion in lateral thalamus or pontine tegmentum)

Common Stroke Localization Patterns — cont'd

Ataxic hemiparesis: mixed contralateral paresis and ataxia with pyramidal signs (lesion in posterior limb of capsule or pons)

10. Lateral thalamic lesions (thalamogeniculate artery occlusions, small lateral thalamic hematomas)

 Contralateral paresthesia or numbness; contralateral hemiataxia, hemichorea, or hemidystonia

11. Lateral medullary lesions (intracranial vertebral artery occlusions, branch circumferential artery occlusions)

 Ipsilateral Horner's syndrome, decreased pain, and temperature loss of the face; hoarseness; palatal and laryngeal palsy; nystagmus; limb and gait ataxia; lateral pulsion of eyes

 Contralateral loss of pain and temperature on trunk and limbs

12. Frontal lobe, caudate nucleus, and anterolateral thalamic lesions (small infarcts or hematomas)

 Abulia; sloppiness; poor organization; poor confrontational memory

---

bleeding is suspected, a careful search during the examination for evidence of systemic bleeding and organ damage associated with bleeding (e.g., of the liver and spleen) is important.

After the examination the initial probabilities listed should be refined and changed depending on the examination findings. Abnormalities unsuspected from the history (e.g., a cardiac murmur, atrial fibrillation, retinal hemorrhages, fever, multiple ecchymoses, weakness on the side opposite the symptoms) should stimulate consideration of etiologic factors not suggested by the history.

Laboratory Evaluation

At this point the hypotheses generated from the history and physical examinations should be tested using both old and new investigative techniques. Testing should begin immediately. Most acute stroke treatments must be instituted quickly to be effective. The window of opportunity is short.[2] Tests should be ordered sequentially rather than all at once because the results of the first preliminary tests clearly affect the selection of subsequent tests.

In the vast majority of stroke patients, it is wise to begin with *neuroimaging* and *blood testing.* Neuroimaging — using CT, MRI, or both — is mandatory in every stroke patient. These studies are noninvasive if performed as they should be — that is, first without contrast-enhancing materials. Both CT and MRI usually are definitive in separating ischemia from hemorrhage, except in some patients with small or old SAHs. When blood is found on the scans, the location and distribution separate subarachnoid, intracerebral, and meningocerebral hemorrhages.[4] In patients with intracerebral bleeding the location, size, and drainage patterns of the hematoma and the presence of accompanying edema, pressure shifts, and hydrocephalus are readily seen on CT scans. These factors determine the etiologic factors, prognosis, and treatment of the hemorrhage. When blood is subarachnoid or meningocerebral, the location of the blood can suggest the presence of an aneurysm or arteriovenous malformation (AVM) at particular sites.[4] MRI can often suggest the presence of old hemorrhages by revealing the imaging characteristics of hemosiderin.

In patients with brain ischemia, CT or MRI can show whether an infarct is present. The location often indicates the vascular territory involved. CT is often ordered immediately when patients are seen in the emergency unit. The most common reasons for this practice are to differentiate between ischemia and hemorrhage and to ensure the absence of bleeding before giving anticoagulant agents. Unfortunately, many brain infarcts are not visible on CT scans taken within the first 8 hours after the onset of ischemia. CT scans taken 1 to 3 days after the onset are more likely to accurately delineate infarcts in patients with persistent neurologic signs. When the clinical diagnosis of ischemia is clear, localization is possible from the clinical findings, and anticoagulation therapy is not planned immediately, delayed CT scans provide more diagnostic and prognostic data. MRI is probably more sensitive but less specific than CT. MRI signal changes are especially useful in imaging brainstem and cerebellar lesions and lesions near the base of the skull. Traumatic basal frontal and temporal lobe hematomas are seen better on MRI than CT. An analysis of flow voids produced by blood moving through arteries on MRI scans and the opacification of basal arteries on enhanced CT scans can each give information about arterial lesions such as aneurysms and occlusions.

The size of the infarct and matching of the extent of the damage seen on the neuroimaging films with the patient's clinical deficit is helpful in prognosticating and planning further investigations and treatment. If the patient's neurologic deficit is more severe than is predicted from the scan, some brain tissue must be nonfunctioning but not irreversibly damaged. Rapid, directed efforts should be made to reverse the ischemic process. A nonfunctioning, reversibly ischemic brain has been referred to as "stunned"; this means it is not normal and not yet dead, but somewhere in between. Often the size, shape, and location of infarcts help predict the etiologic factors[3,4] because lacunar infarcts, watershed border zone lesions, cardioembolic infarcts,[29] and infarcts caused by large artery extracranial and intracranial thrombosis[3,7] all have different and sometimes characteristic imaging appearances.

Blood tests are useful in detecting both hypercoagulable states and bleeding tendencies. At a minimum, screening of every stroke patient should include hemoglobin concentration, hematocrit, platelet counts, prothrombin time (PT), and activated partial thromboplastin time (APTT) studies. These tests can detect most important and severe bleeding diatheses and may suggest hypercoagulability. When indicated, more sophisticated tests of coagulation factors and functions may be ordered, depending on the clinical findings, imaging and vascular testing results, and preliminary results of the hematologic battery of tests. Further coagulation tests include measurements of levels of antithrombin III, proteins C and S, factors VII and VIII, and plasminogen activators and inhibitors and measures of thrombotic and thrombolytic activity and antiphospholid antibodies.

In ischemic stroke patients, noninvasive ultrasound tests nearly always are important and should be performed early in the evaluation. The testing should include ultrasound imaging and Doppler velocity curves and should include both the anterior and posterior circulations and both the extracranial and intracranial arteries. B-mode and color-flow Doppler ultrasound images reliably show in real time the vascular occlusive lesions in the neck.[32] Unfortunately, at present these techniques are applicable primarily to the regions of the origin of the internal carotid and vertebral arteries. The remainder of the cervical portions of the carotid and vertebral arteries can be insonated using Doppler probes; direction of flow and flow velocities can be accurately determined and followed later.

Currently, transcranial Doppler (TCD) ultrasonography allows for the noninvasive detection of severe disease in the large basal intracranial arteries.[19] Special Doppler probes are placed over the orbit, the soft regions of the temporal bones, and the foramen magnum, and arteries are insonated at various depths inward from the skull. The principles of the system can be understood by recalling how a hose is used to wash off a dirty patio or sidewalk. Turning the nozzle of the hose reduces the size of the lumen and increases the pressure and force of the jet of water. The pressure is changed without altering the faucet or input of water. When the nozzle is turned too tightly, the lumen is obliterated and only a dribble or no water comes out of the hose. The velocity of flow is inversely proportional to the diameter of an open artery. Similarly, when an artery becomes narrowed, flow velocity increases. If the artery becomes occluded or severely stenosed, the distal flow velocities fall and no flow may be detected. Severe vasoconstriction caused by SAH usually causes a diffuse increase in flow velocities in a basal artery, whereas a focal region of atherostenosis or embolism leads to a focal velocity change in the affected artery.

The advent of magnetic resonance angiography (MRA) has provided an important advance in the ability to noninvasively image the large extracranial and intracranial arteries and veins.[17] In some centers MRA can be performed immediately after standard MRI brain images have shown the major lesion of interest (e.g., infarct, hematoma, or subarachnoid blood collection). Emphasis can be placed on the neck arteries and the aortic arch or on the major anterior and posterior circulation basal arteries. MRA is a good screening technique for the detection of sizable aneurysms, vascular malformations, and regions of severe arterial stenosis and occlusion. The use of both ultrasonography and MRA make it unlikely that severe occlusive lesions will be missed. The two techniques are complementary. Ultrasonography may detect lesions at sites not imaged well by MRA (e.g., the vertebral artery origin and the tortuous portions of the intracranial carotid and vertebral arteries). MRA can reach areas not shown well by ultrasonography (e.g., the distal basilar artery). At present, MRA is not useful in detecting small distal branch intracranial arterial lesions. The severity of arterial stenosis in the neck is often overestimated. MRA is excellent in detecting and showing occlusions of the intracranial dural venous sinuses.

Cardiac testing is also extremely important.[10,30,31] Perhaps as many as 30% of ischemic strokes are cardioembolic in origin. Cardiac investigations are aimed at detecting potential cardiac sources of emboli and determining the presence of coexistent significant coronary artery disease. Myocardial infarction and sudden cardiac death caused by arrhythmia are common causes of death in patients with occlusive cerebrovascular disease. An electrocardiogram often can show old myocardial infarcts and atrial and ventricular enlargement and may suggest an arrhythmia. Echocardiography, especially using the transesophageal approach, is sensitive to valvular lesions and to atrial and ventricular enlargement. Ventricular contractility and lesions within the cardiac chambers such as myxomas and ball-valve thrombi also are usually well seen. The introduction of saline air bubbles mixed with blood can show shunting of the saline contrast-enhancing material from the right to the left ventricles through atrial and ventricular septal defects, patent foramen ovale, and atrial septal aneurysms. Alternatively, a Doppler probe placed over the cardiac septum during injection of saline air bubbles can detect shunting of blood across the septum. Recently cardiac shunts have been documented by using transcranial Doppler ultrasonography. Air bubbles introduced with saline into an arm vein are audible over the middle cerebral artery by transcranial Doppler imaging in patients with cardiac shunts. Recent studies have begun to show that plaques in the ascending aorta can also be an important source of brain embolism. Transesophageal echocardiography can also show protruding aortic plaques.[1,33]

Ambulatory cardiac rhythm monitoring is useful in detecting arrhythmias. Sick sinus syndrome, characterized by alternating periods of bradycardia and tachycardia, and atrial fibrillation are two common arrhythmias commonly associated with brain embolism. Embolism in patients with atrial fibrillation is more common when valvular disease, left atrial enlargement, cardiac thrombi, and ventricular muscle dysfunction accompany the arrhythmia. In selected patients cardiac exercise testing and radionuclide perfusion studies using thallium and dipyridamole can detect regions of myocardial ischemia. Coronary angiography is necessary in patients whose histories and noninvasive cardiac test results show a high likelihood of potentially life-threatening coronary artery disease.

Review

Thus far the various tests available and the evaluation of patients with suspected strokes and cerebrovascular disease have been described. The various common clinical scenarios are reviewed here to illustrate how the various tests should be used.[9] The first task is to *separate ischemia from hemorrhage*. Neuroimaging can do this by revealing an infarct or blood. When CT and MRI findings are normal and the clinical picture suggests SAH, a lumbar puncture is needed to exclude SAH.

If the lesion is hemorrhage. If the bleeding is subarachnoid, the common causes are aneurysm, AVM, trauma, drug use, a bleeding disorder, and amyloid angiopathy. Tests for bleeding disorders are always indicated. Usually angiography is needed to define an aneurysm. AVMs may be suggested by the MRI appearance of heterogeneous signals and flow void abnormalities representing blood vessels within, adjacent to, and draining the region of hemorrhage. If the clinical picture suggests SAH (i.e., sudden severe headache, vomiting, and cessation of activity without focal signs) and the neuroimaging results are normal, a lumbar puncture is needed to exclude SAH.

If the bleeding is intracerebral, the most common causes are hypertension, AVMs, trauma, drug use, amyloid angiopathy, and meningocerebral bleeding near the base of the brain. Coagulation screening for a bleeding diathesis is always indicated. If the patient is hypertensive and the hematoma is located in the putamen, thalamus, pons, or cerebellum, no other testing usually is needed. The chance of finding another cause is extremely low unless the MRI shows findings that suggest an AVM. If the patient is not hypertensive and the hematoma is superficial or in the cerebral white matter or a ventricle, MRI for an AVM and angiography are usually needed. Multiple small, healed hemosiderin cavities on MRI in an older patient strongly suggest the presence of amyloid angiopathy.

If the lesion is ischemia. The clinical information and imaging appearance of systemic hypoperfusion should be characteristic. There should be a history compatible with circulatory arrest, or the patient may have been discovered unconscious after an interval during which he or she was unobserved and could have had an acute systemic circulatory event. The symptoms and signs should be bilateral. Neuroimaging lesions, when present, should be bilateral and emphasize border zone regions between the major cerebral (anterior, middle, and posterior) and cerebellar (posteroinferior, anteroinferior, and superior) arteries.

If the neuroimaging lesion is a unilateral infarct or if the results of CT, MRI, or both are negative (i.e., show no hemorrhage and no infarct) but the patient has a definite focal neurologic deficit of acute onset, an embolic or thrombotic cause is highly likely. In practice, these processes overlap and are hard to separate. A patient may have a growing carotid artery plaque in the neck with an occlusive thrombus (thrombosis) but have a stroke because of embolism of the clot. I suggest pursuing both etiologic mechanisms at the same time. *First localize the ischemic lesion to either the anterior or posterior circulation.* If the brain ischemia is located within the right anterior circulation, the causative vascular lesion must lie within the vascular pathways leading to that area (i.e., the heart, aorta, innominate artery, right common carotid artery, internal carotid artery, middle or anterior cerebral artery, or anterior choroidal artery, depending on the site of the infarct). If the clinical history included multiple TIAs in the same vascular territory, an arterial rather than cardiac source is more likely. If the patient is a white man, an extracranial internal carotid artery location is probable, especially if a carotid bruit is heard.[13] If the patient is a menstruating women or is black or of Asian descent, an intracranial arterial site is more likely.[13]

If the onset of ischemia was sudden and without warning and if the patient has cardiac disease, the embolism is more likely to be of cardiac than intraarterial origin, although many patients with atherosclerotic heart disease have coexistent extracranial occlusive disease. Cardiac studies (e.g., electrocardiography, transesophageal or transthoracic echocardiography, and rhythm monitoring) and extracranial (duplex scan) and TCD ultrasonography should be performed. The order of cardiac and arterial testing should depend on which is the more probable origin from the demography, clinical features, and associated medical conditions.

If the lesion is within the posterior circulation (brainstem, cerebellum, occipitotemporal lobes), the evaluation should include the heart and posterior circulation arteries. Cardiac testing should be the same as for anterior circulation ischemia because studies show that about one in five emboli are in the posterior circulation.[11] If the lesion involves the medulla, the posterior inferior cerebellum, or both on one side, the causative vascular lesion should lie within the extracranial or intracranial vertebral artery on that side. The extracranial vertebral artery can be studied with ultrasonography using duplex scans, color-flow Doppler, and continuous-wave Doppler in the neck. The intracranial vertebral artery can be well studied using TCD.[19] If the lesion involves the pons, the anterior inferior or superior portions of the cerebellum, or the midbrain, thalamus, or posterior cerebral artery hemisphere territories, both the vertebral arteries in the neck and head and the basilar artery should be studied.

In patients with strokes in either circulation, angiography is ordered if the preliminary tests (CT, MRI, ultrasound, cardiac tests) do not clarify the diagnosis and treatment to be pursued. MRA should be performed first if available.[17] Standard catheter angiography is seldom needed. Blood coagulation tests also should be part of the routine testing of patients with thromboembolic stroke in either circulation. Hemoglobin concentration, hematocrit, platelet count, and PT and APTT studies should always be ordered. In special cases in which hypercoagulability is suspected, antiphospholipid antibodies and various coagulation factors and functions may have to be explored in more depth.

TREATMENT

Space does not allow full, detailed coverage of acute stroke treatment in this text. Acute treatment is discussed in more detail elsewhere.[39,40,47] The principles and basic approach are emphasized in the following. *Treatment depends heavily on the stroke mechanism present in the individual patient.*[38,39]

Subarachnoid Hemorrhage

In general, the main aims in treating patients with SAH are the following:
1. Diagnose and treat bleeding lesions before they rebleed.
2. Prevent and treat complications associated with blood in the cerebrospinal fluid and increased intracranial pressure.

SAH caused by trauma and amyloid angiopathy have no specific controllable bleeding lesions that have a strong potential to rebleed, and these pathologic conditions have no specific treatment. Clearly, if the hemorrhage is due to use of amphetamines, cocaine, or other illicit drugs, the most important prescription is future abstinence. For unexplained reasons, patients with SAH after cocaine use have a high incidence of aneurysms or AVMs (approaching 50%), whereas patients with hemorrhages after amphetamine use do not. Bleeding lesions should be sought and treated in cocaine-related SAH. When SAH is due to a primary bleeding disorder such as hemophilia, thrombocytopenia, or warfarin use, rapid correction of the coagulopathy is the major therapy. To anticipate rebleeding, aneurysms should be treated as soon as feasible. Ordinarily, when the aneurysms are accessible, this is done by surgical clipping using a surgical microscope to aid visualization. Some aneurysms cannot be clipped. These can sometimes be coated and reinforced. Recently, inaccessible lesions have been treated more often using interventional radiography techniques to ablate the lesions. Surgery should be done early in aneurysm patients — as soon as intracranial pressure is controlled and patients are awake and in good condition. Angiomas have a lower rate of acute rebleeding and result in a lower incidence of mortality so that surgery or other ablative therapy is delayed, usually until the patient recovers from the bleeding.

The major complications of blood in the cerebrospinal fluid are the following:
1. Increased intracranial pressure
2. Vasoconstriction
3. Hydrocephalus
4. Cardiac arrhythmias and myocytolysis
5. Hypertension, either primary or secondary to the increased intracranial pressure

Drainage of blood and cerebrospinal fluid by lumbar puncture (or at the time of surgery) helps in monitoring the patient's intracranial pressure, removes some blood, reduces intracranial pressure, and potentially helps prevent hydrocephalus. Blood irritates and blocks pacchionian granulations in the arachnoid membranes, decreasing their ability to absorb spinal fluid. Because spinal fluid continues to be made at the normal rate, fluid accumulates in the subarachnoid space and later in the ventricles. Drainage of cerebrospinal fluid prevents the development of hydrocephalus and reduces intracranial pressure, thus helping to relieve headache.

Hypertension increases the likelihood of rebleeding from aneurysms; thus reducing systolic blood pressure helps to prevent rebleeding. However, antihypertensive treatment must be used and monitored carefully and should be conservative. In some patients the increase in blood pressure is a response to the increase in intracranial pressure. The systemic blood pressure must rise to exceed the intracranial venous pressure to allow for brain perfusion. In these circumstances, a reduction in blood pressure can lead to hypoperfusion of the brain. This is especially likely to occur if the subarachnoid blood has triggered vasoconstriction, thus lowering perfusion either generally or focally. Blood pressure should be reduced to a minor degree while the clinical state of the patient is monitored carefully. Labetalol is an excellent agent for this use.[35] The heart should be monitored for arrhythmia. β-Blockers may help reduce the effect of catecholamines on the heart, the posited cause of the arrhythmias and myocytolysis associated with SAH.

The most important and feared complication of SAH is vasoconstriction of the major basal arteries. Vasoconstriction is due to substances within the blood. The most effective treatment is to increase the fluid volume (hypervolemic hemodilution), which helps maintain blood flow despite vasoconstriction. The degree of vasoconstriction can be monitored by TCD ultrasonography, measuring blood flow velocities.[42] Calcium channel blocking agents may also help reduce or prevent vasoconstriction, but care must be taken against hypotension, which can decrease brain and renal perfusion. Currently research is being pursued to determine whether instillation of recombinant tissue plasminogen activator (rTPA) or other thrombolytic agents might lyse large subarachnoid and cisternal clots within the cerebrospinal fluid and thus reduce the stimulus for vasoconstriction.

Intracerebral Hemorrhage

Hematomas injure surrounding brain tissue as they enlarge, thus potentially increasing the neurologic deficit and morbidity. Large hematomas cause major shifts in intracranial contents and can lead to death by increased intracranial pressure or brain herniations. The aim of treatment is to control the bleeding and the local and generalized increase in intracranial pressure. Rebleeding is less a problem in these patients than in those with SAH. In hypertensive ICH, the patient's blood pressure should be lowered, watching for hypoperfusion-induced worsening of symptoms and signs. Lumbar puncture should be *avoided* in patients with ICH because it can potentiate shifts in intracranial contents. Clearly, if a bleeding diathesis is the cause of ICH, it must be reversed as quickly as possible. In some patients with ICH, especially that caused by trauma and AVMs, secondary disseminated intravascular coagulation can develop and promote further brain hemorrhage.

Surgical drainage of hematomas can be lifesaving. Surgical drainage decompresses the expanding mass. Some hematomas decompress themselves by bleeding into the pial surface cerebrospinal fluid or into the ventricular system. The decision concerning surgical drainage depends on the following:

1. Size of the hematoma
2. Location of the hematoma
3. Clinical signs and whether they are stable, improving, or worsening
4. Imaging documentation of mass effect and pressure shifts

Small hematomas do not increase pressure and do not need drainage. Usually, large hematomas prove fatal, and the damage is already done by the time the patient is brought for medical care. *Medium-sized hematomas in favorable locations for drainage, in patients who are clinically worsening, and that show mass effect and shifts are candidates for drainage.* The most accessible locations are the cerebral lobes, cerebellum, and right putamen. Thalamic and brainstem hematomas are much more difficult to drain. A decreasing level of consciousness and increasing signs of increased intracranial pressure should stimulate consideration of drainage because the prognosis is poor without surgery. Medical treatment of brain edema and increased intracranial pressure using forced hyperventilation and osmotic diuretics or glycerol should be started quickly. Surgery is pursued if these measures do not stabilize and improve the situation. Recently surgeons have begun to use stereotactic surgical drainage with CT or MRI control. This has made the operation more feasible.

Ischemia

The mechanism of stroke is ischemia in 80% of stroke patients. In patients with systemic hypoperfusion, treatment relates to the general circulatory problem. This usually means treatment of the heart disease — that is, control of arrhythmia and restitution of cardiac output — or treatment of acute shock or hypovolemia.

Systemic hypoperfusion nearly always presents with bilateral so-called global ischemia, not focal neurologic signs. When the ischemia is focal, the process is thromboembolic (i.e., either an in situ thrombosis or embolism). In thromboembolic strokes five general types of treatment are important to consider. These are listed in the box on p. 86. Occlusion of a major extracranial or intracranial artery creates two acute problems: (1) lack of blood supply to the region of brain supplied by the artery and (2) a potential source of further thrombus propagation and embolization. Potential ways to *unblock the artery* include direct surgical attack, an infusion of chemical thrombolytic agents, and

---

Treatment of Thromboembolic Ischemic Strokes

Open regions of vascular blockage:
  Surgical (endarterectomy or reconstruction)
  Interventional radiographic (angioplasty)
  Chemical (thrombolysis)
Alter blood coagulability to prevent formation, propagation, and emboliza-
tion of thrombi:
  Agents that alter platelet function, such as aspirin and ticlopidine, are
    used to prevent white platelet–fibrin thrombi.
  Standard anticoagulant agents, such as heparin, heparinoids, and warfarin,
    are used to prevent red fibrin–erythrocyte thrombi.
Augment blood flow:
  Increase fluid volume.
  Maintain or raise blood pressure.
  Decrease blood viscosity (lower fibrinogen or RBC volume).
Increase brain's resistance to ischemia:
  Reduce blood sugar levels and local ischemic brain lactate production.
  Neutralize excitotoxins.
  Decrease brain metabolism.
  Decrease calcium cellular effects with calcium channel blocking agents.
Modify stroke risk factors to prevent further vascular disease:
  Reduce hypertension.
  Reduce hypercholesterolemia.
  Help patient stop smoking.
  Help patient stop drug use.
  Treat heart disease.
  Treat diabetes mellitus.

---

endovascular techniques using instruments and catheters introduced through the vascular system. Clearly time is of critical importance because the longer the brain tissue remains ischemic, the less the chances of reversal of ischemia. In addition, late reperfusion is more likely to cause bleeding into areas of infarction and vascular damage. In general, if the artery is completely thrombosed, surgery and endovascular techniques are not recommended because the occlusive thrombus may be dislodged cranially and mechanical reopening of the artery is unlikely to succeed. Surgical endarterectomy is usually reserved for patients who have not had major infarcts and have some residual lumen and flow in the obstructed artery. Recent randomized controlled trials have shown convincingly the superiority of surgical versus medical treatment in patients with severe carotid artery stenosis in the neck (greater than 70% luminal reduction) when surgery is performed by selected expert surgeons.[20,28] Thrombolysis is potentially useful but currently is in the investigational phase.

At present the most commonly used method of treatment for patients with thromboembolic ischemia is *modification of coagulation factors and functions.* I prescribe aspirin in situations that tend to promote formation of "white" platelet-fibrin thrombi. Platelets agglutinate and adhere to irregular surfaces such as nonstenosing plaques in arteries or on valve surfaces. One or two aspirins a day are given for this situation. Some preliminary studies show that some patients do not get an aspirin effect on platelets at a low dose, and in these patients a higher dose is prescribed. Ticlopidine may also be useful for its effect on platelet function, especially in patients in whom aspirin has not been clinically successful.

I use standard anticoagulant agents in patients with vascular lesions that favor formation of "red" fibrin-erythrocyte thrombi.[36,38] These lesions include severe stenosis of large arteries; recent occlusion of large arteries; cardiac origin embolism from mural thrombi, ventricular aneurysms, and atrial fibrillation; venous stasis in the limbs; and some hypercoagulable states, such as the presence of lupus anticoagulant. When the tendency for thrombosis is persistent, such as in patients with atrial fibrillation and artificial cardiac valves, warfarin is given for an indefinite period. In a number of controlled randomized trials, warfarin has been shown unequivocally to reduce the incidence of stroke in patients with atrial fibrillation.[34] Warfarin therapy is stopped if and when the responsible condition changes so that thrombosis is no longer a major risk. For example, long-term warfarin is used to treat patients with severe inoperable stenosis of the major extracranial and intracranial arteries. If, while under treatment, the stenosed artery occludes without symptoms, the warfarin therapy is discontinued 3 to 6 weeks after the documented occlusion.

When an occlusive thrombus forms, it is poorly organized and does not adhere to the vessel wall. The fresh thrombus poses a major threat of propagation and embolization. Warfarin is given during the 3- to 6-week period during which the thrombus organizes and becomes adherent. Later there is little threat of embolization, and collateral circulation should stabilize. The initial treatment with standard anticoagulant agents should nearly always begin with heparin, which is continued until warfarin increases the PTT to about 1.5 times control levels (about 16 to 18 seconds, International Normalized Ratio of about 1.3 to 1.5). Currently, low-molecular-weight heparin ("heparinoid") is under investigation and may prove superior to heparin.[38,52] The choice of aspirin or another drug that modifies platelet function versus anticoagulant agents depends on the identification of the cardiac and vascular lesions and periodic monitoring of their status. Usually monitoring can be done noninvasively with echocardiography, ultrasonography of the cerebrovascular system, and MRA.

Ischemia, by definition, means a *lack of blood.* It is important to maintain and optimize blood flow to the ischemic zone as quickly as possible. When blood flow to a brain region is reduced, survival of the at-risk tissue depends on the duration and severity of the flow reduction and on reperfusion by opening of the blockage or routing through collateral channels. Brain tissue functions normally when perfused at rates of 40 ml/100 g/min or above. At flow levels of 20 ml/100 g/min, functions stop and the tissue is silent electrically.[52] Blood pressure usually should not be lowered rapidly because a reduction in blood pressure usually causes reduced blood flow unless the pressures were in the malignant hypertension range. Blood pressure levels greater than 210/110 mm Hg may be associated with vasoconstriction and reduced flow. Blood pressure levels in the range of 140 to 180/80 to 100 mm Hg ordinarily should not be lowered rapidly. If the systemic blood pressure remains above this range after a day or more of bed rest, a gentle and carefully monitored reduction of pressure using labetalol is recommended. The blood pressure should not be lowered to the "normal" range; 150 to 160/85 to 95 mm Hg is a good target. When antihypertensive agents are given, the patient's neurologic signs and blood pressure should be closely monitored to avoid worsening of the ischemia. In some patients who have relatively low blood pressures (90 to 130/60 to 80 mm Hg range) ephedrine or another sympathomimetic drug might increase the blood pressure and thus augment brain perfusion. Stroke patients often do not eat and drink normally. Some cannot because of dysphagia; others are ordered not to take anything by mouth; and some are kept away by diagnostic testing at mealtime. Blood drawing is sometimes extensive. Diminished blood and fluid volume can ensue. Every effort should be made to keep the blood pressure, blood volume, and cardiac output at optimal levels. Many patients with acute ischemic events caused by intrinsic atherosclerotic ischemic disease in the feeding arteries or by brain embolism have multiple occlusive lesions. Usually the extent of arterial occlusive disease can be determined by ultrasonography and MRA. Invariably, focal ischemia is caused by a lesion of the arteries directly feeding the ischemic territory, *not by distant remote vascular occlusive lesions* ("ischemia at a distance"). I do not advocate surgical repair of remote lesions as a strategy to improve local blood flow in an ischemic lesion. After the acute stroke, prophylactic treatment of these distant lesions may be indicated to prevent future stroke in the involved vascular territories.

　　More recently, interest has turned to attempts to make the brain more resistant to ischemia. Initial experimental efforts used barbiturates and hypothermia to reduce the energy needs of the brain. Currently, considerable research effort involves investigating various treatments that reduce brain energy requirements and potentially reverse the cascade of acute cellular events leading to irreversible cell death. To understand these potential treatments, clinicians need to become familiar with the cell and tissue pathologic and pathophysiologic changes induced by ischemia. When nerve cells become ischemic, a number of biochemical changes occur that potentiate and enhance cell death. K^+, usually an intracellular cation, moves across cell membranes into the extracellular space.

Ca^{++} moves into cells and compromises the ability of cell membranes to control ion fluxes. The influx of Ca^{++} causes mitochondrial and cell energy failure.[50,56] Normally there is a tenfold gradient between extracellular and intracellular (cytosolic) Ca^{++}.

Decreased oxygen availability leads to production of oxygen molecules with unpaired electrons, the so-called oxygen free radicals. These free radicals cause peroxidation of fatty acids inside cells and in plasma membranes, severely damaging cell functions.[50] Anaerobic glycolysis leads to an accumulation of lactic acid and to a decrease in local pH. The blood level of glucose has an important effect on local tissue metabolism. Increased blood sugar probably leads to more focal production of lactate.[56] Tissue acidosis also impairs cell function and can lead to neuronal death.[50]

Recent interest has centered on the production and release of neurotransmitters. In ischemic areas concentrations of glutamate, aspartate, and kainic acid are significantly increased. Hypoxia, hypoglycemia, and ischemia all cause energy depletion and an increase in glutamate release but a decrease in glutamate uptake. These changes result in toxic exposure of glutamate to vulnerable neurons, enhancing cell death. The neurotransmitters excite the cells and cause increased cell functions and demand for energy (so-called excitotoxic injury).[44] A mismatch develops between the increased activity and demand and the reduced supply, resulting in irreversible cell death. Glutamate entry into the cells opens membranes and increases Na^+ and Ca^{++} influx into cells. Large influxes of Na^+ are followed by entry of Cl^- and water, causing cell swelling and edema.

These local metabolic changes cause a self-perpetuating cycle of changes that increase cell damage and eventually cause cell death. Changes in the ionic concentrations of Na^+, K^+, and Ca^{++}, release of oxygen free radicals, acidosis, and release of excitatory neurotransmitters further damage cells, leading to more biochemical changes that, in turn, cause more neuronal damage. At some point the ischemia becomes irreversible despite reperfusion, which can lead to delivery to the local ischemic site of more Ca^{++}, oxygen free radicals, water, sugar that will be metabolized to lactate, and excitatory neurotransmitters.

The degree of ischemia caused by arterial blockage varies in different zones. In the center of the ischemia, blood flow is lowest and ischemic damage is most severe. At the periphery of the ischemia, collateral flow allows delivery of blood (although at a rate below normal). Metabolism in the center of the ischemic zone may be reduced enough to cause cell necrosis, whereas at the periphery the reduced supply might "stun" the brain, causing function failure but not permanent cell damage. The zone of dysfunctional, but not dead, brain surrounding the central core of infarction has traditionally been called the "ischemic penumbra." Some neurons (e.g., certain areas in the hippocampi) are thought to be more vulnerable to hypoxia and decreased energy and fuel supply than others.

Currently, clinicians and researchers are beginning to test treatment strategies based on a knowledge of these cellular events. Some potential strategies are to decrease blood sugar by giving insulin to reduce lactate production and local acidosis, to use calcium channel blocking agents to block the influx of Ca^{++} into cells, to neutralize oxygen free radicals, to block receptor sites for excitatory neurotransmitters or inhibit these transmitters, and to use agents that solidify or improve cell membrane functions.

Thus far a cascade of events has been described, starting with vascular insufficiency leading to ischemia and neural injury. Such injury can lead to infarction and death of the neural tissue. Intervention can be helpful in limiting the extent of the eventual infarct and thus the degree of impairment. Treatment of the metabolic changes can include limiting the edema surrounding the area of cellular injury. The use of corticosteroids, although widespread, has not been shown to be of benefit in reducing mortality or the degree of impairment in the case of infarction[54] or in intracerebral hemorrhage.[57] The pathogenesis of the edema of an increase primarily in intracellular fluid secondary to cellular injury ("cytotoxic") suggests the preferential use of osmotic diuretics to deal with the effects of increased intracranial pressure.

The effect of a neural injury is impairment in function that is evident on clinical examination. The extent of the impairment may reflect a disturbance other than in the primary area of infarction. These "distant" effects have been described as one component, which has been called "diaschisis." This phenomenon refers to the deactivation of intact brain regions remote from but connected to the site of primary injury.[49] The early return of function is considered to be a different phenomenon from the late return of function secondary to training, which is described in the section on the rehabilitation phase. Diaschisis has been used to explain the rapid restoration of behavioral deficits with the use of pharmacologic agents. The assumption is that drugs exert their effects on intact systems rendered nonfunctional by the primary lesion.

The character of recovery found after subcortical lesions may reflect this phenomenon. For example, with thalamic lesions created by stereotactic thalamotomy, unilateral lesions produce verbal or visual amnesia attributed to cortical dysfunction. These impairments are at a distance from the lesion, and their reversal could explain the remarkable recovery after stroke involving this area, even when initial symptoms are severe. Electrophysiologic data show marked ipsilateral cortical electroencephalographic (EEG) slowing. Positron emission tomographic (PET) and single photon emission computed tomographic (SPECT) studies show a comparable reduction in ipsilateral cortical perfusion. Clinical recovery parallels improvement in these other measures. Mild contralateral cortical metabolic depression can also occur but is transient. Initial and delayed functional improvement following cortical stroke have been viewed as an effect of a partially reversible functional depression of the cortical area surrounding a site of necrotic damage.

Drugs That May Impede Recovery or Reinstate Deficits

Haloperidol
Prazosin
Clonidine
Phenoxybenzamine
γ-Aminobutyric acid (GABA)
Benzodiazepines
Phenytoin
Phenobarbital

In hemiplegic animals some drugs have been shown to accelerate recovery while also affecting cerebral metabolism and neurotransmitter release at sites remote from the primary lesion. For example, unilateral sensorimotor cortex ablation in the rat produced pronounced but transient contralateral hemiplegia. The measurement was based on a beam-walking task. Amphetamine combined with the beam-walking experience enhanced recovery, as compared with control animals. A single administration of the drug given 1 day after injury had beneficial results that were maintained. No effect was seen with the drug when no experience was provided. Haloperidol blocked the activity and delayed recovery, thus implicating the role of catecholamines in recovery. This same effect occurred in the cat. Those with severe hemiplegia responded favorably to delayed but spaced administrations of amphetamine combined with beam walking. The effects have been limited to norepinephrine system agonists but have not occurred with dopamine agonists (DA). For example, the DA uptake-blocker methylphenidate did not promote recovery of motor function.

The application of these findings to humans has been sparse. In a single-blind study, four patients were treated within an average of 6.5 days after stroke with a single oral 10 mg dose of amphetamine with at least a 45-minute session of physical therapy within 3 hours of drug ingestion.[45] A repeat motor examination was carried out the following day. Total motor performance increased substantially, particularly in two of the patients. The difference from the motor function in a control group receiving therapy alone was significant, as measured on the Fugl-Mayer Assessment.

The implications of these studies have an application to the clinical care of persons with stroke in the acute phase. Clinicians may be impeding clinical outcomes in stroke patients with some frequently used poststroke medications.[46] See the box above for drugs that may impede recovery, as determined by animal studies. The frequent use of antihypertensive drugs, especially clonidine and other α-adrenergic blocking agents, and the use of benzodiazepines may be inappropriate.[51]

Stroke patients almost always have risk factors that directly caused or contributed to the stroke. As other acute therapies are instituted, education about modifying these risk factors should begin. Smoking, hypercholesterolemia, and hypertension are probably the most common and important modifiable risk factors. The management of risk factors is described in the section on the rehabilitation phase. As stated previously, hypertension should *not* be aggressively treated during the acute phase of ischemia. However, once the patient leaves the hospital, his or her blood pressure should be carefully monitored and the hypertension treated. During the initial evaluation, risk factors should be sought and systematically investigated. Because some of these risk factors are genetically determined and may be familial, the children should be tested when parents have hyperlipidemia, hypertension, diabetes, or a combination of these. The earlier these risk factors are modified, the better the chances of preventing vascular complications.

PATTERNS OF NEUROLOGIC IMPAIRMENT

Clearly, treatment of the stroke patient must include an attempt to return the patient to as full and complete a normal life-style as possible. Often, the limiting factor in recovery is the nature and severity of the patient's neurologic impairment and his or her ability to adapt to and overcome it. Neurologic deficits, unlike most medical problems, influence all facets of a patient's life, including sitting, standing, walking, turning, speaking, seeing, and thinking. During the initial hospitalization and early recovery period, physicians caring for stroke patients must assess and understand the nature of the neurologic deficits to plan rehabilitation. This section explores the cognitive and behavioral changes that follow stroke. Deficits affecting the sensory and motor system are described elsewhere. The discussion of the deficits is organized according to the usual brain locations involved.

Left Cerebral Hemispheric Deficits

Aphasia. Verbal communication is an essential part of everyday life. Anyone who has been frustrated by the difficulties encountered when visiting a foreign-speaking country will understand what aphasia is like. If one does not speak the language, one cannot understand what is said and is unable to communicate wishes and needs. Only the mood of the person speaking is understandable by gesture and intonation. Because nearly all tests of cognitive function rely on answers to spoken or written questions and directions, language function should always be tested first.

Aphasia can be divided into two large groups: fluent and nonfluent.[63,83] A patient with nonfluent aphasia has obvious difficulty with speech production. The amount of speech is reduced, and often speech is labored and dysarthric and does not have normal rhythm and accentuation. In fluent aphasia, the patient uses an approximately normal amount of speech (sometimes suffering from logorrhea and overproduction of speech, or loquaciousness). Words and phrases are uttered without effort, and words are not slurred or dysarthric. In general, nonfluent aphasia is caused by lesions above the sylvian fissure and involve or are anterior to the central sulcus. The convex superficial and deep portions of the inferior portions of the left lateral frontal lobe are usually involved. In general, patients with fluent aphasia have lesions that are infrasylvian and posterior to the central sulcus, most often affecting the temporal lobe or the inferior parietal lobe. As noted during the discussion of vascular syndromes, clinicians usually identify a type of aphasia by pattern matching — that is, by comparing the patient's pattern of speech and other neurologic findings with that of prototypic patients with typical aphasic patterns.

Broca's aphasia is a nonfluent aphasia characterized by diminished speech output. Words and syllables are uttered with effort, and the mechanics of mouth, lips, tongue, and cheek motor functions are very abnormal. Sounds may be stuttered and dysarthric and are brought forth laboriously. Hemiparesis nearly always accompanies this condition. Comprehension of spoken language is usually preserved, as demonstrated by yes and no types of questions and by the selection of appropriate objects or responses from alternative choices. Most patients with Broca's aphasia are apraxic and do not correctly follow spoken commands even though they understand the meaning of the commands. In these patients, comprehension should not be judged by their ability to follow commands. Similar to speech, writing is sparse and agrammatical, even when performed with the left hand, a typewriter, or a computer. The causative vascular lesion is usually (1) an infarct involving the upper division of the left middle cerebral artery or (2) a deep anterior basal ganglia infarct or ICH.

The other varieties of nonfluent aphasia are *transcortical motor aphasia, global aphasia,* and a minor form of Broca's aphasia. In the transcortical aphasias, speech repetition is preserved despite abnormal speech output, comprehension, or both. Patients with *transcortical motor aphasia* have nonfluent speech with markedly decreased word production. Speech repetition and comprehension are preserved despite the low speech output, separating this clinical syndrome from that of Broca's aphasia. The lesions that cause transcortical motor aphasia are usually in the paramedian frontal lobe in the territory of the anterior cerebral artery involving the supplementary motor area, or they are hemorrhages or infarcts in the anterior portion of the striatum.

A minor and less common syndrome probably represents a minor form of Broca's aphasia and has been referred to as a *"baby Broca's aphasia."*[85] In this syndrome, patients are at first temporarily mute or have markedly decreased speech output. After days to a week or so, they begin to speak but use abnormal speech rhythm and accent (dysprosody). The words spoken are usually correct. The only lasting dysfunction is altered accent and dysprosody. Most patients have at least some transient right facial and hand weakness. The responsible lesion is usually small and limited to the frontal operculum involving the classic Broca's aphasia area. The lesion results from occlusion of one or two small branches of the upper division of the left middle cerebral artery, usually caused by embolus. A small frontal lobe ICH or traumatic contusion could also present as "baby Broca's aphasia."

In *global aphasia,* lesions involve both the frontal and temporal lobes or the temporal lobe and the deep basal gray and subcortical white matter. The parietal lobe is also often involved. At times nearly the entire middle cerebral artery territory is infarcted or there is a large putaminal hematoma. These patients have a nonfluent type of Broca's aphasia and poor comprehension and repetition of language.

In patients with fluent aphasia, there usually is a near normal amount of speech output and words are spoken without effort, mechanical difficulty (no dysarthria), or dysprosody. Usually wrong words, *paraphasic errors,* are used and comprehension of spoken language is defective. In so-called *Wernicke's aphasia* the patient usually makes a great many paraphasic errors, some of which are sound-alike and mean-alike words, *jargon,* nonword sounds, and *neologisms.* Both repetition and comprehension of spoken language are abnormal. Patients are usually not aware that they are speaking nonsense and cannot monitor their own errors and abnormal speech output. Patients with Wernicke's aphasia write with normal penmanship but use many wrong words. Their writing resembles their speech. Reading comprehension is sometimes relatively spared, so that patients do better when shown a written word or phrase than when the same material is spoken.[77] The causative vascular lesion almost invariably involves the temporal lobe, especially the posterior portion of the superior temporal gyrus and its underlying subcortical white matter. Temporal lobar hemorrhages, contusions, and infarcts involving the inferior division of the left middle cerebral artery are the most common causative vascular lesions. Although patients with Wernicke's aphasia usually do not have hemiparesis, they often have a right hemianopia, or an upper quadrantanopia. The limbic portions of the temporal lobes are adjacent to the temporal lobe speech cortex, explaining why some patients with Wernicke's aphasia become irascible, paranoid, and aggressive. I have seen several previously docile, gentle, timid elderly women spit, curse, bite, and kick after experiencing temporal lobe infarcts that rendered them aphasic.

A related speech problem is so-called *conduction aphasia,* which is probably a variant of Wernicke's aphasia.[63,67] Patients use wrong words but are generally able to convey their thoughts and ideas well. Repetition of spoken language is poor, but there is some retention of speech comprehension. The responsible lesions involve the temporal and inferior parietal lobes. Most patients with conduction aphasia have accompanying slight motor and sensory abnormalities in the right limbs.

Two rare but important syndromes also produce severe abnormalities of speech comprehension; however, unlike the situation in Wernicke's and conduction aphasia, speech output is relatively normal. *Cortical deafness* is due to bilateral lesions of the transverse temporal gyri (Heschl's gyrus, the primary auditory cortex). These patients cannot hear but speak, read, and write normally. Brainstem auditory reflex behavior is preserved so that patients with cortical deafness blink when exposed to sudden loud noises. In *pure word deafness,* patients can hear and recognize sounds and music but not language. The causative lesion interrupts auditory input to Wernicke's area in the posterior portion of the left superior temporal gyrus but spares Heschl's gyrus, at least on one side. Lesions can affect the temporal lobes bilaterally or be limited to the left temporal lobe only. Although patients can hear sound, the auditory input does not reach Wernicke's area so that patients cannot understand auditory input as language. They can, however, speak and use written language normally.

Transcortical sensory aphasia is a syndrome of fluent aphasia with preserved repetition of spoken language despite poor comprehension. The cause is usually a temporal lobe infarct in the territory of the left posterior cerebral artery or an infarct or hemorrhage affecting the far posterior portion of the striatum. In *anomic aphasia* the major deficit is in naming objects but speech comprehension and repetition are nearly normal.[76] Often patients use circumlocutory descriptive phrases instead of the desired word—for example, "that thing you wear on your wrist to tell the time" instead of the word "watch."

Acquired disorders of written language. *Alexia,* or *dyslexia,* refers to a defective ability to read and understand written language. The most common cause probably is *aphasia.* No aphasic patient, with the possible exception of some patients with slight anomic aphasia, is able to read and write normally. For this reason, asking patients to write a paragraph is an excellent screening test for aphasia. Children learn to read by reciting the words to themselves, and this behavior is preserved into adult life. Both Wernicke's aphasia and Broca's aphasia[59] are associated with abnormal reading and writing. Another common reason explaining the inability to read is *defective visual perception.* Although it may seem obvious, one cannot read what one cannot see. Ocular and optic nerve disorders, visual field defects and visual neglect, and types of Balint's syndromes (in which things are seen piecemeal) all can cause an inability to consistently read a paragraph of print. When dyslexia is due to defective vision, the patient also has difficulty with non-language-related material. This can be tested by asking patients to describe pictures from magazines or books or the scene they see when they look out the window. Patients should also be asked to trace what they see with their finger, to count the number of objects on the page and point to them, and to copy what they see. When the problem is purely visual, spelling is preserved so that patients can identify words spelled to them and can spell out the letters in spoken words.

The remaining alexic syndromes are usually referred to as *alexia with agraphia* and *alexia without agraphia*. Patients with alexia with agraphia act as if they have become illiterate. They cannot read, write, or spell. The responsible lesion involves the left angular gyrus or its underlying white matter. This is a region through which afferent connections travel from both the auditory cortex in the temporal lobe and the visual cortex in the occipital lobe. Dejerine theorized that the angular gyrus was a specialized zone for written language that developed in humans and was not present in other animals.[69] Some patients with alexia with agraphia also have conduction or anomic aphasia and elements of Gerstmann's syndrome.

In alexia without agraphia, patients can write and spell correctly but they cannot read. Some are able to write a letter but later cannot read back the same. Usually patients with alexia without agraphia (also called "pure alexia" or "pure word blindness") cannot name colors shown to them, although they are able to match colors, tell what colors objects characteristically have, and use crayons or paints to correctly color objects with their customary colors.[73] The usual explanation for this curious syndrome relates to its special anatomy. The responsible lesion usually involves the left occipital lobe and sometimes the adjacent left temporal lobe in the territory of the left posterior cerebral artery. The splenium of the corpus callosum, its adjacent white matter, or both are also involved. Patients usually have a right hemianopia. Visual information must be processed in the right occipital lobe striate cortex, then passed to the language and reading analyzer regions in the left temporal and parietal lobes. The infarct or hemorrhage blocks the afferent input to these zones so that patients cannot name colors and elements of written language. Sometimes they can read individual letters, and often number reading is preserved. Some patients with alexia without agraphia have difficulty naming objects presented to them visually, although they can name the same objects when presented by touch and when described verbally.[64] Amnesia often accompanies the lexical abnormality and can last for as long as 6 months.[64]

Agraphia refers to difficulty with writing. Aphasic patients usually have abnormal writing, which parallels the difficulty in producing correctly spoken language. Patients with Broca's and global aphasia have a greatly reduced writing ability, and their handwriting is poor. Patients with angular gyrus lesions often misspell words although they have no obvious aphasia or alexia. The agraphia is usually associated with other findings that have been linked together under the eponym *Gerstmann's syndrome*. These abnormalities include difficulty with calculations, an inability to name fingers, poor drawing ability, and confusion of the right and left of their bodies and other bodies. Another type of writing abnormality has been called *apraxic agraphia*.[76] In this condition, handwriting is clumsy and poorly formed; at times the patient cannot even hold the pencil or pen properly and can produce little that is legible. Invariably there are other signs of apraxia, with difficulty performing many different motor tasks. Patients with

Wernicke's and conduction types of aphasia often have fluent agraphia — that is, their penmanship is correct, but their words and phrases, similar to their spoken language, are incorrect and may not make sense.

Apraxia. Apraxia is common in patients with left cerebral hemisphere strokes, especially in those lesions involving the left parietal and frontal lobes. The term "apraxia" is used when patients are unable to perform previously learned tasks and the inability is not explained by weakness, aphasia, or sensory loss.[76] The difficulty can be spontaneous and noted during everyday activities (e.g., difficulty with dressing, using utensils, starting the car, turning keys to open doors, and lighting a cigarette). In others the difficulty in performing motor tasks becomes evident when the patient is asked to do something. Apraxia is described according to the body structures used to perform tasks: orofacial, limb, and trunk. Patients with orofacial dyspraxia have difficulty whistling, blowing a kiss, and humming when commanded to perform these and similar activities. Although some patients are unable to protrude their tongues on command, the next moment they may spontaneously stick out the tongue while automatically licking the lips. Patients with truncal apraxia have difficulty performing whole body commands such as standing, turning, and sitting. Usually, limb apraxia involves mostly the hands and arms; for instance, patients fail to show how they would salute, hitchhike, flip a coin, and wave good-bye.

At times apraxia is limited to one side of the body. For example, patients who have lesions involving the left or right medial frontal lobes and the anterior portion of the corpus callosum often have difficulty using the left hand on command, although they are able to perform the same acts normally with the right hand.[24] This lesion is usually due to occlusion of either the left or right anterior cerebral artery.

Apraxia can be best tested in the following three ways[76]:
1. By giving an oral or written command to pretend to do something or to pretend to use an object
2. By using objects placed in front of the patient (e.g., comb, toothbrush, scissors, or hammer)
3. By imitating an action (orofacial, limb, or trunk) performed by the examiner

Although some specialists in higher cortical function abnormalities divide apraxia into ideomotor, ideational, and limb-kinetic types, I do not find these distinctions helpful. In practice, most but not all patients with apraxia also have aphasia. Knowledge of apraxia is important in a practical sense; it helps ensure that clinicians do not falsely diagnose comprehension abnormalities because the patient fails to follow commands normally. In patients with reduced or abnormal speech output, some examiners test comprehension solely by the patient's response to commands. These patients often have right-sided weakness. Failure to follow directions to lift the left hand, put a hand on the stomach, or stick out the tongue may be falsely interpreted as a failure to comprehend the command.

Patients with apraxia often understand but cannot voluntarily control the left hand and orofacial muscles. Tests of comprehension should also include yes and no queries and a chance to select alternatives or objects from spoken directions.

The discussion thus far has centered on so-called left cerebral hemisphere deficits. This assumes that the left hemisphere is dominant for speech — an assumption that is probably correct in more than 90% of right-handed individuals and about 75% of left-handed people. In sinistrals, there is often a mixed dominance so that a lesion on either side can cause an aphasia. The aphasic disturbance is, however, often less severe and less persistent than in patients with speech limited to the diseased hemisphere.

Right Cerebral Hemisphere Abnormalities

The types of dysfunction discussed in the following sections are those ordinarily found in patients with lesions of the right cerebral hemisphere. The lesions are mostly located in the right frontal and parietal lobes and in the right subcortical white matter and basal ganglia in the territory of the right middle cerebral artery. Lesions involving the more posterior portions of the hemisphere in the territory of the posterior cerebral arteries are covered separately.

Although aphasic disorders associated with left hemisphere lesions are obvious, most neurologists have observed that patients with right hemisphere lesions seem to do worse than patients with left hemisphere lesions of the same severity despite preservation of speech. Patients with right hemisphere strokes usually are not able to return to work and often are unsuccessful spouses, parents, and members of society. Their neurologic deficits are less obvious, more subtle, and less easily tested than the deficits discussed in the section on patients with left hemisphere strokes.

Neglect. The term "neglect" is used to describe the act of ignoring one side of space. Neglect can involve only one sensory modality, such as vision, or it can be multimodal and affect visual, auditory, and somatosensory inputs. The term "hemiinattention" is synonymous with neglect and conveys the idea that the individual does not heed or attend to stimuli on one side. Usually the neglect is on the left side of the body and left space, but it can be right sided in some patients with left hemisphere lesions. The neglect can be profound and very obvious (e.g., patients may forget to put their left arm in their jacket or not put on their left shoe), or it can be minor. Ignoring the left side while driving a car is especially serious because this may cause collisions with objects on the left.

Usually neglect is tested by observing patients' behavior and watching the response to various stimuli. When patients are shown a picture or asked to look out the window or around the room, do they observe and describe objects on both sides or merely those to the right? Their eye movements should be watched to see if they have visually explored both sides of space. Patients should also be asked to read a headline or story from a newspaper or magazine. Do the patients begin in the middle or to the right, or are they able to direct their attention to the beginning of the writing on the far left? At times patients misread words by omitting the first letters to the left.

Patients with neglect often omit the *left side of drawings* (e.g., of a clock, daisy, or house) and may fail to copy the left side of the figures. Another useful test is to ask patients to cross off or bisect all of the lines drawn at various angles filling a piece of paper.[58,82] Failure to include the left side is often referred to as *unilateral spatial neglect,* a deficit that can be present without severe hemiinattention.[76,78] Attention to each side of space can also be tested by giving patients stimuli simultaneously to both sides of the body (e.g., wiggling fingers or showing objects in both the right and left visual fields at the same time, touching the right and left limbs simultaneously, or delivering a bilateral simultaneous auditory stimulus from both sides). Some patients are able to detect single stimuli on either side, but they consistently miss one side (usually the left) when rival simultaneous stimuli are given. This phenomenon is usually called *extinction* because the correct response to the single stimulus is extinguished by the rival contralateral stimulus when the two inputs are delivered together. Extinction is one way to detect slight degrees of neglect. However, when a patient cannot correctly perceive a single stimulus on the side of the body contralateral to the stroke, extinction is not a considered diagnosis. Some patients with left hemianopsia do not pick up single stimuli in their left visual fields, and patients with left hemisensory loss may miss a touch on their left arms. Extinction is only used to describe the condition in patients who can reliably and consistently detect stimuli on their left.

At one time, neglect was considered diagnostic of right parietal lobe damage. We now know that neglect can be caused by virtually any large lesion involving the frontal lobe, parietal lobe, deep hemispheric gray and white matter structures, and rostral brainstem. The explanation for neglect differs in lesions in these different loci. The *parietal lobe* is an important receiver of afferent sensory stimuli. Lesions on one side of this lobe mean that input is received mostly in the contralateral parietal lobe from stimuli on the ipsilateral side of the body and space. One heeds what one perceives. If patients see things mostly to the right, they will attend only to the right. The *frontal lobe* is primarily a motor structure, working in conjunction with the caudate nucleus and the anterior limb of the internal capsule. In frontal lobe lesions, although patients receive the afferent input from both parietal lobes, they do not *act* toward the side of space contralateral to the damaged frontal lobe because of the asymmetry of motor function. The right frontal eye fields and right motor, supplementary motor, and premotor cortex all direct behavior to the left side of space. The *rostral brainstem reticular activating system* continuously prods, wakens, and stimulates the ipsilateral cerebral hemisphere. Lesions of the medial midbrain tegmentum and medial thalamus and large lesions of the deep white matter interfere with this alerting system and its distribution to the cerebral cortex. The hemisphere on the affected side is "asleep" or (at least) less vigilant about perceiving or acting on stimuli from the opposite side of the body and space.

Anosognosia. *Anosognosia* is a term used to describe unawareness of an important loss of body function, most often hemiplegia. At times this lack of appreciation can be profound. I have seen many patients with gross, severe left hemiplegia, left hemisensory loss, and left visual field defects who firmly and repeatedly deny that anything at all is wrong with them. At times this problem is not a complete loss of knowledge of the deficit but *failure to appreciate the importance and significance of the deficit* and *failure to be concerned* about the abnormality. The lesion causing anosognosia is usually large.[78] In the past, anosognosia was attributed to right parietal lobe damage, but studies conducted since the advent of CT indicate that the lesions causing this abnormality usually extend into the frontal and temporal lobes and often involve the basal ganglia and deep white matter. Anosognosia is an important organic disturbance and not a psychologic defense mechanism used to cope with a medical disaster. It is not "denial" in the psychiatric sense of willful or unconscious pushing of material out of conscious awareness. Often before examining stroke patients, it is useful to ask them to give a "laundry list" of the dysfunctions and abnormalities that they notice, the parts of the body involved, and the relative severity of the abnormalities. Patients with left hemiparesis who do not mention their weakness should be asked whether both sides, arms, and legs work well and whether they work the same. If the patient still does not mention any loss of left function, he or she should be asked specifically about the left arm and leg. If they have not noticed any loss of function, they should be asked to lift and move the left arm and leg, then asked how these limbs worked. At times, even after complete failure to move the left limbs, the patient still does not verbally acknowledge any dysfunction. In the normal day-to-day function of the human body, the limbs are directed to action, and they respond. Ordinarily, feedback is not required to see if the limbs performed as bid. The stroke patient with left hemiplegia and anosognosia bids the left limbs to move as usual and somehow does not realize that they did not work. Such patients do not have visual and somatosensory feedback from the left side, and many have left-sided neglect. It is not apparent why this abnormality should be limited to patients with right hemisphere lesions.

Dysprosodia. Abnormal appreciation and display of affect is termed *dysprosodia.* Only recently has it become clear that patients with right hemisphere lesions often have abnormalities in detecting the mood and feelings of others and often fail to convey their own feelings. Much communication in life is nonverbal. Facial expression, gestures, and appearance often convey feelings without language. Speech also conveys distinct moods, feelings, and emotions by accent, emphasis, intonation, pauses, accompanying facial expression, and gestures. These nonlinguistic aspects of speech have been termed *dysprosody.*[87] However, the abnormality in patients with right hemisphere lesions is more than just an abnormality in the nonlanguage aspects of speech. The problem is a more global

---

Testing for Dysprosody and Nonlinguistic Speech Abnormalities

Perception of voice affect
  Say or play a prerecorded phrase (e.g., "take the chair"). Speak in a
  happy, sad, angry, silly, commanding, or indifferent voice. Ask the patient
  to identify the mood of the speaker.
Affect of faces
  Show the patient faces with angry, happy, serious, and puzzled expressions.
  Ask the patient to identify affect from alternative descriptors.
Conveying or mimicking affect
  Ask the patient to say the same phrase (e.g., "take the chair") in happy,
  commanding, angry, humorous, and indifferent tones. Ask the patient
  to mime your tone as you say the same phrase.

---

loss of the ability to recognize and send body signals that accurately reflect feelings, emotions, and mood.

Nonlinguistic communication, or body language, is critically important. For instance, when one's wife, husband, or significant other calls and mentions that one should pick up a loaf of bread on the way home, his or her tone and voice usually reflect whether this is an absolute must (i.e., don't come home without it) or not completely necessary (if you get a chance, it would be nice if you got it). The faces and voices of one's boss, spouse, and children readily reveal if they are angry, sad, happy, or indifferent, and one's nonlinguistic behavior conveys a response to that mood. When this ability is lost, it is difficult to recognize and respond adequately to the feelings of others. If patients do not convey their own despair or happiness, it is difficulty for others to respond and help. Similar to the classification of types of aphasia by left hemispheral localization, Ross and others have classified dysprosodia according to the region involved in the right cerebral hemisphere.[74,88] In their view, lesions of the posterior infrasylvian regions of the right hemisphere cause an inability to *recognize* and *comprehend emotional and affective tone of speech*. Recall that temporal lobe lesions in the left hemisphere impair the reception and comprehension of the linguistic aspects of speech. Lesions in the parietooccipital regions of the right hemisphere impair recognition of mood shown by facial expressions and possibly gestures. Parietal lesions may also impair a patient's ability to mimic expressions and the speech intonations of others, a deficit comparable to conduction aphasia in which patients cannot repeat language. Right frontal suprasylvian lesions impair the expression of emotions and affect, just as left frontal lesions impair language output. The evidence for these localizations is not as clear as for localization of aphasic abnormalities in the left hemisphere, but the concept of dysprosody is important in understanding the failure to thrive, relate, and succeed that is so prevalent in patients with right cerebral strokes. The box above outlines bedside testing.

Motor impersistence. Another important right hemisphere deficit has been called motor impersistence.[71] This deficit is also hard to define, but it is important to an understanding of the difficulties many patients with right hemisphere lesions have in returning to work and to normal activities of daily living at home. In this disorder, patients respond to directives, queries, and commands quickly and accurately but impulsively. After the action is quickly performed, just as quickly it is terminated. Patients fail to persist with the activity even if told to do so. For example, when asked to protrude the tongue and keep it there, the patient quickly sticks out the tongue but just as quickly retracts it into the mouth. When asked to hold the arms outstretched, the patient quickly places the arms as asked but drops them quickly, even when exhorted to keep them there. Keeping the eyes shut is nearly impossible for these patients. When testing position sense or the ability to identify objects in a hand, the patient cannot help peeking and looking at the hand even when told firmly and repeatedly to keep the eyes closed. Usually patients are unaware that they cannot keep their eyes closed.

Patients with motor impersistence often answer questions quickly — at times, even before the entire question has been asked. The response is similar to responses in television shows in which the contestants are rewarded if they answer first, even after only a few words of the statement. Instead of thinking and reflecting before replying or doing something, patients with motor impersistence respond impulsively and quickly. In addition, the action is not maintained. In life, many work situations and daily activities require some perseverance. Assembly line–like repetition and persistence are required for many tasks. Restlessness, impulsivity, and a lack of perseverance lead to failure in many simple everyday tasks requiring sustained attention (e.g., setting the dinner table, knitting, cooking a meal, writing a letter, and completing a tax form). The temporal and quantitative aspects of behavior are often more important than the qualitative in determining success. Tests for impersistence include asking the patient to protrude the tongue and hold it there, keep the eyes closed, and keep the hands outstretched. Attention should also be directed to evaluating the speed of the patient's response to any query or command and the patient's ability to persevere with the task.

Fisher originally referred to motor impersistence as associated with left hemiplegia,[71] an indication that patients with this abnormality had frontal lobe or deep lesions that caused contralateral motor signs. I have found that motor impersistence generally occurs in patients with large right hemisphere lesions, usually including the frontal lobe, the basal gray and deep white matter structures, or a combination. Unfortunately, motor impersistence usually lasts, and patients rarely recover.[79]

Constructional apraxia. Difficulty with drawing and copying is termed *constructional apraxia.* The right cerebral hemisphere, especially its posterior

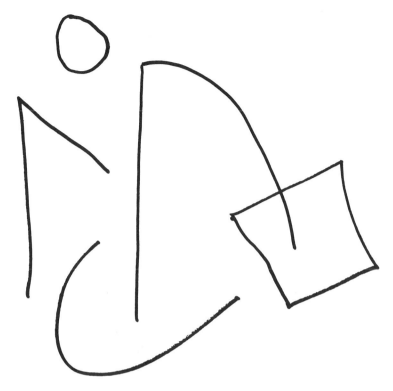

Fig. 5-4   Illustrative diagram that the physician asks the patient to copy.

parietooccipital regions, is known to be specialized for visuospatial functions. Analyzing and conveying the size, shape, angulation, and proportions of objects and their parts are performed best with the right brain, whereas naming and categorizing objects are more left brain functions. Visuospatial function is usually tested by asking patients to draw and copy, using pencil and paper. Because some patients with lesions in the posterior right hemisphere also show unilateral left spatial neglect on drawing and thus omit or distort the left side of drawings, these patients should be asked to draw objects that have general symmetry (e.g., a clock, daisy, or house). They should then be asked to copy a complex figure that cannot readily be described or named (e.g., a figure such as that shown in Fig. 5-4). Instead of using paper and pencil, the patient can copy a figure with tongue blades, cotton swabs, or children's toy blocks. Patients can be asked to orient Kohs' blocks to mimic a diagrammed mosaic.

Drawing and copying abnormalities may result from a variety of brain lesions.[86] Patients with right posterior hemisphere lesions, especially those involving the inferior parietal lobe, usually show left spatial neglect and poor representation of size, shape, angles, and proportions. Copying does not improve their performance. Patients with left cerebral inferior parietal lobe lesions also draw poorly but differently from patients with right-sided lesions. Patients with left parietal lobe lesions usually draw very simple but symmetric figures lacking detail. Angles, shapes, and proportions are preserved. Copying is normal. Patients with frontal lobe lesions often plan drawings poorly, but the visuospatial aspects and relations in the picture are handled normally.

The frontal lobe is involved mostly in planning the picture. Patients with frontal lobe lesions have particular difficulty drawing a floor plan of their own apartment or house. They do poorly when asked to create a floor plan of a "dream house" that would be ideally suited for them and their family. They usually fail to place bathrooms next to bedrooms and misalign the kitchen, dining area, and living rooms. Such a floor plan takes forethought, organization, and planning. Copying of figures is usually normal in patients with frontal lobe lesions since it requires no initiative or planning.

The left brain is specialized for categorization and language functions. Asking patients to draw a house, a bicycle, and a desk or table requires that they first be able to visualize the real object from the name. The resulting pictures are often simplified and rudimentary. Copying requires no conceptualization or categorization and thus is performed normally by patients with left parietal lesions. The defective drawing in patients with right parietal lobe disease relates to their difficulty with visuospatial features. They have little problem with categorization and draw complex figures, but the figures have abnormal configurations, angles, shapes, symmetries, and proportions. Copying does not improve the visuospatial performance.[86]

Abnormalities of the Temporooccipital Lobes

The most important abnormalities found in patients with lesions in the posterior cerebral hemispheres relate to vision, memory, and behavior. The key anatomic components involved are the striate visual cortex (Brodmann's areas 17, 18, and 19) in the paramedian occipital lobes on the banks of the calcarine fissure, the hippocampus and so-called Papez circuit in the medial temporal lobes and medial diencephalon, and the limbic cortex in the medial temporal and inferior temporooccipital regions.

Visual symptoms. Because of the peculiar anatomy of the vertebrobasilar arterial system, an embolus reaching the distal basilar artery moves into the left or right posterior cerebral artery, or fragments may go into the posterior cerebral arteries on both sides. Unilateral infarcts or hematomas in the occipital lobe cause a contralateral visual field abnormality. Visual field loss can be due to involvement of the primary visual cortex along the banks of the calcarine fissure, or it may be caused by interruption of the white matter pathways traveling to the striate cortex. When only the upper bank of the calcarine region (the cuneus) is involved, the patient has a contralateral *inferior quadrantanopia,* whereas lower bank (fusiform and lingual gyri) lesions cause a contralateral *superior quadrantanopia*. When both regions are involved, there is a contralateral *hemianopia*, which includes both the upper and lower portions of the contralateral visual field.

When lesions are restricted to the striate region, there is usually no accompanying visual neglect. Patients are aware that they cannot see to the side, and they compensate for their visual loss by purposefully taking heed of the blind field. When the adjacent parietal and temporal lobes (areas 18, 19) are involved, contralateral visual neglect often accompanies the hemianopia, especially in right-sided lesions.

At times the visual field loss is partial, and patients selectively lose or retain the ability to discern movement, color, or the nature of objects in the abnormal visual field. Visual perception can be abnormal, with objects seen in the preserved field being perseverated into the blind visual field.[66] Flickering, movement, and repetition (palinopsia) of visual objects may occur near the edge of the field defect. Objects may appear too large, too small, angulated, and even inverted. Patients with left-sided lesions that include the splenium of the corpus callosum and the temporoparietal white matter often have alexia without agraphia (described previously in the section on left hemisphere reading abnormalities), an inability to name colors, and elements of Gerstmann's syndrome. Patients with large right-sided lesions in the same regions have left visual neglect and poor drawing and copying skills.

Bilateral visual field loss most often results from embolism to the rostral basilar artery and both posterior cerebral artery branches. At times, severe hypotension produces similar findings by causing ischemia of the middle and posterior cerebral artery border zone regions in the posterior portions of both hemispheres. The visual loss can be severe *cortical blindness,* patchy or limited to the upper or lower portions of the visual fields. Even when there is no conscious visual perception, preservation of the superior colliculi sometimes allows individuals to subconsciously avoid running into objects. For unclear reasons, embolism often involves the lower calcarine bank bilaterally. This causes an upper field visual defect on both sides that is often accompanied by loss of color perception (*achromatopsia*) and loss of the ability to recognize faces (*prosopagnosia*).[68] Color may be completely lost, with all objects appearing black and white, or colors may be blunted or gray. Facial recognition and even matching of identical photographs of faces are often impaired. Farmers often lose the ability to identify their cows. The patient with prosopagnosia only recognizes an individual when he or she speaks. Patients with this deficit usually instruct individuals they are to meet to wear conspicuous hats, dark eyeglasses, or other easily identified apparel to aid recognition.

Bilateral upper bank infarcts most often are due to severe hypotension with borderline ischemia. Patients have bilateral lower visual field defects and usually show features of *Balint's syndrome.*[75,89] Table 5-2 lists the elements of this

TABLE 5-2 Balint's Syndrome

DEFECT	TESTING
Simultanagnosia (piecemeal vision): inability to grasp a visual scene in its entirety; holes or defects in visual perception	Ask patient to: Describe scene or picture Count number of objects or words Identify three objects shown at once
Optic ataxia (poor hand-eye coordination): inability to direct hands using visual control	Ask patient to: Point to noses in a picture Trace with right and left fingers or a pencil over a diagram
Apraxia of gaze: inability to direct gaze voluntarily to desired regions and stimuli	Ask patient to: Look first at clinician's nose, then at clinician's finger on an outstretched hand

syndrome and methods of testing for the individual features that make up the syndrome. The disorder probably is due to defective integration of looking, which is mediated through the frontal and occipital eye fields, and seeing, which is mediated through the striate calcarine cortex. Usually patients also have difficulty localizing objects in space, and they get lost easily.

Amnesia. Memory functions in humans have traditionally been localized to the Papez circuit, a continuous loop from the hippocampi on both sides to the fornices, mammillary bodies, and anteromedial thalamic nuclei and back to the hippocampi.[76,88] Unilateral lesions cause amnesia that can last for as long as 6 months.[62] Amnestic patients cannot make enduring new memories. They often repeat stories or queries just spoken or answered moments before. At times, memories of events that occurred before their stroke are also lost (retrograde amnesia). Some patients confabulate answers for events that they cannot recall. The responsible unilateral lesions usually involve either the lateral thalamus and medial temporal lobe[64] or the medial thalamus.[43] Memory loss can also be found in patients with lesions affecting the basal nucleus of Meynert in the substantia innominata region of the anterior perforated substance. The most common cause of a lesion at this site is bleeding or ischemia associated with rupture of an anterior communicating artery aneurysm.

Patients with amnesia nearly always must rely on lists to remind themselves of data, appointments, responsibilities, and obligations. Memory function should be tested in every stroke patient. This should be done by giving the patient objects, stories, or pictures that they will be asked to recall later. In patients with aphasia, hiding objects around the room should be substituted for verbal information to recall; later the patient will be expected to point to the hiding places of the objects hidden in the room.

Behavior. Lesions of the limbic regions in the amygdala, medial temporal lobes, and fusiform and lingual gyri often cause severe behavioral changes. The same abnormalities also can follow damage to the cingulum and gyrus recti, although strokes in these regions are far less common. *Agitated delirium* is the most common clinical syndrome. Patients are restless, agitated, and speak incoherently with ideas flowing and fleeting from one topic to another. Language usage is correct, but the ideas are often not relevant to the conversation or the events. Yelling, crying out, and aggressive behavior also occur. The most common causes are embolic infarcts in the territories of the unilateral or bilateral posterior cerebral arteries, affecting the lingual and fusiform gyri,[60,84] and infarcts in the inferior division of the middle cerebral artery, especially on the right.[63] Lesions of the rostral reticular formation and the thalami often cause hypersomnolence and diminished activity and interest in the environment.[60]

Frontal Lobe Lesions

The frontal lobe regions have considerable influence on motor behavior, planning, motivation, and personality. Several common, characteristic abnormalities follow damage to the frontal lobes and the deeper structures that interconnect with them (caudate nuclei and anterior thalamus). *Abulia* refers to an apathetic, inactive state in which patients lack spontaneity, have long delays in responding to queries and commands, and fail to persevere with tasks.[72] They sit or lie like blocks of wood and are uninterested and inactive in the environment. This can be tested by asking the patient to count quickly from 20 to 1 backwards or to perform some other task that requires protracted activity (e.g., crossing off all the letter "A"s on a printed page). *Personality changes* include inappropriate jocularity; socially inappropriate, uninhibited behavior; poor insight; and lack of responsibility.[70] Patients are unable to plan for the future and show a lack of concern for others. Some patients become irascible, profane, and aggressive. Patients with frontal lobe infarcts and hemorrhages often perseverate previous responses and seem unable to change subjects or ideas.

Elementary Dysfunctions

Much space has been used here to describe higher cortical function and behavioral abnormalities because they are less familiar to many nonneurologists. The more elementary neurologic abnormalities found in patients with hemispheral and brainstem strokes are commented on briefly in the following sections.

Paresis. Weakness and paralysis are common in patients with stroke and contribute greatly toward disability. The most common deficit is usually termed a *hemiparesis;* yet the weakness is rarely homogeneous in all parts of the affected side. Usually the hand, arm, and foot are more affected than the thigh, leg, and face, but the distribution of weakness varies greatly, depending on the location of the infarct or hemorrhage. Following the pattern of corticospinal innervation, the abductors and extensors of the upper extremity are more involved than the flexors and adductors, and in the lower extremity the flexors and abductors are weaker than the adductors and extensors. The increased extensor tone in the lower extremity allows standing. The flexed, adducted posture of the upper limb facilitates the holding of objects and is much more functional than if the arm were extended by the side of the body. Knowledge of the pattern, distribution, and severity of weakness is important in guiding the restoration of function.

Sensory symptoms. Although sensory symptoms in the form of numbness, paresthesia, and loss of sensibility are common after hemispheric and brainstem strokes, they seldom contribute much to disability unless the sensory loss is severe. Sometimes, delayed-onset central pain develops in the numb limbs and can be a vexing problem to manage. Central pain is important to differentiate from bone and joint pain (e.g., an early "frozen" shoulder caused by immobility) that frequently complicates stroke. Central pain is more diffuse and is usually increased by superficial stimuli such as touch, warmth or cold, and pinpricks, whereas joint-related and musculoskeletal pain is increased by passive and active joint and limb movement.

Hemianopia. This deficit is discussed under visual dysfunctions related to disease of the posterior portions of the cerebral hemispheres. In actuality, hemianopia is seldom a major problem unless there is associated visual neglect. Patients are usually able to accommodate their lives to simple hemianopia.

Nonpyramidal hemimotor syndromes. Many lesions, especially small deep infarcts, affect motor function on the contralateral side of the body without causing appreciable weakness, hyperreflexia, or Babinski's signs. These deficits usually relate to extrapyramidal and cerebellar systems. Slowness, increased tone, dystonic postures, choreic or other adventitious movements, and limb ataxia are found. These may cause a syndrome resembling hemiparkinsonism or hemichorea. Causative lesions usually involve the caudate nucleus,[18] putamen, or thalami.[64]

Dysarthria refers to abnormal speech pronunciation despite normal use of language. This abnormality is found after hemispheric, caudate nucleus, cerebellar, and brainstem infarcts and hemorrhages. Dysarthria caused by stroke is seldom disabling and usually improves when patients are exhorted to speak slowly and deliberately. Dysarthria is prominent and often persistent in patients with bilateral lesions that effect pyramidal and extrapyramidal pathways. These patients with pseudobulbar syndrome also have dysphagia and difficulty in controlling emotional reactions. An examination usually shows increased jaw, facial, and pharyngeal reflexes and bilateral pyramidal tract signs.

Dysphagia is common after stroke and can lead to repeated aspiration and pneumonia.[80,81] Dysphagia is most common, severe, and persistent after brainstem infarcts or hemorrhages. Dysphagia is also a prominent part of the pseudobulbar syndrome described previously. Swallowing abnormalities are also common after large hemisphere strokes, but the abnormality invariably improves with time. The swallowing abnormality in these patients usually is limited to the contralateral pharynx. Dysphagia is especially characteristic in patients with lateral medullary infarcts who have pharyngeal weakness. Food and secretions get caught in the pyriform fossa of the pharynx, and patients often try to extricate the material with a characteristic crowing cough. Evaluation for dysphagia and aspiration using modern fluoroscopic and manometric techniques is important in the majority of stroke patients with motor deficits and is discussed in detail in the section on the rehabilitation phase.[80,81]

Ataxia may involve either the limbs or gait. Most often the limb deficit is a hemiataxia. The involved limbs are hypotonic and show rebound when they are rapidly elevated, then braked quickly. Lurching to the side, veering, and tilting are common after verbal cerebellar infarcts, especially those that involve the territory of the medial branch of the posterior inferior cerebellar artery. Gait training is important in these patients.

Diplopia, dizziness, and ophthalmoplegia. The vestibular system and the nuclear and internuclear components of the oculomotor system are intricately connected in the brainstem to maintain the vestibuloocular reflex, which permits visual fixation during head and eye movements. Dizziness, frank vertigo, angular visual displacement, and tilting are common after vestibular system lesions. Some patients describe oscillopsia, a movement of objects. In patients with diplopia and ophthalmoplegia, covering one eye usually improves the symptoms.

Facial weakness is common after stroke but rarely is a problem unless the CN VII nucleus or its fascicles are involved, causing weakness of eye closure. Failure to shut the eye can lead to corneal ulceration. Facial weakness can also affect the ability to handle food during the oral phase.

In general, strokes occur in older patients who frequently already have many medical problems. Visual loss, hearing loss, arthritis, osteoporosis, neuropathies, and cardiopulmonary disease may all contribute to the disability and are as important to assess systematically as are the neurologic deficits.

REFERENCES

Neurologic Assessment of the Acute Stroke

1. Amarenco P et al: The prevalence of ulcerated plaques in the aortic arch in patients with stroke, *N Engl J Med* 326:221, 1992.
2. Barsan W et al: Early treatment for acute ischemic stroke, *Ann Intern Med* 111:449, 1989.

3. Bogousslavsky J: Topographic patterns of cerebral infarcts, *Cerebrovasc Dis* 1(suppl 1):61, 1991.
4. Caplan LR: Computed tomography and stroke. In McDowell F, Caplan LR, editors: *Cerebrovascular survey report for the National Institute of Neurologic and Communicative Disorders and Stroke (NINCDS)*, revised 61-74, Washington, DC, 1985, NINCOS.
5. Caplan LR: Course of illness graphs, *Hosp Pract* 20:125, 1985.
6. Caplan LR: Of birds, nests, and brain emboli, *Rev Neurol* 147:265, 1986.
7. Caplan LR: Cerebrovascular disease: large artery occlusive disease. In Appel A, editor: *Current neurology*, vol 8, Chicago, 1988, Year Book.
8. Caplan LR: Intracerebral hemorrhage revisited, *Neurology* 38:624, 1988.
9. Caplan LR: *The effective clinical neurologist,* Boston, 1990, Blackwell.
10. Caplan LR: Diagnosis and treatment of ischemic stroke, *JAMA* 266:2413, 1991.
11. Caplan LR: The 1991 E. Graeme Robertson lecture: vertebrobasilar embolism, *Clin Exp Neurol* 28:1, 1991.
12. Caplan LR: Clinical features of spontaneous intracerebral hemorrhage. In Kaufman HH, editor: *Intracerebral hematomas,* New York, 1992, Raven Press.
13. Caplan LR, Gorelick PB, Hier DB: Race, sex, and occlusive vascular disease: a review, *Stroke* 17:648, 1986.
14. Caplan LR, Hier D, D'Cruz I: Cerebral embolism in the Michael Reese Stroke Registry, *Stroke* 14:530, 1983.
15. Caplan LR, Sergay S: Positional cerebral ischemia, *J Neurol Neurosurg Psychiatry* 39:385, 1976.
16. Caplan LR, Stein RW: *Stroke: a clinical approach,* Boston, 1986, Butterworth.
17. Caplan LR, Wolpert SM: Angiography in patients with occlusive cerebrovascular disease: a stroke neurologist and neuroradiologist's views, *AJNR* 12:593, 1991.
18. Caplan LR et al: Caudate infarcts, *Arch Neurol* 47:133, 1990.
19. Caplan LR et al: Transcranial Doppler ultrasound: present status, *Neurology* 40:696, 1990.
20. European Carotid Surgery Trialists Collaborative Group: MRC European carotid surgery trial: interim results for symptomatic patients with severe (70–90%) or with mild (0–29%) carotid stenosis, *Lancet* 337:1235, 1991.
21. Fisher CM, Ojemann RG: A clinico-pathologic study of carotid endarterectomy plaques, *Rev Neurol* 142:573, 1986.
22. Fisher CM, Perlman A: The nonsudden onset of cerebral embolism, *Neurology* 17:1025, 1967.
23. Foulken MA et al: The Stroke Data Bank: design, methods, and baseline characteristics, *Stroke* 19:547, 1988.
24. Geschwind N, Kaplan E: A human disconnection syndrome, *Neurology* 12:675, 1962.
25. Gorelick PB et al: Headache in acute cerebrovascular disease, *Neurology* 36:1445, 1986.
26. Marler JR et al: Morning increase in onset of ischemic stroke, *Stroke* 20:473, 1989.
27. Mohr JP et al: The Harvard Cooperative Stroke Registry: a prospective registry, *Neurology* 28:754, 1978.
28. North American Symptomatic Carotid Endarterectomy Trial Collaborators: Beneficial effect of carotid endarterectomy in symptomatic patients with high-grade stenosis, *N Engl J Med* 325:445, 1991.
29. Raichle ME: The pathophysiology of brain ischemia, *Ann Neurol* 3:2, 1983.
30. Ringelstein EB et al: Computed tomographic patterns of proven embolic infarctions. *Ann Neurol* 26:759, 1989.
31. Signoret JL: Memory and amnesias. In Mesulam M-M, editor: *Principles of behavioral neurology,* Philadelphia, 1985, FA Davis.

32. Sirna S et al: Cardiac evaluation of the patient with stroke, *Stroke* 21:14, 1990.
33. Steinke W et al: Symptomatic and asymptomatic high-grade carotid stenosis in Doppler color-flow imaging, *Neurology* 40:131, 1990.

Treatment

34. Albers GW et al: Stroke prevention in nonvalvular atrial fibrillation: a review of prospective randomized trials, *Ann Neurol* 30:511, 1991.
35. Brott T: Prevention and management of medical complications of the hospitalized elderly stroke patient. *Clin Geriatr Med* 7(3):475, 1991.
36. Cadroy Y, Horbett TA, Hanson SR: Discrimination between platelet-mediated and coagulation-mediated mechanism in a model of complex thrombus formation in vivo, *J Lab Clin Med* 113:436, 1989.
37. Caplan LR: Anticoagulation for cerebral ischemia, *Clin Neuropharmacol* 9:399, 1986.
38. Caplan LR: TIAs: we need to return to the question "what is wrong with Mr. Jones?" *Neurology* 38:791, 1988.
39. Caplan LR: Diagnosis and treatment of ischemic stroke, *JAMA* 266:2413, 1991.
40. Caplan LR, Stein RW: *Stroke: a clinical approach,* Boston, 1986, Butterworth.
41. Caplan LR, Wolpert SM: Angiography in patients with occlusive cerebrovascular disease: a stroke neurologist and neuroradiologist's views, *AJNR* 12:593, 1991.
42. Caplan LR et al: Transcranial Doppler ultrasound: present status, *Neurology* 40:696, 1990.
43. Choi DW et al: Medial thalamic hemorrhage with amnesia, *Arch Neurol* 40:611, 1983.
44. Collins RC, Dobkin BH, Choi DW: Selective vulnerability of the brain: new insights into the pathophysiology of stroke, *Ann Intern Med* 110:992, 1989.
45. Crisostomo EA et al: Evidence that amphetamine with physical therapy promotes recovery of motor function in stroke patients, *Arch Neurol* 23:94, 1988.
46. Dietz MA, McDowell FH: Potentiation of rehabilitation: medication effects on recovery of function after brain injury and stroke, *J Stroke Cerebrovasc Dis* 1:37, 1991.
47. Estol C, Caplan LR: Therapy of acute stroke, *Clin Neuropharmacol* 13:91, 1990.
48. European Carotid Surgery Trialists Collaborative Group: MRC European carotid surgery trial: interim results for symptomatic patients with severe (70-90%) or with mild (0-29%) carotid stenosis, *Lancet* 337:1235, 1991.
49. Feeney DM, Baron JC: Diaschisis, *Stroke* 17:818, 1986.
50. Garcia JH, Anderson ML: Pathophysiology of cerebral ischemia, *CRC Crit Rev Neurobiol* 4:303, 1989.
51. Goldstein LB, Davis JN: Physician prescribing patterns following hospital admission for ischemic cerebrovascular disease, *Neurology* 38:1806, 1988.
52. Hull RD et al: Subcutaneous low-molecular weight heparin compared with continuous intravenous heparin in the treatment of proximal vein thrombosis, *N Engl J Med* 326:975, 1991.
53. Jafar JJ, Crowell RM: Focal ischemic thresholds. In Wood JH, editor: *Cerebral blood flow,* New York, 1987, McGraw-Hill.
54. Norris JW, Hachinski VC: High-dose steroid treatment in cerebral infarction, *Br Med J* 4:292(6512):21, 1986.
55. North American Symptomatic Carotid Endarterectomy Trial Collaborators: Beneficial effect of carotid endarterectomy in symptomatic patients with high-grade stenosis, *N Engl J Med* 325:445, 1991.
56. Plum F: What causes infarction in ischemic brain?: the Robert Wartenberg lecture, *Neurology* 33:222, 1983.
57. Poungvarin N et al: Effects of dexamethasone in primary supratentorial intracerebral hemorrhage, *N Engl J Med* 14:316:1229, 1987.

Patterns of Neurologic Impairment
58. Albert ML: A simple test for neglect, *Neurology* 23:658, 1973.
59. Benson DF: The third alexia, *Arch Neurol* 34:327, 1977.
60. Caplan LR: Top of the basilar syndrome: selected clinical aspects, *Neurology* 30:72, 1980.
61. Caplan LR, DeWitt LD: Aphasia, *MRI Decisions* 1:2, 1988.
62. Caplan LR, Hedley-White T: Cuing and memory dysfunction in alexia without agraphia, *Brain* 97:251, 1974.
63. Caplan LR et al: Infarcts of the inferior division of the right middle cerebral artery: mirror image of Wernicke's aphasia, *Neurology* 36:1015, 1986.
64. Caplan LR et al: Lateral thalamic infarcts, *Ann Neurol* 45:959, 1988.
65. Choi DW et al: Medial thalamic hemorrhage with amnesia, *Arch Neurol* 40:611, 1983.
66. Critchley M: Types of visual perseveration: "palinopsia" and illusory "visual spread," *Brain* 74:267, 1951.
67. Damasio H, Damasio AR: The anatomical basis of conduction aphasia, *Brain* 103:337, 1980.
68. Damasio AR, Damasio H, Van Hoesen GW: Prosopagnosia: anatomic basis and behavioral mechanisms, *Neurology* 32:331, 1982.
69. Dejerine J: Contribution a l'etude anatomo-pathologique et clinique des differentes varietes de cecite verbale, *C R Soc Biol* 4:61, 1892.
70. Eslinger PJ, Damasio AR: Severe disturbance of higher cognition after bilateral frontal lobe ablation: patient EVR, *Neurology* 35:1731, 1985.
71. Fisher CM: Left hemiplegia and motor impersistence, *J Nerv Ment Dis* 123:201, 1956.
72. Fisher CM: Abulia minor vs agitated behavior, *Clin Neurosurg* 31:9, 1983.
73. Geschwind N, Fusillo M: Color-naming defects in association with alexia, *Arch Neurol* 15:137, 1966.
74. Gorelick PB, Ross ED: The aprosodias: further functional-anatomic evidence of the organization of language in the right hemisphere, *J Neurol Neurosurg Psychiatry* 50:553, 1987.
75. Hecaen H, de Ajuriaguerra J: Balint's syndrome (psychic paralysis of visual fixation) and its minor forms, *Brain* 77:373, 1954.
76. Hier DB, Gorelick PB, Shindler AG: *Topics in behavioral neurology and neuropsychology with key references,* Boston, 1987, Butterworth.
77. Hier DB, Mohr JP: Incongruous oral and written naming, *Brain Lang* 4:115, 1977.
78. Hier DB, Mondlock J, Caplan LR: Behavioral abnormalities after right hemisphere stroke, *Neurology* 33:337, 1983.
79. Hier DB, Mondlock J, Caplan LR: Recovery of behavioral abnormalities after right hemisphere stroke, *Neurology* 33:345, 1983.
80. Horner J, Massey EW, Brazer SR: Aspiration in bilateral stroke patients, *Neurology* 40:1686, 1990.
81. Horner J et al: Aspiration following stroke: clinical correlates and outcome, *Neurology* 38:1359, 1988.
82. Kaplan J, Hier DB: Visuospatial deficits after right hemisphere stroke, *J Occup Ther* 36:314, 1982.
83. Kertesz A: *Aphasia and associated disorders*, New York, 1979, Grune & Stratton.
84. Medina JL, Chokroverty S, Rubino FA: Syndrome of agitated delirium and visual impairment: a manifestation of temporo-occipital infarction, *J Neurol Neurosurg Psychiatry* 40:861, 1977.
85. Mohr JP et al: Broca's aphasia: pathological and clinical, *Neurology* 28:311, 1978.
86. Piercy M, Hecaen H, de Ajuriaguerra J: Constructional apraxia associated with unilateral cerebral lesions: left and right cases compared, *Brain* 83:225, 1960.

87. Rolak LA, Rokey R: *Coronary and cerebral vascular disease,* Mt Kisco, NY, 1990, Futura Publishing.
88. Ross ED: The aprosodias: functional-anatomic organization of the affective components of language in the right hemisphere, *Arch Neurol* 38:561, 1981.
89. Tunick PA et al: Atheromatosis of the aortic arch as a source of systemic emboli, *Ann Intern Med* 114:391, 1991.

Additional Readings

Caplan LR, Kelly JJ: *Consultations in neurology,* Toronto, 1988, BC Decker.

Damasio AR et al: Central achromatopsia: behavioral, anatomical, and physiologic aspects, *Neurology* 30:1064, 1980.

Geschwind N: Language and the brain, *Sci Am* 226:76, 1972.

Mesulam M-M: A cortical network for directed attention and unilateral neglect, *Ann Neurol* 10:309, 1981.

Michael EM, Troost BT: Palinopsia: cerebral localization with computed tomography, *Neurology* 30:887, 1980.

Ostergaard JR: Warning leak in subarachnoid hemorrhage, *Br Med J* 301:190, 1990.

Tyler HR: Abnormalities of perception with defective eye movements (Balint's syndrome), *Cortex* 4:154, 1986.

CHAPTER 6

Rehabilitation Management Plan

Nature of the problem
Disorders of sensorimotor control
  Nature of the problem
  Assessment of impairment in the upper extremity
  Prevention of secondary impairments
Efficacy of rehabilitation

NATURE OF THE PROBLEM

Concern for the patient's medical and neurologic stabilization is a priority during the acute phase. At this same time it is also necessary to initiate the plan for alleviating the disabilities that occur as a result of the impairments. The ultimate goal is to enable the patient to perform, as fully as possible, activities of daily living (ADLs) despite continued impairments. This is accomplished by developing alternative means for achieving mobility and other functions. This retraining is the major activity during the subsequent rehabilitation phase. During the acute phase the goal is to maintain the patient's readiness to enter into the retraining and thus to protect the patient from the effects of nonuse of the affected limbs. A major issue is the proper maintenance of position and range of motion (ROM) in those joints in which sensorimotor function has been impaired.

In addition, during the acute phase the degree to which rehabilitation resources should be committed to the patient's retraining must be determined. The decision to allocate resources depends not only on the degree of unimpaired neurologic function (and thus the residual resources of the person) but also on the patient's goals and the outside resources that may be enlisted to enable noninstitutional living. The use of an intensive rehabilitation program reflects the degree to which such a program can be expected to contribute to the development of compensatory strategies in both the person and those who are potential caregivers. In addition, the patient's degree of medical stability must be determined. For instance, it must be decided whether the patient's endurance permits participation in the frequently physically strenuous activities required in more intensive rehabilitation settings.

Determinations must be made about the intensity and extent of retraining, the timing of the retraining, and the most effective location for retraining. In most instances the decision is reduced to the following options: the patient's return home with or without support of various kinds, the patient's transfer to a long-term care facility with or without retraining provided, or the patient's transfer to an inpatient rehabilitation facility that provides both physical care and retraining of a relatively intense, classically interdisciplinary nature. Thus the overall rehabilitation plan must include some determination of the extent of retraining and the resources and type of retraining necessary.

First, committing the appropriate level of resources requires an identification of the degree to which function is compromised, the type of impairment, and the likelihood of a spontaneous recovery sufficient for self-care. To answer these questions, a transformation in the goals of the assessment process must take place. The purpose of assessing neurologic function during the acute phase is to localize the brain and vascular lesions and identify the site and character of the neural injury through the delineation of the impairments. To formulate the rehabilitation plan once neurologic deficits are stabilized, the impairments must be assessed in relation to the patient's eventual life function. The goals of the assessment are changed, as is what is assessed. In the assessment of hemiparesis, for example, the side affected is of concern in terms of the dominant hand and the distribution of impairment between the upper and lower extremities to such a degree that impairments might affect mobility. Instead of assessing primarily the degree of impairment, one must now assess the degree of residual function. For example, the ability to perform hip and knee extension is a good predictor that the patient may be able to stand. One must recognize the opportunities rather than only the problems.

An examination of the sensorimotor system must include the dynamic quality of the system at a particular point in time. At the outset, the findings depend on the degree of injury and the time since injury. In addition to the dynamic of change over time, one must recognize that, at any point in time, the findings depend on the conditions of the examination. For example, motor function in the limbs varies with body position, and sensory findings vary with stimulus strength and the presence of competing stimuli. The performance of the person can be enhanced if the proper conditions are provided. Exploration of those conditions during the assessment period helps to define ways to help the stroke patient learn new skills during the retraining phase.

Second, in addition to determining the level of impairment, the patient's individual goals must be identified in developing a rehabilitation plan. The benefit of retraining also depends on the patient's values and goals. The effects to be achieved and the effort needed to achieve them must be compatible with what the patient wishes.[1]

Third, the degree to which resources are available has an impact on the rehabilitation plan. For instance, the training of family or other caregivers may be the focus of the entire rehabilitation process.

The preceding three factors are more fully developed during the rehabilitation phase itself, when a more complete individual plan is made. Initially, however, one must determine the overall level of resources appropriate for the patient's needs. This decision depends at least in part on the likelihood of benefit and on the availability of resources.

Rationing of health care has become more pervasive. For instance, rationing on the basis of age has been advanced as one criterion for distributing resources.[2] In light of these current concerns about cost of health care there must be far greater emphasis on the outcomes achieved in relation to costs. It is important to enlist the individual in his own retraining to maximize the results achieved in proportion to the resources expended. One way to do this is to increase the degree of involvement of the patient in the treatment planning process. In this way the use of resources is optimized from both an ethical and a utilitarian basis.

DISORDERS OF SENSORIMOTOR CONTROL
Nature of the Problem

A major and common result of stroke is hemiparesis in which the motor control of the affected extremities is impaired as the result of loss of supraspinal effects on the anterior horn cell. The factors hindering functional motor control are not merely weakness but the lack of selectivity of action and coordination at a joint. The balance of motor control that allows agonists and antagonists to work in concert is no longer present. The rapidity of release and contraction of the muscles operating at a joint is frequently compromised. In addition, the upper motor neuron dysfunction impairs selective motor control, which may lead to a mass synergy pattern.[30] Selectivity of normal muscle action is a function of cortical motor control guided by proprioceptive feedback. In the presence of injury to the central nervous system, both the central motor and sensory tracts are disrupted.

During this short-term acute phase the opportunity exists to assess the degree of impairment and its evolution as a prognostic measure to help establish the need for further treatment. During the subsequent longer term rehabilitation phase, the focus is on enhancing motor recovery by various training procedures and on the use of compensatory strategies to address the functional disabilities arising from any impairment that remains. The initial assessment of the degree of motor impairment during this acute care phase requires an evaluation of both strength and the selectivity of motor control and tone. In addition, the assessment should include an evaluation of joint ROM and sensation and perceptual difficulties.

This section describes some of the general principles of assessing motor impairment, then focuses on the assessment of the upper extremities. The affected upper extremity is particularly likely both to remain impaired and to have subsequent secondary impairment caused by improper care during the

---

Six-Stage Motor Recovery Proposed by Brunnstrom

Stage 1   Flaccidity is present, and no movements of the limb can be initiated.

Stage 2   Basic limb synergies or some components may appear as associated reactions, or minimal voluntary movement responses may be present. Spasticity developing.

Stage 3   Patient gains voluntary control of movement *synergies;* full range of synergy components does not necessarily develop. Spasticity increased and may become severe.

Stage 4   Some movement combinations mastered—first with difficulty, then with more ease—that do not follow paths of either synergy. Spasticity declining.

Stage 5   More difficult combinations learned as basic limb synergies lose dominance over motor acts.

Stage 6   Spasticity disappears; individual joint movements possible; and coordination approaches normal.

From Brunnstrom S: *Movement therapy in hemiplegia*, New York, 1970, Harper & Row.

acute phase. Thus it is particularly important that care of this extremity be initiated in the acute phase and continued throughout the life of the person with stroke.

"Patterned motion" refers to the primitive stereotyped synergies of mass flexion and mass extension, which are initiated when the person with hemiplegia attempts to perform a task. The muscles that participate and the strength of their responses are the same regardless of the demand. Particularly problematic is the effect of such a patterned response on the actions of the upper extremity. The functional actions of the upper extremity require considerable flexibility and maneuverability.

In the lower extremity the primitive patterns are discrete and prominent, and most persons with hemiparesis regain considerable mobility. They can initiate the extensor pattern for standing and use the flexor pattern to take steps. The extension and flexion patterns can be used to provide a safe means of walking although the refinements of normal gait are not achieved.[31]

The changes in reflexes and the degree of patterning can make classical conventional testing of muscle strength inappropriate. Following the studies of Twitchell,[37] Brunnstrom described a method to follow the recovery of motor function in persons with hemiplegia.[8] See the box above for the six-stage motor recovery scale, which recognizes the initial loss of reflexes and their return with increasing degrees of motor action selectivity in relation to patterned activities. These patterns vary with the size and location of the brain lesion. In the presence of limitation in selective voluntary action, the effects of posture must also be assessed. For example, in applying these stages of motor recovery to the clinical examination, the Fugl-Meyer Assessment (FMA) is carried out in the upper extremity with the patient in a seated position and in the lower extremity with the patient assuming, successively, the supine, seated, and standing positions, depending on stage of return of motor function selectivity.[17] Functional activation of motor movements in both the upper and lower extremities may vary and is widely dependent on posture, either supine or prone and either sitting or standing.

A number of scales other than the FMA have been developed to measure changes in motor control. These scales were formulated in response to the need for greater simplicity in assessment and for greater relevance to functional outcome. These measurements are described in greater detail in the section devoted to sensorimotor control during the rehabilitation phase. One such measurement is the Rivermead Stroke Assessment developed for use in Britain.[27] Gross function and leg, trunk, and arm functions are sampled. The first category deals with functional movement and assesses a range of movements from sitting and sitting-to-standing to transfers and ambulation. The second category deals with the degree of control of movement. For example, the scale ranges from "rolling to affected side" (i.e., starting from the supine position and moving without the use of the hands) through "standing, step unaffected leg on and off block" (i.e., without retraction of the pelvis or hyperextension of knee) to "lying, dorsiflex affected ankle with leg flexed." The third category of arm movement is more variegated and deals with both motor control and functional movement of the arm. This scale differs from the others; it samples both the degrees of impairment in motor control and the functional aspects in one scale.

Recently, attempts have been made to standardize the assessment of motor impairment in the upper extremity for use in research studies. The aim is to provide a basis for the evaluation of the effectiveness of treatment. See the box on p. 119 for the overall stages and refer to Gowland's article for the specific test items used to explore each stage.[19] The author suggests that the stage achieved along with the weeks after stroke can be used to predict the eventual degree of motor impairment and the subsequent degree of physical disability.

Assessment of Impairment in the Upper Extremity

The recovery of motor control that occurs after stroke varies with the areas of the brain most affected and the severity of the injury. In most instances, in the general order of recovery, the arm remains affected for a longer time than the leg and has a less complete return of function. The classic study carried out by Twitchell was chiefly concerned with the course of recovery in the limbs.[37] An increase in resistance to passive stretch was noted mainly in the flexors and adductors of the upper extremity and in the extensors and adductors of the lower extremity. The first willed movements to return were flexion at the shoulder and

---

Definitions of the Stages of Motor Impairment

Stage 1 This is presynergistic stage. Muscle (i.e., phasic) strength reflexes are absent or hypoactive. No resistance to passive movement (i.e., tonic stretch reflex) is felt. No active movement can be elicited either reflexively by a facilitatory stimulus or volitionally.

Stage 2 Resistance to passive movement is felt. No voluntary movement is present, but active movement can be elicited reflexively by a facilitatory stimulus.

Stage 3 Spasticity is marked. Voluntary movement occurs in synergies (i.e., stereotyped patterns of flexion and extension). Movement results from higher center facilitation of associated reactions or spinal or brainstem reflexes.

Stage 4 Spasticity decreases. Synergy patterns can be reversed if the pattern of movement occurs first in the weakest synergy. Movements combining antagonistic synergies can be performed if the strong components act as prime movers. The synergies lose their dominance; the spinal and brainstem reflexes commence modification and integration by higher centers using more complex neutral networks.

Stage 5 Spasticity waves. Synergy patterns can be reversed even if movement occurs first in the direction of the strongest synergy. Movements using the weak components of the synergies, acting as prime movers, can be performed (i.e., difficult extensor and flexor synergy movements can be mixed.) Spinal and brainstem reflexes become modified and integrated into a more complex network. Most movements become environmentally specific.

Stage 6 Coordination and patterns of movement are near normal. Spasticity, as demonstrated by resistance to passive movement, is no longer present. A large variety of environmentally specific patterns of movement are no longer possible. Abnormal patterns of movement with faulty timing emerge when rapid (ballistic) or complex (ramp) targeted movements are requested.

Stage 7 Normal.

From Gowland CA: *Stroke* 21(suppl 2):2, 1990.

hip. Flexion at the elbow occurred first in conjunction with the shoulder; flexion of the fingers followed as part of an overall flexion pattern of the entire upper extremity. Extensor synergy of the arm begins to appear soon after the flexor pattern. Again, extension appeared first as a movement of the shoulder with subsequent movement of the elbow, wrist, and fingers. Although the common pattern was of movement return first in the proximal muscles, in some cases movement returned first to the hand.

In the stereotyped sets of responses, there is less consistency in the upper than in the lower extremity. However, some consistency was found in the patterned movement of the upper arm involving the scapula, shoulder, and elbow.[11] The pattern is named for the motion at the elbow. A preponderant flexion pattern involves elbow flexion, scapular retraction (adduction and downward flexion rotation), shoulder abduction, and external rotation with forearm pronation or supination. A preponderant extension pattern involves elbow extension and the opposite of the actions previously described. There is scapular protraction (abduction and upward rotation), shoulder adduction and internal rotation, and forearm pronation. Wrist and finger flexion may accompany these other responses. Finger extension is rare. It is important to recognize that there may be considerable variation in the degree to which each component participates.[11]

In another early study, assessment was divided into the proximal, central, and distal segments of the arm.[3] Unlike the pattern described by Twitchell,[37] better recovery was demonstrated at the elbow than at the shoulder and hand. Some shoulder motion tended to return more frequently than hand motion. However, for those patients who did regain full motion, it was more common to find it in the hand than the shoulder. When a comparison is made between agonist and antagonist pairs, there was no difference noted at the elbow. Flexion and extension abilities and supination and pronation abilities were the same in the overwhelming number of patients; in the group in whom differences were present, flexion and extension abilities and supination and pronation abilities were equally affected. However, if one ability predominated in the wrist and fingers, it was more likely to be in flexion. Recall that these studies were concerned only with motion at the several joints and not specifically with strength or functional use of the arm. When evaluating these findings, also keep in mind the effects of the body positions in which the patients were tested.

Other measurement techniques include an assessment of strength with a dynamometer and with the patient in a gravity-eliminated position while performing the middle half of the ROM.[3] A comparison is made with the nonparetic side. Significant differences are found between elbow flexor and extensor abilities (elbow flexors are relatively more affected), between shoulder internal and external rotator abilities (external rotators more affected), and between shoulder extensor and abductor abilities (abductors more affected). This reduced ability to abduct and externally rotate the shoulder is thought to be related to subsequent problems with the shoulder, such as pain and tightness of the capsule.

The time frame in which this pattern evolves varies with the degree of injury and other individual factors. In general, at least a partial return of arm function occurred in about 85% of patients who were followed up to 7 months after stroke. Generally, those who recovered a full ROM experienced an initial return within the first few weeks. Those who recovered a partial ROM had a

---

Arm Function Tests

1. Use both hands to trace a ruled line.
2. Use both hands to open a jam jar.
3. Use affected hand to pick up and release a 2-inch cylinder.
4. Use affected hand to drink water from a glass.
5. Use affected hand to open and close a clothespin.
6. Use affected hand to comb hair.

Modified from Wade DT et al: *J Neurol Neurosurg Psychiatr* 46:521, 1983.

more gradual return, sometimes as long as 6 months after the onset.[3] Other more recent studies continue to show that most if not all motor recovery in the arm can be expected to return by 6 months after onset, with rapid return during the first 3 months.[41] Nevertheless, there is considerable evidence that newer modes of treatment can improve motor control in the upper extremity in those who have not recovered motion more than 6 months after the onset.[24]

The measurement of the degree of arm function impairment can be more directly related to activity.[41] One example of more functional items is described in the box above. The initial score (generally within 3 weeks of onset) was zero in 27% of subjects. Twelve percent received a full score on the initial examination. A bimodal distribution was found after 12 months, with 20% still receiving a zero score but 30% achieving the maximum score. The overwhelming majority of those receiving a full score did so by the end of 3 months, and some subjects who had "partial" scores continued to improve during the successive 9 months until the final assessment at the end of 12 months. Note that poor recovery correlated with the degree of original motor deficit and loss of position sense. Poor recovery did not correlate with a number of other measures, including items that may be considered indicative of the overall degree of severity of the stroke, such as a loss of sitting balance or a degree of motor deficit in the leg. Also note that this study demonstrated ongoing improvement during the period beyond the usual 6 months after onset.

Other attempts at developing "motoricity" scores have been made.[15] One particularly innovative method sought to identify key movements in both upper and lower limbs, combined with a prehension scale to reflect action of the fingers. Based on the rate of motor return found on a sampled population, a weighted score was developed that could be used to predict the ultimate return of specific motor actions. For example, shoulder flexion and elbow flexion along with terminal prehension are sampled in the upper extremity; hip flexion, knee extension, and ankle dorsiflexion are sampled in the lower extremity. Table 6-1 describes the weights applied to the stages on the MRC 0 to 5 scale: 3 signifies

TABLE 6-1   Weighted Scores for Motoricity Scale

STAGE	ALL MOVEMENTS	PREHENSION
0	0	0
1	28	33
2	42	56
3	56	65
4	74	77
5	100	100

From Demeurisse G, Demol O, Rabage E: *Eur Neurol* 19:382, 1980.

movement through a full ROM against gravity, 4 against some resistance, and 5 against full resistance. One may use these weighted scores to develop a specific index for either limb or to measure overall progress.

The assessment of motor control includes not only a degree of selectivity and strength but also an analysis of the degree of abnormal tone affecting the speed and coordination of the agonists and antagonists acting at the various joints. Tone is tested by the patient's reaction to rapid passive motion of all the joint motions of the arm and hand. The required precision and speed of the hand and elbow motion make the smallest degree of spasticity conspicuous. The muscles of the hand and arm rely on the prompt release of their antagonists, rather than on force, so that they can move quickly and with ease. Thus the assessment of this factor is crucial to the achievement of prehensile actions. The assessment should be made with the patient in various body positions because, for example, upper extremity flexion posture is often greater in the sitting than in the lying position.[35]

The analysis ultimately must determine the degree to which functional arm positions can be achieved. The main responsibility of the hand is to perform as a prehensile tool, whereas the arm's role is to place the hand where it is most effective. Placement of the arm must be both versatile and precise. Although the focus is on the extremity per se, the ultimate stabilizing action also requires the selective control of the trunk.[16] For example, for voluntary arm movements to occur while in the sitting position, a forward tilt of the pelvis must initially be present to aid in stabilization. Sitting balance during rehabilitation was highly correlated with performance on functional measures, such as the Barthel Index.[34]

Wrist flexion and extension and finger grasp and release are particularly important for prehensile functions. As a general rule, unless some selective wrist and finger extension is present, the hand cannot be used for functional activities other than as a "paper weight" or passive stabilizer.[35] The term *passive assist,* or *gross assist,* describes actions such as holding a toothbrush while applying toothpaste. When elevation of the upper arm in flexion and adduction, flexion of the elbow, and gross grasp are available, this level of function is possible. If they are present along with extension at the elbow and an active grasp release, the arm is termed a *fair assist* in tasks such as ironing clothes and wrapping packages. With a more facile grasp and release, one may perform such tasks as hanging washed clothes on a line, using a fork, and tying a bow behind the back in dressing, which are termed a *good assist.*[43]

The persistence of a motor control impairment and the greater need for selective motor action make problems in the upper extremity particularly troublesome. During the rehabilitation phase, efforts are made to minimize the patient's disabilities by teaching compensatory strategies for carrying out ADLs. The techniques designed to compensate for loss of motor control in the hand are described in the rehabilitation phase, along with assessment methods more appropriate for measuring the ability to perform ADLs and identifying various training procedures to enhance motor control.

Ultimate performance is affected not only by the degree of motor control achieved; secondary complications, such as pain, and structural impairments, such as contractures, can prevent the optimal use of the upper extremity despite improvement in the degree of motor control. During the acute phase a major effort must be made to safeguard the patient from overstretching or persistent faulty positioning of the flaccid upper extremity to prevent soft tissue injury and subsequent contractures and deconditioning. This minimizes later secondary complications and enables the patient to take full advantage of future motor control.

Therefore it is necessary to assess not only motor function but also the degree to which joints can be passively moved through their arc. These can readily be modified during the acute phase to prevent secondary complications. The ROM is determined by the patient's response to slow careful movements in additional range while avoiding overstretch. Functional ROM is defined as the minimal amount of passive range that a joint needs to make possible the performance of ADLs without pain.[35] See Table 6-2 for minimum functional ranges. These, the minimal goals for the maintenance of range, allow the patient to take advantage of eventual improvements in motor control.

Problems in limiting the useful function of the affected arm are also increased by the degree of concomitant sensory impairment. In one study impairment of sensation to pinprick, two-point discrimination, and vibratory sense (128 cps) was common; one or another was found in approximately two thirds of cases.[38] Failure to recover sensation was correlated with a relatively poor result. A continued problem with two-point discrimination was associated with particularly poor results (as measured by the patient's length of stay). The effect of other sensory loss on the results could not be clearly identified.

TABLE 6-2   Range of Required Motion for Activities of Daily Living

MOTION	MINIMUM RANGE (DEGREES)
Shoulder	
Flexion	100
Abduction	90
External rotation	30
Internal rotation	70
Elbow	
Flexion	120
Extension	30
Forearm	
Pronation	Full
Supination	60
Wrist	
Extension	30
Fingers	
Flexion (metacarpophalangeal)	90
Flexion (proximal interphalangeal)	90
Thumb abduction	30
Thumb interphalangeal extension	Full

In a more recent study with relatively few subjects,[26] somatosensory-evoked responses (SEPs) were derived from the stimulation of the median nerve at the wrist and ankle. In the arm a correlation was found between the degree of motor recovery and both SEP and the clinical examination of position sense. Despite poor motor function in the acute setting, those subjects who had a good somatosensory response regained good function; those with totally absent SEP had a poor prognosis. However, these correlations were not predictive of function in the lower extremity.

Moberg emphasized that the grasping functions of the hand depend not only on mobility, strength, and stability but even more on the sensory input.[28] The fingers must "feel what they are holding, how they are holding it and how strongly they are holding it." Also necessary is an alarm system sensitive to heat or mechanical factors that could cause injury. The ability to differentiate two points at least 10 mm apart has become the criterion for tactile gnosis determining the use of the affected hand. In its absence, the patient achieves bimanual activity only with ongoing visual feedback.[29] The lack of a protective sensibility to heat and pinprick can be significant. However, the converse is not true. The hand that can perceive touch and pinprick may not function well in a precision grip.

Proprioception involves an awareness of limb position while vision is occluded. The effects of proprioceptive deficits require visual feedback about an object's position in space if two-handed actions are to be performed. In addition to impairment in sensation, the patient may have a concomitant perceptual problem associated with disturbances of consciousness and the neglect syndrome. The effects of these perceptual defects are explored during the rehabilitation phase when they can have major consequences on the alleviation of disabilities in managing ADLs.[23]

Prevention of Secondary Impairments

The minimal goals during the acute phase are to safeguard the affected extremities against injury and later impairment caused by pain or contractures. Treatment includes appropriately positioning the upper extremity while the patient is in a wheelchair or bed and safeguarding the arm while the patient is standing during transfers and while carrying out ADLs. Efforts also include attempts to normalize the effects of motor control imbalance caused by reflex mechanisms.

A common impairment is pain in the hemiplegic arm. The incidence varies, depending on the criteria for identifying the pain syndrome.[9] Nevertheless, arm pain is a significant problem for many persons.[20] One recent study defined shoulder pain based on the scale developed by Fugl-Meyer.[6,17] Joint pain in the paretic limb is compared with the nonaffected extremity. A score is assigned based on whether pain occurred during all movement or at the end of the ROM. Severe pain occurred in 32% of subjects; some pain was present in an additional 40%.

Other studies focus on the incidence of the shoulder-hand syndrome (SHS) as a more specific variant of a continuum of pain in the hemiplegic arm.[12] In this syndrome the shoulder is painful, especially on movement, and the forearm and hand are often swollen. In stage I of the syndrome, pain exists along with edema. Pain is assessed on the movement of the fingers, wrist, and shoulders. Again, the degree of pain was scored whether pain appeared only at end of the ROM, presented at mid-range, or allowed little or no movement. The fingers were moved from flexion through 3 degrees of hyperextension at the metacarpophalangeal and proximal interphalangeal joints; the wrist was moved through flexion and extension; and the shoulders were abducted to 96 degrees. Pain was reported as present in 80% of the patients, with edema present in 68%. In this report the severity of pain and its distribution in the various joints are unclear. The overall incidence of SHS was 41%, with a significant relationship between the degrees of upper extremity weakness, proprioception deficit, and visual neglect. If all three variables were absent, the incidence was 7%; if proprioception was impaired, the incidence was 50%; and incidence rose to 61% if visual neglect was also present.

The most severe entity in this continuum is defined as reflex sympathetic dystrophy (RSD), which includes signs of vasomotor instability such as erythema and sweating in addition to edema and pain. The skin, hair, and nails may become atrophic with time. With delayed uptake of radionucleotide in the joints of the hand as the diagnostic criterion, the incidence was about 25%.[36] Metacarpophalangeal tenderness was the most valuable clinical sign of RSD, with a sensitivity of 86% and a specificity of 100%. Swelling of wrist and hand was found in all subjects with RSD but was nonspecific because it was also found in 83% of those without RSD. Hand involvement was more frequent than shoulder involvement both on radiologic scans and clinically. This study suggests that the degree of early vasomotor involvement may be greater than anticipated.

The relationship between pain and edema remains unclear. Caillet identified the painful shoulder as the focus of impairment, with an emphasis on the varied pathogenesis for such pain.[10] The pathogenesis of SHS is a reduction in drainage via the lymphatics and veins from the hand, shoulder, or both.[10] The underlying process may be immobilization of the shoulder or hand caused by weakness. The hand-finger component of the syndrome is manifested as edema of the dorsum of the hand. In turn, this limits the pumping action of finger flexion, and the edema fluid becomes organized and prevents further movement. Subsequent bone changes occur as the result of disuse.

Treatment includes maintaining the patient's ROM and keeping the arm elevated to reduce edema. Active and passive ROM exercises at the shoulder and of the fingers at all joints are advocated. Other physical means of milking fluid from the hand include compression dressings and gloves.[10]

Anteroinferior subluxation of the humeral head is frequently found, particularly with associated weakness of the supraspinatus muscle. This is thought to be a precipitating factor in shoulder pain.[40] An inferior subluxation exists when the humoral head is located below the inferior lip of the glenoid fossa. This is thought to occur when the scapula loses its stability on the rib cage through loss of trunk control or muscle weakness. The resultant downward rotation of the scapula allows the humeral head to "slide down" the more vertically oriented glenoid. Glenohumeral joint stability is maintained mechanically by the angle of the glenoid fossa facing forward and upward by contraction of the supraspinatus muscle and by the scapular stability.[2] Therefore in the early stages of hemiplegia the flaccidity of the supraspinatus muscle may be an important factor in the onset of subluxation. Even when supraspinatus activity returns, the subluxation may persist. With the onset of spasticity the effect on the rhomboid muscles contributes to maintaining subluxation by rotating the scapula downward, and the scapula is internally rotated from pectoral and subscapular muscle spasticity. This concept of the pathogenesis of subluxation has recently been questioned, emphasizing the need for recognizing intersubject variability.[32]

The diagnosis of subluxation can be made clinically when, on palpation, the suprahumeral space is larger than on the other side. Radiographic measurement of subluxation can be another, more objective method.[39] Various supports have been used with radiographic monitoring of their effects on subluxation. The use of a lap board and arm trough and of a Harris hemisling was found to be more effective then the Bobath sling.[7] However, the specificity of such treatment to the presence of pain is unclear. In patients with shoulder pain, radiologic evidence of subluxation was found in approximately only half. No significant difference in pain could be found in those with and those without subluxation, and no correlation existed between the degree of subluxation and the degree of pain.[39]

Alternatively, it is suggested that the actual presence of pain is associated with a reduced ROM of the shoulder. External rotation of the shoulder may be limited as the result of a frequent preponderance of internal rotation.[6] Arthrographic studies in persons with painful shoulders showed adhesive capsulitis in about 75%. None showed rotator cuff or capsular tears.[33] In another recent study of patients with shoulder pain severe enough to interfere with function, moderate to marked relief was achieved by injection of local anesthetic into the subacromial bursa in almost 50% of cases.[22] Thus the author suggests that the source of pain may be related to this structure. The actual pathophysiology of the pain is unclear. However, high concentrations of pain receptors in the capsule and coracohumeral ligament may be affected by the local anesthetic. Pain may also be related to stretching of the tendons of the supraspinatus muscle.[39]

Despite the lack of a clear-cut understanding of the pathophysiology of the pain, it has been suggested that early ROM exercises within a pain-free arc and proper positioning to reduce subluxation will help prevent severe pain in the shoulder.[35] The value of passive ROM exercises (gently done with correct glenohumeral and scapular alignment) was confirmed recently in a study in which more active exercise using an overhead pulley was associated with a significantly greater incidence of pain.[25] In general use are the lap board and the elevated trough wedge to maintain elevation of the arm while in a wheelchair and the sling while ambulating (at a minimum). Early use of a bandage sling in the acute phase prevents tug on the arm during transfers. Early and vigorous treatment with corticosteroids or nonsteroidal analgesics has been advocated.[13,14] Methods such as FES to increase the control of musculature to help hold the head of humerus may also be useful.[42]

In one study the state-of-the-art treatment in acute care hospitals in a metropolitan area did not prevent the appearance of SHS in the presence of impairment in proprioception and visual inattention.[12] The necessity to rely on others for monitoring limb motion and the need for support limit the degree to which this complication can be avoided.

The following case report illustrates the multifactorial nature of pain arising in the hemiplegic arm; in addition, the patient had visual spatial neglect and an injury after a fall. The pain became disabling and the focus of the patient's inability to deal with his stroke. It affected his relationship with his wife to the point that they were considering a trial separation. Treatment with antidepressant medication was ultimately helpful in dealing with the pain; use of protection against further injury and maintenance of ROM at the shoulder were also helpful.

CASE REPORT

R.L. was a 53-year-old, right-handed, white salesman with a history of hypertension and intermittent cardiac arrhythmias who developed a right basal ganglia infarct. Left hemiplegia was complete in his arm; his hip extension was rated as 2/5 when he was seen 10 days after onset. There was no sensory loss to double simultaneous touch stimuli, pinprick, or position sense. In at least one instance the patient fell on his left shoulder while transferring alone, despite his agreement not to do so without supervision. Three weeks after the onset of stroke, R.L. complained for the first time of pain in his left shoulder and arm that interfered with sleep.

Six weeks after the onset R.L. continued to report pain in his left hand and shoulder; some swelling of the hand was present when he kept it dependent. Pain was disabling in that it interfered with sleep, despite use of nonsteroidal analgesics. By this time the patient was dressing independently although he still requiring supervision with bed-to-chair transfers. Although by now independently propelling a wheelchair, he still required cues to compensate for visual spatial neglect.

When R.L. was assessed 8 weeks after onset, hypertonicity was present throughout the left upper extremity, distal greater than proximal, with 1½ fingerwidth of subluxation in left glenohumeral joint. The skin on both hands was similar, with redness noted on all the patient's interphalangeal joints. Mild pitting edema was present in the left hand. Pain was elicited with external rotation of shoulder in the biceps muscle and with shoulder flexion (passive ROM of 0 to 150 degrees), wrist flexion (passive ROM of 0 to 50 degrees), and extension (passive ROM of 0 to 55 degrees).

Ten weeks after the onset of stroke, R.L. continued to complain of pain in his left arm that was almost constant and that worsened after spasms, which occurred as often as 15 per night. The spasms lasted as long as 30 seconds, after which pain appeared that was aching in quality ("like electric needles"). The patient also may have had shaking in the left foot. He refused use of antidepressant medication despite some positive effects on sleep because he felt it made him disoriented the next day. Sixteen weeks after the onset of stroke, pain in the left arm was still troublesome and radiated to the elbow and wrist; the pain started in the shoulder and was almost always constant; the patient described it as stabbing and aching. During the day when the patient was busy with other matters, the pain waned somewhat. The main problem was at night when the pain prevented the patient from falling or staying asleep. Edema in the hand no longer was a problem and was relieved by elevation. R.L.'s wife described her husband's passive ROM shoulder exercises as "easier with less tightness." The patient was using a sling, a Lofstrand crutch, and an ankle-foot orthosis when ambulating. Problems began to occur in the patient's relationship with his wife. They began to sleep in separate bedrooms because the patient's sleeplessness prevented the wife from getting rest. He agreed to the use of a different antidepressant medication.

Five months after the onset of stroke, R.L. reported he no longer had the constant aching pain. He continued to have spasms, which caused transient intermittent pain but which did not interfere with his sleep or his ability to work on his job. There was no edema of hand, and he had full passive ROM of the affected arm. He attributed some of the changes to the use of antidepressant medication, which he found did not cause side effects.

In the acute phase, the goal of managing sensorimotor control is to prevent secondary impairments. In addition to pain, impairments include the effects of muscle action imbalance caused by a preponderant overactivity of the musculature acting at a joint. Problems are not limited to the upper extremity but affect the entire motor system. Attempts are made to influence and control the distribution of muscle tone affected by the brain injury.[21] The goal is to enable the person to regain inhibitory control over abnormal patterns of movement and restored postural control.[21] Particularly relevant are the unopposed actions of the major antigravity muscles—the latissimus dorsi, which brings about internal rotation of the shoulder, and the gluteus maximus which acts as an external rotator of the hip. Unopposed plantar flexion and inversion at the ankle in the acute phase can lead to later difficulties. Maintaining a neutral position in the foot is necessary for later stance. In addition, pressure may be applied to the relatively shallow peroneal nerve.

Positioning of the person in the "antispasticity pattern" is a method to reduce the degree to which these muscles act preponderantly. Therefore the shoulder must be positioned in external rotation and the hip in internal rotation. Extension of the forearm with supination and finger extension with abduction is an associated position. In the lower extremity the knee, ankle, and hip should be positioned in flexion. It is also useful to elongate the trunk on the affected side.

Positioning of the head and body contributes to the antispasticity program. It is important to recall that lying on the back enhances extensor tone and that the prone position enhances flexor tone. The supine position must be used with the greatest care because it encourages the "spasticity pattern." Lying on the side is the most neutral position. Lying on the sound side is a particularly good position. Lying on the affected side is satisfactory, provided the remainder of the limbs are appropriately placed. Johnstone gives a full description of the most appropriate positions.[21]

A case study illustrates the disabling effects associated with improper positioning and a method for alleviating it.

CASE REPORT

R.O. was a 64-year-old man with a history of bilateral cerebral injury following recurrent strokes. He had weakness that affected both upper and lower extremities and that was greater on the right side. He was unable to maintain sitting balance because of a lack of thoracic and lumbar spinal extension. Because of long-standing bed rest, he had lost about 50% of his spinal extension ROM. The patient experienced imbalance with an increase in thoracolumbar and cervical flexion, shortening of the abdominal musculature and anterior chest wall, and hypomobility in spinal extension.

The major management goal was to increase the patient's degree of active trunk control to enable him to sit upright. A bed-positioning program was used to increase the degree of extension. While the patient was in the supine position, folded towels were placed under his back, from T10 to T3. The towels served as a fulcrum over which his body weight stretched his spine into a greater degree of extension. Lengthening of the lower abdominal musculature also occurred. The patient subsequently was able to sit upright with an increased ability to feed himself and to carry out other ADLs in a seated position. He also was better able to stand to carry out transfers from bed to wheelchair.[18]

Hand splints of various sorts can be used to prevent secondary impairments of the upper extremity. Their use should be instituted as early as possible and maintained during subsequent phases. The weakened muscles can cause loss of the palmar arch support, shortening of the flexor tendons with overstretching of the extensor tendons, and possible carpal malalignment or subluxation. The goals are to normalize positioning to prevent these possible problems from limiting later function.

Wrist-hand orthoses include the resting hand splint that is applied on the volar surface. The wrist can be immobilized in 10 to 15 degrees of dorsiflexion because most hand functions are best performed in this range. However, if the finger extensors are selectively weak, the wrist is held in the neutral position or in slight flexion (5 to 10 degrees) to stretch and assist finger extension. Less common is weakness of finger flexion. In these cases, positioning of the wrist in 10 to 20 degrees of extension assists in the ability to close the hand ("tenodesis grip"). In the presence of finger flexor tightness or spasticity, splinting the wrist (even in the neutral position) can contribute to the difficulty. A dorsal splint at the wrist is coupled with a volar finger platform to assist with finger extension.

In recommending a splint, both the pattern of impairment in motor control and the degree of sensory impairment must be considered. The degree of acceptance by the person with stroke to the ongoing use of a splint and the ability to put on and remove a splint are crucial. The use of any splint must be monitored closely. It is frequently necessary to revise the splint as changes occur in the patient's ROM and degree of motor control.

EFFICACY OF REHABILITATION

Of considerable interest is the degree to which intensive interdisciplinary stroke rehabilitation contributes to functional outcome.[46,47,49,65] Justification has long been sought for the relatively costly intensive training programs found in rehabilitation units and free-standing rehabilitation hospitals. In this section the efficacy of retraining is discussed. Several components of retraining are reviewed, including the timing of intervention, the duration of intervention, and patient selection criteria for the highest intensity inpatient stroke rehabilitation.

Retraining does seem to work. Buttressed by recent studies, including random assignment to general medical versus stroke treatment units,[49,69,70] the general conclusion is that gains in functional independence are made particularly by patients admitted soon after the onset of stroke (before 21 days) who commence rehabilitation therapy early and who receive active family and patient education.[68]

Although early treatment is generally advocated at present, considerable evidence exists that intervention can be effective in those whose stroke has occurred months earlier.[73] Indeed, in the absence of random assignment the efficacy of stroke rehabilitation initially was established by relatively late intervention when the effects of spontaneous recovery may be expected to have diminished.[60] However, until quite recently the contribution of early rehabilitation programs (aside from "maturational" effects illustrated by spontaneous recovery) has been difficult to identify.[62]

A major methodologic problem underlying those studies in which random assignment did occur is variation in the selection of patients for whom such efforts would be most useful. One of the studies that did support the effectiveness of stroke rehabilitation was carried out in Scotland.[69] Admittance to the stroke unit was almost immediate (mean of 26 hours after onset), and outcomes were measured at discharge or within 16 weeks after admission if the patient was not yet discharged. Outcomes included the degree of independence in activities such as mobility, toileting and self-feeding. Patient selection was based on the initial presentation on admission of so-called middle-band patients, defined by consciousness at the outset with established or developing hemiplegia.[50,51] The effect of these early selection criteria was to miss some of the "lower band" of persons with stroke characterized by being conscious at outset and able to walk without human assistance. These patients either did not survive or remained dependent but nevertheless would have possibly benefited from being admitted to rehabilitation treatment in the stroke unit. Also excluded was the upper band of persons who were unconscious at outset and already dependent in daily living activities.

A Swedish study admitted all persons with focal neurologic function or transient ischemic attacks after an average interval of 12 hours after onset.[71] The outcomes analyzed included functional status and the need for long-term hospitalization. Thus this study did not preselect those entering into stroke treatment but admitted some of the so-called lower-band patients described previously. When the probability of discharge to the patient's home was assessed, neither age (unless greater than 75 years of age) nor degree of hemiparesis differentiated those benefiting from the stroke unit.[72] It appears that if the prognosis for residual function is good (less severe hemiparesis and less than 75 years of age), stroke unit care accelerates the process of rehabilitation; however, the need for later institutional care is affected to a lesser degree. This may indicate that eventual placement depends not only on the degree of impairment but also on the availability of caretakers. If the prognosis is poor (major hemiparesis and greater than 75 years of age), the ultimate proportion returning home is enhanced. The results of this study suggest that stroke units should be provided to all patients with acute stroke unless comatose on admission.

The effort to select persons who are most likely to benefit from intervention has continued. Still another rehabilitation program in Britain provided either outpatient or inpatient services with referral mainly within 3 weeks after the onset of stroke. This paradigm is somewhat closer to that generally used in the United States, where there is discharge from acute care to rehabilitation facilities after medical stability is achieved. Thus those who died early or who did not require treatment because of an adequate early return of function were selected out. Outcome was measured by Barthel ADL scores 6 months after stroke.[74] The Barthel score at the initial assessment had a fairly high correlation with the score at 6 months. Two other factors adding predictive power were the patient's age (advanced age was negatively correlated with eventual outcome) and the presence of hemianopsia or visual inattention. The Barthel Index was used, in which scores of greater than 61 are compatible with community living.[54] Substantial numbers of patients reached that level, despite varying levels of initial function. However, the time required to reach Barthel Index scores of 61 varied directly with the patient's initial function level.

Attempts to use a subset of the total Barthel Index to predict later performance have also been helpful.[54] Data in one study reflected results of a large-scale multicenter study in the United States, which met criteria for comprehensive inpatient rehabilitation.[52] The average interval from onset of stroke to rehabilitation admission was 19 days. The mean length of stay was 37 days. The outcome measures were a discharge Barthel Index score of 61 or greater; community living status; and participation in household or community activities for those living in the community. In general, maintaining a community living status at 6 months was related to the Barthel Index score. Of those with a Barthel Index score of less than 60, 41% were living in the community; however, of those with a score greater than 61, 85% were living in the community.

A subset of Barthel Index items (B4) included bowel control, eating, bladder control, and grooming. One aim of this study was to determine whether a subset of Barthel Index items would achieve an acceptable level of outcome predictability. Of those who were dependent in all these items at admission, 27% were discharged with a 61 to 100 Barthel Index score; in addition, only 47% of these patients were still living and active in the community at the end of 6 months. In contrast, of those who were independent in all four functions at admission, 97% were discharged with a 61 to 100 Barthel Index score. At follow-up, 93% of the patients were still living in the community and approximately two thirds of them were active in household or community activities.

Therefore it is suggested that assessing merely the four items on rehabilitation admission would be highly predictive of patients' progress during rehabilitation and (particularly) at the 6-month follow-up. However, the total Barthel Index score was far more effective in predicting discharge Barthel Index scores and progress during rehabilitation itself. No cutoff score, for either the total Barthel Index or the B4 subset, is adequately specific or sensitive to be the sole selection criterion for admission. A substantial number of those patients with low scores on admission did benefit sufficiently from rehabilitation to return home. Similarly, discharge scores could not be used as the sole criterion for continued community living at 6-month follow-up. Barthel Index scores of greater than 81 were highly predictive of community living; 95% of those were still living in the community. At 6-month follow-up, however, many patients with far lower scores were also able to live in the community although they were less likely to do so.

Clinical measures of predictability for eventual function also have been sought.[64] Although the use of Barthel Index scores again appeared to be most predictive, the score from arm and leg paresis analyses generally served as a useful predictor. Severe proximal (hip and shoulder flexion) extremity paralysis (less than 2 on the Medical Research Council [MRC] scale) on admission (generally 4 weeks after onset) predicted a poor outcome in functions of the arm and leg, such as feeding, dressing the upper body, and ambulation. Extremity paresis scores of greater than 3 predicted a relatively good functional outcome. Within 14 weeks after onset, 95% of persons reached their highest level of function. Those who recovered completely did so sooner (around 7 weeks) than those recovering incompletely (around 10 weeks). It is interesting to note the lack of significant difference in the "time to maximum extremity function" score between those with less than 2 and greater than 3 MRC scores.

Still another study sought to replicate the patients receiving inpatient rehabilitation in the United States at that time, with an average interval of 30 days after onset to admission.[66] Findings on the clinical neurologic examination were sought as predictors. Because patients could possibly achieve independence in self-care using one-handed techniques, only lower extremity motor strength was evaluated. Proximal leg muscle strength was scored because distal leg weakness could be overcome with assistive devices and bracing. Hip flexion (less than 4) was used as the criterion for existence of a motor deficit. Sensory deficits were measured by hand localization. Field defects were also tested. The patient subgroups identified were those with motor (M) deficits only, those with both motor and sensory (MS) deficits, and those with both sensorimotor and visual deficits (MSV).

The outcome measurement was the Barthel Index. The ability to walk 150 feet with assistance was used as one specific criterion and was eventually met by 90% of all patients. The mean time after stroke for reaching this goal was significantly different for the several groups, as measured by "life table" analysis. The M group reached this criterion 14 weeks after the onset of stroke; the MS group, 22 weeks; and the MSV group 28 weeks.

The overall Barthel Index score of greater than 95 (associated with independence in ambulation and self-care) was likely to be met by both the M and MS groups although the score was reached over significantly different times. The MSV group differed; in that group, most patients had little likelihood of reaching a Barthel Index score of greater than 95. It is also important to note the achievement in this group of a Barthel Index score of greater than 60, which is considered a score of patients consistent with receiving health care management in the home by an aged caretaker trained in hemiplegic dressing, transfer, and ambulation techniques. Approximately 50% of the MSV group reached this goal, although this required a substantially longer rehabilitation unit stay; 70% of the MS group reached this goal within an average stay of 60 days; and 90% of the M group attained this goal within a 40-day stay. Figures for total time since stroke onset were 108 days for the MSV group, 90 days for the MS group, and 67 days for the M group. The duration of treatment was defined by the time required before the patient reached a "plateau." This study further suggests that functional gains in walking with assistance and independence in self-care may be expected for up to 28 weeks after stroke during persistent optimal inpatient rehabilitation.

Thus far the timing of referral and some of the criteria used for patient selection have been considered. The proper selection of patients may relate to criteria other than the severity of the motor impairment. A study from a stroke unit in Nottingham included patients "who had recovered from the acute stage and were in need of rehabilitation but did not require acute medical care."[61] Those "unfit for intensive rehabilitation" were not accepted, but the criteria for that determination was not described. Nearly all referred patients were accepted. A multidimensional assessment served as a predictor. The usual motor function and ADL scales were supplemented by such evaluations as perceptual assessments and language and memory tests. Outcome measures included motor function, place of residence at discharge, and the same ADL scale used on admission. Incontinence in addition to motor function appeared to be the important determinants of outcome. The addition of cognitive measures did not appear to add to the overall predictability.

This study is in contrast to an earlier study in Glasgow by Isaacs, in which rehabilitation services were provided by both physical and occupational therapists (although to a limited extent).[58] Criteria for referral and time of referral were not controlled, although admission to the stroke unit generally occurred after several weeks. The length of stay varied; however, some patients were not discharged (to home or a long-term setting) until as late as 6 months. Outcome was measured by disposition because it is mainly (although not entirely) determined by functional status. Language and perceptual disturbances on clinical examination did not necessarily serve as a barrier to a recovery sufficient to return home. It was a set of cognitive tests that was found to be predictive. These included simple tests of orientation and a "set" test (e.g., questions such as "tell me all the colors you can think of" are asked).

Still another early study in a single center in the United States appears to confirm the relationship between severe cognitive-perceptual difficulties and length of stay.[48] In the study, no screening was done; the average onset-to-admission delay was 38 days; and enrollment in an intensive interdisciplinary treatment model averaged 43 days. Outcome measures were discharge to home or elsewhere, functional status on ADLs (related to level of assistance), ambulation, and length of stay. The presence of dysphasia or a hemisensory defect and age (patients ranged from 40 to 80 years of age) did not seem to affect the outcome. However, adequate cognitive, perceptual, and motor function was relevant. Organic mental syndrome and visual spatial difficulties created poorer results. Despite signs of a poor prognosis, many patients were still able to achieve some degree of independence.

A more recent, thorough study of the effects of comprehensive inpatient rehabilitation in a single center included postdischarge follow-up.[56] This study introduced several new principles for measuring outcome, such as the relation between outcome and length of stay (efficiency) and the degree of discrepancy from 100 on the ADL scale (potential). The criteria used for acceptance to this rehabilitation program were unclear. A modified ADL Barthel Index was used to assess function at admission and discharge. The admission function level was found to be an important predictor of function at discharge although age was not. Age also did not seem to predict the efficiency with which improvements occurred. Efficiency was defined as the difference between admission and discharge scores divided by the length of stay. However, when considered with the level of function on admission, age did appear to affect the degree of achievement of "rehabilitation potential," which was calculated by dividing the difference between admission and discharge scores by the difference between admission scores and 100 (potential improvement). The capacity to achieve some of the rehabilitation potential appeared to be independent of age.

These same measures of the effectiveness of achieving rehabilitation potential and the efficiency of rehabilitation gains were used in a recently completed study in Australia of a comprehensive inpatient rehabilitation program.[67] Transfer from an acute care hospital was generally within 2 weeks after onset for those who were conscious and who were unable to carry out ADLs independently. The timing of transfer is compatible with procedures in the United States although the length of stay in the rehabilitation facility was much longer. The patient selection reflected the middle band, as described previously. The length of stay was determined by "maximum benefit," with a median of 49 days (9 weeks after onset). However, there was a range from 6 to 276 days, with a mean of 61.

A modified Barthel Index was used on admission and discharge. A square of the initial score was the single best predictor of the discharge Barthel Index score. Squaring was found to be useful in recognizing small improvements both in patients with low initial scores and in those with high initial scores. The squaring of the initial score explained considerably more of the variance than the unsquared score although the latter was still the single best predictor. Other variables such as the presence of myocardial infarction and diabetes contributed to the results; each reduced the predicted Barthel Index discharge score by 6 points (although this was distinct from age, which was an independent variable). Some measure of neurologic recovery, particularly hand control, was also helpful in predicting outcomes.

The variation in the length of stay is affected by social and other factors. Thus measures of efficiency and duration of rehabilitation stay do not reflect merely the degree of impairment (however it is measured). For example, the Australian health system is described as having the highest rates of comprehensive inpatient rehabilitation with an extended duration of care. Although it is unclear, it appears that no penalty in the score for efficiency of rehabilitation occurred for an extended duration of stay, affected (as it must be eventually) by the availability of appropriate placement. The achievement of the rehabilitation potential may have been less likely to be directly affected by length of stay, and most scores reflected the effect of the level of function on admission. Nevertheless, only 30% of the total variance in this measure of achievement was accounted for. Other factors significantly contributing to the outcome included age, with each 10 years of age reducing the achieved potential by 9%. Full bladder control increased the achieved potential by 12%, as compared with patients with no bladder control. Each day of delay between the onset of stroke and admission to acute care hospital reduced the achieved potential by 0.5%; each day of delay between admission and the start of rehabilitation reduced it by 0.64%. This factor may reflect the rate with which medical stability was achieved, with longer delays reflecting more severe medical problems. Such medical problems may persist and affect the outcome to some degree.

In one study the application of cost-effectiveness analysis included the relationship between efficiency and effectiveness with actual monetary cost.[14] Changes in the Barthel Index score between admission and discharge were divided by the cost of the stay in dollars. The optimal admission and discharge decision points were established, reflecting the optimal rehabilitation program for those whose Barthel Index scores were neither too high nor too low. Those patients with relatively high functional abilities showed a low rate of improvement because they had already reached a functional plateau; those with very low abilities may not have been able to tolerate the rehabilitation program. Some patients who were admitted with low function levels did not benefit from intensive rehabilitation, whereas others continued rehabilitation after reaching a functional plateau. In neither group were rehabilitation stays cost effective.

A more recent multicenter study reflects the need for an appropriate prospective payment program for rehabilitation in the United States.[63] Excluded from this study were those patients who were eventually discharged to an institutional setting. The Kenney scale and Barthel Index were used. The diagnostic group (DRG 14 for stroke) did not predict costs; however, within a specific category, such as stroke, the severity of illness index (SII) differentiated between costs.[57] Function on admission was not a significant predictor of total charges. It was suggested that this component is subsumed under SII; however, it is more likely that the "3-hour rule" requires all inpatients to receive at least 3 hours of physical or occupational therapy per day regardless of functional level at entry. Preselection of persons able to meet this criterion may reduce the degree to which the functional level at entry is an independent variable. Other criteria, such as medical status expressed as a level of endurance, then becomes the limiting factor.

The recent changes in the speed with which persons with acute stroke enter rehabilitation facilities (secondary to the use of DRGs) have changed the character of rehabilitation programs and created the need for more adequate screening for medical complications.[2] Many of the studies quoted previously reflect an earlier era when patients entered rehabilitation programs later than they currently do in the United States, where the costs of acute care have come under more stringent control. A similar concern with the cost of rehabilitation has brought the proper selection of patients and justifications for lengths of stays under greater scrutiny. Lengthy stays (characteristic of the past) were based on evidence of continued progress ("maximum benefit"). More recently, criteria have shifted to the minimal level of function consistent with placement within a noninstitutional community setting.

In summary, the selection on the basis of degree of neurologic impairment of an appropriate middle band of patients who are medically stable enough to participate in therapeutic exercise is the most useful clinical criterion for optimal efficiency and effectiveness of rehabilitation programs. Efficiency is affected by problems in disposition; effectiveness is explained only in part by the degree of initial impairment or functional level. The effect of age has been interpreted to affect outcome to a differing degree, but it does contribute in several studies. In the largest study currently available, those patients older than 79 years of age did less well, regardless of whether the lesion was on the right or left side.[12] The effects of age and of preexisting limitations and medical problems are still unclear. It is important to emphasize that one cannot exclusively use selection criteria of either a clinical or a functional nature in individual cases. Any of the criteria discussed will inevitably fail to identify persons who could benefit from retraining (false-negatives) and who would not benefit (false-positive).

In the context of increased concern about the relationship between costs and outcome, ethical issues cannot be divorced from professional ones. In some settings, extremely short lengths of stay (ranging from 10 to 14 days) in rehabilitation facilities are the norm—a response to the restrictions in reimbursements during a time when costs of medical and rehabilitation care are rising. Given the evolution of rate of recovery from the acute effects of stroke, a minimal period of time necessary to recover may exist. If costs attributed to hospitalization are to be reduced, an adequate continuum of care levels must be developed, with an increased emphasis on the lower costs of home care and outpatient training. This trend has its limitations. There is a need for an increased commitment of resources for community-based caregiver services enabling persons to live independently. Demographically increasing numbers of elderly persons without families who are able to care for them make such alternatives even more essential in the future. Ultimately, the costs of inadequate rehabilitation may be higher as a result of the increased need for institutionalization and the loss of patient independence.

The following case report illustrates the apportionment of costs that may be less than adequate and the possible value of early intensive rehabilitation.

CASE REPORT

J.D., a 75-year-old, right-handed housewife, lived in an accessible apartment and cared for herself and her son, who was disabled by a cerebral aneurysm. A married daughter lived in the same town with her family, which included two children, 9 and 12 years of age. The daughter worked full time. The patient was in good health, with well-controlled hypertension and hyperlipidemia managed by a low-fat diet. In December, she experienced an ischemic stroke, leading to left-sided weakness. She was hospitalized in an acute care hospital for 7 days, then was transferred to a long-term care facility where she continued to receive physical therapy several times a week. She required a high level of physical assistance and could not be cared for in her daughter's home. In March the daughter was injured in an auto accident and was unable to provide physical assistance to enable her mother to reside at her home. The son, for whom J.D. had been caring, moved to another state where he was cared for by his own daughter, who also had children and worked part time.

By June (6 months after onset) the patient was unable to transfer safely without physical assistance or dress herself. She had become depressed about her status. Another son removed his mother from the long-term facility and brought her to his home in another state. He adapted the ground floor of his townhouse to permit her to have a self-contained apartment in the living room and dining area. Both he and his wife worked full time. Nevertheless, they arranged their shifts so that one or another of them was available to the patient at all times to help her transfer, toilet, and get out of bed. However, with the ongoing need for care, the family had begun to unravel. By July no clear progress had been made despite home physical and occupational therapy.

The patient was admitted to an intensive rehabilitation unit. There was continued evidence of left hemiparesis, with no active movement of the upper extremities but some movement proximally in the lower extremity with hip and knee extension. The patient had an ankle-foot orthosis but not her own wheelchair. She was depressed. There was moderate difficulty with inattention on the affected side and cognitive difficulties with shortened attention span. The patient required physical assistance in moving within her bed, and she needed considerable physical assistance in transfers from bed to toilet and to wheelchair. She was unable to propel herself in the wheelchair or ambulate. She required physical assistance with bathing and dressing.

After about 4 weeks the patient was able to transfer independently and to propel her wheelchair. She became more aware of the need to attend to her affected side and learned to scan her environment to compensate. She was able to ambulate although she needed some physical assistance. She required some supervision but was generally able to dress and bathe herself.

Because of her changes in functional status, she would still be required to stay with her son although it was no longer necessary for her family to be constantly available to provide her with physical assistance. In addition, she had the option of returning to the town where she had previously lived and possibly staying with her daughter, who no longer needed physical assistance herself. Most important was the change in the patient's outlook. She had begun to plan for the future.

The costs of the stroke were high. J.D.'s previous arrangements for her disabled son were disrupted. She was in a long-term care facility for 180 days while receiving rehabilitation of an intermittent and ineffective nature. Her son and daughter-in-law could clearly not continue their support despite their commitment to do so. Her options after more extensive rehabilitation had now increased in that she could stay with either her son's or her daughter's family without placing on them an overwhelming burden of care.

This case illustrates the costs borne for ineffective care and the importance of optimizing the resources to be used in each individual case.

The next section of this book describes an attempt to meet the challenges of expenses and resource allocation during the rehabilitation phase. One must define those characteristics in rehabilitation services, deliverable in a variety of settings, that are indeed helpful in ensuring progress and the optimal use of resources in each individual case.

REFERENCES

Nature of the Problem

1. Jecker NS, Pearlman RA: An ethical framework for rationing health care, *J Med Philos* 17:79, 1992.
2. Jennings B, Callahan D, Caplan AL: Ethical challenges of chronic illness, *Hastings Cent Rep* 18(suppl):1, 1988.

Disorders of Sensorimotor Control

3. Bard G, Hirschberg GG: Recovery of voluntary motion in upper extremity following hemiplegia, *Arch Phys Med Rehabil* 46:567, 1965.
4. Basmajian JV, Bazant FJ: Factors preventing downward dislocation of adducted shoulder joint: electromyographic and morphological study, *J Bone Joint Surg* 41:1182, 1959.
5. Bohannon RW, Andrews AW: Relative strength of seven upper extremity muscle groups in hemiparetic stroke patients, *J Neurorehabil* 1:161, 1987.
6. Bohannon RW et al: Shoulder pain in hemiplegia: statistical relationship with five variables, *Arch Phys Med Rehabil* 67:514, 1986.
7. Brooke MM et al: Shoulder subluxation in hemiplegia: effects of three different supports, *Arch Phys Med Rehabil* 72:582, 1991.
8. Brunnstrom S: *Movement therapy in hemiplegia,* New York, 1970, Harper & Row.
9. Bruton JD: Shoulder pain in stroke patients with hemiplegia or hemiparesis following a cerebrovascular accident, *Physiotherapy* 71:2, 1985.
10. Caillet R: *The shoulder in hemiplegia,* Philadelphia, 1980, FA Davis.
11. Caldwell CB, Wilson DJ, Braum RM: Evaluation and treatment of the upper extremity in the hemiplegic stroke patient, *Clin Orthop* 63:69, 1969.
12. Chalsen GG et al: Prevalence of the shoulder-hand pain syndrome in an inpatient stroke rehabilitation population: a quantitative cross-sectional study, *J Neuro Rehabil* 1:137, 1987.
13. Chu DS et al: Shoulder-hand syndrome: importance of early diagnosis and treatment, *J Am Geriatr Soc* 29:58, 1981.
14. Davis SW et al: Shoulder-hand syndrome in a hemiplegic population: a 5-year retrospective study, *Arch Phys Med Rehabil* 58:353, 1977.
15. Demeurisse G, Demol O, Rabaye E: Motor evaluation in vascular hemiplegia, *Eur Neurol* 19:382, 1980.
16. Fisher B: Effect of trunk control and alignment on limb function, *J Head Trauma Rehabil* 2:72, 1987.
17. Fugl-Meyer AR et al: The post-stroke hemiplegic patient. I. A method for evaluation of physical performance, *Scand J Rehabil Med* 7:13, 1975.
18. Galleli PA: Personal communication, 1992.
19. Gowland CA: Staging motor impairment after stroke, *Stroke* 21(suppl II):II19, 1990.
20. Griffin JW: Hemiplegic shoulder pain, *Phys Ther* 66:1884, 1986.
21. Johnstone M: *Restoration of motor function in the stroke patient: a physiotherapist's approach,* New York, 1987, Churchill Livingstone.
22. Joynt RL: The source of shoulder pain in hemiplegia, *Arch Phys Med Rehabil* 73:409, 1992.
23. Kinsella G, Ford B: Hemi-inattention and the recovery patterns of stroke patients, *Intern Rehabil Med* 7:102, 1985.

24. Kraft GH, Fitts SS, Hammond MC: Techniques to improve function of the arm and hand in chronic hemiplegia, *Arch Phys Med Rehabil* 73:220, 1992.
25. Kumar R et al: Shoulder pain in hemiplegia: the role of exercise, *Rehabilitation* 69:205, 1990.
26. Kusoffsky A, Wadell I, Nilsson BY: The relationship between sensory impairment and motor recovery in patients with hemiplegia, *Scand J Rehabil Med* 14:27, 1982.
27. Lincoln N, Leadbitter D: Assessment of motor function in stroke upper extremity patients, *Physiotherapy* 65:48, 1979.
28. Moberg E: Criticism and study of methods for examining sensibility in the hand, *Neurology* 2:8, 1962.
29. Moberg E: *The upper limb in tetraplegia: a new approach to surgical rehabilitation,* Stuttgart, 1978, Georg Thieme.
30. Mooney V: A rationale for rehabilitation procedures based on the peripheral motor system, *Clin Orthop* 63:7, 1969.
31. Perry J: The mechanics of walking in hemiplegia, *Clin Orthop* 63:23, 1969.
32. Prevost R et al: Rotation of the scapula and shoulder subluxation in hemiplegia, *Arch Phys Med Rehabil* 68:786, 1987.
33. Rizk TE et al: Arthrographic studies in painful hemiplegic shoulders, *Arch Phys Med Rehabil* 65:254, 1984.
34. Sandin KJ, Smith BS: The measure of balance in sitting in stroke rehabilitation prognosis, *Stroke* 21:82, 1990.
35. Savanelli R et al: Therapy evaluation and management of patients with hemiplegia, *Clin Orthop* 131:15, 1978.
36. Tepperman PS et al: Reflex sympathetic dystrophy in hemiplegia, *Arch Phys Med Rehabil* 65:442, 1984.
37. Twitchell TE: The restoration of motor function following hemiplegia in man, *Brain* 74:443, 1951.
38. Van Buskirk C, Webster D: Prognostic value of sensory deficit in rehabilitation of hemiplegics, *Neurology* 5:407, 1955.
39. Van Langenberghe HVK, Hogan BM: Degree of pain and grade of subluxation in the painful hemiplegic shoulder, *Scand J Rehabil Med* 20:161, 1988.
40. Van Ouwenaller C, Laplace PM, Chantraine A: Painful shoulder in hemiplegia, *Arch Phys Med Rehabil* 67:23, 1986.
41. Wade DT et al: The hemiplegic arm after stroke: measurement and recovery, *J Neurol Neurosurg Psychiatry* 46:521, 1983.
42. Waters RL, Wilson DL, Gowland C: Rehabilitation of the upper extremity after stroke. In Hunter JM et al: *Rehabilitation of the hand: surgery and therapy,* St Louis, 1990, Mosby.
43. Wilson D, Caldwell CB: Central control insufficiency. III. Disturbed motor control and sensation: a treatment approach emphasizing orthoses, *Phys Ther* 58:313, 1978.

Efficacy of Rehabilitation

44. Davidoff GN et al: Acute stroke patients: longterm effects of rehabilitation and maintenance of gains, *Arch Phys Med Rehabil* 72:869, 1991.
45. Dobkin BS: Neuromedical complications in stroke patients transferred for rehabilitation before and after diagnostic related groups, *J Neurol Rehabil* 1:3, 1987.
46. Dombovy ML, Sandok BL, Basford JR: Rehabilitation for stroke: a review, *Stroke* 17:363, 1986.
47. Feigenson JS: Stroke rehabilitation: effectiveness, benefits and cost — some practical considerations, *Stroke* 10:1, 1979.
48. Feigenson JS et al: Factors influencing outcome and length of stay in a stroke rehabilitation unit, *Stroke* 8:651, 1977.

49. Garraway WM: Stroke rehabilitation units: concepts, evaluation and unresolved issues, *Stroke* 16:178, 1985.
50. Garraway WM et al: The triage of stroke rehabilitation, *J Epidemiol Community Health* 35:39, 1981.
51. Garraway WM et al: Management of acute stroke in the elderly: follow-up of a controlled trial, *Br Med J* 281:827, 1980.
52. Granger CV, Hamilton BB, Gresham GE: The stroke rehabilitation outcome study. I. General description, *Arch Phys Med Rehabil* 69:506, 1988.
53. Granger CV et al: Discharge outcome after stroke rehabilitation, *Stroke* 23:978, 1992.
54. Granger CV et al: The stroke rehabilitation outcome study. II. Relative merits of the total Barthel Index score and a four-item subscore in predicting patient outcomes, *Arch Phys Med Rehabil* 70:100, 1989.
55. Harasymiw S, Albrecht GL: Admission and discharge indicators as aids in optimizing comprehensive rehabilitation services, *Scand J Rehabil Med* 11:123, 1979.
56. Heinemann AW et al: Multivariate analysis of improvement and outcome following stroke rehabilitation, *Arch Neurol* 44:1167, 1987.
57. Horn S, Sharkey PD, Bertram DA: Measuring severity of illness: homogeneous case mix groups, *Med Care* 21:14, 1983.
58. Isaacs B, Marks R: Determination of outcome of stroke rehabilitation, *Age Ageing* 2:139, 1973.
59. Jongbloed L: Prediction of function after stroke: a critical review, *Stroke* 17:765, 1986.
60. Lehmann JF et al: Stroke: does rehabilitation affect outcomes? *Arch Phys Med Rehabil* 56:375, 1975.
61. Lincoln NB et al: The accuracy of predictions about the progress of patients on a stroke unit, *J Neurol Neurosurg Psychiatry* 53:972, 1990.
62. Lund K: A synthesis of studies on stroke rehabilitation, *J Chronic Dis* 35:133, 1982.
63. McGinnis GE et al: Predicting charges for in-patient medical rehabilitation using severity, DRG, age and function, *Am J Public Health* 77:826, 1987.
64. Olsen TJ: Arm and leg paresis as outcome predictors in stroke rehabilitation, *Stroke* 2:247, 1990.
65. Reding MJ, McDowell FH: Focused stroke rehabilitation programs improve outcome, *Arch Neurol* 46:700, 1989.
66. Reding MJ, Potes E: Rehabilitation outcome following initial unilateral hemispheric stroke: life table analysis approach, *Stroke* 19:1354, 1988.
67. Shah S, Vanclay F, Cooper B: Efficiency effectiveness and duration of stroke rehabilitation, *Stroke* 21:241, 1990.
68. Shah S, Vanclay F, Cooper B: Predicting discharge status at commencement of stroke rehabilitation, *Stroke* 20:766, 1989.
69. Smith ME et al: Therapy impact on functional outcome in a controlled trial of stroke rehabilitation, *Arch Phys Med Rehabil* 63:21, 1982.
70. Stevens RS, Ambler NR, Warren MD: A randomized controlled trial of a stroke rehabilitation ward, *Age Ageing* 13:65, 1984.
71. Strand T et al: Stroke unit care: who benefits? Comparisons with general medical care in relation to prognostic indicators on admission, *Stroke* 17:377, 1986.
72. Strand T et al: A non-intensive stroke unit reduces functional disability and the need for long term hospitalization, *Stroke* 16:29, 1985.
73. Tangeman PT, Banaitis DA, Williams AK: Rehabilitation of chronic stroke patients: changes in functional performance, *Arch Phys Med Rehabil* 71:876, 1990.
74. Wade DT, Skilbeck CE, Hewer RL: Predicting Barthel ADL score at 6 months after an acute stroke, *Arch Phys Med Rehabil* 64:24, 1983.

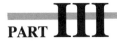
Rehabilitation Care Phase

Edited by
Richard S. Materson

NATURE OF THE PROBLEM

7 **Medical Management**
8 **Prevention of Recurrent Stroke**
9 **Rehabilitation Management: Principles**
10 **Rehabilitation Management: Alleviating Specific Disabilities**

NATURE OF THE PROBLEM

The rehabilitation phase is initiated after the patient achieves medical and neurologic stability. The goals are threefold. First and paramount, alternative strategies must be developed to alleviate the disabilities derived from residual impairments. Second, future impairment must be prevented by protecting the patient from disuse atrophy and contractures and by establishing a plan for dealing with risk factors for recurrent stroke. Third, in the light of the patient's need to participate in relatively strenuous activities, medical stability must be maintained. This phase reflects the duration and goals of what is generally termed medical rehabilitation. It does not necessarily coincide with the patient's stay in an inpatient rehabilitation facility although that was more nearly true in the past. It increasingly extends into outpatient and home settings. The overall character of the rehabilitation phase is that of an educational and therapeutic setting in which persons with stroke are prepared for functioning independent of ongoing assistance and supervision. The intensity of such supervision and intervention may be expected to diminish during the course of retraining. This rehabilitation phase continues until the patient has achieved independent community living and enters into the continuing care phase.

The major goal of the acute care phase is to limit the degree of neural injury with its consequent impairment in such areas as language and motor control. A plan to prevent future impairment also is initiated; its implementation through training continues during this more extended rehabilitation phase. During this new phase, particular attention can be paid to enlisting the person with stroke, the caregiver, or both in the management of risk factors that can affect the likelihood of recurrent stroke or early death from vascular disease. Ultimately, the training during this phase leads to ongoing self-management during the continuing care phase.

The several medical problems frequently associated with vascular disease are significant during this phase, limiting the patient's participation in sometimes relatively strenuous physical activities. Frequently, coexistent diabetes, cardiac disease, or both must be managed. At this time the opportunity exists for the patient, caregiver, or both to be trained in self-monitoring to increase the effectiveness of any treatment program that extends into the continuing care phase.

The focus on impairments during the acute phase shifts during the rehabilitation phase to a focus on diminishing the dysfunctional consequences of those impairments (i.e., managing the resultant disabilities and asset "polishing"). This is the primary goal of the rehabilitation phase. It is crucial to focus on developing adaptation methods, either by training those functions that remain or training the patient to use assistive devices to achieve life goals despite the persistence of impairments.

Recovery of function is the goal. It is essential to define this concept of recovery properly. The functional goals of reentry into life, such as mobility and communication, remain; the actions necessary to achieve these goals may need to change in response to the type and severity of impairment. Training continues both for the person with the injury and for the caregivers, who can then be more responsive to the patient's needs. The interpersonal environment can be an "orthotic" device itself and can assist the patient as well as any physical supports. The design of such supportive environments is part of the work of the rehabilitation phase. Training the person with stroke to interact effectively with such an environment is also a task of this phase. The process by which an optimal environment is designed is crucial to making such a fit effective, and this process of design must involve both the caregivers and the person with stroke as much as possible.

The description of the rehabilitation program in this section illustrates these principles and their application to specific disabilities. The focus is on optimizing the use of resources in each individual case while designing an overall program of comprehensive interdisciplinary rehabilitation.

CHAPTER 7

Medical Management

Nature of the problem
Diabetes
Cardiac disease
  Nature of the problem
  Treatment program

NATURE OF THE PROBLEM

Managing the medical stability established during the acute phase continues during the rehabilitation phase, in which requirements are increased. Intensive inpatient rehabilitation has been defined as the ability to participate in at least 3 hours of therapeutic activities per day. Ongoing medical management is frequently required for such participation. The requirements for participation in a relatively strenuous exercise program are affected adversely by the coexistence of diabetes and heart disease in particular. The endurance required is greater because the energy requirements are increased by the loss of motor control. Unstable cardiac arrhythmia or angina that requires close medical care may be present. The box on p. 147 shows one scale that reflects medical status. With such a scale, the goal during rehabilitation is to maintain an optimal medical status of 4 or above and to achieve a medical status of 6 or above by the time the patient is discharged from an inpatient rehabilitation facility. The level actually achieved determines the patient's eventual living arrangement, which must provide the necessary medical management. The degrees of medical management needed and available are significant factors in the patient's eventual disposition.

The goals during any inpatient rehabilitation process are to minimize the amount of physical illness and the degree to which medical surveillance is required. Preventing physical illness often involves preventing the effects of the usual comorbidities, diabetes and cardiac disease. In addition, the prevention of deep vein thrombosis (DVT), urinary tract infection, and aspiration pneumonia caused by stroke must be ongoing.

The long-term minimization of medical surveillance requires that the patient participate in monitoring his or her own health during the continuing care phase. Training in such self-monitoring can be given during this general

---

Medical Status

The degree to which rehabilitation participation is limited by physical illness:

SCALE POINTS

7. *No problem:* No current medical complications present; medical status allows full participation in therapies and outdoor activities.
6. *Minimal problem:* Resolved (self-limited) medical complications present with no implication for *current* function or participation; medical status allows full participation in therapies but slightly limits activities outside of facility.
5. *Mild problem:* Medical status allows full participation in stable rehabilitation program, but precludes activities outside of facility (e.g., unstable arrhythmia, angina).
4. *Mild to moderate problem:* Full participation in rehabilitation program with ongoing medical management possible (e.g., unstable arrhythmia, angina).
3. *Moderate problem:* Medical problems occasionally limit participation in rehabilitation; patient occasionally misses therapy.
2. *Moderately severe problem:* Medical complications prevent full participation in rehabilitation; patient seen at bedside or for shortened therapy sessions (e.g., poorly controlled diabetes, compromised respiratory status, labile blood pressure, chemotherapy).
1. *Severe problem:* Severe medical complications prevent participation in rehabilitation program; patient is on bed rest and cannot receive bedside therapies. Complications may include decubiti, pulmonary infections, urinary tract infections, deep vein thrombosis, and altered alertness.

From Rehabilitation Institute of Chicago Functional Assessment Scale, Chicago, 1987.

rehabilitative retraining phase. Such training also extends to the management of risk factors that contribute to stroke recurrence and to the morbidity and mortality from more generalized vascular disease.

DIABETES

Three problems can exist in persons with long-standing diabetes with neuropathy who must undergo more strenuous activity. The first is the effect of autonomic neuropathy in limiting the orthostatic response to hypotension; the second is the blunting of some of the signs and symptoms of hypoglycemia in response to exercise[2]; and the third is the effect of long-standing neuropathy in limiting the symptoms of cardiac ischemia. A determination of the degree of impairment in sympathetic autonomic function can be made by identifying the degree to which the Valsalva maneuver brings about normal tachycardia and later blood pressure overshoot.[1] Failure to display these responses can be found soon after the onset of disease but is generally accentuated in those with more long-standing diabetes. The patients most severely affected with resultant orthostatic hypotension are those with combined sympathetic and parasympathetic failure.

In addition to diabetes complicating the ability to participate in exercise, exercise also affects the management of the diabetes. The goal is to maintain the blood sugar level within an acceptable range while minimizing the likelihood of hypoglycemia. Difficulties arise when a person who has been relatively sedentary, with a diet and insulin dosage established for rest, suddenly undergoes exercise.

The following case illustrates the disruption in the usual level of glycemic control caused by exercise; it also describes the effects of such difficulties on the rehabilitation outcome.

CASE REPORT

B.P. is a 74-year-old, obese, right-handed black woman with a 30-year history of insulin-dependent diabetes mellitus, hypertension, and myocardial ischemia. Her diabetes was complicated by nephropathy (a serum creatinine level of 2 with a creatinine clearance of 33 ml/min), retinopathy, and neuropathy (loss of position sense in the feet with absent deep tendon reflexes at the knees and ankles). She was meeting the goal set by her primary physicians of a blood sugar level below 200 mg/dl when tested in the morning and before the evening meal.

The patient experienced a sudden onset of right-sided weakness and slurred speech; the right arm was affected more than the right leg. A head computed tomographic (CT) scan on the day of ictus showed an old left internal capsule infarct. No subsequent head CT scan was done. When the patient was seen 12 days after the onset of symptoms, her medical regimen consisted of enalapril, 10 mg bid; insulin 70/30, 24 units qd in the morning; transdermal nitroglycerin; furosemide, 40 mg qd; and procainamide hydrochloride, 750 mg q6h. In the right leg, hip extension and knee extension against gravity alone was unimpaired, but there was complete plegia of the right arm. Her blood pressure was 160/90 mm Hg. The electrocardiogram showed a first-degree arteriovenous block and a widened QRS; left ventricular hypertrophy was seen on chest x-ray examination.

Throughout her rehabilitation, the patient had considerable difficulty in maintaining her blood sugar below 200 mg/dl. During the first week her blood sugar level ranged as high as 230 to 250 at 4 PM despite as much as 38 units of insulin (Novolin 70/30) in the morning. The patient complained of nausea and experienced bowel impaction during this time. When her blood sugar level fell to the range sought (173 in the morning and 137 at 4 PM), she began to complain of light-headedness. Orthostatic hypotension was also manifest despite a reduction in the dose to 30 units of Novolin 70/30 and cessation of both the enalapril and nitroglycerin. On at least one occasion the patient manifested blood pressure reduction of 30 mm Hg when rising to a sitting position. She complained of light-headedness at the time, and her blood sugar level was 120 mg/dl.

During the last part of her stay the patient again showed elevated blood sugar levels and required increased insulin while manifesting light-headedness and hypotension to exercise. However, she was able to achieve mobility (transferring from a bed to a wheelchair without the need for physical assistance) by the time of her discharge home. The length of her stay in reaching this goal was somewhat longer than the usual — 52 days after onset and 40 days after transfer from an acute care hospital.

This case describes a patient with long-standing diabetes who manifested symptoms of hypoglycemia. Her symptoms occurred with blood sugar levels in the range of 140 mg/dl. Her "set point" thus differed from the usual patient. Complications of diabetes also included orthostatic hypotension. Her difficulties became manifest with increased exercise requirements.

In normal persons, blood glucose levels vary little, even with intense exercise. Hypoglycemia does not occur, and there is preserved function of the central nervous system, which depends on adequate glucose. Glucose use by the working muscle markedly increases. To maintain normoglycemia, the hepatic glucose output must increase. During exercise the plasma concentration of insulin also diminishes.[6] Fig. 7-1 illustrates this interaction.[6]

Problems arise because the normal relationship between exercise and metabolic response has been blunted in persons with diabetes. Ordinarily, insulin production decreases in response to exercise, but this does not occur in the presence of diabetes, with its lack of endogenous insulin from the pancreas. Nevertheless, when a dose of exogenous insulin is given, it enters the circulation at an ongoing or perhaps even increased rate as a result of absorption from active sites. When glucose use is increased by working muscles, the release of hepatic stores of glucose in the muscles also is jeopardized because of the ongoing increased circulating exogenous insulin. Thus hypoglycemia may occur during or following exercise.

The relationship between the presence of diabetes and the response to exercise is affected by the degree of control achieved.[5] In insulin-dependent persons the response to exercise varies with the degree of metabolic control and the ambient level of insulin. In persons whose diabetes is moderately well controlled (150 to 200 mg/dl), exercise causes a moderate decrease in plasma glucose. When these patients exercise regularly, their need for insulin may actually decrease. Changes in the concentration of fatty acids, ketones, and most hormones are similar to those in normal persons. However, patients with poorly controlled diabetes may experience increases in plasma glucose, fatty acids, and ketones during exercise. The deficiency of insulin prevents glucose utilization in the periphery to compensate for the increased blood sugar.

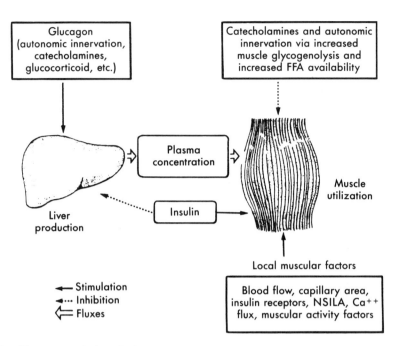

Fig. 7-1 Glucose regulation during exercise and the hormonal and metabolic responses in normal man. (*FFA*, Free fatty acid; *NSILA*, nonsuppressible insulin-like activity.) (From Vranic M et al: Hormonal interaction in control of metabolism during exercise in physiology and diabetes. In Ellenberg H, Rifkin H, editors: *Diabetes mellitus: theory and practice*, ed 3, New York, 1983, Medical Examination Publishing.)

Patients with non-insulin-dependent diabetes also demonstrate a failure to modulate insulin in response to lowered blood sugar levels resulting from exercise. At the termination of exercise, insulin levels are higher than in nondiabetic controls. Hepatic glucose production does not increase.

The presence of autonomic neuropathy further adversely affects the responses to exercise. Exercise-induced increases in catecholamines are depressed. Autonomic neuropathy secondary to diabetes can affect the patient's ability to modulate the relationship between insulin and other hormones. The release of hepatic glucose stores to counteract hypoglycemia is mediated by epinephrine release from sympathetic nerve endings. The increase from hepatic stores is also aided by a reduction in circulating insulin caused by α-adrenergic inhibition of insulin secretion.[4] Both these actions that protect against hypoglycemia may be adversely affected. In addition, the early warning signs of hypoglycemia (palpitations and diaphoresis) may not be present because of the failure of catecholamine release (particularly that of epinephrine).[2]

The set point of the glucose-regulatory system may also be higher in diabetic patients, and therefore they may experience symptoms of hypoglycemia when plasma levels are in normal or even the hyperglycemia range.[5] All these factors impinge on the management of persons with diabetes currently undergoing a more strenuous exercise program.

The goal is to maintain the blood sugar level within an acceptable range. The major focus is on prevention of hypoglycemia. The recommended objective is maintenance of blood sugar levels in the range of 120 to 180 mg/dl, with a mean range of 140 to 150 mg/dl (in light of the possible change in set point). A lesser degree of control of blood sugar level is sought to provide a margin against hypoglycemia.

Hypoglycemia that is severe enough to produce symptoms depends on such factors as the initial plasma glucose level, the duration and intensity of exercise, and the actual plasma insulin concentration. The standard treatment of persons with type I diabetes includes the injection of one or two doses of insulin subcutaneously, creating a slowly absorbable insulin depot; this does not replicate the normal secretion of the pancreas, which can vary acutely, depending on nutrient intake and physical activity. A reduction in the insulin dosage or the ingestion of carbohydrates before or during exercise is required to prevent exercise-induced hypoglycemia. Note that the level of exercise in rehabilitation may be considered to be at least "moderate" in most instances. Table 7-1 describes the relationship between exercise and dietary requirements.[3]

The more strenuous the exercise is, the more glucose dependent the muscle becomes. Thus problems become more salient during strenuous exercise. Hypoglycemia is less likely to occur if exercise takes place at least 4 hours after the injection of short-acting insulin. The increase in counterregulatory hormones (e.g., epinephrine) may offset the concentration of insulin. Glucose levels are more likely to remain stable when there has been a time delay following insulin injection.

Exercise is also contraindicated in the presence of recent vitreous hemorrhage. Those with proliferative retinopathy frequently found in persons with diabetes are at increased risk for such hemorrhage.[3]

Training the person with stroke and diabetes in self-monitoring is an important part of medical management. The goal is to increase the degree to which the person can manage his or her own care. In general, the procedure is to define the goal, clarify the patient's agreement to the goal, and enlist the patient's help in monitoring the degree to which the goal has been met. When applied to diabetes, this procedure has been well established. Blood sugar level self-monitoring devices are widely used; nevertheless, training in self-monitoring can be reemphasized during the patient's stay.

The following case illustrates the opportunity for improving the patient's glycemia control and lessening the need for medical surveillance in the future.

TABLE 7-1   Recommended Increased Intake of Carbohydrates Based on
Plasma Concentration of Glucose Before Exercise and on Type of Exercise*

TYPE OF EXERCISE	EXAMPLE	PLASMA GLUCOSE (mg/dl)	INCREASED CARBOHYDRATE
Light	Walking or leisurely biking for ½ hr	≥ 80	None
		< 80	10-15 g/hr
Moderate	Tennis, jogging, cycling, golfing (walking), vacuuming	> 300	No exercise until control improves
		180-300	None
		80-179	10-15 g/hr
		< 80	Start with 25-50 g/hr then 10-15 g/hr
Heavy	Football, hockey, racquetball, skiing, basketball, strenuous swimming or cycling	> 300	No exercise
		180-300	10-15 g/hr
		80-179	25-50 g/hr
		< 80	50 g initially; monitor blood glucose carefully

Modified from Jensen MD, Miles JM: *Mayo Clinic Proc* 61:813, 1986.
*10 to 15 g of carbohydrate = 1 fruit or bread exchange; 25 to 50 g of carbohydrate = ½ to 1 meat sandwich with a milk or fruit exchange.

CASE REPORT

E.O. is a 64-year-old, obese, black woman with a 45-year history of hypertension that has been treated with various medications; recent control was achieved with diuretics. The patient's non-insulin-dependent diabetes mellitus was treated with 5 mg of glyburide for the past 2 years. The patient had a history of left-sided weakness, which cleared after several weeks, a year before. She experienced a sudden onset of left-sided weakness and dysarthria. A head CT scan showed old right basal ganglia infarcts and an old corpus callosum infarct. The patient's blood pressure initially was 220/110 mm Hg. Right atrial enlargement was seen on three-dimensional echocardiogram; Holter monitor results were negative; and the Venereal Disease Research Laboratory (VDRL) test and antinuclear antibody (ANA) analysis findings were normal. Carotid artery Doppler ultrasonography revealed no stenosis. On admission 12 days after onset, the patient was receiving aspirin, 325 mg, and glyburide, 5 mg qd in the morning. The physical examination showed plegia of the left upper extremity with hip extensors 2/5, a left hemisensory deficit to touch, and position sense errors in the fingers on the left hand. Blood pressure was 160/90 mm Hg. During her hospital stay the patient was familiarized with her blood pressure goal and met the goal without the use of medication. She set a goal of a 10-pound weight loss, which was accomplished 36 days after admission (48 days after onset). Her blood pressure and blood sugar levels remained adequately controlled without medication.

Over the next year the patient received no hypoglycemia medication. During the next year she continued to maintain her weight reduction program, eventually losing 30 pounds. Thus she achieved a weight only 10 pounds above her ideal body weight (IBW). She continued to monitor her blood pressure and meet her goal with low doses of medication.

The training of the patient, family, or both in self-management consists of the following subobjectives:

1. Setting goal
   a. Agreement that the recommended standard of a 120 to 180 mg/dl blood sugar level is desirable
   b. Independent verbalization of the standard
2. Monitoring outcome
   a. Documentation of blood sugar levels
   b. Use of blood sugar level data to take appropriate action
3. Taking action
   a. Receiving regular dose of insulin and knowing type, dose, and administration timing of medication
   b. Arranging for follow-up and knowing the name and telephone number of the physician or clinic

CARDIAC DISEASE
Nature of the Problem

Cardiac disease affects the patient's ability to participate in the relatively strenuous exercise requirements of retraining during the rehabilitation phase. The primary goals are to increase the patient's endurance and tolerance to exercise while minimizing cardiac ischemia. A secondary goal is to minimize the need for medical surveillance after the rehabilitation phase by training the patient in self-monitoring similar to that widely used in cardiac rehabilitation settings.

Cardiac complications are a major problem affecting the patient's ability to function in the rehabilitation setting. In one study there was a 27% incidence of cardiac complications (angina and arrhythmia) requiring acute medical management.[14] Fortunately, death occurred in less than 1%, perhaps reflecting effective screening at admission. This complication rate was significantly greater (3 times) in those with a history of coronary artery disease (CAD) with or without congestive heart failure (CHF) than in those without such a history. Despite a somewhat longer rehabilitation hospital stay, the degree of independent functional status was also less in those with a history of cardiac disease although gains did occur. For example, the discharge score on the Barthel Index is reduced significantly by the presence of a history of myocardial infarction.[15] Particularly noteworthy is the effect of presence of CHF in lessening functional gains. The patient's level of participation is reduced as the result of the precautions necessary to protect against ischemia.

The specific functional gains affected by the presence of cardiac disease are in those activities requiring increased metabolic demands, such as transfers and walking. Wheelchair propulsion, for example, was not as affected, perhaps reflecting the efficiency of wheelchair use. It is well established that myocardial ischemia is affected by specific tasks. The effects generally are greater in leg than in arm ergometry and in dynamic rather than static exercise.[9] Energy expenditures are measured in metabolic equivalents of the task (METs); 1 MET is the basal oxygen requirement of the body in an inactive state (3.5 ml of O_2/kg/min). Table 7-2 describes the energy requirements for some common activities.

In addition to cardiac status, several factors can modify the patient's ability to compensate for the neurologic impairments through therapeutic exercise. Age is one factor. In older persons, light workloads can cause cardiac stroke volumes comparable to younger subjects, but increasing the workload results in lower increases in stroke volume.[10] It has been calculated that persons over 75 years of age can reach energy levels of 2 to 4 METs; those between 65 and 75 years of age can reach levels of 5 to 7 METs. However, with training, athletic older persons have been found to achieve greater than 10 METs. There may also be an increased likelihood of deconditioning for the elderly person, even with short periods of bed rest. Emotional stress from anxiety increases metabolic load. Compensation in response to exercise requirements may be further compromised by polypharmacy. Medication can lead to volume depletion, and hypokalemia from diuretics and β-blocking agents affect the response to exercise.[11] It has been noted elsewhere that patients with diabetes and neuropathy are less likely to experience anginal symptoms. Other neurologic impairments such as aphasia can affect the ability to monitor symptoms.

Factors such as hemiparesis and postural imbalance can increase the intensity of exercise beyond that which can be predicted merely by the overall metabolic requirements by that activity. In these cases efficiency goes down.[7] The metabolic requirements of ambulation by a person with hemiparesis who uses assistive devices are generally greater than those of normal gait.[12] Approximately 3 METs are required for ambulation with a walker or quad cane and ankle-foot orthosis in one's own room. Walking 50 feet at an average pace requires approximately 4 METs.

Treatment Program

One goal is to maintain the patient's heart rate within an acceptable range, achieving increased endurance without causing symptoms or signs of cardiac

TABLE 7-2   Approximate Metabolic Cost of Activities*

	OCCUPATIONAL	RECREATIONAL

1½-2 METs†
4-7 ml O₂/min/kg
2-2½ kcal/min
(70-kg person)
	Desk work
	Auto driving‡
	Typing, electric
	Electric calculating machine
	    operation
		Standing
		Walking (strolling 1.6 km or
		    1 mile/hr)
		Flying,‡ motorcycling‡
		Playing cards‡
		Sewing, knitting

2-3 METs
7-11 ml O₂/min/kg
2.5-4 kcal/min
(70-kg person)
	Auto repair
	Radio, TV repair
	Janitorial work
	Typing, manual
	Bartending
		Level walking (3.2 km or
		    2 miles/hr)
		Level bicycling (8 km or
		    5 miles/hr)
		Riding lawn mower
		Billiards, bowling
		Skeet shooting,‡ shuffleboard
		Woodworking (light)
		Powerboat driving‡
		Golfing (power cart)
		Canoeing (4 km or 2.5 miles/hr)
		Horseback riding (walking)
		Playing piano and other musical
		    instruments

3-4 METs
11-14 ml O₂/min/kg
4-5 kcal/min
(70-kg person)
	Brick laying, plastering
	Wheelbarrow moving (45.4 kg,
	    or 100-lb load)
	Machine assembly
	Trailer-truck driving in traffic
	Welding (moderate load)
	Cleaning windows
		Walking (4.8 km or 3 miles/hr)
		Cycling (9.7 km or 6 miles/hr)
		Horseshoe pitching
		Volleyball (6-man noncompeti-
		    tive)
		Golfing (pulling bag cart)
		Archery
		Sailing (handling small boat)
		Fly fishing (standing with
		    waders)
		Horseback riding (sitting to
		    trotting)
		Badminton (social doubles)
		Pushing light power mower
		Energetic musician

4-5 METs 14-18 ml O₂/min/kg 5-6 kcal/min (70-kg person)	Painting, masonry Paperhanging Light carpentry	Walking (5.6 km or 3.5 miles/hr) Cycling (12.9 km or 8 miles/hr) Table tennis Golfing (carrying clubs) Dancing (foxtrot) Badminton (singles) Tennis (doubles) Raking leaves Hoeing Many calisthenics

Continued.

TABLE 7-2   Approximate Metabolic Cost of Activities — cont'd

	OCCUPATIONAL	RECREATIONAL
5-6 METs 18-21 ml O_2/min/kg 6-7 kcal/min (70-kg person)	Digging garden Shoveling light earth	Walking (6.4 km or 4 miles/hr) Cycling (16.1 km or 10 miles/hr) Canoeing (6.4 km or 4 miles/hr) Horseback riding ("posting" to trotting) Stream fishing (walking in light current in waders) Ice or roller skating (14.5 km or 9 miles/hr)

6-7 METs
21-25 ml O_2/min/kg
7-8 kcal/min
   (70-kg person)
	Shoveling, 10 shovels per min
	   (4.5 kg or 10 lb)
		Walking (8 km or 5 miles/hr)
		Cycling (17.7 km or 11 miles/hr)
		Badminton (competitive)
		Tennis (singles)
		Splitting wood
		Snow shoveling
		Hand lawn mowing
		Folk (square) dancing
		Light downhill skiing
		Ski touring (4 km or 2.5 miles/hr) (loose snow)
		Water skiing

7-8 METs 25-28 ml O_2/min/kg 8-10 kcal/min (70-kg person)	Digging ditches Carrying 36.3 kg or 80 lb Sawing hardwood	Jogging (8 km or 5 miles/hr) Cycling (19.3 km or 12 miles/hr) Horseback riding (gallop) Vigorous downhill skiing Basketball Mountain climbing Ice hockey Canoeing (8 km or 5 miles/hr) Touch football Paddleball

8-9 METs
28-32 ml O_2/min/kg
10-11 kcal/min
   (70-kg person)
	Shoveling, 10 shovels per min
	   (6.4 kg or 14 lb)
		Running (8.9 km or 5½ miles/hr)
		Cycling (20.9 km or 13 miles/hr)
		Ski touring (6.4 km or 4 miles/hr) (loose snow)
		Squash and racquetball (social)
		Handball (social)
		Fencing
		Basketball (vigorous)

TABLE 7-2   Approximate Metabolic Cost of Activities—cont'd

	OCCUPATIONAL	RECREATIONAL
10 plus METs 32 plus ml O₂/min/kg 11 plus kcal/min (70-kg person)	Shoveling, 10 shovels per min (7.3 kg or 16 lb)	Running: 6 mph = 10 METs 7 mph = 11.5 METs 8 mph = 13.5 METs 9 mph = 15 METs 10 mph = 17 METs Tour skiing (8 + km or 5 + miles/hr) (loose snow) Handball (competitive) Squash (competitive)

From Fox SM, Naughton JP, Gorman PA: *Mod Concepts Cardiovasc Dis* 41:6, 1972.
*Includes resting metabolic needs.
†1 MET is the energy expenditure at rest, equivalent to approximately 3.5 ml O_2/kg body weight/min.
‡A major excess metabolic increase may occur as the result of excitement, anxiety, or impatience in some of these activities, and a physician must assess the patient's psychologic reactivity.

decompensation. The stroke rehabilitation program must be combined with a cardiac rehabilitation program. The major focus is on prevention of ischemia. Endpoints, such as general fatigue and dyspnea, are more common than the specific cardiac symptoms, such as angina, and ECG findings, such as ST segment depression and ectopy.[9] The box on p. 158 describes the Rating of Perceived Exertion (RPE), which can be used to establish endpoints. This scale reflects the overall feeling of exertion and physical fatigue. A rating of 6 indicates a feeling of effort when sitting comfortably in a chair; a rating of 11 to 13 is recommended during exercise. Exercise parameters generally are heart rate and systolic blood pressure. The double product divided by 100 has been used as the measure of workload. Generally, parameters are intended to limit progression in the degree of workload if the heart rate is greater than 120 or there is an increment of greater than 20 over resting heart rate. Activity is also stopped if the systolic blood pressure is over 200 mm Hg, or the diastolic blood pressure is over 110 mm Hg, or the patient experiences symptoms of dyspnea, angina, fatigue, and light-headedness.

The criteria used to establish the parameters of an exercise program must be individualized for patients with cardiac disease and brain injury. The presence of impairments in posture and coordination increases the metabolic load, but the degree to which that occurs in an individual varies. Criteria for the selection of patients requiring individual assessment include a history or ECG findings suggesting serious CAD. The usual format for such testing, such as ergometry with ECG monitoring, can be adapted to the person with hemiparesis.[13] Alternately, one may use continuous monitoring for cardiac arrhythmias in coordination with the exercise program.

Rating of Perceived Exertion

6
7 Extremely light
8
9
10
11 Light
12
13 Somewhat hard
14
15 Hard
16
17 Very hard
18
19 Extremely hard
20

A rating of 6 corresponds to an overall feeling of effort when sitting comfortably in a chair. A rating of 19 or 20 corresponds to a feeling of extreme fatigue. A rating of 11 (light) to 13 (somewhat hard) is recommended during exercise.

There is an opportunity to increase functional work capacity by lessening cardiac oxygen cost, even in persons with severely impaired left ventricular function.[2] In persons with a ventricular ejection fraction of less than 27%, an exercise program including both bicycle ergometry and walking and jogging was followed over several months. During the first month, patients exercised at a pulse rate of less than 100 beats. Thereafter, exercise was adjusted to induce 70% to 80% of the patient's symptom-limited maximal heart rate, as established on treadmill testing. There was a significant increase in the ejection fraction at rest, but this did not necessarily correlate with exercise capacity. One patient with an ejection fraction of 25% exercised to only 4.6 METs before fatigue. Another patient with an ejection fraction of 13% achieved 9.5 METs. A substantial percentage of patients showed improved treadmill performance, rising from 6.5 to 9.2 METs. The best measurement of the training effect was oxygen usage. These conditioning effects were not related to an increase in ventricular performance per se, but to improved peripheral oxygen efficiency. Table 7-3 describes a graduated program and the energy requirements of the various stages.[12]

The case report on pp. 159 and 160 illustrates the role of cardiac disease in the proper selection of patients for admission to a rehabilitation facility.

TABLE 7-3 Program for Rehabilitation of Patients with Cerebrovascular
Disease and Associated Cardiovascular Disease

MAXIMAL ENERGY EXPENDITURE	PHYSICAL THERAPY	WARD ACTIVITY
Step 1: 1.1 MET	Passive ROM to all extremities; active plantar or dorsiflexion of ankles several times per day	Feeds self, rolls up in bed at 45-degree angle
Step 2: 2.1 METs	Add passive or active assistive joint ROM on hemiplegic side	Add partial morning self-care, such as washing hands and face and brushing teeth in bed; dangle legs on side of bed
Step 3: 1.8-2.9 METs	Active ROM and progress to minimal resistance with same movements	Add daily self-change of hospital gown; begin to use bedside commode
Step 4: 3 METs	Add ROM with moderate resistance	Sitting in chair for meals; self-dressing, self-shaving, arranging hair for self
Step 5: 3.7 METs	Increase number of times activity is performed, depending on tolerance; stand on toes 10 times; walk 50 ft at an average pace	Begin walking to bathroom; walk in room twice a day; ambulate with hemiwalker or quad cane and brace
Step 6: 4.2 METs	Ergometric stationary bicycle: warm up at 2.4 METs for 3 min, increase to 4.2 METs for 3 min, then cool down	Continue all ADLs required while in hospital; sit up most of day
Step 7: 5 METs	Walk 100 feet	Simplification of techniques and pacing of activities; stress energy conservation
Step 8: 6 METs	Increase exercise rate and intensity	
Step 9: 7 METs	Increase exercise rate and intensity	Begin homemaking activities with instruction in conservation of energy

CASE REPORT

I.B. was a 76-year-old, right-handed white woman with a history of bacterial endocarditis (14 years before), aortic insufficiency, and chronic atrial fibrillation. No obstruction in the coronary arteries was seen on catheterization 9 years previously.

The patient had an acute onset of left hemiparesis. A head CT scan 48 hours after the onset of symptoms demonstrated a right basal ganglion infarct. Carotid artery Doppler ultrasonography showed no significant stenosis; marked cardiomegaly was present on x-ray examination; an ECG showed ventricular response; and echocardiography showed a calcified mitral valve and annulus with a hypertrophied left ventricle and mildly impaired function.

The patient's medical regimen 16 days after onset included digoxin, 0.25 mg; furosemide, 40 mg; coumarin, 2.5 mg qd; and ampicillin, 250 mg qid on 3 days out of 12. The patient showed evidence of respiratory distress when sitting up with bilateral pedal edema. Her blood pressure was 100/60 mm Hg, her heart rate was irregular at 70 beats per minute, and a harsh 3/6 systolic murmur was noted in the left sternal border going to neck. She had flaccid left hemiplegia, but her major problem was hypotension and fatigue, which limited her ability to participate in an exercise program. Despite attempts to increase her cardiac output with rehydration, she was transferred back to an acute care facility.

The following patient illustrates the effects of poor endurance and exercise tolerance in affecting the results achieved. However, the management of her cardiopulmonary disease was successful in permitting her to continue with the rehabilitation program.

CASE REPORT

M.B. was a 87-year-old, right-handed white female with a past history of atrial fibrillation and hypertension. She complained of light-headedness and fell when attempting to stand, sustaining a laceration of the scalp. While in the emergency room, she developed left-sided weakness, starting in her arm and progressing to her leg. The patient also exhibited dysarthria and swallowing difficulties with aspiration pneumonia. The ECG showed an atrial flutter with conversion to normal sinus rhythm following digitalization. The head CT scan obtained approximately 72 hours after onset showed a low-density area in the right basal ganglion area.

The patient's medical regimen at the time of transfer to a rehabilitation facility included digoxin, 0.125 mg qd; verapamil (Isoptin SR), 120 mg bid; and aspirin, 325 mg qd. She was a frail-looking person with a cough productive of yellow sputum. She occasionally experienced extrasystole with a 2/6 systolic murmur at the left sternal border. Flaccid weakness in the left upper extremity was present with trace hip extension and knee extension on the left. The management goals included improved nutritional status (a serum albumin level of 2.6) with weight gain and effective management of the patient's pneumonia.

During her rehabilitation program the patient had major difficulty with endurance and initially required rest periods between therapy sessions. Her endurance was described as an ability to "partially complete ADLs with rest periods and unrestricted time." She complained of intermittent heart palpitations one day while at rest and while on a Holter monitor, which demonstrated very frequent (greater than 30/hour) premature atrial contractions (PACs) with frequent brief runs of supraventricular tachycardia. The patient's blood pressure remained below the goal of 160/90 mm Hg and her antihypertensive medication was reduced initially to Isoptin SR, 90 mg bid. Her appetite was poor, and she complained of difficulty sleeping. She also described her mood as depressed. Therefore she was administered 50 mg of amitriptyline with a subsequent improvement in both mood and vegetative symptoms.

The patient's functional status on admission was low; she required contribution by another person of 75% of the effort necessary to achieve bed mobility, transfers, and dressing and 50% of the effort needed to eat and bathe. After several weeks, her endurance began to improve with a concomitant resolution of the pneumonia. On discharge, her endurance had improved to the extent that she was able to complete ADLs in their entirety although she still required rest periods and unrestricted time. She had gained over 5 pounds, and her serum albumin level had improved to 3. The patient's functional status had improved to the extent that she could transfer with minimal assistance, requiring only 25% of the effort to be provided by another person. She was able to return home to be cared for by her elderly sister with the assistance of a home health aide several mornings a week.

This case illustrates the need for monitoring the patient's medications and the opportunity for significantly improving both endurance and functional status even in those who are elderly.

In patient's with cardiac disease, one of the most important goals is to decrease the degree of medical surveillance necessary after discharge. Patient awareness of the symptoms of angina and ectopy and the methods to counteract them is one aspect. Another method is self-monitoring of the response to conditioning and training by self-measuring the pulse rate. The most effective exercise program to increase the patient's endurance is to define goals collaboratively with the patient.

Eventually the precautions and limitations for exercise are those used by the patient, independent of staff. Criteria are set for bradycardia (a reduction of greater than 10 beats per minute, or a fall below 50 beats) and for tachycardia (more than 120 beats per minute, or an increase of more than 24 beats per minute above the resting heart rate, with a maximum of 120 beats per minute). If aquatic exercise is part of the program, the desired heart rate range should be lowered because ECG abnormalities have been shown to occur at lower heart rates during swimming.[4] Alternatively, the goals can be measured by rating perceived exertion.

The training of the patient, family, or both in self-management consists of the following subobjectives:

1. Setting goal
   a. Agreement that the recommended standard is 70% of the maximal asymptomatic heart rate per degree of perceived exertion
   b. Independent verbalization of the standard
2. Monitoring outcome
   a. Self-monitoring pulse or symptoms such as fatigue, angina, or dyspnea
3. Taking actions
   a. Regular medications and knowing their names, doses, and administration times
   b. Supplemental medications and knowing the criteria for their use
   c. Arranging for follow-up and knowing the name and telephone number of physician or clinic
   d. Knowing the criteria for seeking emergency medical attention

Another goal during the rehabilitation phase is that of managing the risk factors affecting cardiac disease to lessen the likelihood of recurrent myocardial events and possible recurrent stroke. The management of hyperlipidemia by diet, exercise, and medication is discussed in the chapter as part of a more total program of secondary prevention of stroke during the rehabilitation phase.

REFERENCES

Diabetes

1. Ferrer MT, Kennedy WR, Sahinen F: Baroreflexes in patients with diabetes mellitus, *Neurology* 41:1462, 1991.
2. Holdke RD et al: Reduced epinephrine secretion and hypoglycemia unawareness in diabetic autonomic neuropathy, *Ann Intern Med* 96:459, 1982.
3. Jensen MD, Miles JM: The roles of diet and exercise in the management of patients with insulin dependent diabetes mellitus, *Mayo Clin Proc* 61:813, 1986.
4. Porte D et al: Diabetic neuropathy and plasma glucose control, *Am J Med* 70:195, 1981.
5. Richter EA, Rudgerman NB, Schneider SH: Diabetes and exercise, *Am J Med* 70:201, 1981.
6. Zinman B, Vranic M: Diabetes and exercise, *Med Clin North Am* 69:145, 1985.

Cardiac Disease

7. Bard G: Energy expenditure of hemiplegic subjects during walking, *Arch Phys Med Rehabil* 44:368-370, 1963.
8. Conn EH, Williams RS, Wallace AG: Exercise responses before and after physical conditioning in patients with severely depressed left ventricular function, *Am J Cardiol* 49:296, 1982.
9. De Busk RF et al: Cardiovascular responses to dynamic and static effort soon after myocardial infarction loculation, *Circulation* 58:369, 1978.
10. Fitzgerald PL: Exercise for the elderly, *Med Clin North Am* 69:189, 1985.

11. Jackson G, Metcalf J: Common cardiac drugs and rehabilitation, *Int Disabil Stud* 10:138, 1988.

12. Kitkowski VJ: Rehabilitation of patients with cardiac disease and associated cerebrovascular accident, *South Med J* 72:303, 1979.

13. Leach CN, Leach JA: Stroke rehabilitation in elderly patients with coronary artery disease, *Phys Med Rehabil STAR* 3:611, 1989.

14. Roth ED et al: Stroke rehabilitation outcome: impact of coronary artery disease, *Stroke* 19:42, 1988.

15. Shah S, Vauclay P, Cooper B: Predicting discharge status at commencement of stroke rehabilitation, *Stroke* 20:766, 1989.

CHAPTER 8

Prevention of Recurrent Stroke

Nature of the problem
Management of hypertension
  Nature of the problem
  Treatment of hypertension
  Hypertension management program
Management of cardiac factors
  Nature of the problem
  Treatment of hyperlipidemia
  Hyperlipidemia management program

NATURE OF THE PROBLEM

During the rehabilitation phase, the goals initially emphasized during acute care are continued. In acute care the concern is to minimize the degree of neurologic impairment and to develop a plan for preventing future impairment. The assessment made at that time should have led to decisions concerning surgery or medical treatments with antiplatelet or anticoagulant drugs. During the rehabilitation phase the goal is to develop and implement a plan that reduces the likelihood of a secondary stroke frequently requiring a great degree of participation on the part of the person with stroke.

The nature of the population of persons with stroke creates problems in investing resources in rehabilitation. Ultimately, costs must be assessed as "benefit" in terms of dollars saved or "effectiveness" in terms of the level of performance achieved. One factor contributing to a lowering of the ratio between costs and outcome is the usually progressive nature of vascular disease. The cerebral episode is merely a symptom of a more generalized disease process that worsens over time. There is a high likelihood of stroke recurrence and other cardiovascular problems, both leading to early death. Even more serious to many is the recurrence of stroke, leading to more profound impairment with loss of quality of life even if death does not occur.

Most studies of the management of risk factors focus on mortality as the endpoint in defining incidence. Although these endpoints are more easily measured, some measurement of the severity of the functional effects of stroke would provide a more useful measure of the effectiveness of management. Use of this additional factor in measurement makes studies more sensitive to real-life issues, such as the degree of support required. Of particular importance is preventing a substantial reduction in the quality of the patient's life. Institutionalization and the services of caretakers are also expensive. Reductions in the need for such services and improvement in the quality of patients' lives are both measures of success. One way to increase the outcome-to-cost ratio is to increase the payoff period by reducing the likelihood of major impairments affecting both quality of life and mortality from myocardial disease or recurrent stroke.

In a long-term study of a population in Rochester, Minnesota, the stroke occurrence rate for the entire 15-year study cohort was estimated as 27%.[5] Among patients with thrombosis who survived their first stroke more than a month, 10% had a second stroke within a year and 20% within 5 years. Of those who survived the first year, 5% had a stroke recurrence during the second year. Among the survivors of the second year, 5% had a recurrence in the third year. Of those living beyond the initial stroke, over the course of the entire study, approximately 16% died of a subsequent stroke. This number is less than those having a recurrent stroke. Thus it appears that a number of persons with recurrent stroke continued to live. This is also reflected in the number of persons who had more than one stroke recurrence. These recurrences presumably had some effect on function and quality of life.

The survival rate in another study showed a strikingly high mortality rate as compared with the general population. The annual rate of stroke recurrence was 9% for males and 10.6% for females.[4] Such recurrence does not necessarily lead to death. Thus one can infer that, in those who lived yet had recurrent stroke, their quality of life was increasingly affected.

More recently the incidence of stroke recurrence was followed for persons with nonhemorrhagic stroke enrolled in the Stroke Data Bank.[2] The 2-year recurrence rate was 14%, with no difference between blacks and whites. At particularly high risk (24.5%) were those with diabetes and hypertension who had experienced a prior stroke of identified pathophysiologic origins. The incidence was 9.5% for the so-called low-risk group, which contained nondiabetic normotensive persons with no prior stroke and an infarct of nonspecific pathophysiologic cause. However, because it reflects the experience of selected medical centers rather than a more widely based population, this study has methodologic problems.

Ethnic differences in stroke recurrence currently are being delineated, using the experience of one center in the Stroke Data Bank (Fig. 8-1).[7] At the Neurological Institute in New York City, ethnicity appeared to reflect the magnitude of various stroke risk factors in patients with nonhemorrhagic infarcts. The study population was categorized as white, black, or Hispanic. Recurrent stroke, death from stroke by the end of 1 year, or both were most frequent in whites and least frequent in Hispanics. If the effect of the high death rate for whites early in their course of illness is discounted, the differences in rates among

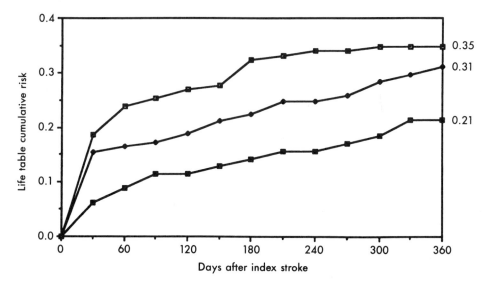

Fig. 8-1 Life table cumulative risk of stroke recurrence or death after cerebral infarction in whites *(top line),* blacks *(middle line),* and Hispanics *(bottom line)* within 1 year. (From Sacco RL et al: *Stroke* 22:305, 1991.)

the several ethnic groups decreased by the end of the first year. Hypertension was somewhat more prevalent in blacks and Hispanics. The incidence of cardiac disease was highest in whites and lowest in Hispanics. The varying effects of individual risk factors in ethnic groups suggests that risk factors should be identified and treated more aggressively, depending on the ethnicity of the patient. For example, Hispanics with nonlacunar infarcts and a history of diabetes had a relatively poorer outcome by the end of 1 year than did other groups.

The most quoted ongoing population-based study was the Framingham study of risk factors for stroke.[8] The most recent finding in this white population continues to indicate that hypertension is the major risk factor for stroke and that stroke incidence is proportional to the level of blood pressure. Other risk factors potentially subject to change are cigarette smoking and cardiac disease, with the latter improved by the treatment of hyperlipidemia and arrhythmia. Recently the use of cocaine and other sympathomimetic illicit drugs has been implicated as another potentially treatable risk factor. Such a connection is not necessarily restricted to young adults although the use of such drugs is more likely in that age group.[6] Tables 8-1 and 8-2 summarize the data derived from the Framingham study, which projects the risk of stroke on the basis of age and the other risk factors and expresses probability as a point system. The number of points can be converted to a 10-year probability for stroke in both men and women. The reader is referred to a more complex method (available in reference 8) to determine the

TABLE 8-1 Probability of Stroke Within 10 Years for Men 55 to 84 Years of Age and Free of Previous Stroke: Framingham Study

RISK FACTOR*	POINTS										
	0	1	2	3	4	5	6	7	8	9	10
Age (yr)	54-56	57-59	60-62	63-65	66-68	69-71	72-74	75-77	78-80	81-83	84-86
SBP (mm Hg)	95-105	106-116	117-126	127-137	138-148	149-159	160-170	171-181	182-191	192-202	203-213
Hyp Rx	No		Yes								
DM	No		Yes								
Cigs	No			Yes							
CVD	No			Yes							
AF	No				Yes						
LVH	No						Yes				

POINTS	10-YEAR PROBABILITY (%)	POINTS	10-YEAR PROBABILITY (%)	POINTS	10-YEAR PROBABILITY (%)
1	2.6	11	11.2	21	41.7
2	3.0	12	12.9	22	46.6
3	3.5	13	14.8	23	51.8
4	4.0	14	17.0	24	57.3
5	4.7	15	19.5	25	62.8
6	5.4	16	22.4	26	68.4
7	6.3	17	25.5	27	73.8
8	7.3	18	29.0	28	79.0
9	8.4	19	32.9	29	83.7
10	9.7	20	37.1	30	87.9

From Wolf PA et al: *Stroke* 22:312, 1991.
SBP, Systolic blood pressure; *Hyp Rx*, under antihypertensive therapy; *DM*, history of diabetes mellitus; *Cigs*, smokes cigarettes; *CVD*, history of intermittent claudication or congestive heart failure; *AF*, history of atrial fibrillation; *LVH*, left ventricular hypertrophy on electrocardiogram.

TABLE 8-2   Probability of Stroke Within 10 Years for Women 55 to 84 Years of Age and Free of Previous Stroke: Framingham Heart Study

RISK FACTOR*	POINTS										
	0	1	2	3	4	5	6	7	8	9	10
Age (yr)	54-56	57-59	60-62	63-65	66-68	69-71	72-74	75-77	78-80	81-83	84-86
SBP (mm Hg)	95-104	105-114	115-124	125-134	135-144	145-154	155-164	165-174	175-184	185-194	195-204
Hyp Rx	No; if yes, see below										
DM	No			Yes							
Cigs	No			Yes							
CVD	No		Yes								
AF	No						Yes				
LVH	No				Yes						

If currently under antihypertensive therapy; add points depending on SBP:

SBP (mm Hg)

	95-104	105-114	115-124	125-134	135-144	145-154	155-164	165-174	175-184	185-194	195-204
POINTS	6	5	5	4	3	3	2	1	1	0	0

POINTS	10-YEAR PROBABILITY (%)	POINTS	10-YEAR PROBABILITY (%)	POINTS	10-YEAR PROBABILITY (%)
1	1.1	10	6.3	19	31.9
2	1.3	11	7.6	20	37.3
3	1.6	12	9.2	21	43.4
4	2.0	13	11.1	22	50.0
5	2.4	14	13.3	23	57.0
6	2.9	15	16.0	24	64.2
7	3.5	16	19.1	25	71.4
8	4.3	17	22.8	26	78.2
9	5.2	18	27.0	27	84.4

From Wolf PA et al: *Stroke* 22:312, 1991.
SBP, Systolic blood pressure; *Hyp Rx*, under antihypertensive therapy; *DM*, history of diabetes mellitus; *Cigs*, smokes cigarettes; *CVD*, history of intermittent claudication or congestive heart failure; *AF*, history of atrial fibrillation; *LVH*, left ventricular hypertrophy on electrocardiogram.

probability of stroke for any 1- to 10-year period for both men and women 55 to 85 years of age.

The following case illustrates the costs of recurrent stroke in human terms and the need to maximize the prevention of such recurrence.

CASE REPORT

M.A., an 85-year-old, right-handed retired salesman, was a widower who lived alone in an accessible apartment building. He walked to a senior center for his lunch but otherwise cared for himself. The patient had two married daughters, one living in the metropolitan area and the other several hundred miles away. The patient's long-standing hypertension was treated with an α-adrenergic antagonist and a daily diuretic. He was also receiving aspirin, 325 mg qd. The patient experienced a sudden "blackout" with loss of consciousness and subsequent left-sided weakness, for which he was admitted to a hospital. A computed tomography (CT) head scan initially showed multiple small infarcts, but 96 hours later it demonstrated a new right basal ganglion infarct. A right carotid bruit was noted with 50% to 75% stenosis. The physical examination findings 3 weeks after onset revealed a frail man with intact cognition but continued slurred speech, left homonymous hemianopia, and left hemiparesis weakness that was greater distally than proximally. On standing, he fell to the left and was unable to walk unassisted. Functionally, he needed some physical assistance in dressing, grooming, and eating. He required minimal to moderate support to propel a wheelchair and appropriately manage footrests and brakes, and he required physical assistance with standing pivot transfers. He had major difficulty in shifting his weight while sitting and standing, often falling to the left.

By completion of his 4-week inpatient rehabilitation program, the patient was independent in self-care activities other than meal preparation. There was particular concern about his safety when using an oven because he tended to become distracted and ignore the left side. He was independent in ambulation. In walking, as with meal preparation, concern still existed because of his attention to the left side. He showed considerable improvement in his ability to handle secretions and swallowing, learned compensatory strategies to avoid aspiration, and was discharged while on a soft diet with thin liquids. He went to his daughter's home where he was able to live with some supervision in activities of daily living (ADLs) and with meals provided.

Several weeks later, the patient returned to his own apartment; his meals were provided initially by Meals on Wheels. He subsequently moved to a facility where his dinner was provided in a congregate dining area, but he continued to make his own breakfast. A home health aide assisted him with bathing several times a week. He eventually returned to taking his lunch at a senior center, but traveled by taxi. He continued receiving blood pressure medication to maintain his blood pressure in the range of 160/90 mm Hg.

Approximately 2 years later, at 87 years of age, the patient began to have difficulty with balance and fell on several occasions. He was eventually taken to an acute care hospital where a head CT scan revealed a new left capsular infarct in addition to the previous one on the right. He had right-sided weakness and difficulty with swallowing. A modified barium-enhanced radiologic examination showed poor pharyngeal peristalsis, pooling in the vallecula, and aspiration; a gastrostomy was required for safe feeding.

On admission to a rehabilitation program 20 days after the latest onset of symptoms, the patient required considerable physical assistance for transfers, ambulation, and ADLs. His gait was unsteady, and he had marked tremor when attempting movement with the right side. His short-term memory was quite impaired, and his progress was limited by an impairment in balance. He continued to require supervision for transfers, bathing, and dressing despite the use of a dressing stick and long-handled sponge. During the course of this second period of inpatient rehabilitation his improvement was less evident. Bursitis in his right shoulder limited his progress in learning adaptive techniques. He was discharged to an intermediate care facility because he continued to require ongoing supervision for all transfers. He was no longer able to return to his own apartment, nor was his daughter able to provide the level of supervision required.

Three months after the onset of this most recent stroke, the patient continued to show progress with eating and was able to receive more than half his caloric intake by mouth. It is anticipated that the gastrostomy will be removed. His gait remains unsteady, but he is able to ambulate with the use of a walker. He forgets to use the walker and requires reminders to do so; he is also unclear about his medications. He has become depressed over his lack of independence, cries easily, and is angry about his need for continued assistance and supervision.

This case illustrates the process of devolution caused by recurrent strokes. Devolution leads to diminished independence with increased requirements for a supportive environment. In this case the period between strokes was a productive one in which the patient, although elderly, was nevertheless able to once again maintain an independent life.

Evidence that the treatment of risk factors can reduce the incidence of recurrent stroke is suggestive although not yet definitive. In one study persons with either ischemic or embolic stroke were followed for at least 3 years, with an average of 5 years of follow-up.[3] Efforts were made to control all known risk factors. For example, the goal in blood pressure control was a systolic pressure of 140 to 160 mm Hg and a diastolic pressure at or near 90 mm Hg. Various antihypertensive drugs and salt restriction were employed. Patients frequently had multiple risk factors, all of which were treated as appropriate. For example, those with a blood hematocrit value greater than 50% were considered "erythrocythemic," and venesection was performed to maintain the hematocrit percentage at or below this level.

Data in this study are difficult to interpret because the incidence of death and recurrent stroke per year rates were not reported. Overall, the stroke recurrence rate during the 5-year period was 16%. The mortality from vascular causes was 17%. Death occurred earlier from myocardial infarction (2.4 years) than from recurrent stroke (4.1 years). A sample group was matched for the time of discharge from the same hospital. Race in the matched group was not defined, and the group was somewhat older. In the matched sample, the incidence of mortality from vascular causes was a minimum of 26%. An additional 7% who died from unknown causes could be possibly attributed to vascular disease. This incidence of mortality (33%) can be compared with the far lower mortality (17%) in the treated group. No estimate of nonfatal stroke recurrence could be made in the matched group. In neither group was the degree of impairment or disability caused by stroke recurrence measured.

Much effort has been devoted to reducing the incidence of stroke and cardiovascular disease through primary prevention. Less attention has been paid to the development of secondary prevention programs in this group, which has a high likelihood of recurrence. It has been pointed out that the subacute rehabilitation period provides a particularly good opportunity to develop a more intensive program for dealing with risk factors amenable to treatment.[1]

Thus one measure of the effectiveness of a rehabilitation program is the degree to which the incidence and the effects of recurrence can be altered. This ultimately translates into a cost-benefit or cost-effectiveness ratio in which increasing rehabilitation lengthens the period for "payoff."

The treatment of risk factors involves a change in patient behavior, necessitating a greater degree of self-management. The treatment program cannot be based solely on prescribed medication. Medication is only a part of a more total treatment program, the implementation of which depends on compliance (or noncompliance) rather than prescription. The process by which the treatment program is designed is crucial to its implementation. The design should be viewed as an opportunity to engender the greatest degree of patient participation compatible with the development of a coherent plan.

MANAGEMENT OF HYPERTENSION
Nature of the Problem

Hypertension is considered the most common and powerful precursor of stroke. Hypertension is the most common predictor of both parenchymatous brain hemorrhage and atherothrombotic brain infarction.[24] The effects of hypertension include an increase in the process of atherosclerosis in the major vessels, intracerebral hemorrhage, and lacunar infarcts. Hyalinization of the muscular walls of the arterioles is thought to be a response to ongoing constriction, as compensation for elevated systematic blood pressure.[21] A fall in blood pressure could lead to inadequate perfusion and consequent tissue ischemia; a rise could cause excessive pressure with resultant hyperemia, edema, and possible hemorrhage. The arteriole is also more liable to occlusion by thrombosis or microemboli. Thus the higher incidence of both lacunar infarcts and hemorrhage may be the result of this change in the character of the small vessels.

Sustained hypertension also accelerates atherogenesis in the larger vessels feeding the brain. The lesions do not differ qualitatively from those ordinarily found in the absence of hypertension, but they show a worsening condition at the usual areas of predilection and an involvement of areas of the arterial tree that are usually spared. The progression of hypertension is further accelerated if the patient's cholesterol level is above 250 mg/dl. The pathophysiologic characteristics of this process result from changes in endothelial permeability and intimal thickening.[24] Therefore it is assumed that treatment of hypertension will retard the progression of an already developed disease process throughout the entire vascular tree.

The effects of hypertension on the incidence of stroke are well established. The incidence was seven times greater in those with hypertension than in those who were normotensive. The risk is proportional to the blood pressure throughout its range. The systolic blood pressure was found to be as good a predictor as any other component.[17] The association with hypertension is particularly significant in blacks in whom the estimated risk of stroke is particularly evident in those below 65 years of age. A recent study continues to document this relationship between hypertension and stroke while emphasizing that the existence of hypertension may not entirely explain the higher incidence of mortality in blacks.[18]

Treatment of Hypertension

Another study followed a group of patients with hemiplegia and hypertension. "Good control" was a mean standing diastolic blood pressure of less than 100 mm Hg. "Poor control" was a mean standing diastolic pressure of greater than 110 mm Hg. Those patients whose hypertension was "well controlled" had a significantly lower likelihood of developing a second stroke during the first 2 years (5% versus 28% with "poor control"). Intracerebral hemorrhage was also prevented, suggesting that the treatment of hypertension reduces the rupture of the small perforating cerebral vessels.[10]

More recent large-scale studies have further supported the effects of reduced diastolic blood pressure in modifying the incidence of both myocardial and cerebral events. It has been further suggested that the blood pressure goal might usefully be lowered beyond what has traditionally been considered the "normotensive" range.[19] The suggested range is a diastolic pressure below 85 mm Hg.[12]

The significance of systolic hypertension, which is far more common in the elderly, has become increasingly evident. The Framingham study found that the stroke incidence was directly related to the level of systolic pressure, even in those whose diastolic pressures had never exceeded 95 mm Hg. For example, the incidence of stroke in men 50 to 79 years of age was 21:1000 with a systolic pressure greater than 160 mm Hg. The incidence was only 5.3:1000 in those whose systolic pressure was below 140 mm Hg.[26] In the Chicago Stroke Study the 3-year incidence of stroke was 2.5 times higher in those with than in those without isolated systolic hypertension. The criterion for treatment was considered to be an average systolic blood pressure of greater than or equal to 160 mm Hg, an average diastolic pressure of greater than 90 mm Hg, or both on three consecutive measurements.

The recent publication of the Systolic Hypertension in the Elderly[22] study more definitely addressed the issue of isolated systolic hypertention (greater than 160 mm Hg with a diastolic pressure of less than 90 mm Hg).[22] The effect of antihypertensive treatment (use of a step 1 diuretic and of step 2 atenolol as indicated) was compared with a placebo in a double-blind study of 5-year follow-up in persons 60 years of age and older. The stroke incidence was the endpoint measured. The incidences of stroke and death from stroke were both reduced in the treatment group, as were deaths from myocardial infarction. The total stroke incidence was reduced by 36% in the treatment group. The magnitude of difference might have been even greater, but 35% of those assigned to the placebo group also took antihypertensive medications. The reduction in the incidence of myocardial events (fatal and nonfatal) was reduced by a similar amount (32%).[22]

Although the importance of managing blood pressure is widely known, some variation exists in the degree of surveillance and intervention. There is evidence that, at least for those with diastolic hypertension, a stepped-up care (SC) group may have significantly fewer episodes of stroke. In one study, the incidence of stroke was 1.9:1000 in the SC group versus 2.9:1000 in the group referred for care by community physicians (RC). The latter group did not entirely achieve the degree of blood pressure control sought (diastolic pressure below 90 mm Hg). The greatest reduction in the SC stroke total took place in the oldest age group (60 to 69 years of age). This study demonstrated the likelihood that stroke can be reduced by a more aggressive treatment program in an elderly population.[15] Stepped-up care in this study consisted primarily of a more uniform and cost-free medication regimen with annual follow-up.

The benefits of stepped-up care can be amplified considerably if the patient participates in such care. Evidence exists that awareness of the degree of control achieved can contribute to a reduction in pressor substances released in the body.[9] Thus a sense that one can be effective in achieving control can lead to a greater degree of control being achieved—knowledge of results can lead to improvement. The availability of relatively reliable devices for the self-measurement of blood pressure can contribute to an ongoing application of a stepped-up care program.[11,20] The benefits include improved cooperation with prescribed treatment.[14] Moreover, such self-measurement outside the medical setting may document a lowered need for medication with decreased cost and fewer side effects.

Hypertension Management Program

Patient participation could be the foundation of a more intensive hypertension management program, particularly for those with a high likelihood of stroke recurrence. In our experience at least two thirds of those entering the rehabilitation phase had a history of hypertension or were receiving treatment at the time of transfer from the acute care setting. The significance of hypertension that occurs during the acute period immediately following a stroke differs from the hypertension present before the onset of the stroke. In one study 84% of stroke patients were hypertensive (blood pressure greater than 150/90 mm Hg when supine) during the first 24 hours after admission.[25] Only one third remained hypertensive 1 week after the onset of stroke. There appears to be a rise in blood pressure with the onset of cerebral ischemia and subsequent restoration of vascular autoregulation. Therefore care should be used in the aggressive treatment of hypertension in this early period.

In the rehabilitation of persons with stroke a program was instituted to develop a stepped-up capability in hypertension management. On transfer to a rehabilitation unit the level of blood pressure control in persons with stroke varied but was generally within the limits ordinarily set. However, the medical regimen on transfer was quite complex, with most patients requiring three to five doses of medication per day. Of those on medication, 70% required more than two doses. Despite a sometimes long-standing history of treatment for hypertension, less than 1% were aware of the goal for blood pressure control or had been encouraged to monitor their blood pressure on a regular basis, despite the ready availability of self-monitoring devices.

The goals were to achieve adequate blood pressure control at the lowest possible cost. Cost considerations include not only the dollar costs of medication but the effects of medication on other aspects of the person's life. The burdens of medication, such as side effects, are particularly problematic in those who are elderly. The fragile physiologic characteristics of the elderly demand particular caution in the use of medication.[23] The ability to maintain a medical regimen can be improved by reducing its complexity, such as reducing the number of different medications and the doses to be administered during the course of a day.

The level of blood pressure control to be achieved was established as 160/90 mm Hg in those 65 years of age or older. Thus those with either systolic or diastolic hypertension were treated. The use of home monitoring devices was encouraged as a means of developing more accurate data about blood pressure under more natural conditions. This information led to treatment being adequate but not excessive. In those below 65 years of age the recommended blood

---

Stroke Prevention and Hypertension Management

The score is based on the extent to which a patient, caregiver, or both demonstrate the ability (1) to state the blood pressure goal; (2) to record blood pressure measurements; (3) to monitor blood pressure; and (4) to state whether or not a blood pressure reading is within an acceptable range.

7. *No problem:* Able to perform independently all four tasks.
6. *Minimal problem:* Able to perform all four tasks using written cues (i.e., using a list of steps, notes, or written instructional materials).
5. *Mild problem:* Requires verbal cues, reminding, or both, or able to perform three of the four tasks.
4. *Mild to moderate problem:* Requires minimal assistance, including supervision, cueing, and instruction to perform two of the four tasks.
3. *Moderate problem:* Requires moderate assistance, including frequent cueing and instruction, to perform two of the four tasks.
2. *Moderately severe problem:* Requires maximal assistance and intense instructional guidance, or able to perform only one of the four tasks.
1. *Severe problem:* Unable to perform any of the tasks.
0. *Not required.*

---

pressure goal was set at 140/90 mm Hg.[16] Rather than establish an arbitrary discontinuity at 65 years of age, the goals were to maintain blood pressure at less than 140/90 mm Hg if the person was 54 years of age or younger, at less than 150/90 mm Hg if 55 to 64 years of age, and less than 160/90 mm Hg if 65 years of age or older.

During the course of the rehabilitation phase, persons with a previous history of hypertension or receiving treatment at the time of transfer were enrolled in this blood pressure management program. The purposes were explained; the specific goal of recommended blood pressure control was agreed upon. Each time the blood pressure was measured, the person with the stroke was encouraged to enter the results in his or her personal log book and the result related to the goals previously set. By the end of the rehabilitation phase, either the person with stroke or the caretaker had been trained with the use of a measuring device and in recording blood pressure and was able to record data in a log book. They were encouraged to bring both to the primary physician at postdischarge follow-up visits. Resting blood pressure was used to ensure standard conditions for testing. The box above describes the scoring of this training program and the assessment of status at admission and discharge.

The degree of medication burden was considerably reduced during this period. The total number of persons on any medication was reduced. Of those who remained on medication, the number of persons on more than two doses was far fewer (30%). Of those on medication, the number receiving only one medication had increased to 63% (Figs. 8-2 and 8-3).

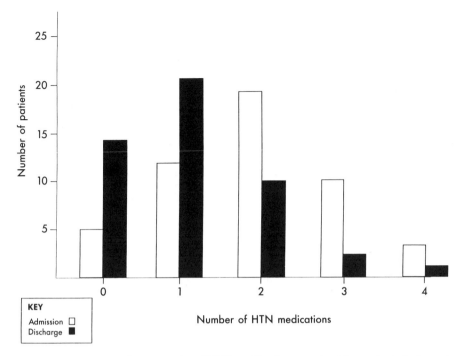

Fig. 8-2 Number of antihypertensive *(HTN)* medications received by patients in hypertension management program.

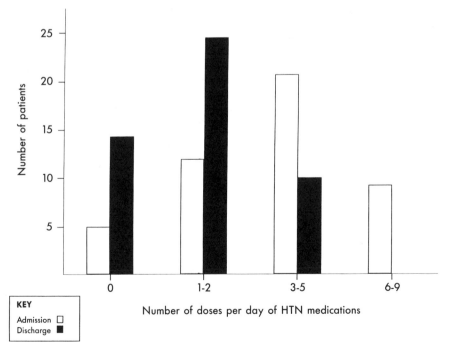

Fig. 8-3 Number of doses per day of antihypertensive *(HTN)* medications taken by patients in hypertension management program.

These efforts were in accordance with recommendations for treatment in the elderly.[23] The particular medication regimen varied with the usual criteria of prudence, using therapy at the lowest possible dose tailored to the individual patient. Particular attention was paid to the avoidance of centrally acting agents in light of evidence that such medications could affect the recovery of motor control.[13] The use of α_1-adrenergic receptor antagonists and α_2-adrenergic agonists (such as clonidine) can cause motor deficits in recovered animals. The α_2-adrenergic agonists decrease the firing of locus ceruleus neurons, thereby influencing the release of norepinephrine at the nerve terminals. The α_1-adrenergic antagonists may block the postsynaptic effects of norepinephrine at receptor sites. A large number of antihypertensive drugs other than clonidine are available.[16]

The following case report illustrates the effects of blood pressure management on the life of the person.

CASE REPORT

R.P. was a 43-year-old, right-handed, black male laborer with a long-standing history of untreated hypertension. He had been noncompliant with a recommended drug regimen. He experienced a sudden onset of left-sided weakness with right-sided headache. A head CT scan showed a large right thalamic and basal ganglion hemorrhage. The patient's blood pressure in the emergency room was 185/120 mm Hg. On transfer to a rehabilitation center 2 weeks after the onset, his blood pressure was recorded to be as high as 190/120 mm Hg during the first 24 hours. On admission the patient's medication included transdermal nitroglycerin 2 inches q6h, labetalol 300 mg bid, clonidine 0.3 mg q8h, and captopril 37.5 mg tid. There was evidence of a left homonymous field defect to finger motion; left-sided weakness of the arm that was far greater than of the leg; and left hemisensory loss to touch, pinprick, and position.

After treatable causes of hypertension were ruled out, major efforts were made to reduce his blood pressure to 140/90 mm Hg. This was accomplished by the time of discharge. Other goals included the use of a simplified and less costly regimen. Another high-priority goal, as stated by the patient, was noninterference with his sexual performance. Ultimately, the medications that obtained blood pressure control were verapamil (sustained release) 240 mg bid, enalapril 20 mg bid, minoxidil 5 mg bid, and hydrochlorothiazide 25 mg qd. The goal for a simplified, relatively inexpensive regimen was met only in part. Selecting medications to require a twice daily regimen helped to meet this goal although only partially. Labetalol, clonidine, and nitroglycerin were eliminated from the regimen in an attempt to reduce the likelihood of impotence and the possible effect on recovery of motor control by centrally acting drugs.

The methods to achieve management of this person's hypertension extended beyond the use of medication. He agreed to his goal and could clearly state it; he agreed to self-monitor the degree to which he met it. He was taught to take and record his own blood pressure readings. In addition, once trained, he began to use relaxation techniques independently. When asked, he attributed the achievement of control not only to the medication but also to his use of relaxation techniques.

When seen at a follow-up visit 1 month after discharge, the patient was meeting his goal and monitoring the results with a blood pressure machine. He was taking his medication. He was able to speak freely about his concerns. He expressed his concerns about his relationship to his mate and how the stroke affected his feelings about himself. During the ensuing months he continued to maintain his medication regimen, met his blood pressure goal of 140/90 mm Hg, and documented this on an ongoing basis. He had difficulty finding a blood pressure cuff that properly fit his arm, but extra Velcro was effective in extending the size of the cuff.

About 12 months after his stroke the patient continued blood pressure monitoring. He kept a record and used the monitor correctly. He found a primary physician who examined him regularly. He continued to take the medication prescribed on discharge. He also found that relaxation procedures were helpful, employing the procedure when experiencing actual feelings of tension.

About 24 months after the stroke the patient was still keeping records and was aware that his blood pressure was out of control. He denied any headache or other symptoms. He had "run out" of medication but had made an appointment with his primary physician to get refills that day. He had acted to get medication refilled on the basis of seeing that his blood pressure was too high. He has remained free of stroke recurrence.

This case report illustrates the value of a total approach to the management of the person with hypertension. The goals included meeting the blood pressure standard of 140/90 mm Hg and several other goals relevant to the individual's specific concerns. These goals could only be defined by the patient's participation. In addition to the use of medication, other means of blood pressure control were used, with an emphasis on enabling the patient to develop his own controls. To achieve the ultimate goal of preventing a future stroke caused by hypertension, the patient must develop a sense of his own power to control his future. He must take responsibility for self-administering medication on a regular basis and for acting in response to the record he is keeping as an example of self-management. In the previous case the patient made an appointment on his own to refill his medications. His requirement for stepped-up care required considerable ongoing support. However, the procedures used to develop a plan for achieving blood pressure control are an important opportunity to empower the patient to deal with the other effects of stroke on his entire life.

MANAGEMENT OF CARDIAC FACTORS
Nature of the Problem

The other major treatable cause of long-term morbidity and mortality in persons with stroke is myocardial disease. In the Framingham study, myocardial disease was a more likely cause of death in persons with stroke than recurrent stroke and was more likely to cause earlier death.[42] A more recent large-scale population study confirms the relative contribution of cardiac factors to the risk of recurrent ischemic stroke. In a group of persons with stroke in the Lehigh Valley study, the combination of "other heart disease" and myocardial infarction was most likely to predict stroke recurrence; it was second only to a history of previous transient ischemic attack (TIA).[44]

A relatively high incidence (28%) of asymptomatic coronary heart disease (CHD) in those presenting with cerebrovascular disease (CVD) illustrates the diffuse manifestations of atherosclerosis.[30] The converse has also been true. The degree of extracranial carotid artery stenosis in persons presenting with CHD is also high.[29] Cardiovascular disease and CVD are specific manifestations of a generalized disease process. Involvement of the larger arterial vessels can occur in both the carotid and coronary circulation. It has been recommended therefore that the existence of coronary artery disease be sought when disease of the cerebral arteries is diagnosed. The use of noninvasive tests of cardiac function, including dipyridamole- and thallium-enhanced scintigraphy, is appropriate for those unable to tolerate exercise.[32,43] Thus the management of the CHD might contribute to a lengthened life span after stroke.

CHD can lead directly to stroke. The effects of heart disease include the development of cardiac arrhythmia, myocardial ischemia, or both as a source of embolic stroke. In persons with chronic atrial fibrillation (AF) in the absence of valvular disease, treatment with warfarin anticoagulant agents has been found to reduce the incidence of primary strokes.[40] In another large-scale study, aspirin (325 mg qd) and warfarin were found to significantly diminish the incidence of primary stroke in persons with nonvalvular atrial fibrillation, as compared with a control group.[46] The incidence of recurrent stroke in the untreated group (8.3% per year) is comparable to that reported elsewhere for stroke recurrence in persons with AF.[28] The relative value of aspirin versus warfarin remains unclear. Because of the association of embolic stroke with recent myocardial infarction, particularly of the anterior wall with left ventricular thrombi, anticoagulant agents are also recommended despite the difficulties in establishing the presence of thrombus.[28]

It is well established that cigarette smoking contributes to the incidence of and mortality from CHD. The relationship of cigarette smoking to cerebral atherosclerosis has been studied in various ways. In those who underwent carotid arteriography for a variety of reasons (mainly for symptoms of carotid insufficiency), the number of years of smoking was most strongly related to the

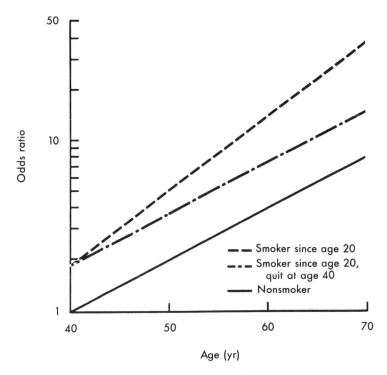

Fig. 8-4 Calculated adjusted odds ratio for likelihood of having severe carotid atherosclerosis as function of age and years of cigarette smoking. Odds ratio of 1 was arbitrarily assigned to 40-year-old person who had never smoked. (From Whisnant JD et al: *Stroke* 21:707, 1990.)

presence of "severe carotid stenosis."[48] The risk of severe carotid stenosis generally increased with age, but the risk increased most steeply for smokers. By 60 years of age the risk for a smoker of 40 years was 3.5 times that of a person of the same age who had never smoked (Fig. 8-4). Smoking cessation limited the accumulation of smoking years and thus the slope of the curve but not the higher overall incidence at the various ages.

The actual incidence of clinical cerebral events such as TIA and stroke was shown to decrease with smoking cessation in the Framingham study.[49] In this group the risk of stroke was related to the dose of cigarettes rather than merely the duration of smoking. It was estimated that the risk of stroke among smokers decreased significantly by 2 years after quitting and reverted to the lower level seen in nonsmokers within 5 years. The effects of smoking may be evident quite early. Particularly noteworthy is the finding in young persons (under 45 years of age) experiencing stroke that both the number of cigarettes per day and the packs per year were significantly higher than a group matched for age and gender.[36]

The process by which smoking contributes to the development of atherosclerosis is unclear. The effects precipitate acute clinical events such as stroke or myocardial infarct. Smoking affects fibrinogen levels in the blood and other factors promoting thrombus formation. Hence the cessation of smoking might be expected to have a relatively rapid effect in reducing the likelihood of clinical events. The origin of the atherosclerotic disease process involving the larger vessels is probably multifactorial. It is advocated that widespread endothelial injury is the precursor of the late fibrous plaques associated with atheromata.[41] This process is thought to be related to the presence of hypercholesterolemia, particularly elevated low-density lipoprotein (LDL), or to direct injury to the endothelium from other risk factors such as hypertension, diabetes, and cigarette smoking. It is postulated that the proliferative response to injury is the result of growth factors such as may be secreted by platelets. The initiation of the proliferation process by deposition of excess serum cholesterol, particularly LDL, is another possible cause.

Conversely the process of atheroma regression depends on a reverse cholesterol transport from atherosclerotic lesions to the liver. High-density lipoprotein (HDL) varies inversely with the incidence of CHD. HDL accepts cholesterol from cells loaded with cholesterol and donates it to liver cells for bile formation and excretion. This activity is apparently connected with macrophage scavenging of excess interstitial cholesterol and LDL. Calcium channel-blocking agents have been found to stimulate this scavenging.[51]

Treatment of Hyperlipidemia

This section discusses the manner in which the treatment of hyperlipidemia contributes to the management of ischemic heart disease and to its reduction as a major determinant of early death in persons with stroke. In addition, reducing the effects of atherosclerosis on the cerebral vessels as a means of preventing stroke recurrence is discussed. As in the management of hypertension, the long-term prevention of recurrent stroke and myocardial infarction by treatment of hyperlipidemia requires a greater degree of patient participation in self-management. The inpatient rehabilitation phase provides an opportunity for changing the patient's life-style and habits, including diet, exercise, and medication regimen.

The effect of significant blood lipid factors is in some dispute. In patients with CVD and thrombotic stroke the serum lipid finding that seemed to be the best predictor was a lowered HDL level rather than elevated total cholesterol (TC) and LDL levels. The latter values correlated better with coronary heart disease.[34] In one study in persons with stroke, blood samples were drawn immediately after admission to a specialized hospital for treatment. The time after stroke when the lipid samples were drawn was important. TC and LDL were found to be reduced in the first week after cerebral infarction, as compared with 3 months after ictus.[39] However, the apparent lipid-lowering effects of cerebral infarction were not found in a more recent large-scale study in Hong Kong.

Rather, there was an initial elevation in TC and LDL levels, as compared with 3 months after stroke.[50] This same study also reported significantly lower lipoprotein (a) levels early as compared with 3 months later. Another study in Austria reported that lipoprotein (a) measured at least 2 months after the onset of stroke was significantly elevated in persons 30 to 60 years of age with ischemic CVD, as compared with healthy controls.[33]

These studies point out the importance of the timing at which blood lipids are measured. The effects of stroke on lipid levels have not yet been finally determined. The return to the "normal" range may be more rapid than anticipated and is still unclear. Our finding is that elevated LDL levels found early after onset persist. If LDL levels are low, repeat assessment should be done several months later to determine the need for intervention. Nevertheless, focusing on the importance of elevated LDL and diminished HDL levels during the postacute phase can help teach the patient an awareness of possible goals and the value of a high-quality diet.

Another study sampled plasma at least 25 days after the onset of new neurologic symptoms to obviate any effects from stroke on serum lipoprotein levels. These levels were correlated with the degree of stenosis on four-vessel arteriography.[38] "Substantial" stenosis was said to be present when the lumen diameter was reduced by greater than one third or when ulcerated plaque was clearly evident. The incidence of hyperlipidemia was significantly higher in those with some degree of extracranial vessel disease as compared with those with purely intracranial vessel disease. The TC level was not as sensitive a predictor as were elevated triglycerides and pre-β_1-lipoprotein.

The relationship between carotid disease and lipids has been explored in a number of studies. In an asymptomatic population (50- to 69-year-old men in the Netherlands), the use of Doppler ultrasound studies of the carotid artery identified 23% with carotid disease; 5% of subjects had a 50% narrowing (group III). Group II was defined as having a normal Doppler ultrasonography result but a history of atherosclerotic disease. Group I consisted of both those with negative Doppler ultrasonographic findings and those with no history of atherosclerotic disease. Table 8-3 describes the data found. Note that those with demonstrated carotid artery disease (group III) had significantly higher TC levels and lower HDL/TC ratios. No significant differences appeared between the two groups with atherosclerotic disease, and both had a significantly lower HDL/TC ratio than the control group (group I).[47] In a similar asymptomatic Finnish male population (between 42 and 60 years of age) the degree of atherosclerosis was estimated by Doppler ultrasonography. The findings ranged from "intimal-medial" thickening of the wall, nonstenotic plaque, and any degree of stenosis.[45] A strong and graded relationship existed between serum LDL levels and the prevalence of carotid atherosclerosis, and the inverse relationship to HDL was confirmed. Another group studied with ultrasonography was those with CHD undergoing coronary

TABLE 8-3   Serum Total and High-Density Lipoprotein Cholesterol Concentrations (mmol/L) and High-Density Lipoprotein: Total Cholesterol Ratio

	GROUP I* (n = 54)	GROUP II[†] (n = 16)	GROUP III[‡] (n = 23)
Total cholesterol	6.02 ± 0.85	6.25 ± 0.93	6.61 ± 1.04‖
High-density lipoprotein cholesterol	1.30 ± 0.39	1.05 ± 0.22§	1.18 ± 0.27
High-density lipoprotein: total cholesterol ratio	0.22 ± 0.06	0.17 ± 0.06§	0.18 ± 0.05§

From Van Merode T et al: *Stroke* 16:34, 1985.
*Group I: Normal subjects ($\bar{x}$ ± SD).
†Group II: Subjects with a positive history of atherosclerosis but without detectable cervical carotid artery lesions ($\bar{x}$ ± SD).
‡Group III: Subjects with asymptomatic cervical carotid artery lesions ($\bar{x}$ ± SD).
‖Significantly higher than in group I.
§Significantly lower than in group I.

angiography who were asymptomatic for carotid artery disease.[29] The HDL concentration was independently and inversely related to the extent of carotid atherosclerosis, whereas the TC and LDL levels did not appear to be significant. Use of the HDL/TC ratio did not appear to improve the ability to explain variabilities in the extent of extracranial atherosclerosis. It appears from these several studies that there is an inverse connection between HDL and carotid atherosclerosis although the relationship to LDL is less clear. Thus intervention leading to an increase in HDL levels may be particularly useful for reducing stroke recurrence. The exercise program described in the previous chapter in the treatment of concomitant cardiac disease provides a possible method for increasing HDL.

Longevity in persons with stroke is affected by myocardial disease and hyperlipidemia. A reduction in myocardial events leads to increased longevity. The guidelines developed for the management of CHD focus on the LDL level as the primary target for modification.[31] It is this focus on CHD that is a basis for intervention in persons with stroke. Based on case findings in the general population, the Expert Panel of the National Cholesterol Education Program established criteria for intervention. These are primarily based on TC levels as a relatively low-cost method of screening populations. In persons who have already had a stroke, it is appropriate to focus more directly on the entire lipid profile rather than on the TC level alone. The goal for reducing myocardial events is to reduce LDL levels. The decision for treatment varies with the existence of risk factors and the level of LDL. The lipid profile requires a fasting measurement of TC, total triglyceride (TT), and HDL levels. The LDL cholesterol level is calcu-

TABLE 8-4 Classification of Low-Density Lipoprotein (LDL) and Cholesterol Levels

CLASSIFICATION (mg/dl)	LEVELS
< 130	Desirable LDL cholesterol
130-159	Borderline high-risk LDL cholesterol
≥ 160	High-risk LDL cholesterol

Modified from National Cholesterol Education Panel: *Arch Intern Med* 148:36, 1988.

TABLE 8-5 Treatment Decisions Based on Low-Density Lipoprotein and Cholesterol Levels

TREATMENTS	INITIATION LEVEL (mg/dl)	MINIMAL GOAL (mg/dl)
Dietary treatment		
Without CHD or two other risk factors*	≥ 160	< 160†
With CHD or two other risk factors*	≥ 130	< 130‡
Drug treatment		
Without CHD or two other risk factors*	≥ 190	< 160
With CHD or two other risk factors*	≥ 160	< 130

Modified from National Cholesterol Education Panel: *Arch Intern Med* 148:36, 1988.
CHD, Coronary heart disease.
*Patients have a lower initiation level and goal if they are at high risk because they already ha
definite CHD or because they have any two of the following risk factors: male sex, family history
of premature CHD, cigarette smoking, hypertension, low high-density lipoprotein (HDL) —
cholesterol, diabetes mellitus, definite cerebrovascular or peripheral vascular disease, or severe
obesity.
†Roughly equivalent to total cholesterol level of < 240 mg/dl or < 200 mg/dl.
‡As goals for monitoring dietary treatment.

lated from these values, as follows: LDL = TC − HDL − TT/5. This equation is useful as long as the TT level is below 400 mg/dl.

Because all patients with stroke have CVD, it is necessary only to identify the second risk factor. A low level of HDL (less than 35 mg/dl) is considered as much a risk factor as hypertension. See Tables 8-4 and 8-5 for criteria for the initiation of treatment based on these interacting variables and the LDL serum level. Note that, in addition to CHD and stroke, risk factors include male sex, cigarette smoking, hypertension, diabetes mellitus, severe obesity, and a family history of premature CHD. Thus, in all cases of persons with already existing stroke and other risk factors, an acceptable LDL level would be 130 mg/dl or below. Initiation of drug therapy is appropriate with dietary therapy if the LDL level is greater than 160 mg/dl. For those with a history of stroke, one of the listed risk factors, and an LDL level between 130 and 160 mg/dl, dietary treatment alone is initially indicated. In any event, treatment with drugs should be an addition to primary dietary therapy in all. TC levels can be used to monitor progress; the test's lower cost and the lack of a need for fasting make it attractive. A TC level of 240 mg/dl corresponds roughly to a LDL level of 160 mg/dl; a TC level of 200 mg/dl corresponds to a LDL level of 130 mg/dl.

In the context of CHD, the value of treatment has been established. A reduction of the TC and, by extension, LDL levels was found to reduce the incidence of CHD as measured by myocardial events, including infarction and death from CHD. Treatment in one large-scale study included the use of bile salt sequestrant to increase the excretion of cholesterol. The degree of reduction in CHD was related to the reduction in cholesterol level. It is projected that a decrement of 10% in cholesterol levels was correlated with a 16% to 19% reduction in the incidence of CHD. Attaining a decrease in LDL levels of 35% (theoretically possible with total compliance with the drug regimen) could reduce the CHD incidence by half.[37]

In the American Heart Association's step 1 diet, the total intake of fat is less than 30%; the total saturated fat intake is less than 10%; and the total cholesterol intake is less than 300 mg/dl. Monitoring of TC levels during the step 1 diet is recommended at the end of 4 to 6 weeks and at 3 months. Adherence to a diet of this sort can lead to an average fall of 10% to 15% in TC levels.[35] Kwiterovitch gives material useful for patient education to help maintain adherence to diet.[35] If the TC criteria are met, the LDL level can be measured to confirm that the LDL goal has been achieved. The goal is an LDL level of less than 130 mg/dl. If unsuccessful, the step 2 diet aims for a saturated fat intake of below 7% and a cholesterol intake of below 200 mg.

To maintain dietary adherence, it is helpful to substitute other food for specific foods high in fat, thus reducing the total fat content rather than aiming for a specific fat target. See Table 8-6 for identifying high fat content foods and selecting substitutes. Table 8-7 gives a list of the total fat and cholesterol content of animal products to aid in selecting those that are lower in those specific components. If the goal is to consume less than 30% of calories from fat, one can calculate the total amount of fat that can be eaten and choose from the alternatives. For example, if the total caloric intake is 1800 calories, the total fat content is about 540 calories on the step 1 diet. Because each gram of fat contributes 9 calories, the total fat content allowed is about 60 g or less. The commonly used 3-ounce serving is easily described as equivalent to the size of a deck of cards.[31]

The use of medication is indicated for those in the high-risk group with a history of stroke and an LDL level greater than 160 mg/dl. The choice of drugs

TABLE 8-6 Recommended Diet Modifications to Lower Blood Cholesterol Levels

	STEP 1 DIET	
	CHOOSE	DECREASE
Fish, chicken, turkey, and lean meats	Fish, poultry without skin, lean cuts of beef, lamb, pork or veal, shellfish	Fatty cuts of beef, lamb, pork; spare ribs; organ meats; regular cold cuts; sausage; hot dogs; bacon; sardines; roe
Skim and low-fat milk, cheese, yogurt, and dairy substitutes	Skim or 1% fat milk (liquid, powdered, evaporated), buttermilk	Whole milk (4% fat): regular, evaporated, condensed; cream; half and half; 2% milk; imitation milk products; most nondairy creamers; whipped toppings
	Nonfat (0% fat) or low-fat yogurt	Whole-milk yogurt
	Low-fat cottage cheese (1% or 2% fat)	Whole-milk cottage cheese (4% fat)
	Low-fat cheeses, farmer or pot cheeses (all of these should be labeled no more than 2-6 g of fat per ounce)	All natural cheeses (eg, blue, Roquefort, Camembert, cheddar, Swiss), low-fat or "light" cream cheese, low-fat or "light" sour cream, cream cheeses, sour cream
	Sherbet, sorbet	Ice cream
Eggs	Egg whites (2 whites equal 1 whole egg in recipes), cholesterol-free egg substitutes	Egg yolks
Fruits and vegetables	Fresh, frozen, canned, or dried fruits and vegetables	Vegetables prepared in butter, cream, or other sauces

Continued.

TABLE 8-6 Recommended Diet Modifications to Lower Blood Cholesterol Levels—cont'd

	STEP 1 DIET	
	CHOOSE	DECREASE
Breads and cereals	Homemade baked goods using unsaturated oils sparingly, angel food cake, low-fat crackers, low-fat cookies	Commercial baked goods: pies, cakes, dough-nuts, croissants, pastries, muffins, biscuits, high-fat crackers, high-fat cookies
	Rice, pasta	Egg noodles
	Whole-grain breads and cereals (oatmeal, whole wheat, rye, bran, multigrain, etc.)	Breads in which eggs are a major ingredient
Fats and oils	Baking cocoa	Chocolate
	Unsaturated vegetable oils: corn, olive, rapeseed (canola oil), safflower, sesame, soybean, sun-flower	Butter, coconut oil, palm oil, palm kernel oil, lard, bacon fat
	Margarine or shortenings made from one of the unsaturated oils listed previously, diet marga-rine	
	Mayonnaise, salad dressings made with unsatu-rated oils listed previously, low-fat dressings	Dressings made with egg yolk
	Seeds and nuts	Coconut

From National Cholesterol Education Panel: *Arch Intern Med* 148:36, 1988.

TABLE 8-7   Cholesterol and Fat Content of Animal Products in 3-Ounce Portions (Cooked)

SOURCE	CHOLESTEROL CONTENT (mg/3 oz)	TOTAL FAT CONTENT (g/3 oz)
RED MEATS (LEAN)		
Beef	77	8.7
Lamb	78	8.8
Pork	79	11.1
Veal	128	4.7
ORGAN MEATS		
Liver	270	4.0
Pancreas (sweetbreads)	400	2.8
Kidney	329	2.9
Brains	1746	10.7
Heart	164	4.8
POULTRY		
Chicken (without skin)		
Light	72	3.8
Dark	79	8.2
Turkey (without skin)		
Light	59	1.3
Dark	72	6.1
FISH		
Salmon	74	9.3
Tuna, light, canned in water	55	0.7
SHELLFISH		
Abalone	90	0.8
Clams	57	1.7
Crab meat		
Alaskan King	45	1.3
Blue crab	85	1.5
Lobster	61	0.5
Oysters	93	4.2
Scallops	35	0.8
Shrimp	166	0.9

From National Cholesterol Education Panel: *Arch Intern Med* 148:36, 1988.

should include a consideration of the value not only of lowering of LDL levels but also of raising HDL levels as a protection against both myocardial disease and stroke. The medications of first choice are bile acid sequestrants, including cholestyramine. Nicotinic acid is the other first-line drug. The latter is particularly useful if there is concurrent hypertriglyceridemia (greater than 250 mg/dl) because bile acid sequestrants tend to increase triglyceride levels. The mode of action of bile sequestrants is to interrupt the bile formation cycle, requiring the liver to process more cholesterol for bile formation. Nicotinic acid reduces the hepatic synthesis of cholesterol. A newer class of drugs includes those acting in the liver to reduce cholesterol synthesis by inhibiting responsible reductase enzymes.[51] A combination of drugs may be necessary if the initial drug chosen is inadequate. Bile acid sequestrant plus either nicotinic acid or a reductase inhibitor can reduce LDL levels by 40% to 50%.[31]

Hyperlipidemia Management Program

In our program, analogous to a hypertension management program in those with stroke, a more intensive effort was made toward reducing LDL (and increasing HDL) levels by increasing patient participation in self-monitoring and planning for modification in diet. The use of drug therapy was minimized. The goal of an LDL level of 130 mg/dl was established. Patients were enrolled in the dietary program with or without medication depending on the initial level. Measurement of the TC level was used to monitor blood lipids in nonfasting specimens. This permitted less complex monitoring procedures and more rapid feedback of results because the facilities for TC measuring are more readily available on follow-up visits after discharge in a physician's office. Once the patient agreed to these goals, the major effort was directed at involving the person with hyperlipidemia in designing the methods by which the goals were to be achieved.

The box on p. 191 describes the continuum of goals and the focus on developing a dietary modification plan than can be scored on admission and discharge. Note that the effect is for the person with hyperlipidemia to participate in a plan to alleviate the problem, including planning goals and means for meeting those goals, with an emphasis on diet.

The plan included having the person with stroke, the caregiver, or both design at least one meal during the inpatient stay that incorporated the agreed on changes. In addition, the patient followed model step 1 or step 2 diet during the inpatient stay. Additional orientation continued under a dietician, nurse, and physician to help develop the patient's commitment to the dietary modification. At follow-up after discharge there was review of agreed-upon dietary changes as well as monitoring of lipid levels.

The following case illustrates the multifactorial relationship of myocardial disease to stroke.

Nutrition Maintenance Knowledge

The score ranks skills related to management of diet, including identifying dietary goals, problem areas in current diet, and diet action steps to meet goals.

7. *Complete independence:* Consistently identifies problem areas, goals, and diet action steps to meet these goals.
6. *Modified independence:* Identifies problems, goals, and action steps but uses assistive device (e.g., a list) or requires more than a reasonable time to complete the identification or action.
5. *Supervision:* Knows goals, problem areas, and action steps. Requires supervision (e.g., cueing or coaxing) to accomplish these skills; achieves them only under stressful or unfamiliar conditions (no more than 10% of the time).
4. *Minimal direction:* Knows goals and problem areas. Successfully performs skills 75% to 90% of the time.
3. *Moderate direction:* Knows goals under all circumstances. Successfully performs other skills 50% to 74% of the time.
2. *Maximal direction:* Accomplishes skills 25% to 49% of the time. Needs direction more than half of the time to identify goals, problem areas, and action steps.
1. *Total assistance:* Accomplishes skills less than 25% of the time. Needs direction nearly all the time, or does not effectively know goals and cannot identify problems and action steps. May require constant one-on-one direction to complete these skills.

CASE REPORT

S.N. was a 50-year-old, right-handed, white male executive with myocardial infarction and recurrent cardiac arrhythmia despite the use of digitalis, flecainide, and nadolol and a quadruple bypass graft. He underwent electrical cardioversion, which was followed 2 days later by a sudden onset of left-sided weakness and slurred speech. A head CT scan 48 hours after onset demonstrated a nonhemorrhagic infarct involving the right middle cerebral artery (MCA) distribution and evidence of mass effect. No intracardiac thrombus was perceived on echocardiogram, but evidence of mild hypokinesis of the anteroseptal wall was seen. The ECG showed sinus bradycardia. The patient was administered anticoagulant agents for the first time and prothrombin time was subsequently maintained at 1.5× control. The presence of hypercholesterolemia had been noted and treated with lovastatin over the past several years.

On admission to the rehabilitation facility 14 days later, the physical examination findings were limited to slurred speech; left hemiparesis of the arm that was greater than of the leg; and hemisensory loss of touch and pinprick. Two weeks after the onset while the patient was receiving lovastatin, 20 mg qd, the lipid profile showed a TC level of 181 mg/dl, an HDL level of 34 mg/dl, and an LDL level of 129 mg/dl. When repeated 3 weeks after the onset with the patient receiving the same dose of lovastatin, the TC level was 150 mg/dl, the HDL was 29 mg/dl, and the LDL level was 104 mg/dl. The LDL level rose to 153 mg/dl 6 weeks after the onset despite the continued administration of lovastatin. Triglyceride levels stayed within normal limits throughout.

Treatment with anticoagulant medication has continued, and patient has remained free of further embolic events despite further episodes of arrhythmia. The concurrent hyperlipidemia was treated by medication and diet. The acute effects of the stroke may have contributed to the relatively low level of LDL and the trough 3 weeks after the stroke. The patient subsequently has noted a rise in his LDL level despite receiving his usual dose of lovastatin.

REFERENCES

Nature of the Problem

1. Goldberg G, Berger GG: Secondary prevention in stroke: a primary rehabilitation concern, *Arch Phys Med Rehabil* 69:32, 1988.
2. Hier DB et al: Stroke recurrence within 2 years after ischemic infarction, *Stroke* 22:155, 1991.
3. Leonberg SC, Elliott FA: Prevention of recurrent stroke, *Stroke* 12:731, 1981.
4. Marquardsen J: The epidemiology of cerebrovascular disease, *Acta Neurol Scand* 57(suppl 67):57, 1978.
5. Matsumoto N et al: Natural history of stroke in Rochester, Minnesota, 1955 through 1969, *Stroke* 4:20, 1973.
6. Sloan MA et al: Occurrence of stroke associated with use/abuse of drugs, *Neurology* 41:1358, 1991.
7. Socco RL et al: One year outcomes after cerebral infarction in whites, blacks and Hispanics, *Stroke* 22:3, 1991.
8. Wolf PA et al: Probability of stroke: a risk profile from the Framingham study, *Stroke* 22:312, 1991.

Management of Hypertension

9. Bandura A: Catecholamine secretion as a function of perceived coping self-efficacy, *J Consult Clin Psychol* 53:406, 1985.
10. Beevers DG et al: Antihypertensive treatment and the course of established cerebral vascular disease, *Lancet*, p 407, 1973.
11. Evans CE et al: Home blood pressure–measuring devices: a comparative study of accuracy, *J Hypertens* 7:133, 1989.
12. Fletcher AE, Bulpitt CJ: How far should blood pressure be lowered, *N Engl J Med* 326:251, 1992.
13. Goldstein L, Davis JN: Restorative neurology: drugs and recovery following stroke, *Stroke* 21:1636, 1990.
14. Haynes RB et al: Improvement of medication compliance in uncontrolled hypertension, *Lancet* 1:1265, 1976.
15. Hypertension Detection and Follow-up Program Cooperative Group: Five year findings of the Hypertension Detection and Follow-up Program. III. Reduction in stroke incidence among persons with high blood pressure, *JAMA* 247:633, 1982.

16. Joint National Committee on Detection, Evaluation, and Treatment of High Blood Pressure: 1988 Report, *Arch Intern Med* 148:1023, 1988.
17. Kannel WB et al: Components of blood pressure and risk of atherothrombotic brain infarction: the Framingham study, *Stroke* 4:327, 1976.
18. Kittner S et al: Black-white differences in stroke incidence in a national sample, *JAMA* 264:1267, 1990.
19. MacMahon S et al: Blood pressure, stroke and coronary heart disease. I. Prolonged differences in blood pressure prospective observational studies corrected for the regression dilution bias, *Lancet* 335:764, 1990.
20. Revised Statement of National High Blood Pressure Education Program: Hunt JC et al: Devices used for self measurement of blood pressure, *Arch Intern Med* 145:2231, 1985.
21. Russell RWR: How does blood pressure cause stroke? *Lancet* 2:1283, 1975.
22. SHEP Cooperative Research Group: Prevention of stroke by antihypertensive drug treatment in older persons with isolated systolic hypertension, *JAMA* 265:3255, 1991.
23. Tjoa HI, Kaplan NM: Treatment of hypertension in the elderly, *JAMA* 264:1015, 1990.
24. Toole JF: *Cerebrovascular disorders,* ed 3, New York, 1984, Raven Press.
25. Wallace JD, Levy LL: Blood pressure after stroke, *JAMA* 246:2177, 1981.
26. Wolf P, Kannel W: Reduction of stroke through risk factor modification, *Semin Neurol* 6:243, 1986.
27. Working Group on Hypertension in the Elderly: Statement on hypertension in the elderly, *JAMA* 256:70, 1986.

Management of Cardiac Factors

28. Cerebral Embolism Task Force on Cardiogenic Brain Embolism: The second report of the Cerebral Embolism Task Force, *Arch Neurol* 46:727, 1989.
29. Crouse JR et al: Risk factors for extracranial carotid artery atherosclerosis, *Stroke* 18:990, 1987.
30. Di Pasquale G et al: Cerebral ischemia and asymptomatic coronary artery disease: a prospective study of 83 patients, *Stroke* 17:1098, 1986.
31. Expert Panel: Report of the National Cholesterol Education Program Expert Panel on Detection, Evaluation, and Treatment of High Blood Cholesterol in Adults, *Arch Intern Med* 148:36, 1988.
32. Hendel RC, Layden JJ, Leppo JA: Prognostic value of dipyridamole thallium scintigraphy for evaluation of ischemic heart disease, *J Am Coll Cardiol* 15:109, 1990.
33. Jurgens G, Koltringer P: Lipoprotein (a) in ischemic cerebrovascular disease: a new approach to the assessment of risk for stroke, *Neurology* 37:513, 1987.
34. Kostner GM et al: Laboratory parameters as discriminators for peripheral atherosclerosis and stroke, *Monogr Atheroscler* 14:119, 1986.
35. Kwiterovich PO: Beyond cholesterol: *The Johns Hopkins complete guide for avoiding heart disease,* Baltimore, 1989, Johns Hopkins University Press.
36. Love BB et al: Cigarette smoking: a risk factor for cerebral infarction in young adults, *Arch Neurol* 47:693, 1990.
37. Lynd Research Clinics Program: The Lipid Research Clinics' coronary primary prevention trial results. II. The relationship of reduction in incidence of coronary heart disease to cholesterol lowering, *JAMA* 251:365, 1984.
38. Mathew NT et al: Hyperlipoproteinemia in occlusive cerebrovascular disease, *JAMA* 232:262, 1975.
39. Mendez I, Hachiuski V, Wolfe B: Serum lipids after stroke, *Neurology* 37:507, 1987.
40. Petersen PG et al: Placebo controlled randomized trial of warfarin and aspirin for

prevention of thromboembolic complications in chronic atrial fibrillation, *Lancet* 1:175, 1989.

41. Ross R: The pathogenesis of atherosclerosis: an update, *N Engl J Med* 314:488, 1986.

42. Sacco RL et al: Survival and recurrence following stroke: Framingham study, *Stroke* 13:290, 1982.

43. Sirna S et al: Cardiac evaluation of the patient with stroke, *Stroke* 21:14, 1990.

44. Sobel E et al: Stroke in the Lehigh Valley: combined risk factors for recurrent ischemic stroke, *Neurology* 39:669, 1989.

45. Solonen R et al: Prevalence of carotid atherosclerosis and serum cholesterol levels in eastern Finland, *Arteriosclerosis* 8:788, 1988.

46. Stroke Prevention in Atrial Fibrillation Group: Preliminary report, *N Engl J Med* 322:863, 1990.

47. Van Merode T et al: Serum HDL/total cholesterol ratio and blood pressure in asymptomatic atherosclerotic lesions of the cervical carotid arteries in men, *Stroke* 16:34, 1985.

48. Whisnant JP et al: Duration of cigarette smoking is the strongest predictor of severe extracranial carotid artery atherosclerosis, *Stroke* 21:707, 1990.

49. Wolf PA et al: Cigarette smoking as a risk factor for stroke, *JAMA* 259:1025, 1988.

50. Woo J et al: Acute and long-term changes in serum lipids after acute stroke, *Stroke* 21:1407, 1990.

51. Yatsu F, Fisher M: Atherosclerosis: current concepts on pathogenesis and interventional therapies, *Ann Neurol* 26:3, 1989.

CHAPTER 9

Rehabilitation Management: Principles

Nature of the problem
Management of the interdisciplinary team
  Nature of the problem
  Possible outcome measures
  Selection of outcome measures
  Making interdisciplinary plans
Neuropsychologic aspects of normal aging and stroke rehabilitation
    WILLIAM GARMOE, ANNE C. NEWMAN, AND JOSEPH BLEIBERG
  Nature of the problem
  Normal aging
    Personality factors
    Psychosocial factors
    Cognitive factors
    Summary and implications for rehabilitation
  Neurobehavioral syndromes
    Lesion characteristics
    Concurrent diseases
    Specific neurobehavioral syndromes: left hemisphere
    Specific neurobehavioral syndromes: right hemisphere
    Specific neurobehavioral syndromes: subcortical vascular disease
    Acute confusional states
  Behavioral and psychologic adjustment to stroke
    Self-esteem and sexuality
    Mood disorders following stroke
    Regression as a model for behavioral disturbances
    Implications for the rehabilitation setting
  Facilitating adaptation and new learning in the rehabilitation setting
    Rehabilitation strategies for neurobehavioral syndromes
    General strategies for the older adult
    Self-efficacy
  Summary and conclusions
Preparing the family for discharge: an interdisciplinary approach
    JANET M. LIECHTY
  Nature of the problem
  Assessment
    Psychosocial assessment framework
    Interdisciplinary team assessment

Interventions
  Programmatic interventions to prepare families for discharge
  Informal team interventions
Conclusion

NATURE OF THE PROBLEM

Thus far the medical issues that may affect the therapeutic exercise program and the development of a more effective plan for reducing the likelihood of recurrent stroke or myocardial death have been discussed. In the rehabilitation phase the major efforts are to enhance the patient's assets and to alleviate by training or use of assistive devices the patient's disabilities.

In the earlier acute phase the rehabilitation plan had its emphasis on the criteria by which persons may be properly selected for retraining and the efficacy of such an approach. In this section we focus on the design and implementation of a comprehensive rehabilitation program for individual patients, recognizing the need to make such planning and treatment meet both ethical and cost considerations.

The outcome measures of such efforts are based on several levels of analysis. The first involves the degree to which a person can live in the least restrictive setting. The option of living alone in one's own home is perhaps the optimal outcome. Physical assistance and supervision for safety are frequently required to achieve this living arrangement. Meeting this goal is the result not only of the rehabilitation of the person with stroke but also of the resources available. The availability of caregiver services varies. Every effort is made to enhance the competence and confidence of caregivers during the rehabilitation process and to maximize their contribution to such an outcome. The compatibility of the environment's physical characteristics with the abilities of the person also varies. An appropriate "environment" must be available and capable of being modified, incorporating both personal care and physical accessibility.

Data from the Framingham study are illustrative.[1] The incidence of institutionalization at 1 year in those surviving 30 days after stroke was 27%. There were significant differences between men and women. For example, a much higher number of women (45%) than men (25%) over 75 years of age were institutionalized. For women, their age and extent of impairment, but not their marital status, were significant variables in predicting institutionalization. However, for men, marital status was the only significant variable. Thus even more severely impaired men might be less likely to be institutionalized if they are married.

The next level of outcome measure is exemplified by the degree to which the person is able to carry out "independently" a specific mobility- or communication-related task. For example, value is placed on a reduction in the amount of physical support, supervision, or both necessary to achieve mobility. These functional outcomes are frequently taken to reflect the effects of the retraining process. During the rehabilitation program, every effort is properly devoted to the retraining of those assets that remain and the proper fitting of assistive devices. However, the degree to which this retraining is accomplished is also determined by both the type and severity of initial impairment and the degree of neurologic recovery.

An additional third level of outcome that can be usefully measured may more directly reflect the actual training program. Supporting the efforts to alleviate disabilities and to promote independent living arrangements is the learning of compensatory strategies — that is, alternative means by which the person may function. For example, a brain injury may lead to the loss of walking as a means of getting around and to the loss of speech and verbal expression as a means of communication. The process of rehabilitation is one of learning alternative techniques to regain mobility and the ability to communicate and to work with caretakers and assistive devices to achieve those activities.

Defining appropriate alternative techniques is a joint process between the professional staff and the person with stroke, along with others in the environment. This third level of outcome is the degree to which the person with disabilities and the caregivers contribute to the design of the compensatory strategies and the degree of independent implementation of the chosen techniques. The patient must learn the compensatory strategies useful in maintaining function despite the impairments; perhaps even more important, the patient must learn that there are a number of such alternatives. Ultimately, the retraining process can lead the person with stroke and the caregivers to generate on their own new compensatory strategies to adapt to the environment. Thus one measure of outcome is the degree to which the patient learns about and uses alternative strategies; perhaps this outcome measurement is even more directly related to the retraining process than are the more commonly measured outcomes of living site and functional status.

Thus the rehabilitation and retraining program is an educational process. The character of the person with brain injury and the type and severity of the injury affect the degree of success. The age and previous educational level of the person are significant variables. Increased age is frequently associated with a reduction in the capacity for new learning. The specific site(s) and degree of brain injury affect the ability to learn alternative modes of achieving life goals. In addition, the health care professional must minimize the risk for depression and learned helplessness often inherent in rehabilitation settings; instead, such professionals must optimize the likelihood of successful learning and the patient's sense of self-worth.

In summary, the patient's possible living arrangements depend both on the degree and type of impairment and on the degree to which compensatory strategies for meeting life needs have been learned. However, dealing effectively with physical and social limitations is not solely the responsibility of the person with disabilities. The restrictiveness of the patient's living environment also depends on the availability of family and other community resources to provide a more independent setting. The availability of accessible transportation, attendant care, and other social systems can affect the patient's outcome regardless of the degree of impairment and changes made through retraining. Thus during rehabilitation, a major portion of the efforts expended is applied to enhancing the fit of the environment's resources to the needs of the person with stroke.

"Independent living" does not merely reflect the degree of support required but the degree to which the patient is able to manage his or her affairs. The goal of retraining must be to enable the person with disabilities to act as independently as possible in managing his or her living situation. It is suggested that the patient's participation in the rehabilitation planning process can become the vehicle for learning to manage new problems. The rehabilitation phase ends when the person with stroke, the caretakers, or both have learned to maximize their resources and to develop compensatory strategies to deal with problems independent of the health professional. The goal is for the patient or caretaker to be an independent problem solver and planner.

The means by which the patient's independence is accomplished is the comprehensive interdisciplinary rehabilitation program described in this section. The approach described here is interdisciplinary, deals with functional disabilities, and uses measurements of outcome intrinsic to the planning process. The principles of developing a learning program for the person with stroke and for caregivers are explored in this chapter. In the succeeding chapter these principles are applied to the major problems of communication and dysphagia, as well as problems in sensorimotor control. The following sections describe specific methods for defining goals and treatment procedures while recognizing the value of interdisciplinary coordination. Maximal patient and caregiver participation dealing with the several specific problems is important to establish the basis for later independent decision making and problem solving in the continuing care phase.

MANAGEMENT OF THE INTERDISCIPLINARY TEAM

Nature of the Problem

The Commission on Accreditation of Rehabilitation Facilities (CARF) has defined rehabilitation programs. See the box on p. 199 for those standards.[2] The activities stated by the CARF are based on the principle that the multidisciplinary team should be organized to support one another throughout

Comprehensive Inpatient Rehabilitation

Comprehensive inpatient rehabilitation is a program of coordinated and integrated services that includes evaluation and treatment and that stresses the importance of the education and training of those served and their families. The program is applicable to those individuals who have severe functional limitations of recent onset or recent regression or progression or who have not had prior exposure to rehabilitation.

The comprehensive inpatient rehabilitation program should have both appropriate rehabilitation services to manage the functional and psychosocial needs of those served and appropriate medical services to evaluate and treat the pathophysiologic processes.

Services should be provided by a coordinated, interdisciplinary team.

A. The team should be the major decision-making body in determining the goals, processes, and time frames for the accomplishment of each person's rehabilitation program.

B. The team should be composed of the treating member of each discipline essential to the patient's accomplishment of the goals.

C. The team should meet on a formal basis at a frequency necessary to carry out its decision-making responsibilities. For each person served, a team conference should occur no less than every other week. There should be interim informal conferences among the members of the team.

D. The program should provide a core group of professionals who comprise the team.
   1. The core members of the team, although not serving every person, should include but not be limited to the following:
      a. Occupational therapist
      b. Physical therapist
      c. Physician
      d. Psychologist
      e. Rehabilitation nurse
      f. Social worker
      g. Speech-language pathologist
   2. The members of the core team should provide therapeutic, educational, and training services consistent with individualized patient needs. This ordinarily occupies most of the day but should not be less than 3 hours per day during a 5-day week for each person served. This is in addition to the contact and the time stipulations for physician and nurse input.
   3. Those served should have the benefit of a consistently assigned staff member from each of the disciplines appropriate to their needs.
   4. Each member of the team should support and enhance the programs being carried out by the other disciplines as part of the rehabilitation plan.

the plan.[8] Such an interdisciplinary effort remains only a goal in many settings,[9] and its cost effectiveness is under attack.[3,7,12] Managing an interdisciplinary planning process requires that staff be concerned with both the process's effectiveness and efficiency. Evaluation of the planning activities is likely to increase such effectiveness.[6]

The making of a rehabilitation plan requires that an individual therapist or other professional interacts with the person with stroke. The goals of the patient and therapist must then be integrated into a more complete interdisciplinary team approach to the patient. The patient-therapist goals may be more effectively reached by coordinating with the various staff. The more effective use of professional resources results from a coordinated approach. The contribution to the planning process of the patient, caregiver, or both must also be maintained in this more complex planning group.

The process is a reiterative one of problem solving over time.[11] A series of planning activities, including an initial assessment and goal setting, are followed by reassessment and further planning. The structure of the planning system is described in Fig. 9-1. Of course, the time frame for this process varies with the person and the severity of the problem. The initial planning session provides the opportunity to identify both the long-term plan relevant to discharge and any short-term goals of high priority that can be well served by the several disciplines working conjointly ("interdisciplinary goals"). At the time of an interim review, generally at weekly or biweekly intervals, both the long-term goals relevant to eventual disposition and the short-term "interdisciplinary plans" can be revised. Frequently, both the person with stroke and those who are to be the caregivers must undergo training. By the time of the discharge conference, goals may be made for postdischarge treatment and other follow-up. This section describes the ongoing assessment and evaluation planning system to achieve interdisciplinary coordination and to maximize opportunities for the person with stroke to participate in the planning and treatment process.

Possible Outcome Measures

Programmatic outcomes range from a return to independent living with or without support to full-time institutional living. Outcomes reflect the degree to which the person with stroke can function without supervision, physical assistance, or both. Ultimately, dispositions can be translated into dollars expended or saved. The type and degree of impairment — cognitive or sensorimotor — are significant variables. However, disposition is not only a result of the achievements of retraining in the use of compensatory strategies to deal with impairments; it also reflects the availability of both family and community resources. The following case reports illustrate the multifactorial nature of the disposition outcome.

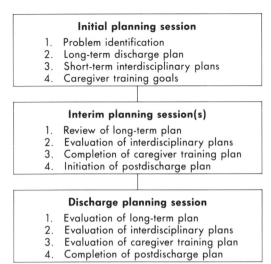

Fig. 9-1 Planning structure.

CASE REPORT

I.B. was a 67-year-old black widower with a previous history of hypertension and peripheral vascular disease. He experienced a sudden onset of difficulty in using the right side of his body and paucity of speech. A head computed tomography (CT) scan showed hemorrhage in the left basal ganglion area with edema of the left parietal lobe. At 17 days after onset the physical examination findings were continued lethargy, paucity of speech, right homonymous hemianopsia, and right hemiparesis. A functional status evaluation showed inattention on the right side and difficulties with mobility and language. The patient initially required "maximal assistance" in all areas of self-care. For example, he required one-on-one supervision for feeding, verbal cueing for taking small bites, and reminders to swallow. Similarly, he required "moderate assistance" in moving in bed and carrying out a squat pivot transfer to a level surface. He had "moderate" oropharyngeal dysphagia with delay in initiating swallowing and with aspiration of thin liquids. He was able to follow simple commands, and his "yes" and "no" responses were considered to be reliable although speech initiation was "moderately affected." His impulsivity and lack of understanding about safety precautions were major problems.

During the course of his rehabilitation (approximately 60 days), the patient began to attend to his right side with minimal cues and became independently mobile with a wheelchair. His impulsivity diminished so that he no longer required constant supervision to remain safe. He could be left on his own for short periods. When transferring from chair to bed, it was helpful for him to verbalize the actions he was about to take. Although he continued to require physical assistance with lower body dressing, he was able to dress his upper body with supervision only. He also was able to initiate a conversation and to speak, although haltingly, and he began to once again read and write his name. He no longer aspirated when swallowing thin liquids.

Despite learning some new skills, this patient continued to require supervision for safety, although not on a constant basis. His children (several sons and two daughters) all worked full time and had limited financial resources. Because of the lack of a mate, returning to his own home was not an option for the patient. Cognitive difficulties limited his progress during rehabilitation. His ultimate admission to a nursing home reflected the inability to enlist family resources to provide the supervision necessary.

CASE REPORT

M.S. was a 75-year-old black widow with a history of communication loss that initially was progressive but had not worsened over the past several years. She could speak only to the extent of saying "yes," "no," and "OK." She would not initiate speech and would respond only to questions. She lived in the basement of her daughter's home and required ongoing supervision from her daughter in carrying out activities of daily living (ADLs) but was able to walk up and down stairs. She experienced a sudden onset of right-sided weakness. A head CT scan yielded negative findings for hemorrhage. The patient showed some improvement in her leg weakness. When examined 10 days after the onset, she showed continued evidence of right-sided weakness, particularly in the arm. She did not verbalize spontaneously and had difficulty in following verbal and demonstrative directions.

Functionally, the patient required supervision and "setup" for safe self-feeding, physical assistance and supervision for dressing, and "maximal assistance" for bathing. She required physical assistance with standing pivot transfers. She was totally dependent in wheelchair propulsion. During the next 30 days, training focused on the family, who would continue to provide her with ongoing continual supervision. The patient also became able to propel a wheelchair with supervision and to transfer to and from a wheelchair with supervision and physical guidance. She was able to return home although she lived on the first floor of her daughter's house rather than in her own private quarters in the basement.

This case illustrates the effects of a severe cognitive impairment present before the onset of motor difficulties. In this case the patient was able to learn compensatory skills that enabled her to regain mobility. The continued availability of family members enabled her to return home despite the need for continuous supervision.

CASE REPORT

E.W. was a 79-year-old white retired widow who had been a government worker and active in community affairs. The patient was found on the kitchen floor in her home with a sudden onset of atrial fibrillation, probable embolic stroke with clearing, and no evident sequelae. The patient was prescribed aspirin and digoxin. Three weeks later she was found on the floor of her home by her son who happened to drop by. A head CT scan showed a left putamen hemorrhage. Right hemiparesis, fluent aphasia, and marked lethargy were present. An echocardiogram showed aortic calcific stenosis and mitral calcification. The patient had hypothyroidism and was started on replacement therapy. On examination 10 days after onset, she had marked fluent aphasia and difficulty following directions. Weakness of the right side of her body was present, with arm weakness equal to leg weakness and with distal weakness greater than proximal weakness. She lacked right-sided sensation in the presence of bilateral simultaneous stimulation. Her proprioception appeared to be intact. She required cues for feeding herself and physical assistance to propel a wheelchair. She could answer "yes" and "no" appropriately. She was able to follow one- and two-step commands. Lethargy and the lack of endurance continued to be major problems.

At the end of 66 days the patient was feeding herself independently. She was able to select her own clothes with verbal cues for locating items. She required prompting for carrying out sequenced tasks. She could complete grooming with supervision after "setup." She was able to ambulate with a walker once she had been assisted to a standing position, although she was unable to climb stairs. She continued to have major difficulty in communicating and required constant supervision. She was unable to return to her own home, which had stairs. Both her sons were successful professionals with greater than usual resources. Neither was able or willing to have his mother move into his home. One son had several children; the other had a wife who worked full time. Therefore a nursing home was the only solution available.

This case once again illustrates the significance of cognitive impairment in the patient's eventual disposition and outcome. These cognitive impairments limit the rate of learning during rehabilitation—even procedural or motor learning. Moreover, persistent cognitive impairments require the patient to be supervised for safety. Thus ongoing supervision is necessary, yet unfortunately it is rarely available in most families in metropolitan areas today.

The availability of family resources in M.S.'s case made possible her return to her daughter's home despite her considerable cognitive impairment. Retraining in motor skills was the factor that enabled her to return. Therefore one may conceivably attribute her return home, at least partially, to the retraining accomplished in the rehabilitation setting. However, the success achieved in wheelchair mobility training was insufficient in the case of I.B., and the mobility achieved via ambulation was also insufficient in the case of E.W. The variables in predicting a patient's return to a home setting or to an institutional one such as a nursing home include not only the type and severity of impairment but also the availability of family support. Such family support is not necessarily a reflection of the family's level of income or education. It may reflect the sex of the patient's children; for instance, M.S.'s daughter was able to provide what E.W.'s sons were not.

Ultimately, the disposition outcome is an important dollar measure of the benefit achieved by rehabilitation. However, in the cases just described, despite considerable improvement in the patients' levels of function, disposition reflected other variables not fundamentally under the control of the rehabilitation staff. Both the type of the impairment and the availability of family resources appear to be the determining variables.

Traditionally, functional skills have been the focus when establishing the range of possible effective outcomes in the retraining process. There are a large number of such scales, with the Barthel Index the prototype.[4] The emphasis has been on items that demonstrate the relative independence of the patient in caring for himself or herself. For example, the Barthel Index consists of two parts, a self-care index and a mobility index. Points are assessed within each of the categories for the various individual skills and the level at which the disabled person functions. For example, "dressing the upper body" is assigned a total possible value of five points. Within the same index, "eating" is assigned a possible total of six points. The total possible score is 100 points, with a score greater than 60 generally signifying relative independence. Within any specific item the highest possible score reflects the person's ability to "do by myself," with variable reductions in scores reflecting the need for assistance. For example, the "dressing upper body" item score is reduced to three (from a possible five) points if it is a task the patient "can do with the help of someone else." The eating score is reduced to zero (from a possible six) points if any help is required.

This same set of principles underlies the more recent Functional Independence Measure (FIM).[5] Its development reflects the need for a uniform data system for medical rehabilitation. Commonality in outcome measures can provide a basis for comparing rehabilitation services in different settings. Measurement at entry and discharge can demonstrate degrees of change during the rehabilitation process. Similar to the Barthel Index, the FIM assesses items particularly relevant to independent self-care and mobility. In addition, sphincter management, communication, and social interaction are assessed. Similar to the

---

Functional Independence Measure (FIM) Items

Bladder management
Bowel management
Social interaction
Problem solving
Memory
Comprehension
Bed-to-chair and wheelchair-to-chair transfer
Toilet transfer
Tub and shower transfer
Locomotion (walking or wheelchair)
Climbing stairs
Eating
Grooming
Bathing
Dressing (upper body)
Dressing (lower body)
Toileting

Barthel Index, the FIM is a measure of disability, not impairment. It measures what the person actually does. See the box above for a list of FIM items.

In the FIM, a seven-point scale is used to reflect the burden of care required in any specific outcome. The burden of care is the "substituted time/energy which must be brought to serve the dependent needs of the disabled individual so that a certain quality of life may be achieved." The underlying rationale for classifying an activity as "independent" or "dependent" is whether another person (a helper) is required, and if help is required, how much. Unlike in the Barthel Index, no item is assigned a specific number of points nor is there variability in score reduction depending on the level of performance. In almost all instances a score of five points reflects need for supervision; a score of four points or less reflects the need for physical assistance. The box on p. 206 illustrates the FIM scale in use.

It is important to recognize that the FIM is not an interval scale. The numbers represent merely a method of recording results. The shift from a five-point (supervision) to a four-point (minimal assistance) score can significantly affect disposition in some settings but not in others. However, once physical assistance is required, the difference in physical assistance required between a four-point score (minimal or less than 25%) and three-point score (moderate or less than 50%) may not necessarily be significant. However, in an individual case the difference in the degree of physical assistance may be quite important. The impact of intervals on the patient's ultimate disposition reflects

---

Burden of Care

7. Complete independence (timely, safely)	No
6. Modified independence (device)	helper
Modified Dependence	
5. Supervision	
4. Minimal assistance (subject = 75% +)	
3. Moderate assistance (subject = 50% +)	Helper
Complete Dependence	
2. Maximal assistance (Subject = 25% +)	
1. Total assistance (Subject = 0% +)	

---

the resources available. However, it is likely that continuous high levels of physical assistance (in the range of >25%) are available only in more institutional settings.

The FIM item concerning stairway mobility illustrates the application of the seven-point scale to a specific item (upper box on p. 207).

The FIM was intended to include a minimum number of items as a basic indicator of the severity of disability. The format of the seven-point scale is retained when broader aspects of rehabilitation are rated. The Rehabilitation Institute of Chicago Functional Assessment Scale (RIC-FAS) is an example of a scale that amplifies the basic FIM.[10] A sample of the RIC-FAS items (in addition to those in the FIM) is listed in the lower box on p. 207. Note the broadening of focus to reflect the characteristics of the entire interdisciplinary team; health, psychologic, and social issues are included. The scale also reflects a new focus on the community integration of functional skills learned in the rehabilitation program. In addition to the major FIM focus on mobility and ADL skills, communication issues have been amplified.

The coupling of the degree of independence achieved on the functional item with the degree to which resources are appropriately available is particularly crucial. The item entitled "continuing care resource availability" is defined as the degree to which postdischarge planning has been successful in developing appropriate resources. For example, if the functional items such as dressing and toilet transfer require physical assistance, the score of this item must reflect the existence of a proper "fit" in that physical assistance is available.

In the design of the outcome measures for the National Rehabilitation Hospital Stroke Recovery Program, the basic FIM items were retained. In large part, RIC-FAS items were used to reflect broadening concepts of rehabilitation. Other new items were added to reflect the relatively unique characteristics of persons with stroke. See the box on p. 208 for a list of items that were generated

Functional Independence Measure — Stairs

Patient climbs up and down 12 to 14 stairs (one flight) indoors:

7. Complete independence — climbs up and down at least one flight of stairs without any type of handrail or support; performs safely
6. Modified independence — climbs up and down at least one flight of stairs, requiring side support or handrail, cane, or portable support; takes more than reasonable time or there are safety considerations

Helper

5. Supervision — requires standby supervision, cueing, or coaxing to climb up and down one flight of stairs
4. Minimal contact assistance — performs 75% or more of the effort required to climb up and down one flight of stairs
3. Moderate assistance — performs 50% to 74% of the effort required to climb up and down one flight of stairs
2. Maximal assistance — performs 25% to 49% of the effort required to climb up and down four to six stairs; requires the assistance of one person only
1. Total assistance — performs less than 25% of the effort required to climb four to six stairs, or requires the assistance of two people, or is carried

Rehabilitation Institute of Chicago Functional Assessment Scale (RIC-FAS)

Medical status
Nutritional status
Chewing and swallowing
Endurance
Depression
Emotional control
Sexuality understanding
Family understanding
Continuing care resource availability
Financial resources
Housing
Transportation
Visual spatial ability
Reading comprehension
Written expression
Meal preparation
Homemaking
Community integration
Vocational plan

Added Outcome Measures Specific to Stroke

Pain management
Nutrition maintenance
Medication maintenance
Stroke prevention
Stroke warning recognition
Continuity of medical care
Substance usage
Awareness of limitations
Adjustment to illness and injury
Vocational and educational planning
Continuing care skills and resource management
Equipment management
Participation in goal setting
Direction of personal assistance
Safety judgment

specifically for use in persons with stroke and that are in addition to those derived from FIM and RIC-FAS. The frequency of medical problems and the contribution of medical risk factors to repeated stroke are highlighted. The "stroke prevention" item exemplifies this major new emphasis during rehabilitation of the stepped-up training in blood pressure management, which is described in Chapter 8. It reflects the extent to which a patient, significant other, or both demonstrate the ability to (1) state the blood pressure goal; (2) record a blood pressure measurement; (3) monitor blood pressure; and (4) state whether or not a blood pressure reading is within an acceptable range.

The significance of the recurrent nature of stroke is reflected in still another item dealing with stroke warning signs. This includes an awareness of early warning signs of stroke and a plan to seek help promptly. These warning signs include numbness or weakness of the face, arm, or leg; difficulty with speech or comprehension; difficulty swallowing; sudden confusion; severe headaches; dizziness or loss of balance; sudden blurred or decreased vision; and sudden changes in mental ability.

The medical issues and patient responsibility for health management are reflected in several additional items. "Nutrition maintenance knowledge" includes skills related to diet management. This includes dietary goals and identification of problem areas in current diet and action steps to meet goals. This item reflects the patient's training in the management of hyperlipidemia, which is described in the section on planning for vascular disease prevention. "Medication maintenance skills" includes patient and caregiver understanding

---

Items Reflecting Patient and Family Participation in Planning

Awareness of limitations
Adjustment to illness and injury
Vocational and educational planning
Participation in goal setting
Direction of personal assistance

---

of medication doses, actions, and side effects and the ability to administer medication effectively. "Continuity of medical care," as measured by the ability to generate a medical follow-up plan, minimizes stroke recurrence.

The importance attached to patient and family participation in the planning process is reflected in a number of items in the box above. Note that the "awareness of limitations" item is defined as the ability of the patient to describe the problem in functional terms (i.e., as disabilities). The patient's participation in setting goals is the next step after problem identification. It is defined as the degree to which an individual can participate in rehabilitation goal setting and treatment planning and can set goals that maximize safe and independent functioning. These two important planning steps — defining problems and goals — are related to procedures outlined elsewhere in this book.

Thus the outcome measures for the Stroke Recovery Program reflect an enlargement of the scope of rehabilitation. Concern with the implications for the continuing care phase places the training or rehabilitation phase in a longer perspective. Prevention of future stroke has become one new focus. Still another is the training of patient, family, or both in health self-management. Responsibility for scoring the various items is with the team members assigned the items, which are primarily within their areas of expertise.

In addition, the goals are not merely to learn new techniques for mobility, self-care, and communication but to fundamentally influence the patient's lifestyle. For instance, not only should the patient learn to achieve mobility but also he or she should learn a process by which problems can be solved as they arise. Initially the planning process requires the patient to identify problems and goals and to assess outcomes and the methods used to achieve those outcomes. Fig. 9-2 describes the order in which these requirements for addressing these key issues can be made in the course of the rehabilitation planning and evaluation process.

The planning structure described in Fig. 9-2 can also reflect the time intervals between discussions of these various issues. Of course, the patient's level of participation in addressing these issues will vary with the skills of the individual involved. The major focus must be on the independent use of the

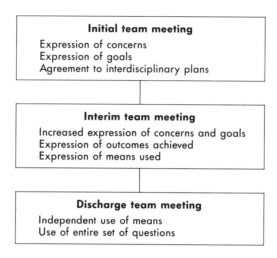

Fig. 9-2   Goals for patient participation.

compensatory strategies that are designed during the rehabilitation process. The degree to which the patient is involved in the design of such strategies can enhance the degree to which they are used in other settings.

Ultimately, the entire set of issues can become questions the person with stroke, the caregiver, or both can use. Asking "What worked?" is particularly important. Learning a specific set of compensatory strategies is merely one aspect of the rehabilitation process. The conditions present in the rehabilitation setting are unlikely to be replicated in the more variegated environment to which the patient must return. Thus the person with disabilities must have a way to generate new strategies in response to unforeseen circumstances. The principle that alternatives exist must be established, and the patient must continue to search for them.

Selection of Outcome Measures

The possible patient outcomes encompass a broad range and reflect the unique characteristics of persons with stroke. Among these possible outcomes, priorities must be established based on the characteristics of the individual person. Problem areas are first identified in functional terms on admission. Priorities reflect an individual's existing disabilities and the projected level of function with retraining and take into consideration the availability of resources to deal with remaining disabilities in the person's environment. Priorities must also reflect the patient's social needs. An important social concern is with optimizing the likelihood that the person with stroke will function outside a long-term care facility. The overall goal is to enable the person and his or her

TABLE 9-1   Status of Patient Transfers from Bed to Chair

	A	G	IG	D
1. Bed mobility				
2. Bed, chair, and wheelchair transfers				
3. Toilet transfer				
4. Tub and shower transfers				
5. Safety judgments				

A, Status of person on admission; *G*, goal or status projected on discharge; *IG*, interdisciplinary goal of high priority; and *D*, status actually achieved on discharge.

family, through training, to maintain the patient in a home setting, which is usually the least restrictive environment. In almost all instances this aim is compatible with the goals of the person with stroke and the family. Once this goal is agreed on, the priority areas contributing to its achievement can become the focus of the coordinated efforts of all who work with the patient.

One priority area that is frequently identified is the patient's ability to transfer safely. Table 9-1 lists items concerning the patient's ability to transfer from a bed to a chair and reflecting the status of the person on admission, the projected status on discharge, the identification of any one or other of these goals as interdisciplinary and of high priority, and the status actually accomplished by discharge.

The priority areas vary somewhat among patients. In almost all instances in persons with stroke, mobility is a major concern. The ability to transfer from a bed to a wheelchair and from a bed to a toilet is fundamental for functioning in the community. For the patient with mobility problems the availability of physical assistance may make it possible to accomplish the goal of home placement, even when a relatively high degree of help remains necessary. The patient may aim for a minimum score of "4," signifying the need for minimal physical assistance. For another patient with an equivalent degree of impairment but less available physical assistance, achieving the goal of being discharged home may require the patient to function at the level of "5," signifying supervision only, without the need for physical assistance.

For example, an obese woman with a recent stroke could be cared for at home by her husband if he were not required to physically assist her in transferring from the bed to a wheelchair. This is impossible for him because his own physical health is compromised as the result of heart disease. However, he is available to help at home because he is retired. Therefore an important early priority is to develop a mode of transfer that the patient can use without the need for physical assistance; it is crucial to her ability to return home.

In another example, a patient with comparable difficulties in transferring lives with her 35-year-old daughter and physically capable adolescent grand-daughter. She could possibly return home, even if physical assistance is still necessary for her to transfer safely. The limiting factor in this instance is her impairment in thinking and in understanding the limitations produced by her brain injury. This patient has difficulty judging safe limits. She has already fallen once when she attempted to transfer on her own. Priorities during the rehabilitation program must focus on training the patient in safety procedures and increasing her awareness of her limitations and the need to ask for help when appropriate. Training of the family members on these issues also becomes a high priority because they will be required to supervise the patient. This same patient has had several strokes over the past several months. Thus another priority for the entire staff is to ensure that the family learns to monitor her blood pressure and other risk factors. It also is necessary for family members to be more aware of the warning signs of stroke. In general, the entire scope of family training has grown in priority in this instance in light of the patient's cognitive impairments and the need for the family to compensate for these impairments through super-vision.

The method for establishing these priorities requires a review of the initial level of functional disabilities and of the resources available in the environment. The difference between the patient's status on admission and that required for a discharge home represents the unmet needs to be remedied by the rehabilitation training program. At the initial team meeting, areas for caregiver training are also identified to supplement those needs that will be unmet through patient training alone.

Making Interdisciplinary Plans

Particular emphasis should be placed on interdisciplinary activities; thus staff resources are fully used to achieve what may not be possible by any one discipline alone within the time allotted. The interdisciplinary team meeting is valuable. When meeting together, involved professionals can facilitate commu-nication about the patient's status and individual service goals. However, if this alone were the goal, their physical presence would not be necessary.[6] The standards of CARF reflect the need for more effective use of team meetings, using the staff members' presence. These guidelines state that "each member of the team should support and enhance the programs being carried out by the other disciplines as part of the rehabilitation plan."

A comprehensive, ongoing system of assessment, planning, and evaluation within a team meeting is described. The format incorporates the possible outcome measures in all the areas of function for persons with stroke. Since each member of the interdisciplinary team has established the status and long-term goals for an assigned area, other members of the team can review the scores. Any discrepancies in scoring can be resolved to ensure a degree of reliability. In addition, the work of the interdisciplinary group is to establish joint interdisciplinary goals.

For example, the speech therapist might develop a set of gestures to be used by a person with communication problems. The content of such a gesture system affects the communication of all those working with the patient. A high priority in an incontinent person is the development of a signal for the need to urinate and defecate that the nurse can use. Similarly, such a gesture must be understood by family members and by therapists working with the person at various times of the day. The consistent use of an effective set of signals is an appropriate interdisciplinary goal.

Similarly, the mode of transfer should be agreed on and understood. For a person with significant problems in safety caused by impulsivity, both the goals to be achieved and the means to achieve them should be agreed upon. For example, it may be helpful for such a patient to verbalize the necessary steps before carrying out motor tasks such as locking the brakes of the wheelchair or standing to transfer. In the team meeting this is shared so that all can hear. Similarly, when mood disturbance limits a patient's performance, it may be beneficial for all caregivers to encourage the patient to state areas of improvement in functioning at the end of each therapy session.

The interdisciplinary goals to achieve priorities need to be made specific enough to be measurable. In generating such goals, the same phraseology as in the more generic outcomes of FIM is used. For example, in a person with visuospatial inattention, the goal may be phrased as "the patient will attend to the neglected side during functional activities with no more than one verbal cue more than 50% of the time." Still another goal in dealing with such visuospatial difficulties could be "the patient will propel a wheelchair between therapy sessions with no more than several verbal cues more than 75% of the time." Thus specificity reflects not only the statement of the goal (e.g., attend to the neglected side) but the context (e.g., during functional activities) and degree (e.g., with no more than one verbal cue and more than 50% of the time). In this manner the questions of what, where, when, and to what degree are answered. One may choose to establish the necessary level of specificity to be sought in writing such interdisciplinary goals.

The interdisciplinary areas can also be broken down into short-term goals that can be evaluated at intervals during the rehabilitation phase. The time frame before such an evaluation and revision is 1 to 2 weeks for most persons with stroke whose hospital stay is in the range of 30 days.

The following is an example of a series of such interdisciplinary goals for the person with communication problems and incontinence:

First goal: Patient will remain dry during the day by pointing to the "toilet" symbol in a communication book when cued.

Second goal: Patient will remain dry during the day by spontaneously pointing to the "toilet" symbol.

One can increase the level of outcome by varying not only the degree of independence but also the technique. For example, use of the call button may be included during the night.

Thus far some interdisciplinary goals have been described. The completion of interdisciplinary *plans* also requires a description of the means (i.e., the activities to be carried out) by which the goals are to be achieved. The involved staff should be assigned as taking the lead role in carrying out the agreed upon interdisciplinary plan and be primarily responsible for monitoring the patient's progress. The lead service staff also take responsibility for initially establishing the patient's and caregiver's agreement with the goals. At subsequent intervals they and others can ensure that the patient also participates in monitoring the outcomes and the means by which the outcomes have been achieved. The following is a plan that was designed for a person with communication difficulties caused by slurred speech:

Goal: The patient's speech will be intelligible greater than 75% of the time when requesting specific items needed for grooming and bathing.

Means: The speech therapist will instruct the patient in the use of a "pacing board" and will gain the patient's agreement with the goal and the use of the pacing board; the speech therapist will co-treat the patient with the occupational therapist and nurse to facilitate the patient's transfer of the use of the technique to other settings.

On subsequent review the plan may be revised, depending on the degree to which the goal has been achieved. In addition to the degree, the means by which the patient achieves the goal can vary as the patient uses the compensatory strategy more independently.

In another example, a plan was designed for a patient with problems in mobility and safety awareness and includes greater detail about the methods to be used and the persons taking responsibility.

Goal: The patient will perform the steps in preparing a wheelchair for safe transfer (i.e., setting the brake and foot rests) with minimal verbal cues.

Means: The physical therapist will identify the steps to be followed and write them on a sheet posted visibly at the patient's bedside and wheelchair. The physical therapist will gain the patient's agreement with the goal. The procedure of the patient reading these instructions aloud will be reinforced by nurses and other staff whenever an opportunity arises for the use of transfer skills.

In the following example, an interdisciplinary plan incorporates the several services dealing with memory problems and the need for knowledge of medication:

> *Goal:* Patient will recall at least 50% of his or her medications and the time for taking them.
>
> *Means:* The assigned primary nurse will gain the patient's agreement with the goal and the use of a log book. The speech therapist will review the schedule with patient. The physician will reinforce the independent use of the log book.

Plans dealing with mood disturbances, which frequently interfere with function, focus on the patient's participation in addressing the planning questions. Note that, in this sample set of plans, the person with stroke initially merely agrees to the plan but functions more independently in assessing the outcome and methods used and that he or she does so to an increased degree over time.

> *First interim plan:* The patient's depression will interfere with function only "to a mild degree" through encouraging the patient to state at least one positive outcome at the end of each therapy session when offered several outcomes from which to select (i.e., multiple-choice responses). This is to be carried out by all therapists, with the psychologist taking the lead in gaining the patient's agreement to the plan.
>
> *Second interim plan:* The patient's depression will interfere with function only "to a marginal degree," with the patient stating at least one positive outcome at the end of each therapy session when asked about such outcomes (i.e., free-choice response). The patient will address the question of what worked in achieving outcomes on a multiple-choice level. The plan is to be carried out by all therapists, with the psychologist taking the lead in gaining the patient's agreement to the plan.

With the preceding plan the structure is in place for defining and evaluating interdisciplinary areas of high priority. Plans need to be revised as priorities change. It is also necessary for plans to be clearly stated so that they can be easily evaluated and revised. Not only must the goals be clearly stated, but they must also detail the means and the degree of contribution by the patient to the entire process. Evaluation and revision of all these aspects are ongoing. In addition to evaluating the outcomes, the review process can include an evaluation of the activities of particular value. In this way the staff and the patient can become increasingly aware of high-priority goals and can increasingly contribute to the means used to achieve them. Such a coordination of staff and patient effort enlists the available resources most cost effectively.

At the time of the patient's discharge a conference is conducted once again to evaluate all areas of the patient's status and to issue a score using the seven-point scale. The status measure can be used to identify ongoing problem areas that will require postdischarge treatment either in the home or in an outpatient clinic. The assessment can also include the degree to which the patient independently implements compensatory strategies. The degree to which caregiver training meets the patient's need for supervision or physical assistance is also assessed.

At the time of the postdischarge follow-up visit a comparable process is carried out. For example, the degree to which a continuity of medical care has been achieved and the degree to which blood pressure control is reliably monitored and adequate blood pressure control is maintained can be assessed. The effectiveness of ongoing physical training for mobility is also assessed, and new plans are made with input from both the team members and the person with stroke, the caregiver, or both.

The following case report illustrates the development of specific inter-disciplinary goals in the context of one patient's pattern of disability and the resources available in her family.

CASE REPORT

P.B. is a 71-year-old, right-handed woman with a history of hypertension. She experienced a sudden onset of right-sided numbness with subsequent right hemiplegia, confusion, and the loss of the ability to recall words. A CT scan showed a large hemorrhage involving the left midtemporal parietal area with surrounding edema. Initially the patient showed some improvement in speech with more fluency and increased movement of her left leg. When examined 14 days after the onset she appeared somewhat depressed. She complained of anorexia and sleep disturbances. She exhibited difficulty in following verbal instructions but did somewhat better when reading instructions. Her speech was fluent with difficulty in choosing words. She had a right homonymous field defect with double simultaneous finger motion. She demonstrated marked right arm weakness that was greater distally than proximally; there was a lesser degree of weakness in the right leg, which again was greater distally than proximally. She made errors in identifying pinprick, touch, and position sense on the right. Although she had good balance when sitting without assistance, she could not stand unassisted.

The patient lived with and cared for her bachelor son who worked full time. Her home had five steps to the front door and five more to the main floor. She lived in a rural area with little home therapy available. Her eldest daughter lived in a suburban area. Although this daughter worked full time, her husband was retired and would generally be available for supervision if necessary. The daughter's home was equipped with a half bath on the main floor and a full bath on the basement level, which was reached by 10 steps with a railing. The patient's other daughters, who lived nearby, were potentially available to help out during the several weeks after discharge. Each of them worked full time, and no one was available at any of their homes for daytime supervision. The patient's preference was to return to her own home and to care for herself there. However, she was prepared to go to her eldest daughter's home at least initially. She was particularly concerned about her ability to get around and care for her own personal needs. She was not particularly concerned about taking full charge of her home and caring for her son.

Problem areas were defined at the time of the patient's entry into the rehabilitation program. Her depression was rated as mild—that is, it impaired functioning and required the patient to have occasional assistance under stress, but it did not interfere with her participation in her rehabilitation program. One major difficulty lay in the area of communication. The patient had moderate problems in understanding both spoken and written language and a comparable level of disability in communicating her needs by the use of gestures. These difficulties interfered with her ability to define her limitations, to participate in goal setting, and to direct her personal affairs. She also had memory problems while performing ADLs. Based on these findings, it did not appear that the patient could be left alone at home. Yet it was unlikely that supervision would be constantly available in any of the home settings available to her. However, supervision was available to a limited degree in the eldest daughter's home where the son-in-law was retired.

The patient's other major area of disability lay in functional mobility. She required moderate physical assistance for all transfers (i.e., bed, chair, toilet, and tub and shower). In locomotion abilities she required minimal physical assistance with a wheelchair; the patient did not contribute at all in ambulation or stair climbing. She required some physical assistance in performing grooming, bathing, and dressing tasks and more assistance in eating. These activities were significantly affected by a moderately severe disability in organizing visuospatial stimuli. She was able to function only in structured situations and with assistance.

In light of the patient's disabilities and the resources potentially available, several short-term interdisciplinary goals were identified as high priority. Major emphasis was placed on enabling her to deal with her feeling of discouragement, on increasing her understanding of spoken language, and on improving her ability to transfer from a bed to a chair and from a chair to a toilet and shower, with particular emphasis placed on her awareness of her right extremities.

In the same areas the long-term goals included reducing the patient's depression so that it interfered only minimally with independent functioning. To help achieve that goal, the patient was required to acknowledge the statement by the therapist about the progress she had made at the completion of each therapy session. The long-term goal in comprehension abilities was for the patient to follow the full range of ordinary conversation, with misunderstanding occurring only when the content was complex or abstract. To achieve this goal, an agreed upon activity was designed in which all therapists encouraged the patient to ask for repetition if she was unable to understand what was being said. The objective was for her to signify in some agreed upon way her failure to understand. This activity also contributed to increasing her "awareness of limitations" and thus to her eventually taking an increased role in setting goals for her own care.

The third area of interdisciplinary activity was for the patient to attend to her right arm and leg during transfers approximately half the time with verbal and gestural cues to be provided by all persons working with her. This activity contributed to the eventual improvement in her visuospatial awareness so that assistance eventually was needed only in specific predictable situations.

At the time of review 1 week later the outcomes of the interdisciplinary goals were evaluated and new plans were made. The patient had made considerable progress in her mood. The new goal was for the patient to independently state positive outcomes when asked, without the need for suggestions or recommendations from various therapists. Her verbal auditory understanding had improved, and she had been signifying any difficulties in understanding. A new goal was established to deal with her ability to express her needs verbally. The phrases to be encouraged were "let me hear it again" and "let me see it written out." The use of these phrases contributed to the patient's long-term goal of being able to converse about almost all everyday situations, with difficulties in fluency and word naming apparent only when less familiar topics were discussed. She had met the goal of attending to her affected side during transfers at least half the time. The new goal was to do so almost all the time with cues. The training of the caregivers focused on their participation in supporting the communication system being established and their understanding of the need for supervision and physical assistance with mobility.

At the time of the patient's discharge to her daughter's home 60 days after the onset, she was able to ambulate independently with the use of a heel cup and to dress herself independently. Her visuospatial ability had improved, but she continued to require assistance even in predictable situations. Major progress occurred in her comprehension of verbal material so that she was able to follow a full range of ordinary conversation, with misunderstanding occurring only when the content was complex and abstract. Her oral expression had improved less; she was better able to communicate about most everyday situations but had difficulty when less familiar topics were discussed. In general, she was able to express her basic needs more than 75% of the time. Writing and reading abilities had not been achieved. The family had been trained to help her use compensatory strategies when dealing with difficulty in finding words and in comprehension. The ongoing speech therapy focused on an increased degree of independence in these strategies. There continued to be concern about the patient's ability to cook safely. For a short time, this was the focus of her work with an occupational therapist on an outpatient basis.

The patient was eager to return to her own home, which she did approximately 5 months after the onset. A "medical alert" system and a telephone programmed for specific emergency numbers were installed because her son worked during the day. "Meals on Wheels" came for a short time, but her son took responsibility for meals aside from lunch, for which she used a microwave oven.

Nine months after the onset, the patient was able to care for her house and remain alone during the day. She spoke well without word-finding problems aside from expressing more complex thoughts. She continued to have difficulties caused by her sensory loss on the right side. For instance, she was unaware of a dishcloth held in her right hand. There was a right-field defect to finger motion on confrontation and extinction of touch on the right hand when stimuli were applied to both hands simultaneously.

This case illustrates the development of interdisciplinary *plans* incorporating both goals and means. The review process focused on evaluating the achieved goals and establishing new goals. The principal efforts during the planning process had been to identify priority areas that would contribute to solving the patient's specific problems—that is, the interaction of her impairments, their functional implications, and the resources available. When addressing goals, it is particularly important for the training program to focus on priority areas to achieve a level of success compatible with the individual's requirements. The patient's long-term goal of returning to her own home was achieved with the aid of several supportive systems, including technical aids and social supports such as "Meals on Wheels." The patient continued to show some sensory impairment, which did not significantly disable her in performing housework and only mildly disabled her in communication and mobility, although some impairment still existed in these areas on neurologic examination.

NEUROPSYCHOLOGIC ASPECTS OF NORMAL AGING AND STROKE REHABILITATION

William Garmoe, Anne C. Newman, and Joseph Bleiberg

Nature of the Problem

Rehabilitation is a learning process. The person with stroke, whose capacity to learn has been affected by multiple factors, is challenged to acquire new skills. Under the best of conditions, such new skills will enable the patient to regain at least some degree of functional autonomy and self-direction, or control, over his or her life. Most often the patient must learn new skills (or relearn old ones) and the surrounding environment must also change to meet the altered capabilities of the patient. Thus both the stroke rehabilitation patient and the environment in which he or she lives must adjust toward the ideal goal of maximizing autonomy and self-direction. Of course, not all patients desire to or are able to direct all aspects of their lives, and more will be said about this later. It is common to consider the challenges faced by the stroke survivor in rehabilitation, but consideration is less often given to the importance of adapting the surrounding (ideally, supportive) environment. The purpose of this section is to discuss the various factors that influence learning in the stroke patient and to consider practical strategies to foster an enhanced learning atmosphere.

To adequately understand and treat the stroke patient who enters rehabilitation, the treatment team must be sensitive to a range of issues. Most stroke survivors are older adults. The aging adult, as part of the normal aging process, faces many developmental challenges. These challenges include an altered role status (resulting from such events as retirement or a change in family structure), loss of friends and family, and an increased frequency of medical conditions. In addition, the normal aging process brings changes in cognitive functioning, which may not be problematic in a familiar, predictable environment but which may complicate adaptation to the demands of the rehabilitation setting. Of course, the neurobehavioral impact of stroke often affects new learning and memory, transfer of learning, communication, spatial-perceptual skills, and the capacity for self-regulation of behavior and affect. Finally, the stroke survivor must also struggle with psychosocial consequences, which can prove to be more limiting than the neurologic syndrome. These consequences include the loss of autonomy, altered self-identity and sexuality, and mood disorders, which are more common following stroke.

To the extent that the rehabilitation environment is able to recognize and respond to issues relating to the normal developmental challenges of aging adults — in addition to the neurobehavioral syndromes and the psychosocial consequences of stroke — the probability of a successful outcome will be greatly enhanced. Lack of appreciation for any of these factors greatly increases the likelihood that the rehabilitation process will be hindered by roadblocks and that the optimal outcome will not be achieved. The following section addresses these issues and discusses strategies to facilitate optimal new learning and adaptation in the rehabilitation setting. The focus of this section is on functional and practical strategies to facilitate the rehabilitation process. Where appropriate, the reader is referred to more extensive conceptual discussions or reviews of the issues outlined here. It should be noted that the emphasis is on the older adult stroke patient; the issues and needs of younger stroke patients are sufficiently different to warrant a separate discussion. In addition, the issue of preexisting psychiatric illness or substance abuse disorders is not addressed.

Normal Aging

Because the risk factors associated with stroke (e.g., hypertension, cardiac disease, atherosclerosis, and endocrine changes) increase with age, the majority of stroke patients are over 65 years of age, with an average age of 72 years.[24,39] Because many of these patients participate in rehabilitation programs to ameliorate the effects of stroke, it is imperative for professionals in the field to understand the normal effects of aging on cognition and personality and the interaction of these factors with the sequelae of cerebrovascular disease. It is also important to appreciate the breadth of psychosocial situations facing the elderly individual and the wide variety of personality and cognitive strengths and weaknesses within the older adult and among the elderly population as a whole.[15]

Personality factors. Although the concept that personality changes occur over one's life span is controversial (because of the many contradictions in the research literature), it is generally agreed that certain developmental theorists have provided valuable approaches to the understanding of the effects of aging on personality and behavior.[45] Erikson's theory of human development provides a particularly useful guide to understanding the evolution of personality as the individual grows older.[33] His theory finds the well-adjusted older adult in a stage of "ego integrity" (versus "despair"), in which successful adaptation to the earlier tasks of living in the areas of work and love leads to a sense of fulfillment and acceptance of the individual's life and death. "The possessor of integrity is ready to defend the dignity of his own lifestyle against all physical and economic threats. . . . In such final consolidation, death loses its sting."[33] This process of integration in aging leads the older adult to engage more in inner reflection versus attachment to objects or to others, such as in earlier stages.[60] The implication for rehabilitation of the elderly is typically in the shift in focus from vocational reintegration and adaptations to external constraints—that is, to assisting the older person in restoring as much functional ability and independence as possible so as to enhance the overall quality of life.[45] More is said about this later.

Psychosocial factors. The elderly person faces a multitude of stressors related to growing old.[24,68] The loss through the death or disability of a spouse or other loved ones is the most obvious source of bereavement and sometimes leads to significant depression, withdrawal, and apathy. Other losses can stem from retirement from one's job and the resulting narrowing of one's professional world and role in society. There may be a sense of emptiness as a parent when children grow up and move away from home to raise their own families. With increasing age, there is the additional burden of physical impairments, including hearing and vision losses, diminished libido, and reduced physical mobility, which can further restrict one's pleasures in living and harm one's sense of identity. Furthermore, cultural prejudices that lead to devaluation of the aging members of society and to restriction of their social, sexual, vocational, and avocational activities can contribute to a sense of profound discouragement regarding the future.

It is unclear how prevalent depression and anxiety disorders are in the elderly,[23,72] but the incidence of suicide clearly increases significantly in older adults. Stoudemire and Blazer report a 5% prevalence rate of clinical depression and a 15% prevalence if one includes the natural grieving response to the proportionately large amount of illness and loss experienced by the elderly.[68] The fact that many older individuals experience some cognitive decline further reduces their resources in coping with the stress of aging and increases their vulnerability to despair. Despite these factors, depression among the elderly often presents with a different group of symptoms than in younger adults, which can make the diagnosis more difficult. Older adults are less likely to report subjective feelings of dysphoric mood. The symptoms that may indicate depression, whether a dysphoric mood is present or not, include multiple physical complaints (for which nothing seems to bring relief); irritability; appetite and sleep disturbances (vegetative symptoms); excessive fatigue and low energy; and even suspiciousness or delusions.[23] Thus it is possible for depression to be evident even though the patient does not report feelings of sadness or dejection.

The diagnosis is further complicated because many medical conditions can cause a prominent depressive disorder. Also, the elderly often take numerous medications, many of which can result in depression as a side effect. Finally, in the elderly patient, symptoms of depression may include prominent cognitive impairment, and it can be virtually impossible to differentiate depression and true dementia. Cummings and Benson use the term *dementia of depression* to refer to patients in whom depression presents with marked cognitive impairment[30] — that is, the level of impairment is such that it fits their definition of dementia, but appropriate treatment results in reversal of the condition.

Another psychiatric disturbance sometimes seen in conjunction with depression in older adults is paranoia.[23] Paranoid delusions can result in part from various sensory losses that often afflict the aged, such as hearing and visual deficits, which decrease effective communication and increase the individual's sense of isolation and alienation.[64] An elderly person's somatic preoccupations, in the absence of physical disease, may also reflect an underlying depression.[23] It has been noted that late onset mania and schizophrenia in the older population are rare.[23]

Of course, because the elderly are often afflicted with a multitude of diseases and receive a variety of medications, psychiatric syndromes sometimes reflect underlying organic states, and it is imperative for the elderly person with abnormal psychologic symptoms to receive a complete medical workup, including a thorough evaluation of the individual's medications and their interactions. In general, psychotherapy with or without adjunctive psychotropic medications is increasingly seen as an important aspect of geriatric services. Psychotherapy provides the opportunity to explore troubling themes of growing older that may exacerbate preexisting "neurotic conflicts" and simply assists in the resolution of normal adjustment problems.

It must be noted that, whereas the events and circumstances that accompany aging are devastating to some, others demonstrate excellent adaptation to the profound changes in their roles and social supports and continue to live highly fulfilling lives. The influence of premorbid personality characteristics cannot be underestimated in predicting the individual's ability to withstand the traumas of aging. A positive outlook and sense of self-worth that are independent of external factors can become invaluable allies in the process of adjusting to the potential assaults on one's self-esteem and security brought on by the aging process. In fact, normal, healthy elderly adults may exhibit an increase in self-esteem caused by the confidence and wisdom resulting from the many achievements of a long life.

Cognitive factors. A number of research studies conducted by neuropsychologists have investigated the effects of aging on cognition, and the results suggest a complex interaction of variables. Factors such as education and socioeconomic status appear to be associated with less cognitive deterioration in the later years. A decline in cognitive functioning does not necessarily accompany aging (in fact, some exceptionally healthy adults, who represent a small minority of the elderly, retain their abilities in most areas of functioning well into the seventh, eighth, and even ninth decades of life). However, specific areas of cognition as seen on neuropsychologic testing appear to be more vulnerable or susceptible to deterioration than others.

For example, in her review of studies of cognitive function in the elderly, Albert noted that no differences have been shown between old and young subjects in the areas of sustained attention (i.e., the ability to maintain one's concentration on a task over extended periods of time) and selective attention (i.e., the ability to ignore stimuli that are not relevant to the task).[16] However, the rate and efficiency of general information processing on both motor and complex cognitive tasks do appear to be adversely affected by age, even in relatively healthy older adults.[16,22,74]

Although naming and verbal fluency tend to decline with age, other aspects of language, such as the ability to use sounds to identify words and to access the physical representation of the word, do not change as compared with younger adults.[16] In fact, in the case of vocabulary usage, conceptual understanding of words sometimes increases with age and experience.[22]

With regard to memory, in contrast to the prevailing view, it appears that older adults are likely to exhibit a disturbance in the ability to freely recall information in secondary, or long-term, and tertiary, or remote, memory.[16,46] On the other hand, studies on sensory memory (the immediate registration of information) and primary, or recent, memory have shown a minimal decline in older adults.[16,46] Recognition and cueing enhance recall in the normal geriatric population but do not completely erase the differences between older and younger adults on memory tasks.[16,46]

Mittenberg et al. explored the hypothesis that age-related changes in normal brains occur bilaterally in the frontal lobes.[59] They point out that elderly individuals not only tend to do more poorly on neuropsychologic tests measuring frontal lobe functions, but they exhibit behaviors consistent with the frontal lobe syndrome, as described by Stuss and Benson,[70] including reduced flexibility, spontaneity, and abstract reasoning and decreased initiative. Other researchers have also found signs of increased frontal lobe dysfunction in elderly versus younger adults, as seen in the use of less efficient strategies for solving problems and an inability to generate alternate solutions when their initial strategies do not work.[74]

An important conceptual approach to the understanding of the differences in new learning between the young and the elderly adult is seen in the model proposed by Craik,[27] which focuses on the environment rather than the type of memory store (i.e., primary versus secondary memory). Craik and his colleagues have shown that differences in learning abilities between elderly and young adults are minimized if the former are given strategies for effective encoding or organization of new information. This led these investigators to the hypothesis that the older normal adult is primarily at a disadvantage in developing and initiating strategies for new learning, which is consistent with the theory of frontal lobe dysfunction in the elderly described previously. Buschke's model of controlled processing, which structures learning situations to include contextual elaborations of new information, reflects a similar approach in understanding and remediating the deficits in memory seen in the elderly.[26]

Some controversy exists about the pattern of normal cognitive decline in aging. Based on the verbal and performance intelligence quotient discrepancies on the Wechsler Adult Intelligence Scale (WAIS) often seen in older adults, it has been hypothesized that right cerebral hemisphere functions decline more with age than do left hemisphere abilities.[54] This theory, however, has been disputed by researchers who explain the differences between verbal and performance intelligence quotient scores on the WAIS as caused by the effects of slower information processing and new learning deficits, rather than a decline in right hemisphere functioning.[17,59] The notion of "crystallized" intelligence (the ability to use well-learned information) versus "fluid" intelligence (the ability to learn and analyze new information)[50] is a distinction that supports this view because fluid intelligence has been found to deteriorate with age and is tapped more by the performance (versus the verbal) subtests of the Wechsler Adult Intelligence Scale–Revised (WAIS-R).

Finally, a caveat is offered. In his review of the literature, Hartke notes the importance of understanding the specific cognitive abilities of the geriatric population in the context of their needs and life situations.[46] For example, it is possible that the test measures used to evaluate the executive or problem-solving skills of older adults may underestimate their abilities to successfully solve real-life problems. In fact, the solutions proposed by older adults should be analyzed for their "age appropriateness" to fairly judge their effectiveness. The distinction between deficits and differences in comparing younger and older healthy adults is being made to assist investigators in more accurately assessing the strengths and weaknesses of the normal elderly by evaluating their abilities in the context of "social/cultural and life-stage demands of older adulthood."[46]

Summary and implications for rehabilitation. The various psychosocial, personality, and cognitive factors described thus far have important implications for the rehabilitation setting, where the older adult is expected to relearn old skills, assimilate new ways of adapting to recently acquired deficits, or both. These alone require significant physical and mental stamina and a sense of optimism about the future. For patients who are depressed about their stroke-related disabilities, the rehabilitation environment (which is removed from the familiar supports of home, represents a separation from other loved ones who may be dependent on the patient, and resembles a school-like approach to learning that is no longer familiar to the older adult) may be an overwhelming experience that offers the potential for further failure.[47] Furthermore, the typically youthful therapy staff, with their emphasis on physical and mental activities and the achievement of goals of autonomy, may sometimes exhibit a lapse in empathy and understanding related to the age differences with their patients. Failure to appreciate differences in the speed of information processing and reaction times in older patients and differences in priorities regarding independence can create unnecessary conflict and distress for both parties.[47]

On the other hand, the rehabilitation setting has the potential to offer elderly patients with stroke-related disabilities an optimal environment for learning by providing a supportive and structured setting for assimilating compensatory techniques and regaining an overall self-confidence, which is invaluable in preparing to return to the community. The critical factor in assisting patients in this process appears to be the recognition of age-appropriate goals and the appreciation of the vast individual difference in patients' external resources, premorbid activity level, and overall capabilities and outlook.

Neurobehavioral Syndromes

Neurobehavioral syndromes are disturbances of mentation and behavior directly related to brain dysfunction. Because stroke potentially can damage any part of the brain, it can affect the full repertoire of human abilities and performances. Comprehensive discussion of the full range of neurobehavioral syndromes can be found in several sources.[56,58,69] The present discussion focuses on those neurobehavioral syndromes following stroke that most frequently challenge the rehabilitation team.

An understanding of stroke-related neurobehavioral syndromes is essential. Studies consistently have implicated neurobehavioral and neurocognitive deficits as the primary causes of poor outcome for stroke patients. In a comprehensive study of factors related to overall outcome in a sample of 300 stroke patients, Ullman concluded that "The most critical determinant is the presence or absence of . . . defects in orientation, memory, judgment, and all aspects of cognitive functioning."[73] In categorizing 45 stroke rehabilitation "failures" on the basis of whether the primary reason for poor outcome was physical disability or cognitive disability, Adams and Hurwitz found that, in over 50% of the cases, cognitive deficits were the primary factor underlying poor outcome, even when recovery of physical function was good.[13] Similarly, in a study of 1506 stroke patients, Adler et al. found that patients with significant neuropsychologic impairment had a dependent outcome irrespective of whether they had good or poor recovery of physical functions.[14] As Lishman summarized, ". . . the mental components of the picture will often be decisive in determining the level of success achieved in rehabilitation."[56]

Lesion characteristics. Although it is widely understood that the location and size of a brain lesion influence its effects, many other features of the lesion also are important. Reliance on a simple lesion location equation proves inadequate for a full understanding of the effects of a particular brain lesion on a given person's behavior and cognitive function. In addition to size and location, Smith[65] and Finger and Stein[37] identify three major categories of neuropathologic process that relate strongly to the behavioral consequences of brain lesions: lesion momentum or velocity, diaschisis, and whether the lesion is evolving or resolving.

Lesion momentum refers to the pace with which a brain lesion evolves.[52] It is well established that rapidly progressive brain lesions produce far greater behavioral deficits than do slowly progressive lesions, a phenomenon referred to as the "serial lesion effect."[37] The influence of lesion momentum, for example, can clearly be seen in the comparison between strokes and low-grade infiltrating tumors damaging the dominant posterior temporoparietal areas. When strokes (high-momentum lesions) produce such damage, the result almost invariably is an immediate onset of aphasia. However, a low-grade astrocytoma can produce substantial damage to the identical region with spared or only mildly disturbed language function. Even within the category of vascular causes, there can be lesions of different momentum and, consequently, of different outcome.

Diaschisis refers to "the radiation of pathologic influences of focal lateralized lesions disrupting the functions of remote, anatomically intact structures not only in the damaged hemisphere, but also in the opposite healthy hemisphere."[65] This means that areas of the brain that were not structurally damaged by the stroke nevertheless may be functionally disrupted, contributing further to the neurobehavioral syndrome. One source of diaschisis can involve the lesion disrupting the physiologic state of remote brain areas, such as when local edema compresses distant structures. Another and probably quite prevalent cause of diaschisis is that most brain areas not only regulate a specific function but also participate as components of functional circuits for a great many additional functions. As Allen notes, most complex tasks require the "cooperative interaction" of distant brain areas within and across hemispheres, with such interaction including parallel and sequential processing and encompassing both excitatory and inhibitory processes.[19]

Evolving and resolving lesions produce different patterns of behavioral stability. This fact led Smith to develop the "principle of inconstancy," which holds that moment-to-moment behavioral inconsistency is a frequent symptom of brain dysfunction.[65] Smith observed that behavioral inconsistency tends to decrease when lesions are resolving and to increase when lesions are evolving. In the rehabilitation setting, inconsistent behavior may be interpreted as poor motivation or cooperation, when in some cases such variability may be the manifestation of evolving or resolving lesions.

Lesion momentum, diaschisis, and inconstancy have several implications for the treatment of stroke patients. Because most strokes are rapid-momentum lesions, behavioral deficits are likely to be in the more severe range of what is expected for lesions of that particular location and size. Diaschisis explains how focal and circumscribed lesions can produce disparate and wide-ranging behavioral consequences. Moreover, given that inconstancy in the patient's performance is a natural and expected feature of the early to middle recovery period, it is important for the staff and family to be appropriately prepared for this so that they do not place unrealistic expectations and burdens on the patient: "You were able to do this an hour ago with your nurse. Why are you unmotivated (uncooperative, noncompliant) with me?"

Diaschisis also is an important concept for understanding the neurobehavioral consequences of subcortical strokes, in which it is not uncommon for small lesions to affect what usually are thought of as cortical functions. Subcortical lesions can have this effect through many mechanisms, including the "disconnection syndromes" described by Geschwind,[42] and through disruption of ascending excitatory tracts whereby the subcortical lesion leaves distal cortical regions unactivated or underactivated, even though the cortical regions involved may be entirely undamaged.

Concurrent diseases. The neuropathologic state of the brain lesion in stroke patients certainly accounts for an important portion of the cognitive and behavioral picture, but it cannot exclusively explain the entire picture. Among the additional factors to consider are the status of the preinjury brain, the cognitive and behavioral consequences of a host of concurrent illnesses, particularly within a primarily older adult sample, and the possibility of dementing illness and processes in addition to stroke.

Symonds is credited with the often quoted statement that "It is not only the type of injury that matters, but the kind of head," and the empirical literature consistently has supported his assertion.[55] These studies, summarized in Bleiberg,[25] show that one of the most powerful predictors of outcome from brain injuries of all types is the quality of the preinjury intellect. In general, overlearned skills and habits are more resistant to loss following brain injury than are less well-learned skills, and people with exceptionally well-rehearsed skills, such as musicians and artists,[41] show more robust retention of such abilities in the face of brain injury.

The stroke that brings a patient to the attention of the rehabilitation staff generally involves sufficient sensorimotor deficit to interfere with independent living skills. The neuropathologic processes underlying these larger, more acutely destructive strokes, however, also can result in less dramatic but nonetheless insidious and severely impairing cerebrovascular diseases. This is particularly true in patients with cerebrovascular disease caused by hypertension, in which the cerebral hemorrhage that brings the patient to the rehabilitation hospital may be merely a more visible sign of much more widespread cerebral damage leading to a multiinfarct dementia. Other systemic diseases that affect the cerebral microcirculation, such as diabetes and atherosclerosis, frequently produce a generalized reduction in cognitive function, in addition to being risk factors for the types of strokes that bring patients to rehabilitation hospitals.

Stroke patients also are at risk for the many nonvascular dementing illnesses that become more prevalent with advanced age, most notably Alzheimer's disease. For some patients, preexisting dementia is first recognized on entry into rehabilitation. Advanced age also carries increased vulnerability to other factors that may result in cognitive impairment, such as sensory deprivation, medication side effects (including overmedication), and nonneurologic systemic diseases. This vulnerability to multiple causes of cognitive dysfunction (in addition to the stroke that may be the focus of immediate attention) argues strongly for the need to perform comprehensive neuropsychologic and neurobehavioral assessments of stroke patients. For example, the condition of two patients, each with equivalently severe aphasia and hemiparesis, can differ sharply by virtue of one having the lesion in an otherwise healthy brain and the other in a brain with widespread and diffuse disease. Clearly, these two patients present quite different rehabilitation problems and challenges.

Specific neurobehavioral syndromes: left hemisphere. The primary neurobehavioral manifestation of left cerebral hemisphere strokes is aphasia, which is treated in detail elsewhere in this volume. Left hemisphere lesions, however, can produce a number of cognitive and behavioral disturbances in addition to aphasia, and these are discussed in the following.

Lesions that affect the deep regions of the left temporal lobe, particularly when including structures such as the hippocampus and amygdala, can produce a significant deficit in the ability to remember and learn verbal information, while at the same time resulting in minimal or no aphasia. Lesions in the left frontal lobe anterior to Broca's area also typically produce minimal or no aphasia, but they can cause substantial impairment in concept formation ability, mental flexibility, verbal abstraction, verbal fluency, and overall verbal facilities.

Left hemisphere lesions usually are not thought of as producing impairments in visuospatial and psychomotor abilities; nevertheless, some important deficits in these areas are often seen. The drawings of patients with left hemisphere disease usually show an intact appreciation for external spatial configuration but an impoverishment of internal detail. A peculiar apraxia of the left hand is seen with lesions that disrupt the anterior corpus callosum. In such cases the lesion produces a right hemiparesis and, at the same time, prevents commands decoded in the left hemisphere from crossing the corpus callosum to the right hemisphere motor areas to activate appropriate responses in the left hand. This apraxia is most frequently seen in patients with Broca's aphasia, who very often show a severe right upper extremity deficit. An understanding of their capacity to mobilize their nonparetic left hand becomes particularly important in the rehabilitation setting.

In general, left hemisphere strokes that do not produce significant aphasia are likely to involve the posterior cerebral artery (PCA) or the anterior cerebral artery (ACA) distributions, with the more prevalent middle cerebral artery (MCA) distribution strokes being the most frequent cause of aphasic syndromes. In addition to the verbal memory deficits noted, left PCA strokes frequently are associated with right visual field disturbances. Left ACA strokes can result in a wide range of cognitive, affective, and behavioral impairments, which are consistent with the diversity of functions subsumed by the dorsolateral, orbital, and inferomedial frontal lobes, the subfrontal white matter with its rich corticolimbic pathways, and the cingulate gyrus.

Specific neurobehavioral syndromes: right hemisphere. Although many symptoms of left hemisphere disease have been well described and studied since the mid-1800s, the appreciation of the contribution of the right hemisphere is more recent and still less than complete.

The aphasias caused by left hemisphere lesions represent various forms of impairment in managing the denotative components of language. It is well established that the right hemisphere supports parallel systems for managing the connotative components of language and communication.[49] Such connotative components of communication include interpreting the emotional tone of verbal and nonverbal communication, generating emotional tone in verbal and gestural communication, using inflection and prosody to add nuance to verbal communication, and accurately perceiving the emotional expression of visually presented human faces. The disruptive potential of such right hemisphere deficits is apparent if one considers that most people have several ways with which to say "yes" and that at least one of these ways actually communicates a very clear message of "no." The patient with such deficits can completely miss the true content of a communication and, indeed, can derive the opposite meaning of what was intended. Given that much of everyday communication relies heavily on gesture, inflection, and other connotative aspects of speech, deficits in this realm are important to identify to help the family and staff understand the need to communicate with the patient in ways in which the denotated content is the truly intended content.

Denial of illness syndromes are among the most striking and disabling symptoms of right hemisphere disease. These syndromes are known by several names, including Babinski's syndrome (denial of hemiplegia), Anton's syndrome (denial of cortical blindness), and anosognosia (denial of illness). Although anosognosia is quite rare following left hemisphere lesions, it is fairly common following right hemisphere lesions, particularly acutely destructive lesions in which the parietal lobe is involved.

Currently it is recognized that the right parietal lobe is involved in regulating attention to both the right and left spatial hemifields and that, with right parietal damage, the ability to allocate attention to both fields is lost. The left parietal lobe can regulate attention within the right hemifield, but unlike the right parietal lobe, it cannot regulate attention throughout both hemifields. Thus damage to the right parietal lobe leaves the person able to allocate attention to the right hemifield but not to regulate attention shifts between the right and left fields; the net result is a disproportionately high allocation of attention to the right hemifield and a low allocation of attention to the left hemifield. Given that much of the obvious manifestation of right hemisphere disease is on the left side of the patient's body, the fact that the left hemifield receives disproportionately less attention can explain, at least in part, why the patient appears to be unaware of the full extent of his illness: the lesion that produced the symptoms on the left side of his or her body also produced an inability to attend well to that side of the body.

The central role of attention allocation processes in anosognosia usually can be seen clearly when such patients are interviewed. General questions such as "How are you?" and "What is wrong with you?" may be met with answers that nothing is wrong, whereas questions such as "What is wrong with your left leg?" (the question itself draws attention to the overt sign of illness) may elicit an accurate response. In general, the examination for anosognosia is based on the examiner starting with questions that do not focus the patient's attention onto the area of deficit and gradually framing questions that increasingly focus the patient's attention. Sometimes the examiner proceeds as far as turning the patient's head so that the hemiplegic left side is in the right visual field, asking the patient to move a left limb, then asking, "Is anything wrong with your left arm (leg)?" Most patients with anosognosia show awareness when given sufficient assistance in attending to the relevant data (the status of the left side of their body), but occasional patients have such dense anosognosia that, when confronted with their hemiparetic limb, they may deny that it is theirs and respond that "I left my good arm home" (or as one patient remarked when he was asked why he was in a wheelchair, "So I'll have something to sit on"). Even when the left arm or leg are not disavowed, it is not uncommon to hear patients talk about their left limbs in the third person and with hatred and depersonalization, such as described by Critchley,[28] whose patient called his left arm "the communist" because it refused to work.

The failure of the patient with anosognosia to attend to the left side of his or her body frequently is matched by an attentional disturbance for the left spatial field outside of the body, frequently termed *left neglect* or *left hemi-inattention*. Left neglect may be seen in all sensory modalities, although it sometimes is present in one but not other modalities. It usually is readily apparent to the rehabilitation team because the patient may dress and groom only the right side of his or her body, may read only the right half of a page, and may run into things with the left side of his or her wheelchair. Consistent with what clinicians recognize, Diller and Weinberg[32] demonstrated that patients with left neglect were more accident prone than patients with left hemisphere strokes.

It should be noted that the above explanation of anosognosia (as resulting from an attention allocation impairment) is consistent with the available evidence but almost certainly is an incomplete explanation. The interested reader can see Weinstein and Friedland[75] and Heilman and Watson,[48] although as Crowne[29] notes, no single model accounts for the entirety of the anosognosia syndrome. Anosognosia and hemi-inattention or neglect are among the most challenging neurobehavioral syndromes with which the rehabilitation team is confronted.

CASE REPORT

H.S., a 71-year-old female, entered rehabilitation 6 weeks following the onset of right middle cerebral artery infarction, which developed following a minor motor vehicle accident. A CT scan following the onset of symptoms revealed a right parietotemporal lobe infarction. Although she was independent premorbidly and cared for her disabled son, family members had noticed episodes of impaired mentation in the months before the onset. She had no prior history of alcohol or other substance abuse.

The woman's initial presentation was significant for marked anosognosia. Left homonymous hemianopsia and severe left neglect were present. She attended to nothing left of midline and watched her roommate's television on the right side of the room rather than her own in front of her. She did not respond to sounds or voices that originated from her left side unless the stimulation was very loud. Written sentences and constructions similarly showed neglect and spatial-perceptual distortions. She showed unawareness of her symptoms, and when attention was directed to her left arm, she reported that it was asleep. She showed virtually no concern or distress about her deficits, although there was evidence that she was depressed. She also displayed severe attention and memory impairment, and at times confusion.

Specific neurobehavioral syndromes: subcortical vascular disease. The subcortical regions of the brain have received increased emphasis in research and clinical studies of behavior. A variety of neurobehavioral syndromes may be seen following focal subcortical lesions, such as memory dysfunction, neglect, mood disorders, and aphasia.[36] Because they involve the cerebral microvasculature, cerebrovascular disease processes such as hypertension and diabetes can also produce bilateral, diffuse damage, typically representing the accumulation of numerous microscopic lesions. The predilection zones for the accumulation of such lesions are the upper brainstem, the midbrain, and the subcortical cerebral white matter. Among the key neurobehavioral syndromes arising from such lesions are the pseudobulbar states and the subcortical dementias. The concept of subcortical dementia is controversial, and an in-depth discussion can be found elsewhere.[57] As with Alzheimer's disease, the rehabilitation setting may be the first time a developing or preexisting subcortical dementia is identified, which will influence the types of goals that can realistically be set with the patient.

Pseudobulbar states arise from damage to the corticobulbar tracts, the most frequent mechanism of such damage being extensive subcortical white matter lesions disconnecting or weakening cortical control over bulbar nuclei. The primary symptom of pseudobulbar states is lability in the outward display of tears, laughter, or both tears and laughter and in the absence of the patient having an equivalent intensity or quality of the actual emotions being displayed. Thus a patient may think about something emotionally neutral or only mildly sad but break into floods of tears or (in rarer cases) laughter. In essence, the lesion creates a discontinuity between the emotions that the patient feels and the emotions that he or she displays. For obvious reasons, pseudobulbar lability of tears frequently is misdiagnosed as depression, and lability of laughter is misdiagnosed as an organic euphoria or denial syndrome. The key to correct diagnosis is always to ask the patient to describe the internal emotional state that accompanies the external emotional display; not uncommonly, patients will relate that their primary emotion during such displays is annoyance (or embarrassment or frustration) and that they are displaying emotions different from those that they are feeling.

Acute confusional states. One final neurobehavioral syndrome that must be considered is the acute confusional state, or delirium. Acute confusional states are common among hospitalized elderly patients, and they can be disruptive and result in significant interference in the management of the patient.[53] Confusional states are not necessarily distinct from the other syndromes discussed previously because the stroke patient may also be in a confusional state. The confused patient is grossly inattentive and disoriented, is unable to sustain meaningful awareness of and interaction with the surrounding environment, and most of the time shows fluctuating alertness and arousability.[69] Cognition is globally impaired, and behavior may be lethargic or restless or may alternate between both. Thought processes can be bizarre, and perceptual disturbances sometimes include hallucinations, delusions, or both.

When recognized, the confusional state can be managed by attempting to address the treatable causes and by structuring the hospital environment so that stimulation is minimized, very basic orientation cues are provided, and a predictable daily routine is established. The rehabilitation setting can actually exacerbate confusion by unintentionally demanding too much of the patient—through a full schedule, frequent travel from one treatment area to another, and a high level of stimulation and expectations for participation. The confused patient responds better if the rehabilitation team is flexible and uses strategies such as shorter sessions, scheduling treatment at times when the patient's attentiveness and arousal are best, avoiding unnecessarily moving the patient from place to place, and establishing a consistent daily routine (including using the same therapists each day).

Behavioral and Psychologic Adjustment to Stroke

Measuring the impact of stroke on the behavior of the patient requires not only consideration of the neurologic syndrome but also careful examination of who the person was before experiencing the stroke. The stroke is imposed on an individual who has a life history, which includes learned patterns of responding to and coping with stress and loss. The behavioral and psychosocial consequences following stroke result from a complex interplay between the type and severity of the lesion, characteristics of the individual, and the response of his or her family and social network. For those individuals who participate in structured rehabilitation programs, the influence of the treatment environment also is of paramount importance. The treatment environment can have both a negative and a positive impact on rehabilitation. Earlier in this section, many of the challenges faced by the aging adult were discussed. An important conclusion that emerges from the literature in this area is that, although certain general tendencies may be observed, the process of adapting to aging and disability is highly individualized.[46] In addition, it is important to cultivate an understanding of the social and developmental issues with which older adults are confronted.

Self-esteem and sexuality. The onset of any type of disability, particularly when the event is sudden and dramatically alters functioning in any way, can result in intense emotional reactions. Although it has been emphasized that reactions to loss and disability vary greatly among individuals, common experiences have been observed.[35,71] These reactions include denial, fear and anxiety, sadness and despair, pervasive depression, anger, and guilt. Not surprisingly, these responses also are often seen following the loss of a loved one[76] and can be viewed as part of a grief reaction. Such reactions may be experienced simultaneously or in stages, depending on the individual. When the patient enters rehabilitation, the neurologic course may have stabilized, but the course of emotional adjustment is often only beginning. As a result, emotional reactions and displays can be intense and variable, even when such responses are adaptive or a healthy part of the grieving process. In addition, in those stroke patients for whom self-regulation of affect is disturbed, a behavioral display of emotion can be even more intense and confusing, with the outward expression not necessarily correlated with the mood state.

Disability onset often represents a strong assault on self-esteem, relating to an altered sense of self-control or autonomy, self-image (including body image), and sexuality. In any individual the maintenance of positive self-esteem depends on many factors. If a key component of one's self-concept involves being an autonomous person who is capable of handling the physical and mental challenges of life, the onset of stroke represents a strong challenge to such self-perceptions. Even healthy elderly adults are confronted with the likelihood of loss of autonomy or independence in at least some areas of life,[47] but these changes happen to the stroke victim in a sudden and dramatic manner. Essentially, the abilities and skills that were important aspects of positive self-esteem and that brought gratification and reinforcement in interpersonal interactions are partially or totally lost, leaving the person feeling less competent and adequate. How each individual experiences and adjusts to such changes varies greatly. The following case example is illustrative:

CASE REPORT

A.D., an 84-year-old widow, was admitted for rehabilitation following a left cerebral infarct that resulted in right hemiparesis, Broca's aphasia, and ideomotor apraxia. Since the time of her husband's death, she had redirected her energies to platonic social relationships and church activities, and sexuality did not represent an issue for her following her stroke. However, she was distressed by the paralysis in her arm and leg because of her loss of autonomy. Her self-identity in recent years had centered around her ability to be completely independent, and the threatened loss of such autonomy was overwhelming for her. Other impairments, such as her language disorder (which did begin to improve rapidly) and hemifacial paresis, were less distressing to this patient, even though they affected social communication and personal appearance.

A final area requires brief mention here. The stroke patient often experiences altered sexual functioning. This may result directly from the neurologic sequelae of the stroke, from altered physical and cognitive capabilities, and from psychosocial factors. A commonly held view about older adults is that they become (or should become) asexual.[23] This view probably reflects many factors, including outdated theories of physical drives, ageism, and the anxiety that many younger adults feel about their elders and parents being sexually active. For the stroke patient the medical, physical, and cognitive limitations can be compounded through a loss of intimacy and privacy in the hospital setting, subtle communication of disapproval about sexual behavior from staff and family, and lack of knowledge about how to address or overcome problems with sexual functioning. In addition, there may be denial of the problem, manifest as reluctance on the part of staff and the patient to address sexuality issues as part of rehabilitation. However, to ignore changes in sexuality and sexual functioning can be a disservice to many patients.

Mood disorders following stroke. Mood disorders represent a significant problem for individuals who suffer stroke, with the most prevalent diagnosis being depression. Other types of psychiatric morbidity are uncommon (e.g., mania) and are not discussed here. The identification of depression following stroke is critical for several reasons. First, it is a common disorder following stroke, and one that often can be treated successfully. Second, depression often is manifest in behavior through loss of motivation, paucity of energy and heightened fatigue, failure to cooperate with (or invest oneself in) the rehabilitation program, and failure to achieve goals that seem to be within the patient's capacity. In this manner, depression can serve as a mediating variable that can limit the potential success of the rehabilitation effort.

For the purpose of this discussion, the definition of depression is consistent with the *Diagnostic and Statistical Manual of Mental Disorders* (DSM-III-R) used by the American Psychiatric Association.[20] Depression involves a constellation of symptoms, including depressed mood or marked loss of interest and pleasure in usual activities; appetite and sleep disturbances (vegetative symptoms); psychomotor agitation or retardation; and possible suicidal ideation. For a diagnosis of depression these symptoms must be present and prominent for at least 2 weeks. Significant interference typically is seen in disrupted daily functioning, and the severely depressed person may not even be able to summon the mental and physical energy to arise from bed during the daytime.

CASE REPORT

J.B., a 59-year-old male, was admitted for rehabilitation approximately 3 weeks after a cerebellar stroke, which required a craniotomy and surgical resection of an arterial venous malformation. His premorbid history included glaucoma and severe alcohol abuse, but he had been abstinent for the past 7 years and was very active in Alcoholics Anonymous. His mentation was essentially globally impaired, with arousal, orientation and memory, mental flexibility, and spatial-perceptual abilities all affected. He acknowledged a persistent dysphoric mood, feelings of discouragement, and sleep disturbance. He also tended to be irritable and felt anger at the demands placed on him throughout the day. His energy level was diminished, and he typically returned to bed as soon as he was allowed to do so. He denied experiencing thoughts or urges to harm himself, and he showed no evidence of delusions or hallucinations.

Depressive disorders in the rehabilitation setting often take the form of an adjustment disorder. An adjustment disorder involves a maladaptive reaction to a clear psychosocial stressor, occurring within 3 months of the event but not lasting beyond 6 months. Maladaptive responses are defined as involving significant disruption in occupational, social, or family roles in excess of what would be expected in response to the stressor. It can be difficult to define what constitutes a maladaptive reaction because a major stressor can lead to a temporary disruption in social or occupational functioning as part of the normal adaptation. The important point for the rehabilitation therapist is to recognize that a difficult adjustment may be identified with a variety of diagnostic labels. The term *adjustment disorder* sometimes is used by mental health professionals to avoid the unfair labeling that can result from a diagnosis of major depression.

The diagnosis of clinical depression must be distinguished from the normal or expected types of mood disturbance following stroke (or any significant trauma). Patients can be expected to experience periods of sadness and grief following stroke, which for some individuals can be intense. As noted earlier, reactions to the loss experienced with stroke may include sadness and despair, fear and anxiety, anger, depression, guilt, and denial. It is important to recognize that these reactions are common and can represent a healthy response to loss. Of course, not all patients display an intense grief reaction; some may show only mild distress or even seem unconcerned. It is beyond the scope of this chapter to explore the issue of abnormal or maladaptive grieving, and there are detailed discussions of this issue elsewhere.[76] In such cases close involvement of a mental health professional is essential to facilitate the patient's adjustment to rehabilitation. For the patient who is displaying genuine, strong emotional reactions, it is important not to overreact, which can cause the patient to feel even more distressed and anxious. Often, a coordinated, empathic response from team members will help the patient to grieve, while also devoting energy to rehabilitation goals.

In the stroke patient the ability to identify depression may be further complicated by disordered emotional regulation and expression. Emotional lability is a common problem following stroke and may result from a variety of lesions. The regulation, perception, and expression of emotion are complex phenomena that defy explanation on the basis of left versus right hemisphere stroke. Both cerebral hemispheres, the frontal lobes, and subcortical and limbic structures influence the regulation of emotion.[49]

It is not uncommon for members of the family and rehabilitation staff to respond to the patient who is emotionally labile as though he or she were depressed. This can result in a great deal of confusion and frustration for the patient and the person with whom he or she is interacting. Careful questioning and observation of the patient will help reveal whether the outward expression of emotion is disconnected from the internal mood state. For many patients, the tearfulness (or, less commonly, laughter) may indicate a general state of emotional arousal, and the patient needs to be questioned further to assess what the inner mood or emotional state is at that time. Erroneous assumptions can also be made when the labile patient is truly distressed, but the outward display of emotion is much more intense than the inner mood experience. Again, the patient must be questioned in a careful and supportive manner; it can be helpful to have the patient rate the intensity of his or her subjective distress. Similar difficulties can be encountered in patients who present with flattened affect or apathy as part of the neurobehavioral syndrome. The subjective inner mood state may not be highly correlated with the outward expression (or lack thereof), which can result in overestimates or underestimates of the prevalence and intensity of depression.

CASE REPORT

H.S., a 71-year-old female (introduced earlier as an example of anosognosia), was admitted for rehabilitation following a right cerebral artery infarction. She also showed symptoms of depression. Her affect was markedly flattened, but the few spontaneous comments she made had a depressive tone. Significant psychomotor retardation was evident. She rarely initiated conversation, sighed at several points during the initial interview, and acknowledged loneliness and depression since the death of her spouse (whom she sometimes spoke of in the present tense). A discussion with family members revealed that before her stroke the patient had been seeing a counselor for prolonged struggles with grief related to the loss of her spouse.

In this case the diagnosis of depression was difficult because flattened affect, reduced spontaneity and initiation, and poor attention and memory all can be seen as characteristics of both stroke and depression. In this case the depressive statements and recent history indicated that depression, in addition to stroke, was a factor.

In medically healthy adults, severe depression can produce a dementia syndrome with marked cognitive impairment.[30] Even in less severe depression, attention, memory, and the speed and efficiency of mental functions often are affected. Some evidence suggests that cognitive impairment is more severe in stroke patients with depression than in those who are not depressed, when controlling for the size and location of lesion in the brain.[67] In the Starkstein et al. study, it was unclear whether depression led to deterioration of cognitive functioning or whether greater cognitive impairment contributed to more severe depression. Quite possibly the relationship between these two variables is not causal, but instead also involves other factors interacting in a complex manner.

The relationship between stroke, depression, and severity of cognitive impairment remains unclear at this point. In either case at least one study concluded that patients with depression achieve lower scores on ADL measures as long as 2 years after stroke.[61]

Estimates of the incidence of depression following stroke vary depending on the source cited and the criteria used in diagnosis. In addition, the incidence of depression following stroke must be interpreted within the context of the base rate for older, normal adults. Base rate refers to the incidence with which the problem occurs among all older adults. Although there is disagreement about how prevalent depression is in normal older adults,[23,72] it is clear that the problem occurs more frequently in stroke victims. Robinson and his colleagues asserted that approximately 50% of stroke victims show symptoms of depression (diagnoses of major depression and dysthymia added together) within 2 weeks of their stroke, and rates rise to 60% within 6 months.[63] Others have suggested a somewhat lower prevalence of 30% to 40% following stroke.[38] In a series of studies, Robinson and his colleagues concluded that poststroke depression, when left untreated, may last 6 months or longer and continues to be a problem for many patients as long as 2 years following the onset of stroke.[61] Although researchers must investigate this issue further, it is clear that depression represents a major problem for stroke victims and that the prevalence exceeds what would be expected in a normal elderly population.

Poststroke depression probably involves the interaction of multiple etiologic factors, including psychologic stressors and the loss experienced, neurologic mechanisms related to altered neurotransmitter functioning,[67] and possibly the premorbid coping style. Robinson concluded that strokes that produce lesions in the left anterior regions of the brain are most likely to produce depression. Other studies have not supported the association between lesion location and depression, and the question continues to be examined.[51]

Finally, the preceding discussion provided several examples of factors, both neurologic and psychological, that often complicate an accurate identification (and thus treatment) of depression. The costs of either failing to identify depression or erroneously concluding that it is present can be significant. In the former instance the patient will be left to suffer with a condition that usually is treatable and may not achieve rehabilitation goals that would otherwise be attainable. In the latter instance the patient may be treated with medications that can have significant physiologic and cognitive side effects (including confusion). In the attempt to enhance the reliability of diagnosis, one avenue that has been researched involves the search for a neurochemical marker of depression, such as the dexamethasone suppression test (DST). However, research to date has failed to consistently support such an approach with stroke patients.[43] The diagnosis of depression continues to rely on self-report and behavioral observations by mental health professionals familiar with stroke syndromes.

Treatment intervention for poststroke depression is most efficacious when a combination of pharmacotherapy (if appropriate), psychotherapy, social supports, and coordination of team efforts work in conjunction. Antidepressant medications can be effective with stroke patients when factors such as age-related changes in absorption and metabolism of drugs and the impact of polypharmacy are recognized. The accurate diagnosis of depression, ruling out other etiologic factors, and consultation with a psychiatrist skilled in geriatric practice are critical steps in choosing appropriate medications. Even with such resources, it may take some time to find the most effective medication and the optimal dosage, and this process often lasts beyond the period when the patient is an inpatient. When depression is so severe that the patient cannot participate in rehabilitation in a productive manner, transfer to a psychiatric facility may be required.

Psychotherapeutic interventions vary depending on the nature of the problem and the background of the clinician. The depressed stroke patient will continue to struggle with issues of loss, grief, and adjustment to altered abilities after discharge from inpatient rehabilitation, and ongoing psychotherapy and medication management is appropriate for such individuals. Often, the focus of intervention during rehabilitation involves helping the patient motivate himself or herself to persist in treatment, derive reinforcement from gains made, and begin the process of grieving and accepting the loss that has been experienced. The rehabilitation setting also offers the opportunity for less traditional psychotherapeutic interventions, involving all treatment team members, such as the following case illustrates:

CASE REPORT

A.D., an 84-year-old female with a left middle cerebral artery infarct (introduced in an earlier example), presented with right hemiparesis, Broca's aphasia, and depression. Treatment strategies included antidepressant medication and psychotherapy. The patient was reluctant to allow members of her treatment team to perform a home visit or contact friends from her church, who were a source of strong support. She typically asserted that she would do well at home, without being able to share realistic plans for how she would manage. On a few occasions the patient took risks and placed herself in potentially unsafe situations while attempting to be independent in daily self-management. In psychotherapy sessions it became clear that her self-esteem had suffered severely; she was overwhelmed by her loss of autonomy and, in particular, the subjective meaning that she attached to such loss (i.e., that she was now an invalid and a burden).

Psychotherapeutic interventions focused on helping the patient to acknowledge her loss and fears about possibly not being able to return to her home independently and helping her to accept the loss of function of her arm (return of function in her leg was relatively good) and speech. Psychotherapy also focused on reframing her thinking so that acceptance of help from others was viewed as facilitating her return to autonomy (which was a realistic goal), rather than indicating that she was a burden to others.

Physical, occupational, and speech therapy sessions also provided supportive but challenging treatment. Rather than attempting to force the patient to allow therapists to contact friends, the patient and team developed visual aids on how to assist with stair climbing, which could be used to communicate with others. She also practiced communicating such needs to unfamiliar staff who volunteered to play the role of a friend offering help.

Over the course of her 1-month rehabilitation stay, the patient showed improvement in her affect, motivation, and self-esteem. She also was able to meet her goal of returning to her home, even though she remained reluctant to accept the level of assistance recommended by the team. The treatment was effective because the treatment team worked closely together on strategies specifically addressed at enhancing the patient's perceived autonomy and self-esteem and alleviating her depression. The benefit of medication, psychotherapy, or coordinated team goals alone would certainly have been less effective than the coordinated approach with close communication.

Regression as a model for behavioral disturbances. The experience of stroke represents a severe psychologic trauma: The event is unexpected and sudden; the prior history does not prepare the victim to cope with the situation; and the consequences or results are undeniable (i.e., deficits following stroke are usually obvious and often permanent). Gunther applied the concept of regression to help understand the behavioral disturbances frequently seen in patients who have suffered a stroke.[44] For many stroke victims the reality of what has happened is overwhelming, and they are unable to cope with their loss. Similar to the grief reaction following the death of a loved one, feelings of shock and numbness may describe the patient's experience; in effect, the death of oneself has occurred because the old self has been lost. Gunther describes several stages that may characterize the adjustment of the patient at such times. Initially the patient may become passive and dependent, relying heavily on others and not actively participating in decisions about such issues as medical care. Although such behaviors may in part reflect the direct metabolic and neurologic effects of the stroke (e.g., reduced initiation and active cognition), they also help the patient to deny the reality of what has happened to avoid overwhelming emotional pain and to maintain a sense of control.

Although the passive-dependent style may be adaptive during the acute poststroke period, entry into rehabilitation leads to a confrontation of this self-protective posture.[25] The rehabilitation setting entails the continual confrontation of deficits and limitations because therapists focus each day on affected limbs or mental abilities. In addition, the rehabilitation setting places a strong emphasis on compensating for deficits in behavior and cognitive functioning. The patient receives "frequent, obvious, and entirely compelling exposure to the consequences" of his or her stroke.[25] The patient is confronted with the reality that his or her self-perception is no longer consistent with the evidence encountered in daily activities. In other words, those abilities and skills that used to provide the individual with self-esteem and identity may have been lost. The patient may also lose all confidence in his or her ability to influence recovery and return to independence (e.g., helplessness and hopelessness). At this point the patient experiences what Gunther calls the depressive crisis.[44] His or her coping mechanisms are overwhelmed, and personality functioning becomes brittle and oftentimes rigid. When a person's self-esteem and self-perception are destroyed, the ability to meet the challenges of rehabilitation is severely reduced.

Faced with the depressive crisis, the patient seeks to restore personality stability and self-esteem. Ideally the patient finds adaptive means to restore self-esteem and stability of personality and emotional functioning. To do so, the patient needs to be able to accept the loss of the former self and to reconstruct a new self-identity based on the capabilities, skills, or roles that are altered from the past or that are perhaps entirely new. The rehabilitation team is important in this process, not only in helping the patient to learn new skills, but also as a supportive therapeutic network providing affirmation and reinforcement. If the patient is not able to accept the loss and to work toward developing a new sense of self, the result may be a pathologic attempt to balance self-perceptions with the current reality. Under such conditions the patient may display strong denial or a distortion of reality, blaming and directing his or her anger toward treatment staff and caregivers. Patients who are overwhelmed in this manner sometimes show irrational or magical thinking about their abilities or the expectation of recovery. When such behavior persists, rehabilitation falters and a sense of anger and helplessness can develop in the patient and the staff.

Implications for the rehabilitation setting. The impact of the rehabilitation setting often is overlooked when assessing the behavior and cognitive functioning of patients and when developing treatment goals and plans. The term *rehabilitation environment* refers to the physical facilities, organizational factors, and interpersonal dimensions that interact in an effort to help the patient maximize his or her level of functioning. Without careful consideration the rehabilitation environment may actually interfere with, rather than facilitate, learning and adaptation. Such unintended negative effects can occur in many ways. The rehabilitation setting may place excessive expectations on the cognitive functioning of the older adult. The patient may perceive a loss of control and autonomy in the setting. In addition, there may be unintended effects relating to the value system of rehabilitation and complications of the interpersonal relationships between treatment staff and patients. Thus, although patients are placed in explicit settings for the purpose of skills acquisition (e.g., therapy sessions and education groups), many less obvious conditions may interfere with the establishment of an optimal learning environment.

Consider the tasks that confront the stroke patient (or any patient) on entering rehabilitation. In many ways the acute care setting is different from the rehabilitation unit or hospital. It has been pointed out that the acute medical care setting tends to reinforce passive and dependent behavior.[40] In addition, as discussed earlier, passive emotional and behavioral responses may represent an early coping strategy in the face of trauma. Most adults have at least some experience with acute care hospitals so that they have expectations about how they should act (irrespective of whether such expectations are adaptive). On entering rehabilitation the patient can no longer rely on prior experience to guide behavior. Expectations that the patient become more physically active and begin to engage in self-care, transfers, and mobility may be very different from what was experienced during acute care.

A further challenge involves the many different professionals with whom the rehabilitation patient interacts. Possibly the patient has never been in contact with many of the professions that are represented on the treatment team. The distinctions between different professions may not be salient to the patient, and when such distinctions are lacking, it is more difficult for the patient to learn the identities of individual therapists. These illustrations are not meant to provide an exhaustive catalog of the demands placed on the patient that can interfere with new learning and adaptation. However, rehabilitation therapists who work with stroke patients need to be sensitive to the potentially overwhelming challenges faced by patients.

Earlier in this section a brief review of age-related changes in cognitive functioning suggested that older adults show altered abilities in many areas as compared with younger adults. In particular, age-related decline has been noted in the rate and efficiency of information processing and new learning skills. In addition, mental flexibility for novel problem-solving situations declines as a function of age. Such changes in cognitive functioning often are not problematic because the life-style of the older adult tends to be routine or consistent, with well-learned patterns and activities and a relatively low level of novel situations. However, the rehabilitation setting often is structured in a manner that unintentionally assaults the cognitive and physical vulnerabilities of older adults. The pace is fast, and patients may find themselves scheduled for 6 to 8 hours of treatment, with multiple location changes throughout the day. It is not uncommon for patients to comment that they feel as if they have returned to school or work (or in the case of one patient, to boot camp). Thus treatment settings may be characterized by high levels of stimulation, a large volume of new information to integrate, and rapid and frequent changes in treatment settings and activities. Many patients struggle to maintain the mental and physical stamina for such demands, and this may be expressed through emotional reactions. Most stroke patients enter rehabilitation with notable cognitive impairment in the areas of attention, memory, speed and efficiency of information processing and new learning, and mental flexibility, which may further affect the ability to adapt to the demands of rehabilitation.

CASE REPORT

J.M., a 53-year-old female, was admitted to the stroke program of a rehabilitation hospital following a recent, large, left middle cerebral artery stroke. She presented initially with severe nonfluent aphasia, impaired new learning and recent memory, and right homonymous hemianopsia. Her behavior also suggested that she experienced at least a mild loss of awareness of the extent of her physical and cognitive deficits. She was married, had a graduate-level education, and had no prior psychiatric history. Her premorbid medical history included cardiomyopathy, for which she had been a transplant candidate at the time of her stroke. During the first 2 to 3 days she showed strong emotional lability, intense pain and emotional responses to range-of-motion exercises and transfers, and increasing reluctance to participate in treatment sessions. She acknowledged periods of sadness, but denied experiencing a persistent dysphoric mood. On observation it was clear that the patient was overwhelmed by the physical and cognitive demands being placed on her. Within 2 days after admission the patient had been scheduled a full day of treatment sessions, with few breaks and frequent changes of location and tasks.

Hartke conceptualizes entry into the hospital for the older adult as a "dual admission."[47] The admission has literal and psychologic meaning. The psychologic meaning derives from the reality that can no longer be denied; it involves "admission to oneself that an illness is serious, perhaps life changing or life threatening." Perhaps the most frightening life change experienced by many older patients entering rehabilitation is the potential loss of independence or autonomy, which can also be conceptualized as loss of control. The patient has experienced a loss of physical and cognitive self-control as a result of the stroke. Most likely the patient has also lost his or her ability to control finances and home management, and his or her role in the family also has changed. These losses are temporary for some patients, until they are able to return to their prior life-style. However, when impairments require that significant changes in life-style or living situation be made, the loss of autonomy and increased dependence can be demoralizing.[47]

The rehabilitation patient must also submit to institutional rules and procedures, with an implicit and sometimes explicit expectation or pressure to comply with hospital practices concerning activities that previously were under the patient's control. Examples include decisions about when patients should be awakened and go to bed and what activities and outings are best for the patient. The patient also loses control over privacy, with personal space in the patient's room frequently entered by others without warning or permission. Many patients are not able to make certain decisions or judgments by themselves, as a result of their cognitive impairment or lack of knowledge about rehabilitation settings. However, the treatment team needs to be continually sensitive and guard against automatically making decisions in the patient's best interests when the patient may be capable of being an active participant.

The work of rehabilitation is carried out as an interpersonal process. The acquisition of new skills is accomplished largely through interaction with therapists, who teach skills, support patients (both emotionally and physically), and encourage or reinforce the attainment of goals. Stroke patients typically are much older than most members of the treatment team. The treatment team often is composed of professionals who are young and energetic and who derive satisfaction from working hard to reach challenging goals (e.g., many have a graduate degree or specialized training). Whereas rehabilitation professionals may be motivated by challenge, patients tend to be motivated by success. The rehabilitation setting often communicates a value system suggesting that, to succeed, patients should expect to delay pleasure and exert hard work and that gratification should come from stepping up to challenges. Many older adults value comfort over independence, and even healthy elderly people often are confronted with their changing capacity to be independent in all aspects of life.[47]

The age difference between patients and members of the team can also influence behavior and relationships in other ways. All humans react emotionally in their relationships with others. These reactions may be more pronounced in the rehabilitation setting because patients have experienced significant losses and may be anxious and fearful about the future. At times the emotional reactions of one person to another may be influenced by factors or issues that exist in an entirely separate relationship. For example, the stroke patient may respond to the rehabilitation therapist as though she were a daughter or niece. To the extent that the patient has positive or negative feelings toward the daughter or niece, these may be played out in the relationship with the rehabilitation therapist.

This is not to suggest that all behavior is the result of how the patient feels toward other significant people in his or her life. However, when the patient interacts with members of the team in a very negative, angry, or manipulative manner, he or she may be responding to issues that have carried over from past experience. At such times the patient usually is not deliberately or consciously acting in such a manner. The patient may not recognize how past issues are affecting present behavior and also may not appreciate the intensity of the reactions directed at team members. Such difficult patient relationships can be highly stressful, and staff should not feel responsible for fully understanding the depth of the patient's motivations or intervening to change the patient's behavior. Consultation with the mental health professional on the team will facilitate understanding of the patient, lead to generation of alternative ways of interacting with the patient, and help therapists to feel supported in their difficult task.

Facilitating Adaptation and New Learning in the Rehabilitation Setting

In the most general sense the goals of rehabilitation focus on the learning of new skills and the facilitation of psychologic adaptation to disability. A discussion of ways to facilitate new learning and adaptation in the rehabilitation environment introduces an irony. A critical step in the pursuit of such goals is to tailor the treatment package and environment to the individual needs of each patient, and to develop a set of general strategies for doing so seems contradictory. In actual practice, however, a balance can be struck between general interventions that benefit almost all patients and specific strategies tailored to each individual. It is a reality that deliberate, individualized attention to issues of new learning and adaptation often is prompted by the onset of problem behaviors — that is, problem behaviors in rehabilitation often serve as a cue that changes need to be made in the treatment being provided. The ideal situation involves preventive measures, through the development of conditions that support skills acquisition and psychologic adjustment.

Rehabilitation strategies for neurobehavioral syndromes. It is beyond the scope of this chapter to provide an in-depth discussion of the strategies for specific neurobehavioral syndromes. However, it is essential that the rehabilitation team develop a thorough understanding of the pattern of cognitive strengths and impairments as they are present in a particular patient. Although this may seem an obvious point, the intense demands on time and resources in many rehabilitation programs can result in uniform treatment approaches that may not accommodate the cognitive limitations of many patients. Similarly, the use of numerical rating scales applied to all patients, although valuable for research and program evaluation, can miss important information about how an individual patient with a specific syndrome can be helped to learn new skills.

In developing strategies for specific patients, it can be helpful to think of cognitive deficits and strengths on two levels. This approach is adapted from Alexander's conceptualization of assessing patient competence.[18] The value of this conceptual framework is that strengths and deficits are evaluated in terms of their impact on the patient's ability to compensate. Some deficits, although having a significant impact on functioning, can be circumvented through a reliance on other preserved cognitive abilities, possibly including the use of compensatory tools or techniques. Alexander refers to these as "operational deficits." For example, the patient with focal memory impairment but preserved judgment and self-awareness probably can learn to use a log book or appointment calendar to overcome the deficit. Similarly, many patients with aphasia are able to use augmentative strategies to circumvent their communication impairment. However, other types of impairment, which Alexander refers to as "general deficits," may disrupt or interfere with all areas of mental function and thus cannot be circumvented through the use of other cognitive skills. When careful evaluation reveals deficits that cannot be circumvented, rehabilitation strategies need to focus on environmental resources, such as family members, structured and supervised settings, and (when such impairment is severe) institutional care.

There is no clear dividing line between the two types of conditions, and assessing a patient's capacity to compensate for or circumvent significant cognitive impairment represents a major challenge for the team. Consideration of this issue requires an evaluation of the neurobehavioral syndrome, placed within the context of the demands presented by the environment in which the patient lives. For example, the consequences of mild left neglect and attention disturbance may be different for the stroke patient who is retired and lives with his spouse as compared with the patient who lives alone and takes frequent trips in his car. This approach suggests that the impact of most types of cognitive impairment is relative rather than absolute.

Ideally, each stroke patient would be able to learn compensatory skills that would allow for maximal self-management in daily life. However, stroke syndromes that present with prominent hemispatial neglect, attention and self-awareness disturbances (anosognosia), or impaired judgment related to disinhibited or poorly motivated behavior are least likely to be able to be circumvented through skills acquisition and compensatory strategies; the rehabilitation efforts typically need to address environmental supports and training of family members. Prominent memory syndromes also are likely to be difficult to circumvent, but such strokes usually also involve other significant impairments. Severe aphasic syndromes also usually result in impairment that cannot be circumvented. Within all of these categories the presence of a severe affective disorder may limit the patient's ability to compensate for or circumvent the impact of cognitive deficits. This is not to suggest that stroke patients with deficits in the mentioned areas are incapable of significantly improving or benefiting from rehabilitation. In addition, many patients who initially present with an impairment that cannot be circumvented improve to the point that they can use other cognitive functions in a compensatory manner. However, early identification of such impairments will help the team to focus their energies in the most efficient and productive manner for each patient.

Assessment within this framework should be multidimensional, including formal neuropsychologic evaluation and observation of functioning in real-life situations (or simulated real-life situations). Data from both sources represent different, although overlapping, aspects of patient functioning, and together they contribute to a clarification of the overall clinical picture. Thus, when formal testing and observations of functioning in daily activities seem inconsistent, the team should not question which source of data is correct, but rather how the two sources of information complement each other and contribute to a full understanding of the patient's abilities and limitations.

Assessment practices must also keep pace with new discoveries about cognitive functioning. Perhaps the best illustration of this involves the research over the past decade into procedural memory. Procedural memory refers to the skills acquisition or improvement that can occur in patients irrespective of explicit or declarative memory of having learned the task[66] — that is, a patient with severe memory impairment may be able to learn a new skill or activity (generally thought of as involving perceptual-motor or pattern-analyzing skills) and improve performance with practice, even though he or she does not remember having done the task previously. Procedural memory has been demonstrated in populations such as alcoholic Korsakoff's syndrome and brain-injured adults still in posttraumatic amnesia.[34] The possibility that procedural learning can be deliberately facilitated in rehabilitation to increase functional skills is exciting. (It may be that rehabilitation therapists have long been training procedural skills without realizing it.) However, much still needs to be learned about this concept, including understanding which neurobehavioral syndromes spare such learning and whether practical strategies for rehabilitation can be derived from the present knowledge of procedural learning.

General strategies for the older adult. Many practical strategies can help the rehabilitation setting become more supportive of the older adult's attempts to regain the maximal level of independent functioning possible, given their particular situation. Hartke emphasized that early education about the rehabilitation program and what to expect can help the patient become oriented and feel more secure.[47] In addition, patients can be encouraged to participate in the process of identifying and negotiating important goals, to the extent that their cognitive and psychologic functioning permits. This can be beneficial in several ways. Most patients will be more likely to assume ownership of goals they have helped set. In addition, having the patient help to identify and set goals provides subjective information about what he or she considers to be important for recovery and a high quality of life, which may be different from what the treatment team identifies. Having the patient participate in developing goals can also build rapport between the patient and therapist and may provide early information about possible motivational or adjustment issues. The types of responsibility offered to patients can also include the opportunity to decide for oneself when to wake up and go to sleep and when to take rest breaks (within reason, of course). Goals should be as concrete and measurable as possible and should be written in the language of the patient. This will help the patient monitor his or her own progress toward goals that he or she helped to develop.

Several simple strategies can be used to help the rehabilitation setting accommodate the age-related changes that affect new learning in the older adult. Older adults are likely to learn more effectively if the pace of rehabilitation is less demanding and if treatment settings do not have excessive levels of noise and distraction. This could involve establishing a slower pace on a daily basis, perhaps by reducing the number or length of treatment sessions, and providing rest periods.

CASE REPORT

J.M., a 53-year-old female with severe nonfluent aphasia following a left middle cerebral artery stroke (described in an earlier case example), displayed marked lability, intense pain and emotional reactions to therapy activities, and increasing reluctance to participate over the first several days of her rehabilitation stay. Intervention involved reducing the number of treatment sessions each day, scheduling specific rest breaks, and reducing the level of verbal demands or directions presented to her. The change in her behavior was almost immediate. Within 2 days she was able to participate in most sessions, showed an increase in functional activities, and, although continuing to display emotional lability and pain reactions, was more able to persist in treatment despite such discomfort.

New information to be learned can be presented in smaller bits, with increased amounts of rehearsal and practice time. It is also helpful to plan for a generalization of skills by practicing new skills in multiple settings, which are similar in nature to the situations in which the patient ultimately will be living. These and many more strategies that experienced therapists have discovered require a rehabilitation setting and team that is sufficiently flexible to accommodate the needs of individual patients. This can require greater efforts but is more likely to produce the fruits of successful rehabilitation outcomes.

Self-efficacy. Self-efficacy refers to the expectations that individuals have about how well they can master a difficult situation.[62] The concept was introduced by Bandura in the behavioral treatment literature for the treatment of psychologic disorders but is applicable to rehabilitation.[21] Bandura pointed out that people develop a sense of how well they can cope in problem situations (expectations of effectiveness). Research has shown that individuals are able to use such expectations to accurately predict how well they will be able to master difficult challenges. Thus self-efficacy refers to the internal self-statements and expectations a person holds about whether he or she possesses the skills needed to succeed in a situation. To master a situation that provokes avoidance and anxiety or fear, a person must believe first that a particular skill or behavior will be effective and second that he or she is capable of carrying out that response.[21]

Self-efficacy is applicable to rehabilitation in several ways. First, to increase the likelihood that patients will actually apply the skills and strategies taught, attention must be paid to their sense of self-efficacy. If the patient does not believe that the skill will be effective or that he or she is capable of applying the skill, training efforts are less likely to succeed. The self-efficacy model emphasizes participant learning over vicarious learning. This means that people learn to master difficult situations better if they learn in a hands-on manner rather than through observing others without actually participating. One of the strengths of stroke rehabilitation programs is that the majority of learning does involve hands-on experience and thus is a positive force in building self-efficacy.

A sense of self-efficacy also is essential for the generalization of new skills to novel or naturally occurring situations. Of course, this represents one of the greatest challenges of rehabilitation because skills are useless unless they are applied outside of therapy. Self-efficacy attributions can be powerful mediating variables, influencing whether a patient will apply skills learned in therapy to other situations. It cannot be assumed that skills learned in the physical therapy gym will generalize to other settings. Generalization may not occur for reasons such as the impact of cognitive impairment (e.g., memory and mental flexibility) and differences between the situation in which the skill was learned and in which it needs to be applied. New skills are more likely to be applied in situations that are similar to that in which learning occurred. To the extent that the patient's self-efficacy attributions can be increased, he or she is more likely to carry over skills to novel settings and to persist in using the skill.[31]

Self-efficacy attributions can be encouraged in many ways. They can be enhanced or even directly targeted as part of a psychotherapy process, which can be closely coordinated with the goals being pursued in rehabilitation. However, this is by no means limited to formal psychotherapy treatment with a mental health professional. For most patients the daily contact with physical, occupational, and speech therapists becomes a critical source of support, encouragement, and positive regard. The relationship with a supportive but challenging therapist who has confidence in the patient's ability to learn and apply new skills cannot be underestimated as a catalyst toward increased self-efficacy. In addition, as mentioned earlier, hands-on, or participant, learning, is one of the most effective strategies for enhancing self-efficacy.

It might seem obvious that providing patients control over as many aspects of rehabilitation as possible also enhances self-efficacy. However, too strong an emphasis on such an approach can backfire. It is more important to help patients take control of or responsibility for their rehabilitation at a level that is consistent with their beliefs and attributions.[47] Some patients may feel a greater sense of mastery or control when important decisions or issues are delegated to others.

CASE REPORT

J.B., a 59-year-old male (introduced in an earlier case report), was admitted for rehabilitation following a cerebellar stroke and subsequent craniotomy. He had a history of severe alcohol abuse but had been abstinent for the past 7 years. He displayed depression characterized by persistent dysphoric mood, feelings of discouragement, irritability and anger, reduced energy and initiation, and sleep disturbance. He was treated with a combination of pharmacotherapy, individual counseling, and moderation of rehabilitation goals. He responded well to treatment; his symptoms began to decrease within 10 days and after 3 weeks caused minimal interference. However, J.B. did not want to be closely involved in setting goals and making important treatment decisions. He felt that he needed to have others do so, and he resisted attempts by team members to give him such responsibilities. At times he became dissatisfied with this arrangement because family members and staff did not always act in the way he wished. Despite such times, he was most comfortable having others make key decisions and remained motivated for treatments, and this fit his needs with regard to self-control.

Summary and Conclusions

This section attempted to provide an overview of the multitude of factors influencing cognitive, psychologic, and behavioral functioning following stroke. The intent was not to offer an exhaustive review of the areas covered, and many of the topics introduced would require a full text to discuss in detail. A central theme is that effective rehabilitation can proceed only when the team is sensitive to issues of normal aging as they influence psychologic adjustment and learning, to the psychosocial consequences of stroke specifically and disability in general, and to the neurobehavioral syndrome resulting from damage to the brain. This includes considering the impact of the stroke within the context of the life situation of the patient. A second theme is that rehabilitation is most successful when the learning of compensatory skills occurs in a context that promotes self-efficacy because patients must believe that they have the ability to carry out the skills the team is helping them learn. Finally, rehabilitation efforts are enhanced dramatically when the group of individuals involved with the patient work as a team, coordinating the development of goals aimed at enhancing patient functioning and psychologic adjustment. It is when these three areas are appropriately addressed that the patient benefits most and that the treatment team feels most gratified in their efforts.

PREPARING THE FAMILY FOR DISCHARGE: AN INTERDISCIPLINARY APPROACH

Janet M. Liechty

Social workers have been practicing in hospitals since the early 1900s, assisting patients and families with the practical and emotional transitions between hospital, home, and community.[83] This endeavor to prepare and assist patients and families to develop realistic plans for continued care has persisted through this century as a vital contribution of social workers in health care settings.[85] Commonly referred to as discharge or continued care planning, this task requires knowledge and expertise in human behavior, family systems, health care delivery systems, and community resources. Historically, social work has been grounded in a systems approach to problems whereby an individual is viewed within the context of his or her family, culture, and society.[110,112]

Although the central focus in stroke rehabilitation is the patient and his or her progress, in actuality, it is both the patient and the family who are required to compensate for newly acquired impairments through learned techniques and skills after discharge. As the volume of literature indicates, rehabilitation specialists working with people with strokes and other brain injuries are showing an increasing interest in the family, including family assessment,[79,80,86,120] family intervention,[87,108,118] family functioning and coping,[91,101,102,106] family participation in the rehabilitation process,[88,104,116,121] and the impact of family variables on patient outcomes.[90,91,95]

As the rehabilitation team expands its concept of the consumer and its treatment focus from the patient alone to the patient and family or caregivers, the clinical expertise of the social worker is increasingly useful to facilitate the team's family treatment approach. Team efforts with families must be based on a thorough family psychosocial assessment to ensure that the goals and treatment are therapeutically appropriate and realistic given the family's biopsychosocial resources, capacities, and limitations. Moreover, interdisciplinary interventions with families must be based on the available research about caregivers, family functioning, and patient outcomes.

This section illustrates interdisciplinary team efforts within a rehabilitation setting to assess and prepare the family to appropriately accommodate the stroke survivor on discharge. Following a discussion of the nature of the problem, a model of family psychosocial assessment and a structure for team assessment are presented. Programs for interdisciplinary interventions with families are illustrated, and recommendations for maximizing the therapeutic benefit of informal team contacts with families are outlined.

The term *interdisciplinary* is used throughout this section and is distinct from the term *multidisciplinary*.[105] The multidisciplinary team refers to numerous distinct and autonomous disciplines represented on a team. The interdisciplinary team also refers to numerous disciplines represented on a team, but this team functions collaboratively to achieve common objectives. In the latter, discipline-specific goals are integrated into a larger scheme that "is greater than the simple sum of the activities of each individual discipline."[105]

Nature of the Problem

The nature of the problem that families of stroke survivors face in the rehabilitation setting is twofold: (1) The patient typically cannot return to the same, unmodified living situation he or she was in before the stroke because of altered physical capabilities, and (2) often either the patient and family are unaware of options for modifying and selecting an appropriate environment or they experience practical and emotional barriers to implementing their options. The term *family* is defined here as the pool of actual or potential caregivers after discharge. Although typically this refers to a nuclear or extended family, it may include a significant other, a neighbor, or a friend. However, it has been noted that, in contrast to relatives, non–kin assistance tends to be less intensive and to subside over time.[82]

The problem families face in the rehabilitation process is unpreparedness. Ordinarily, a family has not anticipated the occurrence of a stroke and so is unprepared to manage its effects, assuming that the stroke resulted in a set of impairments and caregiving needs that did not exist before the stroke. Rehabilitation is a means of specialized and systematic preparation. Although acute treatment is oriented toward a cure, rehabilitation is oriented toward (1) improving functioning so that the patient can return to the community as independently as possible, (2) minimizing the disability resulting from physical impairment, and (3) improving the patient's quality of life. In this way the entire interdisciplinary rehabilitation process prepares the patient and family for discharge: return to home life, adequate continuing care, and community reentry.

The continued care planning process is guided by several basic principles. The first is that *discharge should be to the least restrictive setting available* that meets patient needs. Ideally, this is a return to the patient's home or premorbid environment, assuming it was the least restrictive situation available at that time. The qualifier of "available" in the preceding principle is crucial; the efforts of the most experienced continued care planner are circumscribed by the internal resources of the family and patient and by the external resources within the community and society. In some cases the home environment or caregivers are not able to meet the patient's needs. In these instances nursing home placement may be desirable and appropriate. Contrary to popular opinion, a study showed that nursing home placement does not necessarily lead to poor adjustment or irreparable family disruption.[94]

The second principle is that of *the patient's right to self-determination*. Considered a basic tenet of democratic societies,[77] this principle refers to the patient's right to make choices and to direct his or her own life. It requires that the team members refrain from imposing their values and personal biases on the patient's and family's decisions. Specifically, this might include a patient's choice to move to a nursing home or the right to refuse a certain treatment. More broadly, it refers to a fundamental commitment on the part of the professional to respect the patient's capacity for self-direction and decision making based on the patient's own values, beliefs, and ethnic or cultural preferences.[97] This level of respect results in the professional taking a learning and information-seeking posture with and about the patient and family. The professional who is mindful of self-determination not only tolerates but tries to maximize the patient's and family's influence on the rehabilitation goals, treatment priorities, and continued care plans.

CASE REPORT

M.L. was a 64-year-old stroke survivor who was capable of progressing to a level at which she would need minimum assistance for all self-care and mobility tasks. However, she and her husband insisted that he provide maximum assistance for all her survival needs. This was difficult for the team because they saw this as inhibiting her progress and their rehabilitation goals.

After substantial education, training, and counseling efforts with the family, it became clear that the patient's and spouse's choice was to teach the spouse to carry out the patient's care needs rather than to teach the patient to do so independently. Although this went against the values about independence within the rehabilitation field, the team eventually had to put aside its values, respect those of the patient and family, and provide treatment that was consistent with the patient's and family's decision.

The third principle is that of *active participation on the part of the patient and family in the continued care planning process.* Research has repeatedly demonstrated that the family plays a pivotal role in the rehabilitation outcomes of stroke survivors.[98,113,122] Approximately 80% to 90% of health-related caregiving is provided by families rather than by formal support programs,[82] and families provide an array of services to stroke survivors, including companionship, shopping, transportation, home maintenance, financial management, personal care, and homemaking.[78] Families also function as care managers, problem solvers, and decision makers regarding care provisions[121] and are a primary source of affection, concern, and emotional support for the patient.[82]

Family members are indispensable participants in the lives of stroke survivors and contributors to the continued care preparation and planning process. Research implies that integration of patients and families into the decision-making aspects of team care and planning is efficacious to rehabilitation outcomes.[92] Active participation is also a fundamental component of empowerment models of intervention,[103,108] and it supports the role of the patient and family as decision makers.

It is imperative that family involvement not replace patient involvement. The patient, regardless of the degree of impairment, should be informed and included in treatment planning to the fullest extent possible. As Brody states, "Some families, with the best intentions, tend to infantilize the disabled or older adult and to take over too much. Any implication that control over [the patient's] life has been transferred to others can be detrimental to the patient's rehabilitation, intensifying feelings of helplessness, hopelessness, negative self-image, and loss of autonomy, all of which already have been stimulated or intensified by the loss of function."[82]

The fourth principle is to *maintain a focus on what the patient and family will need to know, perform, and manage in their discharge environment.* The range and number of potential physical, social, and emotional rehabilitation goals is endless and necessitates setting priorities and maintaining a focus on a select number of goals. These goals must be realistic, relevant, valued by the patient and family, and appropriate to the patient's projected life demands after discharge.

The demands after discharge differ from the demands within the hospital setting. The patient will encounter a much greater variety of challenges (e.g., uneven surfaces, increased sensory input) and variations in the complexity of challenges (e.g., answering the phone while cooking and caring for a child) in the home or community than what the hospital presented. She or he will make the transition from a predictable, regulated setting to an unpredictable, sometimes chaotic environment.

A patient's success within the hospital does not necessarily guarantee success in the home or community.[115] Therefore rehabilitation and continued care planning must attempt to identify and orient the patient toward the projected demands of the discharge environment to promote a transfer of skills and to prepare the patient and family to meet specific discharge demands, both physically and emotionally.

The principles guiding care planning and preparation are the following: (1) ensure that discharge is to the least restrictive setting available; (2) respect the individual's right to self-determination; (3) maximize active participation on the part of the patient and family in the continued care planning process; and (4) maintain a focus on what the patient and family will need to know, perform, and manage in their discharge environment.

Assessment

Each stroke survivor's family has its own unique set of life circumstances, its own preferred style of learning, its own ways of coping with crisis, its own distinctive display of opinion and will, and its own wisdom about appropriate solutions to discharge dilemmas. Preparing patients and families for discharge is a different venture with each family. The rehabilitation team can contribute most effectively to family adaptation when its members learn about and begin to understand normal family processes and the salient uniqueness of each particular stroke survivor's family.[87] Gathering and communicating this information is a primary objective of the rehabilitation social worker's psychosocial assessment.

Psychosocial assessment provides the foundation for the broad task of formulating a continued care plan with the family. It is the meaningful integration and synthesis of facts, observations, and information regarding the individual, his or her environment, and the relationship between these variables. This information is gathered from the patient, family, and interdisciplinary team through observation, interviews, and consultation.[117]

An additional method of gathering information is an empiric assessment such as the McMaster Family Assessment Device.[89] Empiric family assessment methods are increasingly used by social workers and family therapists in rehabilitation settings in conjunction with clinical assessment. The advantages and disadvantages of empirical assessment are discussed in the literature.[79,80]

Psychosocial assessment for the purpose of continued care planning keeps these interrelated spheres in simultaneous view: (1) the care needs of the patient (i.e., what is physically, socially, and emotionally required for a safe discharge and adequate adaptation); and (2) the patient, family, and environment's physical, social, and emotional will and capacity to meet these care needs. The assessment is not static; it is dynamic. It is made at the time of admission and continually revised based on the patient's functional progress, evolving care needs, available community resources, and patient and family emotional status. The patient's capacity for independent survival can fluctuate on a daily basis, as he or she gains self-care skills, greater mobility, or improvements in language and cognition. Similarly, the will and capacity of the family and environment to meet the care needs of the patient can change on a daily basis as the patient obtains approval for or is denied public benefits, as family members agree on how to meet care responsibilities, and as families change their minds about what actions to take.

Given the time constraints of an inpatient setting and the need to set achievable goals for the patient's stay, it is important for the social worker to focus on evaluating patient and family functioning as it pertains to the course of rehabilitation, adjustment to disability, and continued care planning. Psychosocial assessment in nonhospital settings makes use of the family's presenting problem as the starting point of therapy. In rehabilitation the de facto presenting problem is the practical, social, and emotional sequelae of the stroke, which includes the challenge of continued care. Of course, the patient and family may present with additional premorbid problems, such as alcohol abuse, marital conflict, or poverty. These problems are seen as comorbidities to the presenting problem and are addressed in that context.

Thus marital conflict certainly could be addressed in the rehabilitation hospital but is most appropriately addressed in the context of the couple's psychosocial adaptation to the stroke and the decisions concerning continued care planning. This period of crisis affords the family and the social worker a unique window of opportunity to observe marital and family relationship patterns otherwise indiscernible. The social worker may refer the family to outpatient counseling services after discharge for problems requiring longer term intervention.

CASE REPORT

L.C. is a 35-year-old, recently married male who survived a left-sided cerebrovascular accident, which resulted in hemiparesis and severe aphasia. Before the stroke he held three jobs (two part time), had received numerous citizenship awards for his community volunteer efforts with troubled youth and the homeless, and spent a great deal of time with his family of origin. His wife of less than 2 years traveled extensively for her corporation, and the couple rarely spent time together. The event of the stroke completely disrupted their pattern of infrequent communication and a primary focus outside of the marriage. Although married and attracted to each other, cohesion in their relationship had not yet developed. Their primary emotional attachments were still outside of the marriage, and they were hesitant and unfamiliar with operating as a team. Central to the couple's ability to make concrete decisions about plans for L.C.'s continued care was the patient's and wife's need to face issues of commitment, priorities, investment of time and energy, expectations of each other, and the future of their marriage. These issues emerged spontaneously in the course of continued care planning counseling and challenged the couple to work on their relationship in a way that might otherwise not have occurred. Enough positive resolution was achieved to make a safe discharge plan, and the couple readily accepted a referral for outpatient marital counseling services to continue the work they began in the rehabilitation setting.

Psychosocial assessment can be conceptually organized in a variety of ways. The unifying concept is that the patient does not exist as a psychologic being apart from his or her surroundings (e.g., family, work, economics, religion, culture, and society); nor is a person solely the product of his or her social environment. Instead, it examines the person in interaction with the environment; it is a complex relational model. The psychosocial approach to assessment enables the practitioner to gather data, observe, and evaluate both psychologic and social dimensions to functioning; and it provides a conceptual model to examine the relationship between these and other significant life variables.

A framework for psychosocial assessment is presented as a means of illustrating the scope of factors considered relevant in rehabilitation and to lend perspective on which areas are amenable to interdisciplinary interventions and which areas are most appropriately addressed by the trained mental health professional (e.g., social worker, psychologist, and family therapist). A tool for structuring interdisciplinary patient and family assessment findings is also outlined.

Psychosocial assessment framework. Romano delineates four major areas of psychosocial inquiry for assessment within a rehabilitation setting: (1) situational information; (2) cultural information; (3) interactional information; and (4) personal information.[117] In addition to these four categories, this author adds three other areas — (5) environmental resource availability; (6) family emotional unit information; and (7) family caregiving potential.

It is important to note that the data gathered and the information solicited are influenced greatly by the particular social worker's theoretic framework (e.g, family systems, cognitive-behavioral, psychodynamic) and that theory guides assessment. The amount of information a social worker can elicit is infinite; theory guides what information is important and how the facts and observations are synthesized into a coherent assessment.

Assessment of situational information. Romano includes in this category the "factual data about the patient's living situation, source and amount of income, resources, expenses and outstanding debts; type and extent of health insurance coverage; level of education and type of employment; avocational interests and activities prior to [stroke]; and the family group, including persons residing with or available to the patient."[117] This category includes structural accessibility of the home.

Assessment of cultural information. Romano includes in this category the "data on ethnocultural and religious identity, both that with which the patient was raised and that to which he still subscribes. However emancipated from one's background one believes oneself to be, people maintain shadows of ethnocultural values and belief systems, which affect their response to crisis."[117]

Assessment of interactional information. Romano includes in this category the "anecdotal and observational data on the patient's interpersonal relationships and about significant others' knowledge and understanding of the impairment and its implications. Noted here would be current and past marital issues, parent-child relationships, nature and extent of friendships, repertoire of social skills, sexual functioning, experiences and abilities in negotiating with complex social systems, relationships with pets, and so forth. Wherever possible, it is helpful to obtain behavior-specific information, e.g., by asking how the patient's family handles decision-making, how they communicate, how they fight, how they resolve conflict, and who has what jobs within the family."[117]

Assessment of personal information. Romano includes in this category "how the person has dealt with stress in the past, what the person's understanding is of the impairment and its implications, whether the person has an internal or external locus of control (that is, a belief that the person's actions can influence subsequent events as opposed to the belief that the person is a victim of circumstance or beneficiary of luck), the patient's personality style, self-image, rewards, habits, coping mechanisms, and emotional state."[117] In addition, information reflecting the person's health behaviors, adaptability, cognitive status, learning style, creativity, resourcefulness, and problem-solving abilities is useful personal data. Bishop and Miller, summarizing from several studies, suggest that cognitive disturbances in patients, more so than physical impairments, are associated with the impaired family functioning of caregivers.[80] Thus assessing the impact of a patient's cognitive deficits on family functioning is critical.

Assessment of environmental resources. This category, an addition to Romano's formulation, considers the availability and limitations of resources, benefits, programs, and services on the local, state, or national level that exist outside of the patient's nuclear or extended family unit. While the locus of the first four categories is the patient and family, this category highlights the options and potential for assistance outside of the patient and family resources. This can include both practical (e.g., a homemaker) and emotional assistance (e.g., a stroke support group) available after discharge.

The availability of environmental resources will vary depending on the patient's geographic location, age, income, and local or state provisions. The lower the situational, cultural, interactional, and intrapersonal resources and strengths of a patient and family, the greater their need for environmental resources to buttress them and assist them through the transition. Overall, families make modest use of formal support systems and do so when they have exhausted personal options and support resources.[82] Environmental resources typically fall into the following categories:

1. Financial (e.g., disability pension, public assistance, food stamps)
2. Health coverage (e.g., private health insurance, Medicare, Medicaid)
3. Social and emotional (e.g., support groups, friends, clubs)
4. Physical accessibility (e.g., transportation, architectural structures)
5. Educational opportunities (e.g., vocational retraining, library services to homebound)
6. In-home rehabilitation therapies (privately and publicly funded)
7. Home health aide or personal care aide assistance (privately and publicly funded)
8. Community programs and services (e.g., Meals On Wheels, senior centers, emergency call services, community case management, child-care services)

Environmental resources refer to the availability of any of the above to a particular patient and family. Environmental limitations might include a lack of state Medicaid nursing home beds, a lack of affordable transportation, cutbacks in senior services, an absence of local stroke support clubs or groups, and prevalent social ills such as ageism, handicappism, and racism.

To make use of environmental resources, the social worker must be able to inform and refer patients to appropriate services while simultaneously screening for eligibility, affordability, and accessibility based on patients' unique financial, geographic, and functional needs profile. The evaluator continually consults a mental contingency chart when screening a patient and family for benefits and community resource options. In recent years there has been a growth in municipal efforts to develop on-line computerized listings and descriptions of local, state, and federal social programs, self-help groups, and private sector services, but the majority of social workers must rely on their own experience and knowledge in this area and on dated directories, files, and lists.

Information about the family emotional unit. This category, also an addition to Romano's formulation, considers the overall social, emotional, and physical functioning of the family in which the patient participates. This category requires that the practitioner take a wide-angle view of the family emotional field. It puts the individual and his or her dyadic relationships in the context of a larger emotional system, the nuclear and extended family. The theory that facilitates this view and guides the gathering and use of the data is the natural family systems theory developed by Bowen.[81]

In this area the social worker gathers select information on each member of the patient's nuclear and original family, including birth; death; marriage and divorce; geographic location; sibling position; summary and dates of any emotional, physical, and social illnesses experienced; nature of relationship patterns to manage family anxiety (i.e., conflict, distance, accommodation, and emotional projection) and fluctuations over time; presence and activity of emotional triangles; family leadership over time; level of acute and chronic anxiety within the family system; and degree of emotional contact or isolation present between the various family members. The curious reader should refer to the literature on natural family systems theory for further exploration.[81,96,99,109]

A relationship between caregiver anxiety and stroke outcomes has been established. One study found that caregiver anxiety was the variable most strongly associated with patient maladjustment.[93] Another study found that anxious caregivers were less likely to report depression in the stroke survivor.[93]

Caregiver potential. This category is fundamental to family assessment in a rehabilitation setting. It includes the family's current experience and skill to carry out needed caregiving tasks, skill-learning potential, availability of time, practicalities of alternate living arrangements, physical capacity to lift or transfer the patient, number of potential caregivers in a family, preexisting responsibilities of family members, capacity for flexibility in roles, and emotional capacity and willingness to function as caregivers. Brody points to potential family conflicts around caregiving issues, such as who assumes the caregiving role, how to divide responsibilities, the type and place of care, and intergenerational problems when a patient moves into an adult child's home.[82]

Prolonged life span, the aging of the "baby boom" generation, and a decreased birth rate have resulted in radical demographic changes that affect stroke survivors and caregivers. The number of elderly people is rising and the number of young people declining, which puts more potential caregiving responsibilities on fewer individuals. As Brody states, "In short, all of the evidence indicates that nowadays more adult children provide more care to more older people over longer periods of time than was ever the case in the past."[82]

Families may attempt to provide care at the expense of their own goals, jobs, social lives, or well-being. Macnamara et al. summarize the findings of numerous studies, reporting the following symptoms of caregiver strain: guilt, somatic complaints, fatigue, anxiety, depression, sleep disturbances, social withdrawal, marital disturbances, and decreased employment.[102] In light of these issues it is imperative that the social worker and team collaborate with the family to carefully assess their caregiving potential, build in social support buffers[95] and preventive treatment, and, most important, respect the family's ability to know its own limits and make decisions aimed at preserving the entire family's well-being.

CASE REPORT

G.B. was a 69-year-old widowed stroke survivor who, at discharge, required moderate physical assistance with toileting and other personal care, transfers, and homemaking. Although her cognition enabled her to use good judgment and remain safely alone, she required an attendant for physical assistance. Extended-family members initially made generous offers to be available to G.B. on a 24-hour basis, and she gladly agreed to this arrangement because it averted nursing home placement. However, as discharge neared, it became clear this plan would not work.

Despite good intentions and herculean efforts, the family members were not able to attend family training sessions because of their work schedules and family responsibilities nor were they able to find time to take G.B. home on an overnight pass or to attend crucial therapy and planning sessions with the social worker. The reality gradually became clear: The family was emotionally willing to provide care but practically unable to do so. Although this family may have risked job losses and abdicated other responsibilities to care for the patient in the first few days or weeks after discharge, this care plan would not have been sustainable. The family's insufficient compliance highlighted a major discrepancy between their intentions and their capacity to provide care after discharge. After exploration of the contributing factors in a family counseling session, the assessment was revised to reflect the family's caregiving potential more accurately.

The entire team contributes directly or indirectly to the ongoing psychosocial assessment. The first assessment category (situational) is gathered by a variety of team members. The second category (cultural) is primarily assessed by the social worker, who is responsible to assist the team in understanding cultural variations and how these may have an impact on the patient or family's roles, perceptions, and expectations. The third (interactional) and fourth (personal) categories are assessed formally by the social worker and psychologist but are linked closely to the entire team's observations, insights, and input. The fifth (environmental) and sixth (family emotional unit) assessment categories are assessed primarily by the team social worker, who communicates pertinent findings, changes over time, and treatment implications to the team.

The seventh and final category (caregiver potential) is assessed by the team members who observe and work directly with family members in hands-on training situations (e.g., nursing, physical, occupational, and speech therapies) and the social worker. The team members evaluate for physical capacity, learning potential, and safety, and the social worker evaluates for the family's availability, dependability, and emotional capacity to assume the caregiving role. The physician often contributes to this part of the assessment, particularly when the family has selected the physician as the team member with whom they want to discuss difficult placement issues. Often, the family seeks reassurance that the decision they are making is medically necessary for the patient or family members, which typically indicates a high degree of perceived caregiver burden in the family.

This overview of a model of assessment illustrates the scope of family psychosocial assessment pertinent to rehabilitation and the areas in which the interdisciplinary team contributes significantly to the family evaluation. A structure for standardizing the team's assessment is considered in the following.

Interdisciplinary team assessment. If much of the family psychosocial assessment is based on interdisciplinary observation, the question becomes how to facilitate the exchange of information and findings across disciplines. In addition to verbal exchange in regularly scheduled team conferences, a structure can be employed to make salient aspects of each discipline's evaluations available to the entire team. The continued care planning process is unequivocally contingent on knowledge about the patient's functional status. To summarize these team findings in an orderly and usable manner and to facilitate the exchange of team members' information and assessments, a multiuser functional status rating form is needed. The Functional Status Report (FSR) serves this purpose.[107] The FSR incorporates functional rating scales from the Functional Independence Measure,[114] the Rehabilitation Institute of Chicago Functional Assessment Scale,[111] and the Functional Assessment Measures.[119]

The FSR is an interdisciplinary tool used to document (1) patient and family levels of functioning at the time of admission and discharge and (2) the rehabilitation goals. The FSR customized for use in the Stroke Recovery Program at the National Rehabilitation Hospital is a set of 70 behaviorally based items to be evaluated and scored on a predefined seven-point scale from independence to dependence on tasks such as self-care skills and cognitive functioning. The FSR does not provide or assume interpretation of the data. The use and interpretation of these data are the charge of each team member within his or her own assessment model and theoretical framework.

Once completed by the team, the FSR is a useful visual aid, providing a broad interdisciplinary view of the patient's overall functioning and the family's functioning on selected scales. Although the FSR items do not do justice to the depth of evaluation team members from each discipline conduct with the patient and family, it provides a standardized summary of team members' findings. It is also a visual cue to consider the interrelatedness of all data and team members' efforts.

For example, although the social worker is not trained to rate a patient on ambulation or dysphagia, these data are crucial in assisting the family with developing a safe discharge plan. Similarly, it is not the physical therapist's expertise to evaluate family dynamics, but information such as the availability of family members to provide patient care has significant implications for the type of education and goals addressed in physical therapy.

Although responsibility for rating each item is assigned to a specific member(s) of the team (e.g., expressive communication to the speech therapist), all team members are free to contribute observations and opinions on rating any of the items. It requires role release, which is the temporary suspension of team members' unique perspective, to generate a cooperative assessment about problems facing the patient or family. Role release is the deliberate, time-limited surrender of discrete, discipline-defined boundaries for the purpose of improved collaboration and assessment. It exemplifies interdisciplinary (versus multidisciplinary) evaluation.

The FSR also facilitates realistic and objective assessment and goal setting because it requires team members to use a standardized measure of functional status and expected gains. This helps reduce the likelihood of team members' subjectivity influencing their prognosis for improvement. Families can unwittingly pressure therapists to present idealistic promises of recovery, and therapists require objectivity to remain realistically hopeful. The team process can also be self-correcting; if one team member's FSR rating of cognitive status and prognosis is unrealistic, the probability is good that another member will challenge it and move the team toward a more objective appraisal.

In summary, the FSR facilitates a team assessment in several ways. First, it provides a visual cue for the team to focus on the gestalt of patient functioning and family variables rather than on discrete functional tasks taken out of context. Second, it provides a structure around which role release can occur to foster contributions across the lines of each unique discipline. Third, the FSR facilitates realistic and objective team assessment and goal setting through the use of standardized measures and the process of self-correction within the team setting.

CASE REPORT

A.J., a 67-year-old energetic and extremely independent widow, survived a severe left cerebrovascular accident with hemiparalysis. Her primary concern was to return to her rural trailer home in a nearby state about 100 miles from the hospital. She had only one daughter who lived in the same city as the hospital and had no other relatives. The closest neighbors to her trailer were 2 miles away, and none were home during the day.

At the time of the rehabilitation hospital admission, the patient required maximum assistance with all mobility, transfers, and self-care functions. She also showed severe cognitive deficits with impaired memory, insight, judgment, and safety skills. Her progress in rehabilitation was minimal, influenced by the severity of the impairment, low cognitive and learning potential, and chronic levels of family anxiety. Even so, she insisted on returning to an independent life in her trailer and vehemently refused the idea of going to live with her daughter and family. She reacted even more negatively to the idea of a nursing home in her own town or near her daughter.

The anxiety level in the family was quite high, with a history of conflict and unresolved emotional issues between the patient and her daughter. The daughter, highly ambivalent and unable to clarify her own opinion regarding the discharge placement, could not openly disagree with her mother's wishes despite the significant cognitive problems interfering with the patient's judgment and planning.

The daughter was a single parent who worked full time and had health problems of her own, including back problems. Her physical and practical ability to meet the needs of her mother in her home was dubious, yet she asserted that she would take her mother home. The patient's daughter briefly considered a nursing home placement, but with this option came feelings of guilt and the worry of increased conflict with her mother. The option of the patient applying for Medicaid was traumatic because it meant the patient would need to sell her land and home before qualifying.

The potential for the rehabilitation team to become mired in the strong emotional currents of this family was high. In the absence of realistic goals and planning on the part of the patient and her daughter, the team had to rely on its own judgment about appropriate discharge options based on the FSR and patient's rate of progress. Although the patient and family applied intense pressure to the team to set unrealistic goals so that the family could reassure the patient she would return home independently, the team was able to stay anchored in a factual assessment reflected in the FSR. One of the team members reacted strongly and negatively to the idea of the patient being discharged to a nursing home, although it seemed as though there were no other viable option. In reaction to this, he temporarily found himself overestimating the patient's ability to be independent and the daughter's ability to provide hands-on care, but with team input and his own FSR ratings before him, he was able to regain objectivity.

The FSR data also helped the team to focus on the composite of factors rather than on one particular discipline's area of expertise. A.J. showed maximum dependence on mobility, self-care, and transfers; severe cognitive impairments of judgment and safety; and no availability of home health aide resources in the rural area from which she came. Although any one of these deficits may not have rendered the patient's goal impossible, the aggregate data did. The FSR provided an interdisciplinary-based anchor in assessment that assisted the team in making a calm, unified recommendation about a continued care plan in a highly anxious family field.

This case report demonstrates three ways in which the FSR facilitates a team assessment: (1) as a visual cue for the team to focus on the gestalt of patient functioning and family variables; (2) as a structure around which role release can occur; and (3) as a set of measures that promotes objectivity and allows for self-correction within the team setting.

A.J.'s case highlights the need to assess the two spheres mentioned earlier: the care needs of the patient (what is physically, socially, and emotionally required for a safe discharge and adequate adaptation) and the patient's, family's, and environment's physical, social, and emotional will and capacity to meet these care needs. A thorough family psychosocial assessment provides the basis for interdisciplinary team interventions with families, as described below.

Interventions

Assessment and intervention are not discrete activities in actual practice; they are interdependent, and one informs the other over time. The team cannot make an appropriate assessment and plan without input from the patient and family; and the very process of seeking their input and participation begins preparing the family for change. Developing the continuing care plan and intervening effectively with the family to prepare them for discharge is a complex endeavor. Each patient and each family member has individual goals, survival needs, and responsibilities. These competing agendas and possible family dysfunction may produce emotional or practical barriers to carrying out a plan. It has been shown that stroke survivors of poorer functioning families have poorer treatment adherence after stroke than those of better functioning families.[94]

The rationale for including families in the rehabilitation process has been offered previously in this section and is considered to be a basic principle by which continued care planning is carried out. There is a growing consensus in the literature that families must be full participants in the rehabilitation process, that systematic family intervention and treatment is needed, and that family variables do affect patient outcomes. Much of the family research focuses on the effect of disability on families, such as describing characteristics of caregiver strain,[102] caregiver burden,[101] or marital adjustment after an injury.[106] Other studies examine potential mitigating variables to poor family adjustment following disability, such as social support.[95,100]

An area of study that is particularly relevant to the rehabilitation field is that of family functioning variables as predictors of stroke outcomes. In one study, family variables were better predictors of patient adjustment and days of rehospitalization than typical clinical variables such as mood, age, or side of lesion.[91] Another study found that family functioning positively influences adherence to treatment, but that patient functional capacity has no significant impact on family functioning.[92] Family functioning has been shown to predict some clinical variables, but the reverse is not true. Contrary to popular assumptions, this suggests that the family may influence the condition more than the condition influences the family. If this finding persists, it has profound implications for the focus of treatment in rehabilitation.

In establishing the goals of family intervention, it is important to delineate which family variables have been found to be associated with patient adjustment and outcomes. The family variable of affective responsiveness (i.e., the ability to respond with an appropriate quality and quantity of feelings) consistently predicted reduced rehospitalization time the year after stroke.[92] In another study the following variables were found in families that adhered to treatment after stroke: communication (clarity and directness of information exchange), problem solving (ability of the family to solve problems effectively), and affective investment (the interest family members invest in each other).[92]

Successful stroke care at home 1 year after the onset has been associated with families in which the caregiver (1) demonstrates more knowledge of stroke care than other caregivers in the study; (2) is less depressed initially; (3) is married to the survivor; (4) is more likely to have attended a stroke education class; and (5) reports healthy family functioning.[90] Successful psychosocial adjustment has been linked to the availability of social support, the patient's satisfaction with social supports, the support of a significant personal relationship, the support of close friends, and the support of those in one's community.[95] Stroke education and practical caregiving rehearsal have also been associated with successful outcomes, and the benefits of this type of education were found to be sustained and enhanced by concurrent family counseling.[92]

These findings suggest that training, education, and counseling interventions with families should attempt to develop or enhance the characteristics associated with successful outcomes. Thus reasonable and prudent goals for family intervention include the following:

1. Enhance communication skills (clarity and directness of information exchange) between family and patient.
2. Reduce caregiver depression.
3. Increase family's knowledge about stroke care.
4. Increase family's practical skills in stroke care.

5. Minimize family dysfunction.
6. Enhance appropriate levels of affective responsiveness and investment.
7. Increase the likelihood of families participating in stroke education classes.
8. Teach or enhance family problem-solving skills.

Outlined below are team programmatic interventions that encourage family participation and collaboration with the team to prepare for the patient's discharge and that respond to the implications for treatment found in the literature. Finally, recommendations for maximizing the therapeutic benefit of informal team contacts with families are outlined.

Programmatic interventions to prepare families for discharge. In a rehabilitation setting, families often have occasion to participate in a variety of classes, educational and support groups, hands-on training, and structured activities planned by hospital staff. Ideally, these programmatic interventions are coordinated within an overall plan.

One model for such a plan is the Caregiver Education Program, such as the Stroke Recovery Program that the National Rehabilitation Hospital is currently developing. This is an education, training, and family counseling program for stroke patients and their caregivers and is integrated into the total rehabilitation program. The Caregiver Education Program provides a framework for structuring, coordinating, and implementing all aspects of caregiver and family involvement in the rehabilitation process. The Caregiver Education Program aims to empower caregivers and families with information, skills, choices, and attitudes that will increase the likelihood of successful home care, family adjustment, and community reentry.

The Caregiver Education Program may be structured around a timeline from admission to discharge and assignment of responsibilities to specific team members. For example, on the day of admission, the basic goals are to begin establishing a rapport between the family and patient and the key team members (primary nurse, physician, and social worker) and to communicate the structure and expectations of the program. The family and patient also receive an educational packet with materials on orientation, educational groups, stroke prevention, rehabilitation expectations, and stroke and caregiver community support group information. Components of the Caregiver Education Program are outlined and described in the following.

Orientation seminars. Seminars are offered once a week or more to introduce new families and patients to the rehabilitation philosophy, typical schedules, expectations, descriptions of the different team players, and how and when to use each. The orientation group may also provide initial emotional support to new families who have questions and uncertainties about this next stage of stroke treatment.

Family support groups. Participation in hospital stroke support groups is sometimes limited to current patients and families or may also include former patients and families. The "buffering effect" of social support on stroke survivors' and families' potential adjustment problems has been documented.[95]

Family training. Families are scheduled to participate in an agreed on number of therapy hours (usually 3 to 9 hours) to learn safe and effective mobility, communication, and self-care techniques with the patient. During training, families are exposed to what the patient is capable of doing independently, and this knowledge decreases the likelihood of either exaggerated or inadequate assistance given by the family to the stroke survivor.

Training helps the family move toward a more realistic and factual appraisal of the patient's capabilities, progress, potential, needs, and limitations. One or two training sessions can also contribute greatly to the team's evolving assessment and formulation of an appropriate discharge plan. Training equips the family with the skills and techniques that will be needed in the discharge environment and highlights those skills that need further development.

Family and patient health and nutrition education. A nurse or physician may lead classes or individual instruction on stroke prevention, medication, hypertension, and diabetes management. Dieticians may counsel families regarding nutrition, weight loss, or dietetic restrictions.

Day pass assignments. A day pass assignment is "homework" given to the patient and family, which they are to complete away from the hospital during a planned outing of several hours. Day passes are designed to give the patient and family the opportunity to practice targeted skills in a realistic life setting that the patient is likely to encounter after discharge. Specific goals are set for each day pass, and the family and patient report back to the team on their return. Day passes help to clarify and refine rehabilitation goals, test if the patient's and family's new skills can be generalized within the community, and promote realistic discharge preparation and planning.

Community reentry group. The community reentry group is a 3-week series of community outings with a different focus each week. Each week the therapeutic recreation specialist collaborates with a different team member (speech therapist, occupational and physical therapists, and social worker) to address issues in a community setting (communication, mobility, and emotional adjustment, respectively). Families are encouraged to participate. This experience provides the patient and family with a chance to apply newly acquired compensatory skills to situations in the community and offers useful feedback to the team about the patient's and family's transference of training and learning. It also gives the staff an opportunity to model appropriate levels of assistance to the stroke survivor and to model assertive behavior, such as informing a store manager about inaccessible corridors. The outings give the staff natural opportunities to collaborate with the family on problem-solving issues of accessibility for the disabled, dealing with the public, and community mobility.

Family conferences. Family conferences are held 1 to 2 weeks after admission, and the primary purpose is to facilitate clear and accurate communication between the patient, family, and team. Family conferences provide the family and patient with an opportunity to hear about progress and recommendations from each member of the team and how each part relates to the whole. It is also a time for families to ask questions and have their concerns heard and addressed by the team. Clear and accurate communication between team members and families is crucial to the families' ability to make informed and wise decisions about continued patient care. Communication problems between rehabilitation consumers and professionals have been cited as a cause of anger and stress in patients and families.[84]

Family conferences provide the patient and family an opportunity to witness the teamwork in action, whether through agreement or constructive disagreement between the team members. This is typically the only chance the family has to view and speak with the entire team at once, and it can be a powerful experience that helps patients and families synthesize what they have learned into a coherent whole. Families sometimes feel they are given conflicting messages by team members, and the conference provides a time to clarify what was meant and what was heard.

The physician's presence and participation are central to family conferences. Families often want reassurance that the team has informed, concerned, and involved leadership from the physician, and families may look to the physician for verbal and nonverbal indications about the competence and trustworthiness of other team members. When families watch differences of opinion between team members handled constructively and respectfully, it sends an empowering message that they too have permission to disagree with the medical establishment without apprehension. As the team leader, the physician sets the tone for the entire conference.

Social activities. Evening and weekend activities planned by therapeutic recreation specialists, such as movies or social events, can provide important opportunities for the family and patient to interact with each other and with others at a normal social gathering. Such events can help decrease the focus on the "sick" member and promote normalization. Similar to community outings and day passes, these events challenge the patient and family to rehearse their skills at managing newly acquired limitations (e.g., compensating for left sensory neglect or use of a wheelchair).

Interdisciplinary goals. Interdisciplinary goals are identified as early as possible, usually at the initial team conference, and can be geared toward the patient or the family. The team selects three or four interdisciplinary goals that are either priority rehabilitation issues for the patient or priority discharge planning issues for the family and that can be appropriately addressed by a variety of disciplines.

For example, the physician, nurse, and speech pathologist may collaborate on the patient's goal of medication management because it entails education about the type and reason for medications, monitoring of the patient's reliability in self-administration, and development of cognitive strategies for drug recognition and maintaining a schedule. Another interdisciplinary goal might be for the patient to initiate the daily use of his or her communication log with each therapist.

Family-oriented interdisciplinary goals might include (1) increasing the family's confidence with using the patient's communication device by overseeing the family's use of the device with the patient during two family-training or therapy sessions per week or (2) improving the family members' ability to deal with the patient's emotional lability by practicing one of several learned techniques (redirection, relaxation cuing) with the patient once each day during training or visits. Family interdisciplinary goals should have the overall aim of increasing the family's competence and confidence to meet the challenges presented by caring for the stroke survivor.

CASE REPORT

L.M. was a 44-year-old male with diabetes whose cerebrovascular accident rendered him partially blind, nonambulatory, emotionally labile, and cognitively unimpaired. He was a high-level professional speechwriter at the peak of his career. In their earnest desire to "cheer up" their loved one, the family profusely showered the patient with gifts, and unrequested helpfulness. He resented it and told the team that he felt patronized and pitied. However, he was initially unable to express this to his family. He became tearful when he tried to do so, to which the family anxiously responded with increased displays of helpfulness, and this made him more frustrated and labile. L.M. agreed with the rehabilitation philosophy, which was to do as much for himself as possible, but his family had difficulty watching him struggle with his emotional control and daily self-care tasks. Their caring instincts resulted in them taking over for him, thus preventing the patient from dealing with his new limitations.

In this case the team interventions with the family included (1) meeting with the patient and family to improve communication; (2) assisting the family to structure their interactions with L.M. by establishing guidelines regarding the help offered to the patient; (3) monitoring adherence to these guidelines during family training and observation on the unit and in family therapy sessions; (4) teaching the family how to deal effectively with the patient's emotional lability and having them practice these skills during visitation hours and outings; and (5) problem solving with the family about how the family could redirect their zeal to be involved in more constructive behaviors that enhanced rather than impeded the patient's progress.

Cotreatment and collaboration between the patient, family, and team was highly beneficial in this case. The social worker and psychologist cotreated the family and patient in family counseling, which was useful because the social worker was particularly attuned to the family's perspective and the psychologist to the patient's. The social worker and physical therapist collaborated during a therapy session to help the patient learn techniques for increased emotional control (e.g., relaxation, distraction) and ways in which to apply these strategies when his lability interfered with physical therapy. The occupational therapist and nurse collaborated on teaching and applying self-care skills and worked with the family in training sessions and on the unit to increase their understanding of what the patient could do if given the opportunity.

Family counseling. Although the purpose of this section is to illustrate the interdisciplinary aspects of work with families in rehabilitation, it is important to note that family counseling has been shown to enhance and sustain the benefits of educational interventions, which otherwise tend to diminish 6 months to 1 year after the patient's stroke.[93] Through the social worker's time-intensive role with the family as a continued care planner, a therapeutic alliance is typically established. In addition to collaborating with the family on continued care planning, it is recommended that the social worker meet with the family for regularly scheduled family counseling sessions. In the continued care planning role, the social worker has substantial opportunity to observe family dynamics, communication patterns, leadership and hierarchy structures, decision-making styles, problem-solving skills, and alliances, which can provide an excellent clinical base on which to engage the family in effective short-term therapy.

When indicated, the social worker may also collaborate with a psychologist or other team member to provide family counseling. If the patient is aphasic and the family is having technical difficulty communicating about psychosocial issues, the speech therapist and social worker may cotreat the patient and family. If there is considerable family conflict about return-to-work issues, the social worker may request that the vocational specialist cotreat the family in one or several of the family sessions. Cotreatment between social worker and physician in select family counseling sessions can be productive when families are having difficulty accepting the medical prognosis or making major medical decisions. The authority of the physician's position can be used to help families begin to accept a permanent disability and to support the family interventions of other team members.

The social worker as continued care planner and family therapist helps the family integrate the input from all of the team members and synthesize the discrete recommendations into a coherent whole. The social worker provides the family with a therapeutic context in which the necessary learning, problem solving, and adaptation can occur. The family's relationship with the social worker enhances interdisciplinary efforts. As primary liaison to the family, the social worker helps ensure that the family is hearing the team's messages accurately and that the team is aware of the family's main issues, concerns, and goals. The therapeutic relationship may employ one or all of the following interventions: education, family and individual psychotherapy, problem-solving training, information and referral, cognitive-behavioral interventions, crisis intervention, communication training, emotional support, practical guidance, or skills development.

Preparing the family for discharge is approached by the team on two levels. The first level involves the practical task of identifying, educating, training, and securing the presence of the necessary assistive devices, family members or friends, professionals, and community referrals for the patient to leave the hospital safely. This is the "what" element and is the level at which most rehabilitation programs solicit family involvement.

The second level is the therapeutic task of engaging the patient and family in the continued care planning. This is the "how" element. It involves the therapeutic process of empowering patients and families to become their own care planners, managers, problem solvers, and advocates and enabling them to identify and manage their unique emotional response to a crisis so that they can move on with their lives.

If the task of preparing families for discharge is not approached at this second therapeutic level, psychosocial adjustment and treatment adherence outcomes are compromised, and the continued care plan may or may not be suitable for or sustainable by the family. Family counseling involves the family at a personal level, validates their unique experience of and response to the event, and individualizes psychosocial treatment to ensure its relevance to their particular situation. Just as the rehabilitation patient is encouraged and required to put compensatory skills and techniques to use beyond the therapy hour, so is the family carefully guided to learn and apply problem-solving skills to their real-life discharge dilemmas and emotional adjustment issues.

Informal team interventions. In conjunction with programmatic components of the Caregiver Education Program, the interdisciplinary team has myriad opportunities to positively affect family functioning and adaptation in the course of routine interactions with families. Some guidelines for team members are outlined in the following, but it is beyond the scope of this chapter to explore this important subject in detail.

Team members of all disciplines have contact with family members, and every interaction sends overt and covert messages to the family about the patient and the rehabilitation professionals. Each team member is responsible for his or her part of the interaction and the messages his or her behavior conveys. This creates countless opportunities during the patient's treatment for staff to use their interactions with the family in a therapeutic and team-coordinated manner. It is the responsibility of the social worker to enhance the team's understanding of family dynamics to facilitate coordination of the team's approach with families.

There is a tendency in the helping professions to become too narrowly focused on techniques and elaborate schemes to induce change in another individual. A feverish focus on interventions is often a reflection of staff anxiety and may neglect a more fundamental ingredient of therapeutic success—the professional's use of self. Although techniques and specific interventions can be helpful, of far greater importance is the helper's level of emotional maturity, self-awareness, and respect for families. Some guidelines may be useful for team interactions with families to maximize family strengths and competence and minimize family and team anxiety and reactivity.

1. Treat the family as a unit capable of making decisions and solving problems. There is no place for patronizing behavior toward families within the successful rehabilitation team.

2. Ask questions that stimulate the family to think of options and challenge unrealistic plans on their own rather than give premature advice or argue with them.

3. Withhold value judgments and allow families to make decisions and choices that they, not the team, can live with. Recognize and respect cultural variations and, whenever possible, capitalize on the strengths of the family's background. For example, if the family's culture mandates a high level of involvement, help them to do so in as responsible and effective a manner as possible.

4. Respect and use the family's vast knowledge about the patient. Next to the patient, the family is the team's greatest resource. They hold the information about premorbid functioning and personality and can help the team ascertain what the patient's most pressing rehabilitation needs are.

5. Recognize when one's own anxiety (manifested in such ways as dislike, excessive worry, team conflicts, taking sides with or against the patient, and overzealous caring) is heightened. Seek to manage and contain one's own anxiety and not allow it to infect the patient or family. Family members can think and problem solve better when anxiety levels are low.

6. Cultivate objectivity on the team members' parts. Objectivity is not synonymous with being impersonal or disconnected; it involves making contact in a calm and nonanxious manner. Subjectivity, on the other hand, is heightened

by anxiety. It constantly enters in relationships with families and must be acknowledged and minimized. Subjective team behavior usually reveals more about the helper than the family. Subjective behavior includes biases and prejudices, overinvestment in a certain patient's outcome, finding oneself in a desperate attempt to change the patient's mind, or becoming overly attached to a patient.

7. Avoid taking sides in patient-family-team conflicts. Team members, similar to any human in an emotionally charged situation, may be pressured to take sides with or against patients or with or against other team members. Complaints are best resolved by redirecting the anxiety back to the original parties at odds. When handled constructively, complaints offer an opportunity to improve services and to clarify misunderstandings.

8. Assess the family's cognitive and intellectual levels and learning styles, and capitalize on their learning strengths. For example, some families need everything written down to assimilate all the new information; for others this is intimidating, and they prefer hands-on demonstrations.

9. The team must put into practice between its own members what it espouses to do with families and patients. If the team values the consumers' opinions and seeks to empower them to be successful after discharge, it must also respect each colleague's professional opinion and seek to empower its members to be successful with patients and families. The consumers will learn as much about a team's capacity for tolerance and respect by observing the team in action as by a team's polished words and behavior with the patient. The team member's emotional maturity, self-awareness, and respect are perhaps best revealed by his or her unrehearsed interactions with other staff.

10. Learn to be comfortable with not knowing the answers. Patients often put health care professionals in the untenable position of experts, so that the team member may feel obliged to fulfill this expectation, whether it is warranted or not. No one is an expert in every area; team members do themselves and patients a service by acknowledging this.

Conclusion

An interdisciplinary approach to preparing families for discharge is anchored in a commitment to collaboration, respect, and communication between team members, the patient, and the family. Psychosocial family assessment is conducted by the social worker while drawing extensively on each team member's contributions to the understanding of the family. This ongoing assessment is the cornerstone of interdisciplinary family intervention. Preparation of the family for discharge is facilitated through interdisciplinary assessment, team goals, programmatic interventions, and therapeutic use of informal team contacts with family. These team efforts are designed to empower patients and families to face the challenges presented by the stroke with confidence and competence after the team is discharged from their lives.

REFERENCES

Nature of the Problem

1. Kelly-Hayes M et al: Factors influencing survival and need for institutionalization following stroke: the Framingham Study, *Arch Phys Med Rehabil* 69:415, 1988.

Management of the Interdisciplinary Team

2. Commission on Accreditation of Rehabilitation Facilities: *CARF standards manual for organizations serving people with disabilities,* Tucson, 1992, The Commission.
3. Diller L: Fostering the interdisciplinary team, fostering research in a society in transition, *Arch Phys Med Rehabil* 71:275, 1990.
4. Granger CV, Hamilton BB: Measurement of stroke rehabilitation outcome in the 1980s, *Stroke* 21 (suppl 2):II46, 1990.
5. Granger CV et al: Stroke rehabilitation: analyses of reported Barthel Index measures, *Arch Phys Med Rehabil* 60:14, 1979.
6. Hart T, Hayden ME, McDowell J: Rehabilitation of severe brain injury: when you stick to the facts, you cut the losses. In Miner ME, Wagner KA, editors: *Neurotrauma,* vol 2, Boston, 1990, Butterworth.
7. Keith RA: The comprehensive treatment team in rehabilitation, *Arch Phys Med Rehabil* 72:269, 1991.
8. Melvin JL: Interdisciplinary and multidisciplinary activities and the ACRM, *Arch Phys Med Rehabil* 61:379, 1980.
9. Melvin JL: Status report on interdisciplinary medical rehabilitation, *Arch Phys Med Rehabil* 70:273, 1989.
10. Rehabilitation Institute of Chicago: *Rehabilitation Institute of Chicago Functional Assessment Scale,* Chicago, 1987, The Institute.
11. Wade DT: Stroke rehabilitation and long-term care, *Lancet* 339:791, 1992.
12. Wood-Dauphinee S et al: A randomized trial of team care following stroke, *Stroke* 15:864, 1984.

Neuropsychologic Aspects of Normal Aging and Stroke Rehabilitation

13. Adams GF, Hurwitz LJ: Mental barriers to recovery from stroke, *Lancet* 2:533, 1963.
14. Adler E et al: *Stroke in Israel, 1957–1961: epidemiological, clinical, rehabilitation and psychosocial aspects,* Jerusalem, 1969, Polypress Limited.
15. Albert MS: General issues in geriatric neuropsychology. In Albert MS, Moss MD, editors: *Geriatric neuropsychology,* New York, 1988, Guilford Press.
16. Albert MS: Cognitive function. In Albert MS, Moss MD, editors: *Geriatric neuropsychology,* New York, 1988, Guilford Press.
17. Albert MS, Heaton RK: Intelligence testing. In Albert MS, Moss MB, editors: *Geriatric neuropsychology,* New York, 1988, Guilford Press.
18. Alexander MP: Clinical determination of mental competence: a theory and a retrospective study, *Arch Neurol* 45:23, 1988.
19. Allen M: Models of hemispheric specialization, *Psychol Bull* 93:73, 1983.
20. American Psychiatric Association: *Diagnostic and statistical manual of mental disorders,* ed 3, Washington, DC, 1987, The Association.
21. Bandura A: Self-efficacy: toward a unifying theory of behavior change, *Psychol Rev* 84:191, 1977.
22. Bayles KA, Kazniak AW: *Communication and cognition in normal aging and dementia,* Boston, 1987, Little, Brown.

23. Berezin MA, Liptzin B, Salzman C: The elderly person. In Nicholi AM, editor: *The new Harvard guide to psychiatry,* Cambridge, 1988, Belknap Press.
24. Binder LM, Howieson D, Coull BH: Stroke: causes, consequences, and treatment. In Caplan B, editor: *Rehabilitation psychology desk reference,* Rockville, Md, 1987, Aspen Publishers.
25. Bleiberg J: Psychological and neuropsychological factors in stroke management. In Kaplan D, Cerullo L, editors: *Stroke rehabilitation,* Boston, 1986, Butterworth.
26. Buschke H: Control of cognitive processing. In Squire LR, Butters N, editors: *Neuropsychology of memory,* New York, 1984, Guilford Press.
27. Craik FIM: Age differences in remembering. In Squire LR, Butters N, editors: *Neuropsychology of memory,* New York, 1984, Guilford Press.
28. Critchley M: Misoplegia or hatred of hemiplegia, *Mt Sinai J Med* 41:82, 1974.
29. Crowne DP: The frontal eye field and attention, *Psychol Bull* 93:232, 1983.
30. Cummings JL, Benson DF: *Dementia: a clinical approach,* Boston, 1983, Butterworth.
31. Davidson PO: Issues in patient compliance. In Millon T, Green C, Meagher R, editors: *Handbook of clinical psychology,* New York, 1982, Plenum.
32. Diller L, Weinberg J: Evidence for accident-prone behavior in hemiplegic patients, *Arch Phys Med Rehabil* 51:353, 1970.
33. Erickson EH: *Childhood and society,* ed 2, New York, 1963, WW Norton.
34. Ewert J et al: Procedural memory during post-traumatic amnesia in survivors of severe closed head injury: implications for rehabilitation, *Arch Neurol* 46:911, 1989.
35. Falvo DR: *Medical and psychosocial aspects of chronic illness and disability,* Gaithersburg, Md, 1991, Aspen Publishers.
36. Filley CM, Kelly JP: Neurobehavioral effects of focal subcortical lesions. In Cummings JL, editor: *Subcortical dementia,* New York, 1990, Oxford University Press.
37. Finger S, Stein DG: *Brain damage and recovery,* New York, 1982, Academic Press.
38. Finkelstein SP et al: Antidepressant drug treatment for post-stroke depression: retrospective study, *Arch Phys Med Rehabil* 68:772, 1987.
39. Funkenstein HH: Cerebrovascular disorder. In Albert MS, Moss MB, editors: *Geriatric neuropsychology,* New York, 1988, Guilford Press.
40. Gans JS: Facilitating staff/patient interaction in rehabilitation. In Caplan B, editor: *Rehabilitation psychology desk reference,* Rockville, Md, 1987, Aspen Publishers.
41. Gardner H: *The shattered mind,* New York, 1974, Vintage Books.
42. Geschwind N: Disconnexion syndromes in animals and man, *Brain* 82:237, 1965.
43. Grober SE et al: Utility of the dexamethasone suppression test in the diagnosis of poststroke depression, *Arch Phys Med Rehabil* 72:1076, 1991.
44. Gunther M: Psychiatric consultation in a rehabilitation hospital: a regression hypothesis, *Am J Psychiatry* 12(6):572, 1971.
45. Hartke RJ: Introduction. In Hartke RJ, editor: *Psychosocial aspects of geriatric rehabilitation,* Gaithersburg, Md, 1991, Aspen Publishers.
46. Hartke RJ: The aging process: cognition, personality, and coping. In Hartke RJ, editor: *Psychosocial aspects of geriatric rehabilitation,* Gaithersburg, Md, 1991, Aspen Publishers.
47. Hartke RJ: The older adult's adjustment to the rehabilitation setting. In Hartke RJ, editor: *Psychosocial aspects of geriatric rehabilitation,* Gaithersburg, Md, 1991, Aspen Publishers.
48. Heilman HM, Watson RT: Mechanisms underlying the unilateral neglect syndrome. In Weinstein EA, Friedland RD, editors: *Advances in neurology.* Vol 18. *Hemi-inattention and hemispheric specialization,* New York, 1977, Raven Press.

49. Heilman KM, Bowers D, Valenstein E: Emotional disorders associated with neurological diseases. In Heilman KM, Valenstein E, editors: *Clinical neuropsychology,* ed 2, New York, 1985, Oxford.

50. Horn JL, Cattell RB: Age differences in fluid and crystallized intelligence, *Acta Psychol* 26:107, 1967.

51. House A et al: Mood disorders after stroke and their relation to lesion location: a CT scan study, *Brain* 113:1113, 1990.

52. Jackson JH: On affections of speech from disease of the brain, *Brain* 2:323, 1879.

53. Kirshner HS: *Behavioral neurology: a practical approach,* New York, 1986, Churchill Livingstone.

54. Klisz D: Neuropsychological evaluation in older persons. In Storandt M, Stiegler IC, Elias MF, editors: *The clinical psychology of aging,* New York, 1978, Plenum Press.

55. Lezak M: *Neuropsychological assessment,* ed 2, New York, 1983, Oxford University Press.

56. Lishman WA: *Organic psychiatry: the psychological consequences of cerebral disorder,* London, 1978, Blackwell Scientific.

57. Mandell AM, Albert ML: History of subcortical dementia. In Cummings JL, editor: *Subcortical dementia,* New York, 1990, Oxford.

58. Mesulam MM: *Principles of behavioral neurology,* Philadelphia, 1985, FA Davis.

59. Mittenberg W et al: Changes in cerebral functioning associated with normal aging, *J Clin Exp Neuropsychol* 11:918, 1989.

60. Neugarten BL: Adaptation and the life cycle, *J Geriatr Psychiatry* 4:71, 1970.

61. Parikh RM et al: Two-year longitudinal study of post-stroke mood disorders: dynamic changes in correlates of depression at one and two years, *Stroke* 18(3):579, 1987.

62. Rimm DC, Masters JC: *Behavior therapy: techniques and empirical findings,* ed 2, New York, 1979, Academic Press.

63. Robinson RG, Star LB, Price TR: A two year longitudinal study of mood disorders following stroke: prevalence and duration at six months follow-up, *Br J Psychiatry* 144:256, 1984.

64. Schienle DR, Eiler JM: Clinical intervention with older adults. In Eisenberg MG, Sutkin LC, Jansen MA, editors: *Chronic illness and disability through the lifespan: effects on self and family,* New York, 1984, Springer.

65. Smith A: Principles underlying human brain functions in neuropsychological sequelae of different neuropathological processes. In Filskov S, Boll T, editors: *Handbook of clinical neuropsychology,* New York, 1981, Wiley & Sons.

66. Squire LA: *Memory and brain,* New York, 1987, Oxford.

67. Starkstein SE, Robinson RG, Price TR: Comparison of patients with and without post-stroke depression matched for size and location of lesion, *Arch Gen Psychiatry* 45:247, 1988.

68. Stoudemire A, Blazer DG: Depression in the elderly. In Beckman EE, Leber WR, editors: *Handbook of depression,* Homewood, Ill, 1985, Dorsey Press.

69. Strub RL, Black FW: *Neurobehavioral disorders: a clinical approach,* Philadelphia, 1988, FA Davis.

70. Stuss DT, Benson DF: Neuropsychological studies of the frontal lobes, *Psychol Bull* 95:3, 1984.

71. Sutkin LC: Introduction. In Eisenberg MG, Sutkin LC, Jansen MA, editors: *Chronic illness and disability through the lifespan: effects on self and family,* New York, 1984, Springer.

72. Trezona RR: Assessment and treatment of depression in the older rehabilitation patient. In Hartke RJ, editor: *Psychological aspects of geriatric rehabilitation,* Gaithersburg, Md, 1991, Aspen Publishers.

73. Ullman M: *Behavioral changes in patients following strokes,* Springfield, Ill, 1962, Charles C Thomas.
74. Van Gorp WG, Mahler M: Subcortical features of normal aging. In Cummings JL, editor: *Subcortical dementia,* New York, 1990, Oxford University Press.
75. Weinstein EA, Friedland RP: Behavioral disorders associated with hemi-inattention. In Weinstein EA, Friedland FP, editors: *Advances in neurology.* Vol 18. *Hemi-inattention and hemispheric specialization,* New York, 1977, Raven Press.
76. Worden JM: *Grief counseling and grief therapy: a handbook for the mutual health practitioner,* New York, 1982, Springer.

Preparing the Family for Discharge: An Interdisciplinary Approach

77. Abramson M: Ethical dilemmas for social workers in discharge planning, *Soc Work Health Care* 6(4):33, 1981.
78. Anastas JW, Gibeau JL, Larson PJ: Working families and eldercare: a national perspective in an aging America, *Soc Work* 35(5):405, 1990.
79. Bishop DS, Evans RL: Family functioning assessment techniques in stroke, *Stroke* 21 (suppl 2):II50, 1990.
80. Bishop DS, Miller IW: Traumatic brain injury: empirical family assessment techniques, *J Head Trauma Rehabil* 3(4):16, 1988.
81. Bowen M: *Family therapy in clinical practice,* Northvale, NJ, 1978, Jason Aronson.
82. Brody EM: Informal support systems in the rehabilitation of the disabled elderly. In Brody SJ, Ruff GE, editors: *Aging and rehabilitation: advances in the state of the art,* New York, 1986, Springer.
83. Cannon IM: *Social work in hospitals,* New York, 1913, Russell Sage Foundation.
84. Carberry H: Communication problems between head injured patients, their families and rehabilitation professionals, *J Cognitive Rehabil* 10(2):24, 1992.
85. Davidson KW: Evolving social work roles in healthcare: the case discharge planning, *Soc Work Health Care* 4:43, 1978.
86. DePompei R, Zarski JJ, Hall DE: A systems approach to understanding CHI family functioning, *Cognitive Rehabil* 5(2):6, 1987.
87. DePompei R, Zarski JJ, Hall DE: Cognitive communication impairments: a family-focused viewpoint, *J Head Trauma Rehabil* 3(2):13, 1988.
88. Durgin CJ: Techniques for families to increase their involvement in the rehabilitation process, *Cognitive Rehabil* 7(3):22, 1989.
89. Epstein NB, Baldwin LM, Bishop DS: McMaster Family Assessment Device, *J Marital Fam Therap* 8:171, 1983.
90. Evans RL, Bishop DS, Haselkorn JK: Factors predicting satisfactory home care after stroke, *Arch Phys Med Rehabil* 72:144, 1991.
91. Evans RL et al: Prestroke family interaction as a predictor of stroke outcome, *Arch Phys Med Rehabil* 68:508, 1987a.
92. Evans RL et al: Family interaction and treatment adherence after stroke, *Arch Phys Med Rehabil* 68:513, 1987b.
93. Evans RL et al: Family intervention after stroke: does counseling or education help?, *Stroke* 19(10):1243, 1988.
94. Evans RL et al: Caregiver assessment of personal adjustment after stroke in a Veterans Administration medical center outpatient cohort, *Stroke* 20(4):483, 1989.
95. Friedland J, McColl MA: Social support and psychosocial dysfunction after stroke: buffering effects in a community sample, *Arch Phys Med Rehabil* 68:475, 1987.
96. Friedman EH: *Generation to generation,* New York, 1985, Guilford Press.

97. Hollis F, Woods ME: *Casework: a psychosocial therapy,* ed 3, New York, 1981, Random House.
98. Kane JN: Compliance issues in outpatient treatment, *J Clin Psychopharmacol* 5:22S, 1985.
99. Kerr ME, Bowen M: *Family evaluation,* New York, 1988, Norton.
100. Kozloff R: Networks of social support and the outcome from severe head injury, *J Head Trauma Rehabil* 2(3):14, 1987.
101. Livingston MG, Brooks DN: The burden on families of the brain injured: a review, *J Head Trauma Rehabil* 3(4):6, 1988.
102. Macnamara SE et al: Caregiver strain: need for late poststroke intervention, *Rehabil Psychol* 35(2):71, 1990.
103. Mayer JB et al: Empowering families of the chronically ill: a partnership experience in a hospital setting, *Soc Work Health Care* 14(4):73, 1990.
104. McKinlay W, Hickox A: How can families help in the rehabilitation of the head injured?, *J Head Trauma Rehabil* 3(4):64, 1988.
105. Melvin JL: Interdisciplinary and multidisciplinary activities and ACRM, *Arch Phys Med Rehabil* 61:379, 1980.
106. Moore AD et al: Family coping and marital adjustment after traumatic brain injury, *J Head Trauma Rehabil* 6(1):83-89, 1991.
107. National Rehabilitation Hospital: *NRH program evaluation system: functional status report guide,* Washington, DC, 1992, National Rehabilitation Hospital.
108. O'Hara CC, Harrel M: The empowerment rehabilitation model: meeting the unmet needs of survivors, families, and treatment providers, *Cognitive Rehabil* 9(1):14, 1991.
109. Papero DV: *Bowen family systems theory,* Boston, 1990, Allyn & Bacon.
110. Perlman HH: *Social casework: a problem solving process,* Chicago, 1957, University of Chicago Press.
111. Rehabilitation Institute of Chicago: *Rehabilitation Institute of Chicago Functional Assessment Scale,* Chicago, 1989, The Institute.
112. Reid WJ, Epstein L: *Task centered casework,* New York, 1972, Columbia University Press.
113. Reiss D, Gonzales S, Kramer N: Family process, chronic illness and death: on weakness of strong bonds, *Arch Gen Psychiatry* 43:795, 1986.
114. Research Foundation, State University of New York: *Uniform data system for medical rehabilitation,* Buffalo, 1990, State University of New York.
115. Rohe DE: Psychological aspects of rehabilitation. In DeLisa JA, editor: *Rehabilitation medicine principles and practice,* Philadelphia, 1988, JB Lippincott.
116. Romano MD: Ethical issues and families of brain-injured persons, *J Head Trauma Rehabil* 4(1):33, 1989.
117. Romano MD: Psychosocial diagnosis and social work services. In Kottle FJ, Lehmann JF, editors: *Krusen's handbook of physical medicine and rehabilitation,* Philadelphia, 1990, WB Saunders.
118. Rosenthal M, Young T: Effective family intervention after traumatic brain injury: theory and practice, *J Head Trauma Rehabil* 3(4):42, 1988.
119. Santa Clara Valley Medical Center: *Functional assessment measures,* Santa Clara, Calif, 1986, Santa Clara Valley Medical Center.
120. Schwentor D, Brown P: Assessment of families with a traumatically brain injured relative, *Cognitive Rehabil* 7(3):8, 1989.
121. Smith VJ, Messikomer CM: A role for the family in geriatric rehabilitation, *Top Geriatr Rehabil* 4(1):8, 1988.
122. Strand T et al: Non-intensive stroke unit reduces functional disability and need for long term hospitalization, *Stroke* 16:29, 1985.

CHAPTER 10

Rehabilitation Management: Alleviating Specific Disabilities

Communication disorders
PAUL R. RAO
  Nature and extent of the problem
  Assessment of left cerebrovascular accidents
    Aphasia
    Apraxia of speech
    Agnosia
    Dysarthria
  Right hemisphere communication impairment
  Multiple-infarct dementia
  Comprehensive assessment and diagnostic therapy
    Diagnostic therapy
    Conceptual framework
  Development of a treatment plan
    Establishment of an interdisciplinary communication care plan
  Treatment (philosophy and implementation)
    Coaching
    Patient education
    Continuous quality improvement
Dysphagia and its management
THERESE M. GOLDSMITH AND CHRISTINE R. BARON
  Normal swallowing function
    Models of swallowing and ingestion
    Physiology and sequence of normal swallowing
    Neural control and regulation of swallowing
  Characteristics of dysphagia in the stroke population
    Neuropathology
    Clinical manifestations
    Course of recovery
    Special considerations
  Assessment
    Dysphagia screening
    Clinical evaluation

Specialized diagnostic procedures
Acute phase concerns
Texture modification
Nonoral feeding alternatives
Rehabilitation phase
Dysphagia goal setting
Dysphagia therapy techniques
Continuing care issues
Enhancing motor function
Nature of the problem
Assessment of plasticity
Treatment procedures
Training in activities of daily living
CHRISTINE BIRD AND REBECCA C. MAHONEY
Nature of the problem
Assessment
Activities of daily living performance
Activity analysis
Sensorimotor components
Cognition
Perception
Home evaluation
Equipment assessment
Driving assessment
Work evaluation
Goal setting and treatment planning
Treatment approaches
Retraining of performance skills
Compensatory strategies
Adaptive equipment
Environmental adaptation
Treatment applications
Feeding
Dressing
Grooming and hygiene
Home management
Training in mobility
RICHARD S. MATERSON AND MARK N. OZER
Nature of the problem
Assessment
Analysis of gait
Treatment of mobility disorders

Identification phase
In-bed phase
Sit-up phase
Stand-up phase
Step-up phase
"Step-out" phase
Special problems of patients with poor neurologic return

COMMUNICATION DISORDERS

Paul R. Rao

Nature and Extent of the Problem

America was dramatically introduced to stroke and aphasia by Koppit's 1978 award-winning play *Wings,* in which Edith Stilson, a former aviatrix, is portrayed as having had a stroke with resultant aphasia.[2] When her doctor asks what happened to her, Ms. Stilson turns to the audience and responds, "Near as I can figure it, I was in my brain and crashed." What a stark definition for stroke — a brain crash! Stroke, or a cerebrovascular accident (CVA), is the most frequent cause of injury to the nervous system.[20] According to the National Institute of Neurological Disorders and Stroke, stroke is the nation's third leading killer, with nearly a half-million Americans stricken annually when blood flow to the brain is interrupted and nerve cells are damaged and with a resultant 150,000 deaths annually from stroke-related causes.[23] Current stroke survivors number 2.5 million Americans. According to the American Heart Association, most strokes occur in people over 55 years of age, with the average age about 70 years. Because of improved poststroke medical management, nearly 80% of stroke patients survive their first CVA, and the 10-year survival rate is approximately 50%. According to Sahs et al., the recovery levels for 100 survivors of acute stroke are as follows[30]:

Postacute Stroke Status	
10*	Return to work with virtually no impairment
40	Retain mild residual disability
40	Remain so severely disabled that special service or assistance required
10	Require institutional care

Based on the preceding figures, 80% of persons with stroke are candidates for a rehabilitation regimen that may enhance communication abilities. Rosenbek et al. extrapolated from Sahs' data the statistical projections for com-

---

* Number at this level per 100 stroke survivors.

munication disorders: over 1 million Americans will suffer left CVAs annually, and 80% of those survivors will exhibit aphasia, apraxia, or both, whereas an equal number of persons will suffer right CVA annually with a majority of those survivors exhibiting some cognitive-communication impairment.[29] Left and right CVAs and brainstem strokes also may result in dysarthria. Hence, the cumulative effects of stroke may result in an impairment of any of the following communication abilities: voice, speech, language, fluency, and cognition. There is mounting evidence that "brain crash" has a life-shattering impact on a person's communication abilities.[7,17,29]

The stroke survivor may experience a communication disorder defined as "any impairment in communication . . . and the focus is on the individual's capacity to exchange thoughts and information clearly and plausibly rather than on speech, hearing, or language deficits."[34] Thus *functional communication* "is the ability to receive a message or convey a message, regardless of the mode, to communicate effectively and independently in a given environment."[2] The emphasis is less on the various systems or components of speech and language and more on the gestalt or holistic perspective of communication. How, when, what, where, and why does a person affected by stroke need to communicate? Asking for a drink, watching television, telling a joke, selecting from a menu, and listening to a sermon are all challenges to the person with a communication impairment. According to Sarno, "the impact of a verbal impairment on interpersonal interactions, on the use of verbal activities for leisure, on the ability to receive employment, on the overall effect on the quality of life, and on the patient's ability to compensate and/or circumvent the deficits all play a part in the patient's effectiveness as a communicator."[31] The current rehabilitation focus is on functional communication. If a person with stroke is unable to relate his phone number, he may be able to find it in his wallet and display it or be able to write it, dial it, or even look it up in the phone book. The crux of the clinician's role with the person with a communication disorder is to first establish the primary problem, then to problem solve with the patient, attempting to determine the most effective, efficient, and reliable method(s) for breaking the silence barrier. The underlying assumption is that a barrier (handicap) for one person with stroke is not a barrier for another. The preceding definition of functional communication suggests that communication wants and needs vary among individuals and for the same individual in different environments.[10] Contrast the communication needs of a highly educated scientist with those of an individual with limited educational and vocational attainment. Consider the communication challenges at work or school versus those found in a home or nursing home. For these reasons functional communication must be individually defined for each stroke person, and as outlined by Aten, one "must consider the severity of the communicative disturbances, the premorbid life-style of the patient, and the setting in which that person will ultimately reside."[4]

The intent of this section is to stress functional communication, whatever the specific impairment, to arm the patient, significant others, and the rehabilitation team with the requisite knowledge, skills, and abilities to enhance functional communication. I have attempted to make the assessment and treatment phases of adult communication disorders user friendly to foster enhanced training in the use of compensatory techniques. An underlying assumption of this approach is that, by increasing the opportunities to learn and observe the dynamics of communication intervention, the family can increase their therapeutic involvement (cotherapy) and thereby expedite the patient's goal attainment and timely, optimal disposition. Finally, the following treatment approach espouses an interdisciplinary, cotreatment model in fostering generalization of functional communication strategies so that activities of daily living (ADL) needs are met both in and out of the hospital.

Assessment of Left Cerebrovascular Accidents

The communication problems most common after a left CVA are aphasia, apraxia, agnosia, and dysarthria. The definition of each adult neurogenic communication disorder that may occur after a stroke can be found in Table 10-1. Reference to these definitions is helpful when completing a thorough assessment of the prominent symptoms and underlying communication impairment following a left CVA. In a standard assessment the diagnostic search concentrates on the primary deficit (i.e., the communication problem chiefly responsible for disrupting the process by which the patient communicates or gets a need met).

The key concept in aphasia is language; in dysarthria, motor speech; in apraxia, motor programming of speech; and in agnosia, recognition. These are the four unique communication impairments that may result singly or in combination following a left CVA. The assessment is conducted to ascertain the presence or absence of a communication impairment following a stroke. The traditional clinical assessment considers neurologic data that identify primary signs and symptoms consistent with the probable etiologic factor and locus of lesion. Thus, if a dextral person suffers a left-sided middle cerebral artery (MCA) infarct to the frontal lobe with resultant hemiplegia, the diagnostician can rule out a number of neurogenic communication disorders (e.g., right hemisphere communication impairment, dementia, and dysarthria) and thereby conduct a further differential diagnosis to determine whether the underlying communication impairment is aphasia, apraxia, or both (refer to Table 10-2 for a decision tree on neurogenic communication disorders).

The second type of assessment the rehabilitation team undertakes is the *functional communication assessment,* which can be defined as follows[2]: assess the extent of the patient's ability to communicate with others in a variety of contexts, considering environmental modifications, adaptive equipment, time required to communicate, and listener familiarity with the client; special accommodations of

TABLE 10-1 Definitions for Six Neuropathologic Conditions of Speech, Language, or Both

NEUROPATHOLOGIC CONDITION	DEFINITION
Agnosia	Impairment of the ability to perceive and differentiate stimulus patterns although the sensory mechanism is intact; the most frequently seen types: auditory, visual, and tactile recognition disorders[27]
Aphasia	An acquired impairment of language processes underlying receptive and expressive modalities; caused by damage to areas of the brain that are primarily responsible for the language function[9]
Dementia	An organic syndrome demonstrating decline of memory and other intellectual functions in comparison with the individual's previous level of function; determined by the history of decline in performance and by abnormalities noted from clinical examination and other tests[13]
Apraxia of speech	An articulation disorder resulting from impairment caused by brain damage to the capacity to program the positioning of speech muscles and the sequencing of muscle movements for the volitional production of phonemes; no significant weakness, slowness, or incoordination of these muscles in reflex and autonomic acts; prosodic alterations possibly associated with the articulatory problem, perhaps in compensation for it
Dysarthrias	A group of speech disorders resulting from disturbances in muscular control—weakness, slowness, incoordination—of the speech mechanism caused by damage to the central or peripheral nervous sytem or both; term encompasses coexisting neurogenic disorders of several or all the basic processes of speech: respiration, phonation, resonance, articulation, and prosody[8]
Right hemisphere disorder	An acquired disorder in the expression and reception of complex, contextually based communicative events resulting from disturbance of the attentional and perceptual mechanisms underlying nonsymbolic, experiential processing[21]

the communicative partner to either receive or enhance reception must be considered. This definition takes into consideration a wide range of communication needs. Frattali points out that it is also stated positively by addressing ability rather than disability.[10] This positive orientation contrasts markedly with more traditional clinical assessment tools focusing on the identification of deficits. This section attempts to consistently include the positive "functional" perspective when discussing impairments following stroke. It is the functional communication assessment that refrains from fragmenting the realm of communication into its various component processes. Thus voice, speech, fluency, language, and cognition are integrated into a holistic framework of communication. The team rates the patient's functional communication, not the patient's aphasia or apraxia. However, the impairment must also be addressed.

Aphasia. As can be seen in both Tables 10-1 and 10-2, aphasia is defined as a language disorder and commonly occurs after a left CVA. The most notable aphasia classification systems (reviewed by Tonkovich[35]) are as follows:

- Severity (e.g., mild, moderate, severe)[9]
- Modality (e.g., receptive versus expressive)[37]
- Behavioral (e.g., simple aphasia, group I)[33]
- Statistical (e.g., Porch Index of communicative abilities)[25]
- Syndrome (e.g., Boston Diagnostic Aphasia Examination)[14]

The most commonly adopted aphasia classification system is the syndrome approach. At a team conference, one is most likely to hear about a person with Broca's, Wernicke's, or anomic aphasia. The syndrome approach is useful because it describes a given type of aphasia in terms that are understood by most rehabilitation disciplines. Clinicians in neurology, neuropsychology, physiatry, and speech and language pathology commonly employ the syndrome classification approach when describing persons with aphasia. Three particularly discriminating patient language behaviors helpful in classifying aphasia by syndrome are *fluency, comprehension,* and *repetition. Fluency* is useful in determining whether a person with aphasia is nonfluent (telegraphic [e.g., in Broca's aphasia]) or fluent (paragrammatic [e.g., in Wernicke's aphasia]). Patients who are nonfluent typically have a lesion anterior to the central sulcus, whereas persons with fluent aphasia typically have a lesion posterior to the central sulcus. Thus fluency is a binary anterior and posterior decision. A patient with Broca's aphasia might request something to drink by asking, ". . . Ah . . . me . . . ah water," whereas a patient with Wernicke's aphasia might ask, "If you could velly please when the glass is full, thank you," and a patient with anomic aphasia might ask, "Could I please have a, you know, not a plate, a cup, yes a cup, no a glass of something to drink." Different content, fluency, and style are seen in these three exemplars of the three classic aphasia syndromes. The second differentiating language behavior is *comprehension.* The patient with oral language comprehension difficulties typically has suffered a lesion somewhere in the MCA distribution (frontal, temporal, or parietal area), whereas a patient with a reading comprehension difficulty typically has suffered a lesion somewhere in the posterior cerebral artery (PCA) distribution (occipital area). Finally, *repetition* distinguishes patients with MCA infarcts (lesions to the language cortex) and those with anterior cerebral artery (ACA) or PCA infarcts. A person with aphasia who has a repetition difficulty most likely had an MCA lesion, whereas a person with aphasia who is fairly facile at repeating words or phrases

TABLE 10-2 Decision Tree for Adult Neurogenic Communication Disorders
Following Stroke

ETIOLOGIC FACTOR	BRAIN LOCUS	IMPAIRMENT AND SYMPTOMS
Single infarct	Left side, right side, or brainstem	Motor speech impairment: affecting coordination and/or control of speech production anywhere along the speech system of respiration, phonation, articulation, resonance, and prosody, resulting in a "simplification" disorder
	Left side of brain	Recognition impairment: affecting information processing in either visual, auditory, or tactile modalities
		Language impairment: affecting linguistic components of semantics, syntax, phonology, and/or pragmatics
		Motor speech impairment: affecting the ability to program the speech musculature, resulting in a "complication" disorder
	Right side of brain	Cognitive-communication impairment: affecting linguistic, extralinguistic, and nonlinguistic aspects of communication, primarily caused by a disruption of the attention mechanism
Bilateral infarct	Left and right sides of brain	Motor speech impairment: same as for single infarct
Multiple infarct	Cortical, subcortical, and axial	Intellectual impairment: affecting judgment affect, memory, cognition, and orientation to at least some degree

MCA, Middle cerebral artery; *ACA*, anterior cerebral artery; *PCA*, posterior cerebral artery.

COMMUNICATION DISORDER	CLASSIFICATION	LOCALIZATION
Dysarthria	Flaccid	Lower motor neuron
	Spastic	Upper motor neuron
	Ataxic	Cerebellar system
	Hypokinetic	Extrapyramidal system
	Hyperkinetic	Extrapyramidal system
	Mixed	Upper and lower motor neuron
Agnosia	Visual	Occipital lobe
	Auditory	Temporal lobe
	Tactile	Parietal lobe
Aphasia	Broca's	MCA, frontal lobe*
	Wernicke's	MCA, temporal lobe
	Conduction	MCA, arcuate fasciculus
	Anomic	MCA, angular gyrus
	Global	Massive MCA, multilobes
	Transcortical motor	ACA, prefrontal
	Transcortical sensory	PCA, parietooccipital
	Isolation	ACA/PCA, watershed area
Apraxia of speech	N/A	MCA, Frontal lobe
Right hemisphere communication disorder	Linguistic Extralinguistic Nonlinguistic	Right hemisphere, nonlocalizing
Dysarthria	Spastic	Upper motor neuron (pseudobulbar palsy)
Dementia	Multiinfarct dementia	Cortical, subcortical, and axial

TABLE 10-3 Aphasia Syndrome Decision Tree

FLUENCY	COMPREHENSION	REPETITION
NONFLUENT Transcortical motor Broca's Isolation Global	**GOOD COMPREHENSION** Transcortical motor Broca's	**GOOD REPETITION** Transcortical motor
		POOR REPETITION Broca's
	POOR COMPREHENSION Isolation Global	**GOOD REPETITION** Isolation
		POOR REPETITION Global
FLUENT Anomic Conduction Transcortical sensory Wernicke's	**GOOD COMPREHENSION** Anomic Conduction	**GOOD REPETITION** Anomic
		POOR REPETITION Conduction
	POOR COMPREHENSION Transcortical sensory Wernicke's	**GOOD REPETITION** Transcortical sensory
		POOR REPETITION Wernicke's

(APHASIA)

Modified from Davis GA: *A survey of adult aphasia*, Englewood Cliffs, NJ, 1983, Prentice-Hall.

TABLE 10-4 Basic Classification of the Aphasia Syndromes

SYNDROME	FLUENCY	COMPREHENSION	REPETITION
Nonfluent			
Broca's	−	+	−
Global	−	−	−
Transcortical motor	−	+	+
Isolation	−	−	+
Fluent			
Wernicke's	+	−	−
Transcortical sensory	+	−	+
Conduction	+	+	−
Anomic	+	+	+

−, Impaired; +, relatively intact.

probably has a lesion outside the language cortex. Table 10-3 provides a decision tree that takes into consideration the above three discriminating language behaviors in arriving at the most likely aphasia syndrome for a given patient.

Once the language disorder of the patient with a left CVA is determined, the degree of impairment is ascertained by reviewing the patient's overall functional communication abilities. Table 10-4 summarizes the impairments in the various aphasia syndromes under the categories of fluency, comprehension, and repetition. This review takes into consideration the pretrauma status and posttrauma needs and communication options of the person with aphasia.

Some degree of difficulty in listening, talking, reading, and writing is common to all persons with aphasia. In short, to one degree or another, stroke persons with aphasia have difficulty processing symbols receptively and expressively. Receptively, the person with aphasia may have minimal or massive difficulty comprehending written or spoken words, phrases, sentences, and paragraphs. Expressively, the person with aphasia may have difficulty expressing himself in writing or speech. His spontaneous speech may include paraphasias or slips of the tongue. Verbal or semantic paraphasias are word substitutions (e.g., "pen" for "pencil"), whereas literal or phonemic paraphasias are sound substitutions (e.g., "fen" for "pen"). Thus the person who has word-finding difficulty (anomia) may produce a word or sound substitution when striving to label an object correctly. When the patient's verbal response is unintelligible, it is termed *jargon* or *neologistic jargon.* Hence, the patient with Wernicke's aphasia who asks for a "fwerple" when he means to say a "pen" has resorted to non-English jargon. One final output characteristic of severe left hemisphere damage that relates directly to aphasia is the phenomenon of perseveration, repeating a word over and over when no longer appropriate to the stimulus. Thus the listener, caught up in conversation with a person who has aphasia, is first struck by the fluency of his speech and thereafter by the paucity, relatedness, or both of his verbal attempts. Hesitations, self-corrections, paraphasias, jargon, perseveration, and silence are present — a true loss of words. This is the essence of aphasia. A language spill that forces the listener to put the pieces of the communication puzzle together in concert with the person who has uttered the puzzle. Perhaps the context that best resembles the language breakdown seen in aphasia is the common scenario experienced by a native speaker in a foreign country; he knows what he wants, but his listeners just do not understand.

Apraxia of speech. Because a lesion in Broca's area may disrupt the ability to plan and implement coordinated motor activity, it is not surprising that apraxia of speech (AOS) is a common, related impairment that often occurs with aphasia. The most distinguishable characteristic seen in persons with apraxia of speech is the marked difference in performance between volitional and automatic tasks.[16] The person with AOS typically has significant difficulty counting backwards from 10 to 0 (a volitional, purposeful task), whereas counting from 1 to 10 is usually a simple task (an automatic nonvolitional task). According to Wertz et al., the four most salient clinical characteristics of apraxia of speech are as follows[36]:

1. Effortful, trial and error, groping articulatory movements, and attempts at self-correction
2. Dysprosody unrelieved by extended periods of normal rhythm, stress, and intonation
3. Articulatory inconsistency on repeated productions of the same utterance
4. Obvious difficulty initiating utterances

This cluster of behaviors is useful in differentiating the nonlanguage problem of AOS from the telegraphese of Broca's aphasia and the literal paraphasic speech of Wernicke's aphasia. The person with apraxia of speech might ask for something to drink as follows: "Ah, ah, I want a kuh, kuh glass of water." Initiation difficulty and sound substitutions (phonology) are common in the context of normal grammar (syntax) and content (semantics). The assessment of suspected apraxia of speech includes a language screen and an extensive battery of speech production tests that elicit simple to complex volitional utterances under varying conditions (imitation, oral reading, spontaneous speech). The case of H.B. was an unusual one, referred for an augmentative communicative device by the patient's family physician.

CASE REPORT

Following a CVA in the left MCA, H.B. was mute with no significant motor signs. She was treated at home by a visiting therapist for several months without notable benefit, according to both the patient and the spouse. Three months after the CVA, H.B. was evaluated for a "global aphasia" and the accompanying reports detailed therapy plans based on simple "yes" and "no" questions and the development of a simple communication book. The pertinent finding was that H.B. had severe apraxia of speech and only mild residual mixed aphasia. What accounted for the earlier global aphasia in the light of the discovered apraxia of speech? H.B. was able to write about her basic needs accurately and appropriately. When her spouse incredulously asked H.B. why she had not written in the past 3 months, she wrote, "You didn't ask."

Agnosia. Agnosia is a prelinguistic problem that is fairly simple to diagnose but also fairly uncommon. If a person is suspected of having more than one agnosia, he more than likely has aphasia because agnosia is, by definition, an impairment affecting only one modality. Thus the person with pure word deafness caused by a focal lesion in the temporal lobe between Heschl's gyrus and Wernicke's area hears sound but does not recognize what is said. In this sense, it is a prelanguage deficit; the person cannot recognize the similarities and differences of sound (e.g., "pot" and "bought" may sound the same) and therefore is in no position to begin to comprehend these sound strings as meaningful words. However, the person with an auditory agnosia may be able to read, write, and talk (i.e., the other three channels [modalities] of communication may still be operational). Hence, a person may have an auditory, a visual, or a tactile agnosia. If more than one of these channels is involved, the person probably has aphasia, not agnosia. One patient referred by an audiologist for a suspected central deafness "could hear, but could not understand." A comprehensive evaluation revealed that the patient had pure word deafness; she could read, write, and talk much as before but could make no sense of what was being said to her. She exhibited a classic auditory-verbal agnosia with no aphasia.

Dysarthria. Another common sequela of a left CVA lesion is a mild concomitant dysarthria, a motor speech problem that can be differentiated from apraxia of speech both in volition and phonetic complexity. As already mentioned, the person with apraxia of speech has more difficulty with volitional tasks, whereas the person with mild dysarthria (usually right facial palsy and tongue deviation) caused by a unilateral left CVA produces more intelligible speech on volitional tasks. The second area of divergence between apraxia of speech and dysarthria is phonetic complexity. The person with apraxia of speech tends to make numerous substitutive attempts at the initial target phoneme (e.g., "fen, sen, ten, puh, puh, pen"). The person with mild dysarthria tends to make a single distorted attempt at the whole word (e.g., "hen" for "pen," as a result of the patient's inability to close the lips sufficiently to build up the intraoral pressure to make the plosive "p"). The person with mild dysarthria either omits or distorts words and typically does not substitute. Hence, the person with apraxia of speech complicates speech production, whereas the person with dysarthria simplifies speech production. The only appropriate dysarthria classification scheme appropriate for this type of upper motor neuron disease caused by a unilateral left CVA is one of severity (i.e., mild, moderate, or severe). Finally, the person with dysarthria but no aphasia has intact language and therefore is able to understand spoken or written language and to produce written or verbal language as well as before the stroke. The person with dysarthria may not be perfectly intelligible, but his word use (semantics), word order (syntax), and sound selection (phonology) are correct. Perhaps the best analogous situation is the person whose speech is sluggish (less articulate) immediately on leaving the dentist with the residual effects of a local oral anesthetic agent. The oral muscular control and coordination are lost, and therefore the person's speech may be unintelligible.

Right Hemisphere Communication Impairment

Fifteen years ago, persons with right hemisphere damage were not typically enrolled in a communication treatment program unless they exhibited a severe motor speech impairment (dysarthria). In the late 1970s, however, with the interest in pragmatics blossoming in aphasiology, attention was also directed to the communication impairment found in patients with right CVAs. Despite the typical characteristics of left neglect, flat affect, and impulsivity (a triad of symptoms often occurring with problems in pragmatics), patients with right-sided CVAs simply were not being referred for communication problems. Myers' seminal work in this area provided a rationale and framework for the assessment and treatment of persons with communication disorders caused by right hemisphere damage.[21] This area of research is still in its infancy, and the efficacy of rehabilitation in this population is surely less well documented than the century-old literature on aphasia. As Myers and Mackisack confess, we are only beginning to understand the effects of right cerebral hemisphere damage on communication capacity.[22] At present, treatment tasks tend to focus on the "behaviors" that cause problems in communicating in context and not typically on the underlying processes. Thus right hemisphere communication impairment (RHCI) goals stress compensation of deficits rather than recovery of function. Nevertheless, much progress has been made in assessment, classification, and treatment of persons with RHCI.

According to Myers and Mackisack, the communication deficits associated with RHCI are divided into three broad categories: linguistic, nonlinguistic, and extralinguistic.[22] Despite the linguistic descriptors employed, it is important to note that the person with left CVA and aphasia has an underlying linguistic problem. In fact, Myers and Mackisack attribute the majority of the RHCI problems to the underlying perceptual and attentional deficits found in this population.[22] If the person with RHCI suffers from impulsivity, neglect, and

TABLE 10-5   Selected Communication Problems Seen in Persons with Right Hemisphere Communication Impairment

AREA OF DEFICIT	PROBLEMS
Linguistic	Confrontation naming
	Word fluency
	Auditory comprehension of complex material
	Dysgraphia caused by substitutions, repetitions, and/or omissions
Nonlinguistic	Left neglect
	Visuospatial deficits
	Impaired processing in context
Extralinguistic	Topic maintenance
	Impulsivity of response
	Literal interpretation
	Insensitivity to communication situation
	Interpreting and producing affective facial expression
	Interpreting and producing prosodic features of verbal messages

Modified from Myers P, Mackisack L. In LaPointe L, editor: *Aphasia and related neurogenic language disorders*, New York, 1990, Thieme Medical Publishers.

flattened affect, it is little wonder that the patient is unable to attend properly to the complexities of a fast-paced conversation, an editorial page, or a physician informing him of the need for further tests. In patients with RHCI, the ability to appreciate the importance, relevance, or even the existence of what is happening in context is often seriously impaired. A menu of communication problems seen in RHCI can be found in Table 10-5.

In summary, according to Tonkovich, right hemisphere lesions give rise to a number of communication disorders and associated deficits that may interfere with normal communicative interactions.[35] The nature and theoretical causes of these disorders are not thoroughly understood because neurologic organization in the right hemisphere makes localization of these symptoms difficult. Nevertheless, at least a classification schema and workable theoretical model for assessment and treatment of persons with RCHI are currently available.

CASE REPORT

S.W., a Ph.D. in microbiology who had had a right CVA, was referred to the speech-language pathology department for evaluation of his "writing problems." On completion of an extensive language and cognitive battery, the patient was found to have a moderate RHCI characterized by moderate left neglect, prosopagnosia (problems in facial recognition), aprosodia (little prosody in expressive speech), reduced divergent language (written and verbal), and autotopagnosia (lack of awareness of illness or impairment). Writing was the least of his problems, and his spouse and family were frankly struck by how "this was not the man we knew" even though he could "talk pretty well." This is the type of patient who could easily fall through the rehabilitation referral cracks because no clearly overt communication impairment was present. Once the team, spouse, family, and patient became aware of the constellation of communication problems and consequent compensatory strategies that could work for S.W., an aggressive cotreatment regimen resulted in a favorable outcome. S.W. is currently a grants manager for the federal government. By his own admission, had he not been referred for his "writing problem," the course of rehabilitation would not have resulted in his successful vocational reentry.

Multiple-Infarct Dementia

Dementia resulting from multiple infarcts amounts to nearly 25% of all dementias. This intellectual impairment is differentiated from all of the previously mentioned stroke-induced disorders by its cause (multiple infarcts), course (decline), and constellation of symptoms (decrements in judgment, affect, memory, cognition, and orientation). It is differentiated from Alzheimer's disease by the presence of neuroradiologic and neurologic findings consistent with multiple infarcts. Thus persons with multiple-infarct dementia (MID) typically have a history of chronic high blood pressure, atherosclerosis, and ministrokes. The diagnostic dictum is that persons with MID must demonstrate a deficit in each of five macro areas—judgment, affect, memory, cognition, and orientation (JAMCO)—and demonstrate neuroradiologic findings consistent with multiple infarcts. Person with MID typically are not amenable to classic rehabilitation, but they do require assessment to rule out a pseudodementia or an exacerbation of aphasia, apraxia, or other communication disorders.

CASE REPORT

A.G., a retired physician with a previous history of left CVA with aphasia, was referred for an evaluation of his communication status following a recurrent stroke with an exacerbation of aphasia and other residual complications such as irritability, confusion, mood changes, and incontinence. The reevaluation of A.G. following this most recent neurologic episode revealed a marked decrement in the patient's judgment, affect, memory, cognition, and orientation and suggested that the patient was exhibiting an intellectual impairment as a result of multiple infarcts. It was thought that the deterioration in language (the aphasia) was not the primary deficit, but that intellectual abilities were dampened across the board. A referral to a psychiatric gerontologist confirmed the assessment, and A.G. and his family were immediately involved in summoning the available community resources to cope with MID.

Comprehensive Assessment and Diagnostic Therapy

Diagnosing, putting the label on the problem, has two primary purposes: providing a prognosis and indicating appropriate mànagement. Thus far we have defined and assessed the various neurogenic communication disorders and discussed differential diagnoses. Table 10-6 provides a comparison of 11 relevant areas in poststroke speech, language, and cognitive-communication disorders.[5] Having honed in on a diagnostic label, the diagnostic-specific assessment process that results in a treatment plan is outlined in the box on p. 297.

On completion of the comprehensive assessment, the clinician is expected to arrive at a communication diagnosis (Table 10-2) and prognosis. The prognostic exercise may involve a behavioral,[33] statistical,[26] or variable approach.[29] Table 10-7 summarizes the research and prognostic variables important in aphasia and related neurogenic communication disorders following stroke. Obviously, the medical and speech and language variables are more potent than the subject or other variables. The prognostic challenge is to estimate the potency of these various factors and make the best clinical estimate about the patient's overall prognosis. In formulating a prognosis, the team asks the following three queries:

1. Prognosis for what?
2. Which factors are positive?
3. Which factors are negative?

Although the correspondence is not one-on-one, the clinician does get an impression as to what are the "best odds." Once a determination is made that the patient's overall prognosis is good, fair, or poor for a given level of functional communication, the clinician must estimate the patient's response to treatment:

1. Will treatment help?
2. If so, what modalities should be treated and in what order?
3. What type of treatment should be used?

Diagnostic therapy. At National Rehabilitation Hospital the average length of stay (LOS) for stroke has declined steadily from a high of 48 days (1985) to a low of 28 days (1992). Acute medical rehabilitation continues to ratchet down on a continuing basis, with the only end in sight being no inpatient rehabilitation stay for most persons with stroke. Although that extreme scenario is unlikely, it

TABLE 10-6 Poststroke Speech, Language, and Cognitive Communication Disorders Compared on Eleven Relevant Dimensions

DIMENSION	SPEECH DISORDERS	LANGUAGE DISORDERS	COGNITIVE-COMMUNICATIVE DISORDERS
Auditory comprehension	Intact	Impaired	Difficulty with subtle, complicated, or sequenced communication
Verbal language	Intact	Paraphasia, impaired word order	Intact
Reading	Intact	Impaired	Left neglect, inattention to detail
Writing	Intact	Impaired	Left neglect, omission, perseveration, and substitution
Speech	Slurred	Intact	Impaired
Memory, attention, and concentration	Intact	Intact	Impaired
Orientation	Intact	Intact	Impaired
Analysis and problem solving	Intact	Intact, nonverbal	Intact verbal
Behavioral style	No change	Slow, cautious	Quick, impulsive
Insight into effects of stroke	Intact	Varies	Impaired
Motor involvement	Left or right	Usually right	Usually left

From Baron C: Poststroke speech, language, and cognitive-communication disorders contrasted according to eleven relevant dimensions. Table produced as part of National Rehabilitation Hospital SLP Student Training Lecture Series, 1988.

is likely that the average LOS for stroke in a rehabilitation facility will continue to decline. Even a 3-week period does not leave the treatment team sufficient time for a comprehensive evaluation. Current inpatient therapists must hit the ground running on the second day of a stroke patient's admission. The team must already have determined from preadmission and medical records data the subjective complaint and rehabilitation goals of the patient; the pertinent biographic, medical, and behavioral information concerning the stroke patient's candidacy for rehabilitation; and the necessary neurologic and neuroradiologic findings that permit the assigned therapist to be eclectic in the tests and diagnostic approaches to be undertaken.

Areas of Comprehensive Assessment

A comprehensive diagnostic test protocol should consist of the following areas of assessment:

- Subjective complaint and reason for referral
- Background information, including medical biographic and behavioral history
- Sensorimotor screens (e.g., hearing and vision test results)
- Oral motor examination of structures and function of the speech and swallowing mechanisms
- Standard voice and speech evaluation: examining pitch, quality, and intensity of voice and speech intelligibility for words, phrases, and sentences, noting sound distortions, omissions, and substitutions
- Standard language evaluation, examining spontaneous speech, auditory and reading comprehension, repetition, naming, and writing
- Standard cognitive screen, examining orientation, memory, language, writing, and calculation
- Functional status assessment of communication
- Patient and family participation and contribution
- Environmental prosthetic and device inventory
- Pragmatic performance and potential, examining the use of language in context and reviewing the patient's use of substitution and compensation strategies

TABLE 10-7 Prognostic Variables Important to Aphasia and Related Neurogenic Communication Disorders Following Stroke

SUBJECT VARIABLES	MEDICAL VARIABLES	SPEECH AND LANGUAGE VARIABLES	OTHER VARIABLES
Age at onset	Etiologic factors	Severity of disorder	Months after onset
Education	Site of lesion	Classification and type of disorder	
Intelligence	Extent of lesion		Motivation
Handedness	Coexisting medical problems	Coexisting communicative impairment	Stimulability
Monolingual or multilingual		Memory and attentional deficits	Environment
		Sensorimotor and perceptual deficits	
		History of earlier treatment	

Modified from LaPointe L: Aphasia therapy: some principles and strategies for treatment. In Johns D, editor: *Clinical management of neurogenic communication disorders*, ed 2, Boston, 1985, Little, Brown.

Five years ago the treatment team had the luxury of at least a week to complete a thorough, even scholarly, diagnostic workup. Currently, one must short-circuit the comprehensive approach and determine immediately the most pressing communication problems and the most promising approaches to functional remediation. Thus the results of a "yes" and "no" battery of questions do not provide the clinician with merely a percentage of "yes" and "no," reliability but with diagnostic therapy data as well, such as:

- The best input channel or combination of channels
- The variables that optimize success and minimize failure
- The most stimulable content and methodology

Hence, for example, diagnostic therapy does not only tell the clinician that Mr. Jones scored 45/60 on the Western Aphasia Battery's "yes" and "no" subtest but also that, given more time and a repeated stimulus, his accuracy was enhanced; in addition, although several errors were noted as the result of impulsivity, the patient did self-correct at least once. This type of data helps the team at the initial team conference to decide on the most effective means of getting the message across so that the patient and significant others can follow the critical training in self-care, ambulation, and other areas. In summary, diagnostic therapy is the clinician's follow-up effort at finding an immediate, practical application for the test results. According to Rosenbek et al., the diagnostic and prognostic treatment approach is intended to determine whether a patient can learn, generalize improvement on treated stimuli to untreated stimuli, and retain what has been accomplished, as well as whether the patient is willing to practice.[29] This information is invaluable to the team, patient, and family as they move together toward achieving the rehabilitation goals. The diagnostic instrument and diagnostic therapy should not just label behavior but assist the team, patient, and family to reap benefit immediately from the prognostic and prescriptive elements. A sound diagnostician not only attempts to find what the stroke survivor can or cannot do, but more important, he or she attempts to discover the most fruitful approach for enhancing functional communication and achieving the best possible outcome.

CASE REPORT

B.H., who had had a left CVA with severe Broca's aphasia and apraxia of speech, was enrolled in an interdisciplinary rehabilitation program involving physical and occupational therapies and SLP. The initial speech and language workup revealed an extremely supportive, intuitive, and involved spouse who was prepared to become a cotherapist. Although B.H. had a severe communication impairment and a marked hemiplegia that limited ambulation and completion of his own ADLs, the team jointly agreed with B.H. to involve his spouse in all aspects of his treatment. Diagnostic therapy determined that gesture and other nonverbal approaches were the optimal avenues of communication and that frustration and poor endurance could be circumvented by brief rest periods and resumption of the treatment activity. The spouse became the common denominator of all three therapies, carrying over each interdisciplinary goal to each session and practicing each of the day's activities with B.H. in the evening and on weekends. The aggressive interdisciplinary cotherapy paid off, with the patient achieving the selected goals that permitted him and his spouse to enjoy a quality of life after stroke that empowered them to do for each other what they both now knew they were capable of as a team.

Conceptual framework. The level of outcome should be thought of across a continuum. Wilkerson conceptualized three levels of outcome – micro, middle, and macro.[38] For example, word-finding ability (micro level) leads to functional communication (middle level), which leads to independent living (macro level). Frattali[11] notes that these levels parallel the World Health Organization (WHO)[39] model of consequences of pathology: impairment (dysfunction at the organ level), disability (functional consequences of impairment that affect performance of daily tasks), and handicap (social disadvantage resulting from an impairment or a disability).

According to Frattali, each level requires a different approach to measurement:

> Our traditional diagnostic tools are known to measure impairment. They are useful for differential diagnosis and identification of specific speech, language, swallowing, or hearing deficits, and strengths. Functional assessment tools measure ability to communicate in natural environments. Quality of life scales or handicap inventories measure handicaps. Measures of handicap capture physical, psychosocial, technologic, and economic barriers that create dependency or suppress quality of life.[11]

The crucial clinical query at this stage is at what level intervention gives the consumer the "most bang for the buck." Our diagnostic tools, outcome measures, and handicap inventories must be used adroitly to optimize the team's diagnostic assessment and treatment and (as a result) to deliver the most appropriate, desired, and functional outcome as efficiently and effectively as possible. One of the important variables in the current rehabilitation equation is the dyad of the patient and significant other as comanagers of their own rehabilitation destiny through expanding options and minimizing the handicap.

Development of a Treatment Plan

The treatment discussion can be put in the intersecting context of three models: the WHO's model of consequences of pathology[39]; Wikerson's model of outcome[38]; and Lubinski's model for intervention.[19] Table 10-8 attempts to capture this confluence of thought and organize the treatment discussion. Traditional treatment might focus on the impairment, which corresponds to

TABLE 10-8   Models of Consequences of Pathology, of Outcome, and, of Therapy

WORLD HEALTH ORGANIZATION'S[39] MODEL OF CONSEQUENCES OF PATHOLOGY	WILKERSON'S[38] MODEL OF OUTCOME	LUBINSKI'S[19] MODEL FOR INTERVENTION
Impairment	Micro	Skill approach
Disability	Middle	Effectiveness approach
Handicap	Macro	Opportunity approach

Wilkerson's micro level[38] and Lubinski's *skill approach.*[19] The skill approach focuses on improving the specific speech, language, or hearing disorder in the communicatively impaired adult, such as teaching a person with dysarthria to use an intrusive schwa sound to say a word that contains a consonant blend [kuhlutter = clutter]. The functional communication approach to treatment focuses on the person's disability and targets the middle level of outcome, employing the effectiveness approach.[4,19,38,39] In contrast to the skill approach, the effectiveness approach stresses improving the individual's ability to receive and transmit messages through any means possible with the aid of a trusted, facilitating communication partner. The listener of a person with dysarthria knows a hierarchy of strategies for improving speech intelligibility (e.g., asking for a repeat, a rephrase, the first letter of word, and a spelling of the word). Finally, the handicapping condition of stroke warrants addressing the macro level of outcome, wherein the patient strives for independent living. It is at this level that Lubinski espouses the opportunity approach.[19] In the patient's own milieu, the opportunity approach to communication therapy is premised on the philosophy that, for communication to occur, the stroke patient must want (1) to communicate and (2) to live in an environment that stimulates and reinforces communication.

In the community the person with dysarthria may minimize the handicap by having a communication book or a speak-and-spell prosthetic device that might expedite and/or augment speech intelligibility in as many and varied contexts as the patient was accustomed to before the stroke.

CASE REPORT

R.J., a 64-year-old microbiologist with lingual dystonia caused by microvascular disease, was fitted with an oral prosthesis and realized a fivefold increase in speech intelligibility at the word level. In addition, a marked improvement in self-confidence and success at work was accompanied by an enhanced style and rate of speech communication and consistently employed communication repair strategies. R.J.'s family and immediate circle of employees at work were educated and trained about his communication repair strategies. According to the patient, even with only moderate speech intelligibility, he has resumed family and work activities with only a minimal social handicap.

The team completes a "site visit" and prepares an "environmental impact statement" detailing the components of the physical and social environment that might either facilitate or reduce communication opportunities. Once the barriers to communicate are identified, the clinician, patient, family, and (if applicable) employer jointly address how to eliminate or circumvent these barriers.

Establishment of an interdisciplinary communication care plan. A point that has been emphasized throughout this book is that interdisciplinary goal planning must involve the key member of the team, the *patient,* in targeting the outcome of rehabilitation. The speech and language pathologist is also an integral member of the team and brings to the first team conference a wealth of information about the communication diagnosis; the functional status report, using appropriate outcome measures; the results of diagnostic therapy that can arm the team with targeted functional communication strategies; the prognosis for eventual functional communication; and the suggested approach to individual treatment, group treatment, and cotreatment. However, therapy does not occur with the patient in a vacuum. The rehabilitation goals must be tempered not only by the individual's prognostic variables but also by the exigencies of the length of stay, the 3-hour rule (in which physical and occupational therapies may command at least 3 hours of treatment time per day), census (in which stroke admissions may be higher than projected), and the speech and language staffing level (there may be six or seven other prime speech and language treatment candidates). However, none of these factors is as paramount to meeting rehabilitation goals as is the patient's own involvement, agreement to, and input in the interdisciplinary treatment care plan.

The steps to establishing this communication care plan are logical, sequential, and participatory. The first step is to identify the problem (e.g., the person with stroke has a mild anomic aphasia) and what the patient sees as his or her major communication problems. This question leads to an investigation of the potential solutions by identifying micro, middle, and macro goals.[11] The speech and language pathologist must obtain the patient's and family's input. In Ozer's structure of the planning process, the team essentially seeks the answer to four questions[24]:

1. What are your concerns?
2. What is your greatest concern?
3. What are your goals?
4. What are your specific goals?

These questions move from the general to the specific and may involve varying degrees of patient participation in the planning process, from independence to no choice at all.[24] Obviously, by definition, significant communication impairment hinders the patient's involvement in this planning process, but a keen family advocate can speak on the patient's behalf. The speech and language pathologist can assist with this goal-setting process in a variety of ways. The approach I have found most user friendly and fruitful is to provide the patient, family, or both with a menu of skills and abilities (micro and middle level of outcomes) grounded in daily living categories. It is unrealistic to simply ask a person with aphasia what his or her concerns are. A more productive approach is to provide a list of skills and abilities and ask the patient, family, or both to rate the daily living skills (DLS) list according to the following rating system:

0   Cannot do as well as before the stroke but do not need to work on just yet

+   Can do as well as before the stroke

◇   Cannot do as well as before the stroke but would really like to be able to do this (i.e., want change)

The team may compose its own communication skills menu or select tools such as the Functional Life Scale,[32] the Rehabilitation Indicators,[6] or the Communication Effectiveness Index.[18] The patient and family need *structure* to respond to the goal-setting questions.

Once the goals are set, the next step is to identify the resources needed (e.g., a high-technology communication device) or other means or methods to accomplish the patient- and team-driven goals. For example, the speech and language pathologist might report to the team that a patient with severe Broca's aphasia is resorting to Amer-Ind Code[28] to get his message across. The team should know that the patient's list of core gestural signals (communication repertoire) will be maintained on a card in his pocket and that the patient and team should consult this list when striving to encourage the use of gesture to problem solve and get needs met. In addition, the patient has been trained to request repetitions if he is unsure of what was said, and the team has been encouraged to use gestures liberally with verbal instructions and to be prepared to repeat or rephrase instructions for the patient.

Once the patient has set goals with the team and the team has outlined a plan and any potential barriers, the agreed on goals should be mapped chronologically on a time line, as shown on p. 303.

When possible, the team goals should be tied to the functional status report, wherein each interdisciplinary goal is tied to a specific outcome measure. Obviously this allows the team to measure patient progress and team effectiveness in real terms by measuring the final outcome at discharge. If real progress is not made toward increasing independence (and minimizing the handicap of the stroke condition), the interdisciplinary goal was not met.

Day one of admission

Problems identified and a functional status report made

Goal identified and a team meeting held

Resources and barriers identified

Family conference held and outline of skills effectiveness and opportunities made

Interim meeting held on goals: status report given

Discharge team meeting and funtional status report made

Day 28— discharge

CASE REPORT

R.J., a 72-year-old dextral male, suffered a left CVA with global aphasia 5 years earlier. He received several years of unproductive treatment and, for the past 3 years, has lived at home in Florida with a housekeeper and received no rehabilitation. At his daughter's request, R.J. was evaluated at National Rehabilitation Hospital and found to be a candidate for a short-term intensive rehabilitation stay (2 weeks) to be followed by a 1-month outpatient regimen. As a result of the joint planning of the team, daughter, and patient, the major interdisciplinary goal was identified: R.J. would convey ADL needs via gesture, drawing, or both in all therapy contexts. R.J. quickly developed a repertoire of 30 gestural signals. This repertoire was listed on a name tag, so that each person encountering R.J. would be aware of what gestures might be elicited such as "eat and drink" at lunch and "shave and wash" in the morning. The daughter became actively involved in the treatment program, watching the day's speech and language session (captured on video) with her father in the evening and practicing the signals with him. In only 2 weeks the main interdisciplinary goal was accomplished; in addition, R.J. acquired 30 Amer-Ind Code signals[28] and attained 90% accuracy on a standardized aphasia reading and "yes" and "no" battery. R.J. returned home with the ability to get his needs met and, more important, the power of initiative in developing his own ADL plan.

Treatment (Philosophy and Implementation)

A simple definition of handicap is "a limitation of choice." The impairment (aphasia) results in a disability (language disorder) that causes the stroke patient to experience a handicap (prevents the person from resuming his pretrauma familial, vocational, or avocational status). The prescription for stroke rehabilitation is to attempt to maximize the stroke patient's options—that is, to provide the handicapped person with more societal choices. In the context of a poststroke communication disorder, the following three rehabilitation approaches can be employed to minimize the handicap by maximizing options:

- *Enhance functional capacity:* by helping the person with aphasia change behavior through rehabilitation strategies
- *Reduce demands of the environment:* by minimizing the penalty on the person with aphasia, such as removing competing signals (turning off the television) and optimizing transmission of signals (having pencil and paper available)
- *Provide assistive devices:* by determining a menu of core needs, then fabricating a communication board that pictures or lists these same needs for the adult with a communication disorder to be able to convey wants and needs

Thus the speech and language pathologist joins the patient, family, and treatment team in arriving at the most pragmatic plan to achieve functional communication goals in an efficient and effective manner.

Coaching. Ylvisaker and Holland chose a sports analogy to clarify executive functions to both clinicians and head-injured young adults.[40] Specifically, they employed the image of an internalized coach to represent to patients their role in governing their own actions. Ylvisaker and Holland found that understanding the functions of a coach enables many patients to use the concrete goal of becoming a good self-coach in their own rehabilitation.[40] The executive or coaching functions they considered in the treatment of cognitive-communicative disorders were as follows:

1. Self-awareness: being cognizant of one's own strengths and weaknesses and factors that affect one's functioning
2. Goal setting: setting goals that are realistic, meaningful, and challenging
3. Planning, preparing, and training: putting oneself in a position to complete a task effectively
4. Self-instruction: giving oneself specific appropriate directions about how to carry out a task effectively
5. Self-motivation: "getting going" and "shutting down" when appropriate
6. Self-monitoring: attending to one's performance and factors that interfere with success
7. Problem solving and practical reasoning: taking stock of one's performance and modifying goals, plans, or strategies in response to obstacles[40]

This coaching analogy is also applicable to many individuals in the stroke population for whom goal setting, self-monitoring, and problem solving are crucial components in effectively getting a message across or solving a problem. Thus the clinician serves as a coach and mentor to the stroke patient who is engaged in a game of life.

CASE REPORT

C.R. was a 37-year-old who experienced stroke with aphasia nearly 1 year earlier. His stroke recovery was surprising in its breadth and depth. His initial status was severe in all vital spheres. He could not walk, talk, or bathe and toilet. The prognosis was fairly grim for such a bright young man with a wife and two young children. C.R. desperately wanted to get better and at the outset was assertively a part of the team's planning and implementation process. C.R., an avid sports fan, moved from "yes" and "no" questions and a single communication book, then later to an alphabet board, and finally to self-motivated internal coaching to arrive at his message and intent in a complete, coherent, and cogent manner. Four days per week, he puts into practice the above-mentioned seven-step coaching model in his work reentry as a customer service agent for a major U.S. airline. One day per week, C.R. attends a vocationally focused rehabilitation program, where physical, occupational, and vocational therapist and a speech and language pathologist review and refine the prior week's successes and debrief and detail the failures to ultimately ensure success so that C.R. can resume his prior highly competitive job.

An initial period of diagnostic therapy provides the team and the patient with additional "coaching intelligence" to strategically plan how to attack a problem and how to succeed at getting a need met. According to Ylvisaker and Holland, diagnostic treatment involves the systematic exploration of the effects on learning and general adaptation behavior of the following*:

1. Learning environment (e.g., what is the level and pace of activities?)
2. Patient endurance, persistence, and initiative (e.g., does the patient attempt to communicate with strategies?)
3. Alternate cueing systems (e.g., do gestures facilitate verbalization?)
4. Type of task presented (e.g., processing difficulty and interest factor — does avocational interest [sports, politics] foster enhanced communication?)
5. Types of reinforcement, density of success, explicitness of rules, and instruction (e.g., does the patient perform an established routine [self-cueing hierarchy] when confronted with a communication breakdown?)
6. Use of compensatory strategies and the ability to generalize and maintain the use of strategies (e.g., does the patient use a pacing board to slow the rate of his dysarthric speech?)
7. Adaptability to revised educational or vocational goals (e.g., following a pilot regimen at work, is the patient amenable to retraining for another position?)

In summary, the philosophy of stroke treatment promoted in managing communicatively impaired adults is to empower the patient to become more involved in his own care — that is, to foster in the patient the desire to increasingly become his own case manager. Once the patient is apprised of this rehabilitation charge and affirms involvement, the patient may enroll in a rigorous training regimen. Of particular importance in this training program is the engagement of the patient as a planner, and the question of what the patient wants to accomplish

---

* Modified from Ylvisaker M, Holland A: In Johns D, editor: *Clinical management of neurogenic communication disorders,* ed 2, Boston, 1985, Little, Brown.

and how he can accomplish it should be foremost. An array of executive functions is systematically tapped by the coaching team to enhance outcome.[40] The initial phase of training and self-coaching is preoccupied with diagnostic therapy or exploring the candidate's strengths and weaknesses, liabilities and assets, with an eye toward teaching the most effective strategy to communicate and determining from the patient what works best under different circumstances (for a list of important variables to consider in the selection and training of compensatory strategies, see Ylvisaker and Holland's article[40]).

Whatever the poststroke disorder, this philosophy and the approaches discussed can provide the framework for ameliorating or compensating for the communication disability. Ancillary, but no less important, interventions are patient education and continuous quality improvement monitoring.

Patient education. For each disability the team provides the patient with whatever learning resources are necessary for him or her to understand the following:

• The nature and extent of impairment
• The pitfalls and prognosis
• The potential treatment approaches
• The prospective frequency, intensity, and duration of treatment

A plethora of information-laden books, films, articles, and fact sheets are available from numerous agencies and associations (e.g., the National Stroke Association, the American Heart Association, the American Speech-Language Hearing Association, the National Aphasia Association, and the Alzheimer's Disease and Related Disorders Association). These materials can be borrowed and perused by the patient, family, or both. The rehabilitation environment should resemble less a medical setting and more an educational milieu in which a laboratory, a library, and a lounge are populated and practiced in equal proportion. In this way, the team is in a position to recommend to the patient a given medium relevant to his current communication problems. One of the premises of an educational approach to rehabilitation is that, before the individual can actually ask the right questions, he or she must learn a corpus of information about the topic. In short, the patient must learn what to ask. Thus learning resources should be available to enlighten the patient about his communication options. Once the patient is primed for learning and empowered to become his or her own case manager, the coach can move to a mentoring role, which may involve a number of activities, such as role playing and discussing, brainstorming, and game playing.

A group that facilitates generalization of the fruits of coaching and mentoring is the Stroke Club, "where stroke survivors find the understanding and motivation they so badly need to keep up the struggle to improve their lives."[3] There are more than 1200 such clubs throughout the United States, most operating in networks maintained by the American Heart Association, the Easter

Seal Society, the Courage Stroke Network, and the National Aphasia Association. According to Ammirato, Stroke Clubs offer vital support (educational and social) and self-help to more than 50,000 stroke survivors and family members.[3] The club's goal is to lessen the isolation of the stroke survivors by channeling them into an active peer group that undertakes a wide range of activities. This "supportive" club milieu is ideal for fostering risk-taking communication that is a crucial next step to striving to communicate in the community. The club consists of peers who not only are willing listeners but, more important, are empathetic proponents of overcoming a handicap. Although formal therapeutic intervention does not occur in a stroke club, the clubs still can have therapeutic effects: "The survivor is never done with his or her rehabilitation. They can experience improvement five or ten years down the road . . . . The survivors are hungry for information about the latest technology, therapy, and social benefits."[3]

Thus the merits of a stroke club or other peer group are undeniable; it affords persons with stroke an opportunity to unabashedly be themselves, to not have to "pass" as nondisabled, and to never have to say they are sorry for having a stroke.

Continuous quality improvement. Obviously the rehabilitation team is charged with attempting to deliver the best outcome in a reasonable period of time at a reasonable cost. In addition to documenting the patient's progress (weekly for inpatients and monthly for outpatients)—for which the clinician notes the status of each short-term goal (whether the criterion was met) in measurable, functional terms—the speech-language pathologist must also document appropriate test and retest data that reflect progress toward the patient's goals. Integral to this dual documentation of test results and goal attainment is the ongoing monitoring of the patient's involvement in the program. The speech-language pathologist should decide whether to provide the patient and family with regular opportunities to add input to therapy goals and to rate the patient's functional communication.[6,18] The speech-language pathologist must also decide whether to provide consumers (e.g., the patient, family, payor, physician) an opportunity to rate their satisfaction with the speech-language pathologist, the environment, and the program.[12] The premise of a continuous quality improvement (CQI) program is that one can always do better—that is, render therapy more effectively, efficiently, and professionally. The litmus test is not the progress note, not the functional outcome score, and not the cost. The litmus test of a satisfactory speech-language pathology intervention is a satisfied customer, a stroke survivor who feels that rehabilitation had a significant impact on his or her life and that the dollars, time, and effort were worth the investment. Another means of obtaining consumer input is to request the patient and family to maintain a daily log wherein the parties are requested to highlight or list daily communication accomplishments, failures, or both.

The diary approach provides invaluable insights about what are viewed as "problems" and "successes" by the patient and family. The historical consumer report of communication struggles may then become the treatment focus, wherein the speech and language pathologist attempts to problem solve with the patient and family about what worked, what did not work, and what could be done better next time. Role playing various scenarios that have already transpired provides a fruitful opportunity for discovering optimal communication repair strategies. If the consumers (in this case the patient and family) are not regularly invited to provide input on goals, progress toward goals, and overall satisfaction with the program, the team has not really engaged in CQI.

In closing, two letters from R.J.'s daughter, who was delighted with his brief rehabilitation stay, are presented. Recall that it has been 5 years since R.J.'s CVA and that, following a brief rehabilitation stay, he became communicative via a combination of gestures and drawing.

Letter 1   **August 23, 1990**   **Re: R.J.**

This is to keep you abreast of how dad has sustained his progress since working with you.

He has initiated "letters" to his son in California who writes to him every week. He also has written to me several times and enclosed a bird's-eye view drawing of his neighborhood with the streets labeled correctly and the route of his daily walk marked in red. His salutation and signature are correct, but the words in the text of the letter are copied randomly from books. Nevertheless, the letters are extremely heartwarming to receive and make us feel more connected to him.

He is able to negotiate his medication with housekeepers and relatives now. As you know, most of his medication was withdrawn and so now he sometimes feels pain from his arthritis. Previously he would have panic attacks if he noticed any change of medication routine. Now he is able to trust that he is communicating (both sending and receiving) accurately enough to adjust his own pain medication.

At his son's wedding in Chicago, his brothers and sisters-in-law noted that he seemed more relaxed, happy, and healthy. He indeed gestured and drew pictures for them and clearly indicated that he was happy with the results of his hospitalization.

I gave him a VCR when he left here. He now indicates to his housekeeper through drawing that he wants a National Geographic, opera, or drama video rented for him. He also communicated with a drawing to my aunt that he needed a new razor.

I can't tell you how full of gratitude my heart is toward you and everyone who worked with us at the hospital. Bless you and thank you.

Sincerely, K.J.

Letter 2   **February 11, 1991**   **Re: R.J.**

Here's a cc of a letter I received today from Dad. In it he tells me he is still walking, where, how far, and how long it takes him. He acknowledges receiving the 50th wedding anniversary card I sent (had mother lived, they would have been married 50 yrs Jan 18 and I knew he would be thinking about it). He tells me his brother, FJ, will arrive the a.m. of Feb. 21 and that he received and thanks for ("truant an") the Victor Borge video I had sent to him. How's that for communication!

Best Wishes, K.J.

DYSPHAGIA AND ITS MANAGEMENT

Therese M. Goldsmith and Christine R. Baron

Dysphagia, or impairment in swallowing function, is a frequently occurring and potentially serious consequence of stroke. Prevalence studies suggest that between 25% and 45% of people who sustain a CVA experience dysphagia.[58,62,110,111] In fact, stroke has been implicated as the most common neurologic cause of dysphagia.[47,89]

The impact of dysphagia on an individual's homeostasis, course of rehabilitation, and quality of life should not be underestimated. Medical complications that may result from dysphagia include aspiration pneumonia, malnutrition, dehydration, and asphyxiation caused by airway obstruction.[43,83,108] Swallowing dysfunction has been associated with a higher mortality in stroke patients.[111] Barer demonstrated an inverse correlation between swallowing impairment and functional ability at 1 and 6 months following stroke, after controlling for other indicators of overall stroke severity, and concluded that dysphagia may "lead to complications which hamper functional recovery."[44]

The maintenance of safe, adequate alimentation and hydration can obviously contribute to recovery following stroke. Perhaps less obvious but no less critical a factor for many stroke survivors is the enhancement of quality of life provided by the ability to safely and comfortably consume food and liquid by mouth. In recent years, evidence has increasingly suggested that the early identification and management of dysphagia can facilitate the resumption of safe, efficient, and pleasurable oral feeding, thereby enhancing functional recovery and quality of life.[61]

This section provides an overview of normal swallowing function, describes identifying characteristics of dysphagia and special considerations in the stroke population, discusses dysphagia assessment and therapy techniques, and addresses issues pertinent to the acute, rehabilitation, and continuing care phases of recovery from stroke.

Normal Swallowing Function

Models of swallowing and ingestion. Three-, four-, and five-stage models of deglutition or ingestion have been proposed in the literature. A preliminary "anticipatory stage," which includes decisions regarding initiation of the feeding process, dietary selection, and regulation of rate and quantity of ingestion, has been described.[76,88] Logemann[85] and others[72,105] describe a subsequent oral preparatory phase during which mastication, salivary lubrication, and cohesive bolus formation are achieved. Many investigators agree on the final three phases of swallowing: (1) the oral phase, during which the solid or liquid bolus is transferred from the mouth to the pharynx; (2) the pharyngeal phase, which begins with the initiation of the swallowing reflex and proceeds with transport of the bolus through a relaxed cricopharyngeal muscle into the proximal esophagus; and (3) the esophageal phase, during which the bolus is transported through the esophagus and lower esophageal sphincter into the stomach.*

Physiology and sequence of normal swallowing. A brief review of the physiology of the oral preparatory through the esophageal phases of swallowing is presented in the following. More detailed descriptions of the physiologic process and its anatomic correlates have been published elsewhere.†

Oral preparatory phase. On introduction of food or liquid substance into the oral cavity, a labial seal is generally formed and maintained to prevent leakage. In the case of liquids or foods of a puree or paste consistency, the bolus may be held between the tongue and the anterior hard palate in preparation for its transfer to the pharynx. Alternatively, some individuals may manipulate this material within the oral cavity before initiating a swallow.[83,204] Foods requiring alteration in particle size and texture before a bolus can be formed are masticated, using rotary, three-dimensional movements of the mandible and tongue.[72,83] During this process the food is moistened and chemically altered by saliva secreted from the parotid, submandibular, and sublingual salivary glands.[91] The masticated material is then collected in a midline depression formed by the dorsum of the tongue in preparation for swallow initiation.[101] In some cases of normal swallowing function a portion of the bolus may extend into the oropharynx before the swallow is actively initiated.[81,83]

Oral phase. With the bolus in its preparatory position, the voluntary oral phase of swallowing begins. Respiration reflexively ceases. The tongue is retracted and elevated against the hard palate in an anterior-to-posterior fashion, squeezing the bolus into the superior portion of the pharynx. The levator and tensor veli palatini muscles contract, elevating the velum and placing it in contact with the posterior pharyngeal wall, thereby preventing nasopharyngeal leakage or regurgitation.[54]

---

* References 46, 47, 72, 80, 91, 105.
† References 45, 54, 72, 83, 90, 91.

Pharyngeal phase. The pharyngeal phase of swallowing is a reflexive, complex series of motor events that in the normal adult are completed in approximately 1 second.[45,53,94] This phase is initiated as the bolus stimulates sensory receptors in the anterior faucial arches,[93] or alternatively in the tongue, soft palate, pharyngeal walls, epiglottis, or larynx,[72,83,107] thereby triggering the swallowing reflex.

Once this reflex is triggered, a series of nearly simultaneous events occurs. The hyoid bone and larynx are pulled upward, and the latter moves forward as the result of contraction of the extrinsic laryngeal musculature. The vocal, vestibular, and aryepiglottic folds are firmly adducted in an inferior to superior sequence.[83] Tilting of the epiglottis to a transverse position provides additional airway protection. Elevation of the velum and contraction of the posterior and lateral pharyngeal walls result in initiation of the pharyngeal peristaltic wave.[72] The bolus is subsequently propelled through the pharynx by a stripping action produced by the pharyngeal constrictor muscles. The cricopharyngeal sphincter relaxes, allowing the bolus to pass into the upper esophagus.

Under normal circumstances the bolus is transported smoothly and completely through the pharynx. Minimal, if any, residue is observed at the level of the valleculae, pyriform sinuses, or cricopharyngeal muscle on completion of the swallow.

Esophageal phase. The esophageal phase of swallowing begins when the bolus enters the proximal esophagus through the cricopharyngeal sphincter. A series of peristaltic waves carries the bolus through the proximal, medial, and distal esophagus to the gastroesophageal sphincter. The bolus passes through this relaxed sphincter and into the stomach. The lower esophageal sphincter then closes to prevent reflux of stomach contents. Normal esophageal transit time varies from 8 to 20 seconds.[83]

Neural control and regulation of swallowing. Neural control of mastication is thought to be provided by a neural pattern generator in the reticular formation of the brainstem. Peripheral sensory feedback provided by intraoral receptors and transmitted via the trigeminal nerve is believed to play a role in the initiation and ongoing modification of this process.[98] Lower motor neuron innervation for the muscles of mastication is provided by the trigeminal nerve, whereas the labial and buccal musculature is supplied by the facial nerve (cranial nerve [CN] VII) and the intrinsic lingual musculature by the hypoglossus (CN XII).

Triggering of the swallowing reflex generally occurs on transfer of the bolus to the oropharynx, at which time CN VII, IX, and X transmit afferent messages to the swallowing center in the reticular substance of the medulla from sensory receptors in the faucial arches, tonsils, velum, base of the tongue, and posterior pharyngeal wall.[54,56] Lower motor neuron innervation of the pharyngeal and laryngeal musculature originates in the ipsilateral nucleus ambiguus and travels through CN IX, X, and XI.

Neural control of the esophageal phase is independent from that for the preceding phases and involves interaction between central and peripheral neurons.[90] The striated muscles of the upper one third of the esophagus are supplied by the lower motor neurons of the nucleus ambiguus, whereas innervation of the smooth muscle of the more caudal end of the esophagus is believed to involve parasympathetic pathways originating in the dorsal motor nucleus of the vagus nerve.[92]

Characteristics of Dysphagia in the Stroke Population

Neuropathology. Because of the bilateral upper motor neuron innervation of most of the cranial nerves involved in swallowing, it is sometimes assumed that neurogenic dysphagia results only from bilateral damage to the cerebral hemispheres or from a lesion in the brainstem, where bilateral descending pathways are in close proximity. Although dysphagia may be more frequently encountered, or in some cases be more severe following brainstem or bilateral cerebral strokes, dysphagia following unilateral cerebral infarcts is a well-documented phenomenon.* Specifically, lesions in the most inferior portion of the precentral gyrus or the posterior portion of the inferior frontal gyrus in either hemisphere appear to be associated with the development of swallowing difficulty.[87,95]

Clinical manifestations. Although definitive differential profiles of dysphagia characteristics corresponding with the site of lesion have not been identified, some preliminary observations have been made. These are highlighted in the following discussion of the clinical characteristics of swallowing impairment that may be present following stroke.

Anticipatory phase. Impulsivity with regard to regulation of rate and amount of food and liquid intake is not uncommon in the stroke population and seems to be particularly prevalent in individuals with right hemisphere damage. This "stuffing" of material into the oral cavity, which frequently occurs in conjunction with ongoing verbalization, has obvious implications regarding increased risk for choking episodes. Conversely, reduced initiation of food or liquid intake may also occur. This behavior, not uncommon in persons with bilateral frontal lobe damage, poses a challenge in terms of maintenance of adequate oral nutrition and hydration. Such a challenge is illustrated in the case described below.

CASE REPORT

B.S., a 62-year-old female, was admitted to an acute care hospital following the sudden onset of right-sided weakness and loss of speech. A computed

---

* References 42, 58, 67, 87, 95, 110.

tomography (CT) scan of the head revealed an area of hypodensity in the left posterior parietal region, suggestive of a left middle cerebral artery ischemic event. Observation of swallowing difficulty was also reported in the patient's acute care medical record, and a surgical gastrostomy was performed. One month after the CVA, B.S. was admitted to the National Rehabilitation Hospital. Her feeding status on admission was nothing by mouth (NPO); all nutrition and hydration were provided via a gastrostomy tube. The results of interdisciplinary clinical evaluations were suggestive of an unusual adynamic condition that severely compromised the patient's ability to initiate any voluntary movement. When voluntary movement was initiated following repetitive multimodality cueing, that movement became stereotypical in nature, with the patient unable to shift to a different movement pattern. The patient was mute, and a significant aphasia was suspected, although the precise nature and severity of the language impairment were difficult to determine in the face of the patient's motor initiation impairment.

Intensive interdisciplinary treatment efforts yielded some improvement in the patient's ability to imitate and initiate limb movements. A limited clinical dysphagia evaluation was attempted with small amounts of pureed food and revealed that, once food was introduced into the oral cavity by the clinician, B.S. appeared able to transfer and swallow the bolus with only a mild delay. A videofluoroscopic modified barium swallow study confirmed a delay in bolus formation and pharyngeal contraction and revealed a small amount of pooling in the valleculae. However, no laryngeal penetration or aspiration of the bolus was evident on any of the food or liquid textures administered (thick and thin liquids, purees, and mechanical soft items).

Once it was confirmed that B.S.'s "swallowing difficulty" was primarily attributable to a motor initiation problem, her oral intake was gradually increased through the therapeutic feeding efforts of the patient's speech-language pathologist, occupational therapist, and nurses. Her gastrostomy tube was removed 5 weeks after her admission to the rehabilitation facility, and nutrition and hydration were successfully maintained on a mechanical soft and thin-liquid diet.

Oral preparatory phase. During this phase, difficulty may be encountered in achieving or maintaining an adequate labial seal, resulting in leakage of food or liquid from the mouth. This leakage is frequently seen contralateral to the site of lesion in patients with unilateral cerebral infarcts and may pose an even more severe problem for persons who have sustained bilateral hemispheric or brainstem damage. Prolonged, ineffective mastication or difficulty initiating and coordinating oral manipulation of the bolus was most often associated with left hemisphere damage in Robbins and Levine's study.[95] Pocketing of residual food in the cheek of the affected side is also frequently encountered in patients with unilateral cerebral damage and is especially prevalent among patients with right hemisphere damage. Xerostomia (dry mouth) sometimes occurs in the stroke population and may be a side effect of some pharmacologic agents. This lack of sufficient saliva may interfere with the ability to adequately break down food substances and to form a cohesive bolus.

Oral phase. Poor lingual control may interfere with the ability to achieve effective posterior transfer of the bolus and has been observed in subjects with right, left, and bilateral cerebral lesions and with brainstem strokes.[110] Ineffective valving of the velopharyngeal port, resulting in intrusion of the bolus into the nasopharynx and potential leakage through the nose, is sometimes encountered in persons with bilateral or brainstem damage.

Pharyngeal phase. In recent studies between 30% and 70% of stroke patients selected for videofluoroscopic evaluation of swallowing function have demonstrated aspiration of foreign material below the level of the true vocal folds.[65-67,80,110] Delayed initiation of the swallow reflex and reduced pharyngeal peristalsis with resultant residue in the valleculae and pyriform sinuses were observed across lesion sites by Veis and Logemann[110] and more frequently in subjects with right than left cortical CVA by Robbins and Levine.[95] Both of these conditions are associated with an increased likelihood of aspiration. Limited or absent laryngeal excursion during the swallow may result in reduced airway protection and inadequate generation of the pressure variations that facilitate passage of the bolus through the pharynx. Poor lingual–to–posterior pharyngeal wall contact at the initiation of the swallow may also have an adverse effect on the ability to generate adequate pharyngeal pressure variations. Incomplete vocal fold adduction, observed only in brainstem lesion subjects by Veis and Logemann,[110] also increases the risk for aspiration. Finally, cricopharyngeal dysfunction may prevent or limit the passage of the bolus into the upper esophagus, resulting in an accumulation of residue in the pharynx, which may subsequently be aspirated (Figs. 10-1 and 10-2).

Esophageal phase. Stroke has not generally been found to produce functionally significant esophageal motility disorders. However, preexisting esophageal disorders in the stroke population are not uncommon and may complicate the clinical manifestations of dysphagia. For instance, the ability to safely manage esophageal reflux caused by a hiatal hernia may be compromised by pharyngeal motility disorders or reduced effectiveness of airway protection mechanisms. This is particularly true in patients positioned in the supine or semireclined position.

Course of recovery. Although dysphagia has been found to be prevalent following stroke, several studies suggest that in many cases this condition resolves within 1 to 2 weeks.[44,58] In the interim a prophylactic program designed to minimize the risk of aspiration and asphyxiation while maintaining adequate alimentation and hydration should be employed. Such a program may involve nonoral feeding alternatives; modification of dietary textures; close supervision during meals; regulation of bolus size and rate of intake; compensatory postural

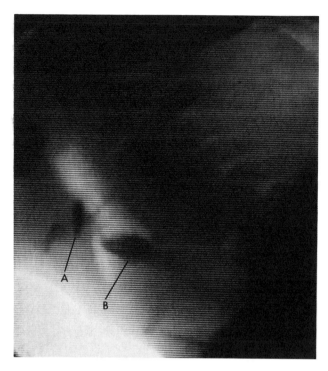

Fig. 10-1   Videofluoroscopic visualization of residue in the valleculae (*A*) and pyriform sinuses (*B*) after patient has swallowed barium-enhanced foodstuff.

adjustments to protect the airway during swallowing (see the discussion of acute phase concerns); or a combination of these. When dysphagia is a persistent problem, more intensive and extended efforts to rehabilitate swallowing function are often indicated.

Even in those patients with initially severe dysphagia, the prognosis for eventual oral feeding is often favorable. In a series of recent investigations, Horner and her colleagues found that more than 80% of a sample of brainstem stroke patients and nearly 90% of the samples of bilateral and mixed stroke populations were able to resume oral feeding.[65-67]

Special considerations

Aging. Because the incidence of stroke is higher among the elderly than in other age groups, it is important to be aware of changes in swallowing function that may occur as a normal consequence of aging. Before stroke, these changes may go undetected as the result of personal compensation. Combined with stroke-related changes, however, their effects may become clinically significant.

One of the most well-documented changes in swallowing function associated with aging is an increased delay in the elicitation of the swallowing

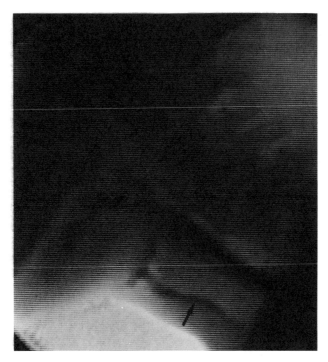

Fig. 10-2 Videofluoroscopic visualization of aspiration while patient swallows barium-enhanced liquid.

reflex. Tracy et al. found that, in one group of normal elderly adults, laryngeal elevation did not occur until the bolus reached the level of the valleculae.[109] Others have reported a reduced elasticity of pharyngeal tissue resulting in increased pharyngeal residue.[55,100] Increased aspiration caused by a reduction in epiglottic tilt has also been reported.[100] Sheth and Diner described poor dentition or loose dentures caused by alveolar ridge degeneration and an increase in cricopharyngeal dysfunction and gastroesophageal reflux in normal elderly adults.[100]

In addition to changes in swallowing function that may occur with aging, it is important to note that the nutritional needs of the elderly are quite different from those of younger adults.[52,59] Their special needs should be taken into consideration in dysphagia management.

Medications. Some medications have been found to have an effect on swallowing function. Antihistamines and anticholinergic, diuretic, antidepressant, and antihypertensive agents are known to reduce saliva production, whereas phenothiazines may create oral motor disturbance.[105] The effects of these drugs should be carefully monitored when treating poststroke dysphagia.

Tracheostomy tubes. Tracheostomy tubes are sometimes placed after stroke when upper airway integrity is compromised. In these cases the management of dysphagia should proceed with special care because of the existing respiratory compromise and potential for aspiration if the patient is dysphagic. The presence of a tracheostomy tube does offer clinicians the added benefit of monitoring tracheal secretions for potential aspirate during or after trial feedings. This monitoring technique is generally conducted using brightly dyed food substances to maximize the ability to differentiate aspirated food material from tracheal secretions. Although sometimes clinically useful, this technique is not always a reliable indicator of the presence, amount, or cause of aspiration.

Assessment

The quality of the dysphagia assessment following a stroke directly affects the efficiency with which appropriate treatment can be initiated. Assessments should be carried out with precision and in-depth knowledge of normal and abnormal anatomy and physiology of the swallowing mechanism.[70] The dysphagia assessment should result in accurate diagnosis of the nature and extent of the swallowing problem and should provide the specific information needed for the formulation of a treatment plan.[92]

Dysphagia screening. Because of the prevalence of swallowing problems after stroke (see the discussion on prevalence on p. 310), all stroke patients should be screened for dysphagia. Although nurses are frequently designated to perform dysphagia screens, any professional who has been trained to recognize the warning signs of dysphagia is qualified to conduct a screen. A dysphagia screen should begin with a careful review of the patient's medical history. Specific information suggestive of dysphagia includes a history of pneumonia or other pulmonary problems, sparse food and liquid intake, signs of dehydration or weight loss, and cranial nerve dysfunction (CN V, VII, IX, X, and XII). After the medical history is obtained, the patient should be observed briefly (for 15 to 30 minutes) while eating a meal. Behaviors suggestive of dysphagia are recorded, and referral for further dysphagia evaluation is made if significant behavioral observations or the medical history suggests dysphagia may currently exist. Criteria for passing or failing a screen should be set within each institution to ensure proper and consistent identification of high-risk patients (see the box).

Clinical evaluation. When a dysphagia screen is failed, the suspicion of dysphagia must be confirmed or ruled out by more in-depth evaluation. A speech-language pathologist is frequently designated to conduct this evaluation or to coordinate an interdisciplinary evaluation with the attending physician, occupational therapist, nurse, dietician, respiratory therapist, or a combination of these.[88]

The interdisciplinary model has certain advantages because it allows for coordination of the effort of multiple professionals during evaluation and

---

Components of a Dysphagia Screen

ORAL-MOTOR

Drooling
Coughing
Choking
Throat clearing
Wet voice
Difficulty chewing
Pocketing food in cheek
Difficulty keeping bolus in mouth

COGNITION

Neglect
Impulsivity
Rate
Initiative

SELF-FEEDING

Difficulty cutting food
Difficulty opening containers
Difficulty using utensils
Incoordination
Difficulty moving food to mouth
Poor positioning

---

supports a team management of treatment. Because stroke can affect many systems that have an influence on swallowing and feeding, this team approach is often ideal in managing dysphagia after stroke. Responsibility for various aspects of the clinical evaluation is determined by the constellation of the interdisciplinary team and the expertise of individual team members.

Case history. The clinical evaluation should begin with a detailed case history.[50] A medical record review and direct questioning of the patient or family should focus on the patient's subjective complaints, history of the swallowing problem, eating habits, respiratory symptoms, vocal changes, current medications, adequacy of intake, weight gain or loss, history of pneumonia, neurologic history, and results of previous swallowing examinations.

Physical examination. After a case history is obtained, physical examination of the patient should include a thorough oroperipheral examination by the speech-language pathologist.[104] Mandibular, labial, and lingual range and strength of movement are assessed. Oral sensation is tested. General dental condition is noted. This information may be used in predicting the adequacy of oral preparatory and oral phase bolus management. Assessment of the gag reflex, volitional cough, laryngeal elevation during dry swallow, and vocal quality are helpful in predicting adequacy of the pharyngeal phase of swallowing.

Language, cognition, visuomotor skills, and upper extremity functioning should be screened to the extent that they will influence feeding and swallowing ability. Adaptations to the examination process should be made if problems in these areas are observed to allow for maximal patient participation.

Clinical swallowing examination. Observation of the patient while eating provides information concerning functionally integrated swallowing abilities. Patients are given foods and liquids of various textures, frequently in the context of an actual meal, and in-depth observations of behaviors screened earlier are recorded (see box on p. 319). Potential compensatory strategies can be introduced as needed to maximize safety and adequacy of intake. Results of the evaluation are recorded and an interdisciplinary treatment plan is formulated. Often the treatment plan is accompanied by a recommendation for further specialized diagnostic workup, such as videofluoroscopy.

Value and limitations. The results of careful clinical evaluation are used to identify dysphagia and make preliminary determinations about its nature and severity. The potential effectiveness of compensatory strategies, including the patient's ability to execute the strategy, can be observed. Based on the results of a clinical evaluation, an initial treatment plan may be formulated, recommendations for further specialized studies may be made, or both. Clinical evaluations are not reliable in predicting certain specific dysphagic characteristics (e.g., pharyngeal weakness or reduced airway protection). Logemann reported that 40% of patients who aspirated were not identified during the bedside examination.[83] Studies of neurogenic dysphagia attempting to delineate reliable clinical predictors of aspiration have met with variable results. Abnormal gag reflex and wet-hoarse voice[80]; dysphonia[67]; and abnormal volitional cough, abnormal gag reflex, or both[66] have been related to aspiration.

At the same time an absent gag reflex was reported to be of limited prognostic value in detecting aspiration because it was seen with almost equal frequency in aspirating and nonaspirating stroke patients.[67] Silent aspiration, or aspiration without overt signs of difficulty, was found to occur in 28% of one group of stroke patients referred for dysphagia evaluation.[67] Specialized studies, such as videofluoroscopy, must be conducted to reliably detect aspiration, especially silent aspiration, and are widely used following careful clinical evaluation.*

Specialized diagnostic procedures. Many specialized diagnostic techniques have been developed for or applied to the evaluation of dysphagia. Cinefluoroscopy,[71] scintigraphy,[102] sonography,[99] manofluorography,[86] videofluoroscopy,[77] fiberoptic endoscopy,[74] and most recently the Exeter Dysphagia

---

* References 61, 66, 78, 83, 88, 105, 106.

Assessment Technique[96] have been described in the literature. Although use of each technique has inherent benefits and limitations, videofluoroscopy is the most popular procedure for the evaluation of dysphagia.[105]

Videofluoroscopy. A videofluoroscopic modified barium swallow procedure is well suited for the evaluation of dysphagia following stroke. Based on results of the clinical evaluation, the study can be planned and conducted to meet the patient's individual needs. Patients are seated upright, often in a specialized chair designed for maximal comfort and ease when positioning changes are needed. Barium-impregnated foods and liquids of various consistencies are given to the patient in controlled amounts (or patient-regulated amounts if appropriate).

Although such studies are most often conducted by a speech-language pathologist and a radiologist, other interdisciplinary team members sometimes participate in the evaluation process. For example, a physical or occupational therapist may participate to achieve optimal patient positioning for the purposes of the study. Studies are recorded on videotape to allow for careful analysis; to educate the patient, family, and other team members; and to use for comparison with future studies.

Although a popular technique, videofluoroscopy does involve a certain degree of radiation exposure and is sometimes limited in the degree to which it is able to replicate — and therefore investigate — clinical symptoms. Because these studies capture only a brief snapshot of actual performance, dysphagia management decisions based on their results should be verified by further observational evaluation.

With these limitations in mind, the values of videofluoroscopy remain impressive. It allows for a careful examination of the nature and extent of dysphagia, including identification of the physiologic components responsible for clinical signs and symptoms. It provides the opportunity to visualize if and under what conditions aspiration occurs. It is an objective means of evaluating the effectiveness of compensatory treatment techniques. Perhaps most important, it provides the information needed to develop a safe and effective treatment plan.

Acute Phase Concerns

During the period immediately following a stroke, the primary concern in management of a patient with dysphagia should be the assurance of safe and adequate alimentation and hydration. Failure to manage a patient's oral intake adequately at this stage could result in serious complications, such as aspiration pneumonia, malnutrition, or dehydration. These sorts of complications necessarily lead to prolonged acute hospitalization and the delayed initiation of intensive rehabilitation and recovery.

Although a thorough interdisciplinary assessment is the best method to guide clinical dysphagia management, many stroke patients may not be able to tolerate or participate in such an assessment during the acute poststroke phase. Furthermore, some acute care settings are unable to provide such a workup because of the lack of either qualified personnel or diagnostic equipment. Therefore the acute determination of whether or not a dysphagic patient is capable of safely receiving an adequate oral intake may be based on more limited information than is afforded those making a similar decision later in the rehabilitation process.

The acute dysphagia assessment should focus specifically on whether the patient can maintain safe and adequate alimentation and hydration on a regular (texture) diet with thin liquids. If this is not possible, texture modification, provision of nutritional supplements, or both are considered to preserve the oral intake. If these steps are not sufficient to preserve a safe oral intake, nonoral feeding methods must be considered.

Texture modification. Based on the results of a dysphagia assessment, stroke patients exhibiting signs of dysphagia should be placed on a diet that will allow safe oral intake. In general, thickened or gelled liquids are less likely to be aspirated after stroke than are thin liquids.[60] Likewise, purees or formable solids (e.g., applesauce or mashed potatoes) are usually safer than foods requiring excessive chewing and oral manipulation or multiply textured food (e.g., stir fry).[92] It is crucial, however, to keep in mind that these generalities do not apply to every patient. Only an individual dysphagia assessment can determine the appropriate texture modifications for a given patient. Texture modification is a common method for dysphagia management after stroke. The cited advantage of this approach over nonoral feeding alternatives is that it allows the continued use of the swallowing mechanism during feeding, thereby providing an opportunity for neuromuscular facilitation and reducing the likelihood of disuse atrophy.[79] The ability to modify the diet texture appropriately depends on the availability of skilled professionals to perform the assessment, make texture modification recommendations, and provide the recommended diet on a consistent basis. When the patient is receiving a texture-modified diet, careful and frequent medical monitoring for signs of aspiration, malnutrition, and dehydration is advised. If a texture modification plan is developed without the benefit of videofluoroscopic assessment, the importance of such monitoring is even greater. When patients cannot maintain adequate and safe alimentation and hydration while receiving a texture-modified diet, partial or complete nonoral feeding methods should be implemented in a timely manner.

Nonoral feeding alternatives. Nasogastric tube feeding is the method of choice when the need for enteral feeding is expected to be temporary (2 to 4 weeks). It may also be used as long as tolerated for patients who are unable to undergo or who refuse placement of other enteral tubes.[51]

Percutaneous endoscopic gastrostomy (PEG), surgical gastrostomy, or jejunostomy is recommended for patients who are expected to require long-term enteral feeding. Since its development in 1980,[57a] the PEG has experienced growing popularity because of its low complication rate relative to other types of enteral feeding methods. Each method, however, possesses relative risks and benefits, which have been described elsewhere.[103] The method appropriate for any patient should be individually determined.

In conclusion, because the risks of not managing dysphagia appropriately during the acute phase after stroke are relatively great, decision making during this stage tends to be conservative. When doubt exists about the patient's swallowing abilities, texture-modified diets or enteral feeding tubes are often prescribed. This is appropriate, and it ensures that a healthy patient will enter the rehabilitation process.

Rehabilitation Phase

Dysphagia goal setting. During the rehabilitation phase the emphasis is placed on reducing the actual swallowing impairment, ameliorating the functional disability resulting from that impairment, or both. Rehabilitation goals relative to dysphagia may range from the resumption of full and efficient oral feeding to the establishment of safe oral consumption of small amounts of texture-modified foods or liquids as a supplement to tube feedings. In either case, enhancement of the quality of life is the ultimate goal.

In many settings the establishment and achievement of rehabilitation goals relative to feeding and swallowing abilities are an interdisciplinary endeavor. The physician, rehabilitation nurse, clinical dietician, speech-language pathologist, and occupational therapist are among the professionals most often involved in this process, with their respective roles defined within the context of the particular program. Regardless of specific role definitions, however, the participation of each member of the team is vital to the successful management of the dysphagic stroke patient.

As with any aspect of the medical rehabilitation process, the involvement of the patient and his or her family is critical to the development of appropriate feeding and swallowing goals. In certain family situations the ability of a family member to eat and drink independently is a significant factor in decisions concerning discharge disposition. For some persons with severe dysphagia the ability to resume even small amounts of oral feeding is of paramount importance to their quality of life. For others, improvement of swallowing ability is less of a priority.

Persons with dysphagia who have not been involved in the ongoing establishment of their swallowing rehabilitation goals are less likely to understand and subsequently to adhere to recommendations or compensatory procedures established by the rehabilitation team. This potential for a breakdown in communication is demonstrated in the following case description.

CASE REPORT

F.T., a 56-year-old male who had sustained a right hemisphere CVA, was admitted to a rehabilitation facility following a 1-week stay in an acute care hospital. He was receiving a regular diet. The clinical dysphagia evaluation (conducted within 24 hours of the patient's admission) was suggestive of oral- and pharyngeal-stage dysphagia. Moderate aspiration of thin liquids and pharyngeal pooling of more solid food substances were confirmed by videofluoroscopy the following day. A modified-texture diet of mechanical soft foods and thickened liquids was recommended, and therapeutic feeding was initiated.

The nursing staff reported that, despite the speech-language pathologist and primary nurse having informed the patient and his spouse of this change in recommended diet levels, the patient's wife continued to bring her husband's favorite carbonated beverage from home for him to drink. She reportedly reasoned that, because soft drinks had been offered to her husband in the acute care facility, she could see no reason why he should not continue to receive them. Further discussion with the patient and his wife made it clear that neither understood the rationale for the team's recommendation of a modified diet.

The speech-language pathologist and attending physician subsequently conducted a review of the patient's videofluoroscopy study with both the patient and his spouse. An effort was made to highlight the aspiration that could be seen to occur when the patient drank thin liquids, and the treatment plan for improving the patient's ability to manage thin liquids was outlined. Following this educational session, compliance with diet recommendations and treatment protocols was markedly improved. The clinical dietician's development of an appropriately thickened form of the patient's favorite carbonated beverage also enhanced the patient's and spouse's satisfaction and patience with the dysphagia therapy process.

Dysphagia therapy techniques. Dysphagia therapy techniques may be directed toward stimulating improved physiologic functioning, or they may be compensatory in nature. Compensatory techniques may take the form of a modification of the external environment or task, or they may require internal modifications of the specific behaviors that compose the swallowing act. In addition to stimulation exercises and behavioral or environmental compensatory procedures, some aspects of dysphagia may be managed surgically, prosthetically, or pharmacologically.

Swallowing is a highly complex, coordinated, and interdependent act. It must be understood that modification of one aspect or component of the process may result in changes at other points within the system. With this in mind the following discussion of specific dysphagia management techniques takes place within the framework of the previously described phases of the feeding and swallowing process.

Anticipatory phase. One must be alert and reasonably attentive to consume food and liquid safely and efficiently. Oral feeding during periods of lethargy should therefore be avoided. Minimizing environmental distractions is sometimes helpful in enhancing the attention of an easily distracted patient.

Close supervision of patients who are impulsive or who demonstrate poor judgment is recommended. Verbal cues and a highly structured feeding regimen may be required to facilitate initiation and continuation of the feeding process. To the extent possible, attractive presentation of an individual's preferred foods at appropriate temperatures is suggested to encourage participation in the feeding process and to stimulate production of saliva.

Appropriate regulation of bolus size and rate of intake may be achieved through direct clinician control of rates and amounts, provision of external cues, or use of adaptive utensils that assist the patient in independently controlling the amount of food or liquid introduced into the oral cavity at any one time.

Oral preparatory phase

Stimulation. Inadequate lip closure during the oral preparatory phase of swallowing may be addressed by direct attempts to stimulate improved functioning of the labial or supporting mandibular musculature or both through active or active-resistive exercises. The proprioceptive neuromuscular facilitation (PNF) techniques described by Farber may be helpful in achieving improved labial closure and in inhibiting the primitive oral reflexes that may emerge in the patient with diffuse bilateral cortical damage.[57] For some patients the simple, consistent provision of a verbal cue (e.g., "lips tight") is sufficient to eliminate leakage of material from the mouth. Ideally the patient ultimately internalizes this cue and no longer requires external prompting by the clinician.

Techniques to stimulate improved mastication abilities may include direct lingual and oral manipulation exercises. The latter involves oral manipulation of a moist swab or other object that can be easily controlled by the clinician. This oral manipulation proceeds from simple lateralization to a more complex rotary pattern simulating normal chewing.[83]

The provision of sour foods or juices at each meal may stimulate saliva production for patients with xerostomia. Investigation of the patient's medications may implicate one of these as the cause of the patient's dry mouth (see the discussion on medications on p. 317). When possible, substitution of an alternative medication may alleviate the problem.

Compensation. A compensatory approach to impairments in the oral preparatory phase may involve modification of diet levels to include substances that are more easily broken down and controlled. For patients with impaired oral sensation, placement of food on the less involved side of the mouth or use of foods and liquids that provide maximal taste, temperature, or textural sensory input may enhance oral manipulation and control. "Pocketing" of residual food substances on the hemiparetic or sensory-impaired side of the oral cavity may

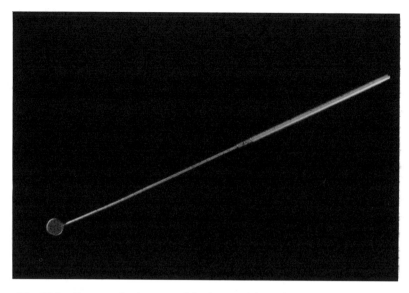

Fig. 10-3 Laryngeal mirror used in the provision of thermal stimulation.

also be reduced by strategic placement of the bolus. The provision of external cues to train systematic lingual searching for residual food also may be beneficial.

Compensatory approaches to inadequate labial closure include placement of the food or straw on the stronger side of the mouth or, in the case of someone with a concomitant facial hemisensory deficit, cues to wipe away food that has leaked from the involved side of the mouth after every few bites. In extreme cases of bilateral flaccidity of the mandibular musculature, a chin strap is a prosthetic approach that may be used to achieve labial and mandibulomaxillary approximation.

Oral phase. Active and active-resistive lingual exercises may be employed to improve the lingual-palatal contact necessary for successful propulsion of the bolus to the pharynx. An alternative or adjunct for some stroke patients is the use of an oral prosthesis, which reshapes the contours of the hard palate to facilitate lingual-palatal approximation.[83]

A prosthetic approach to the management of velopharyngeal incompetence during swallowing involves the fabrication and employment of a palatal lift. This appliance maintains the velum in an elevated position, thereby facilitating closure of the velopharyngeal port.

Pharyngeal phase

Stimulation. To stimulate improved physiologic function for the patient with vocal fold paralysis, the vocal fold adduction exercises of pushing, pulling, and coup de glot voicing may be used.[83] Thermal stimulation of the anterior faucial arches with an iced laryngeal mirror, as described by Logemann,[83] has been demonstrated to be successful in achieving more prompt elicitation of the swallow reflex for several subsequent swallows[75] although further investigation of more sustained effects of this technique is needed (Fig. 10-3).

Compensation. A number of internal and external compensatory techniques for impairments in the pharyngeal phase of swallowing exist. For persons with delayed initiation of the swallowing reflex, a flexed head position has frequently proved to be helpful. This position enlarges the vallecular space, thereby providing an additional "safety net" in which the bolus may rest until the swallow reflex is triggered (Fig. 10-4).[83]

Selley described an oral prosthesis, or "palatal training appliance," which appeared to facilitate elicitation of the swallowing reflex by providing additional sensory stimulation to the oropharyngeal region.[97] Modification of thin liquids to a more thickened consistency is another technique that may provide heightened sensory input and greater control of the bolus while awaiting a delayed swallow reflex. Groher demonstrated that patients receiving a mechanical soft and thickened liquid diet had significantly fewer episodes of aspiration pneumonia than patients on a pureed and thin-liquid diet.[60]

Some individuals with reduced pharyngeal peristalsis spontaneously compensate for this impairment by reducing bolus size or swallowing multiple times to clear the pharynx of residue.[48] Coughing or throat clearing with subsequent swallowing of pharyngeal residue is also sometimes observed. Patients may be taught to consciously incorporate these techniques into a set of individualized compensatory swallowing maneuvers, employed as protection against potential aspiration. Logemann suggested that alternating liquid and solid boluses may also be helpful in clearing the pharyngeal residue that often results from reduced pharyngeal peristalsis.[83]

Logemann discussed a number of specific swallowing techniques that may be used to compensate for impaired pharyngeal and laryngeal function. Among the most commonly used are the supraglottic swallow, head-turning and head-tilting postural adjustments, and the Mendelsohn maneuver. The supraglottic swallow is a volitional airway protection technique that requires the patient to consciously hold his or her breath (thereby adducting the vocal folds) while swallowing. This is generally followed by a volitional cough, intended to clear the pharynx or laryngeal vestibule of any residual material.[83] Use of this technique may be beneficial for patients with vocal fold paresis, reduced laryngeal elevation during the swallow, reduced pharyngeal peristalsis, or a combination of these.

In the case of unilateral pharyngeal or laryngeal impairment, turning the head toward the affected side has been found to divert the bolus down the side of the pharynx that is intact.[73,83,85] *Tilting* the head toward the *unaffected* side accomplishes this same objective.[83] Use of either of these techniques may reduce

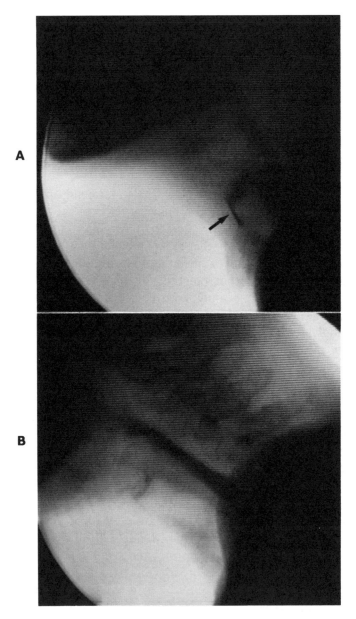

Fig. 10-4 Aspiration is observed when liquids are swallowed by, **A,** patient in neutral posture, but, **B,** not with compensatory neck flexion.

pharyngeal residue and the risk for aspiration. The functional exclusion of the impaired side of the pharynx, which is accomplished by the head-turning maneuver, has also been found to reduce upper esophageal sphincter tone, which may facilitate passage of the bolus through the cricopharynx.[85]

The Mendelsohn maneuver is a technique "designed to improve cricopharyngeal opening during swallowing by voluntarily prolonging and accentuating laryngeal upward and forward movement."[82] The patient is asked to feel his or her larynx digitally while swallowing and to attempt to prolong the period of maximal laryngeal elevation. It should be remembered that these types of behavioral compensatory techniques may be more difficult to implement with individuals who have language or cognitive deficits.

In the event that behavioral compensatory measures are unsuccessful, cricopharyngeal dysfunction may be managed by repeated esophageal dilation procedures or through cricopharyngeal myotomy. These techniques are generally not attempted until at least several months after the CVA to allow for the spontaneous recovery of muscle function or a determination about whether compensatory interventions may be effective.

Esophageal phase. Generally, comorbidities of esophageal function in the stroke patient are surgically or pharmacologically managed because no evidence exists that either stimulation exercises or compensatory maneuvers are effective with these conditions. In some cases it may be appropriate to recommend reflux precautions, such as elevation of the head of the bed; avoidance of dyspeptic foods; ingestion of smaller, more frequent meals throughout the day; and fasting for 2 to 3 hours before retiring.[49,69]

Continuing Care Issues

An appropriate dysphagia treatment plan maximizes recovery while providing safe and adequate alimentation and hydration. It is the responsibility of the treatment team to ensure that the patient (and the family, when available) understands and can potentially implement the plan at home. As a patient nears discharge from a rehabilitation setting, other factors must be considered in the treatment plan that relate to long-term management.

First of all, the extended plan for dysphagia management must incorporate the environment to which the patient will be discharged. For example, when a patient is discharged to a nursing home, preparation and careful monitoring of a texture-modified diet may be difficult. Nursing homes have a large proportion of patients who require assistance with eating, and the potential for too few or poorly trained personnel is sometimes high.[63]

Similarly, for a patient being discharged home, the ability and desire of the patient, family, or both to implement the treatment plan may be enhanced or diminished over time. For example, when diet preparation and compensatory technique use are time consuming, especially if recovery is slow, the patient and family may opt for nonoral feeding methods or may choose to rearrange their daily schedule to adapt to a longer mealtime routine.

Whatever the possible modifications to treatment plans at discharge, patients should receive follow-up evaluations at intervals during which change is likely to be observed. For most patients, this is monthly during the first 4 to 6 months after stroke, with the frequency diminishing thereafter. Only through follow-up evaluations can treatment plans be kept current and effective.

CASE REPORT

Acute Phase

S.F., a 74-year-old dextral male, was admitted to an acute care facility with a sudden onset of bilateral weakness in his extremities (greater on the left side than the right). A diagnosis of brainstem CVA was made, and no hemorrhage was identified. The patient was prescribed a course of heparin, but gastrointestinal bleeding developed and the heparin was discontinued. Severe difficulty with speech and management of oral secretions was evident, and a tracheostomy was performed. A gastrostomy tube was also placed, and the patient was given NPO orders. At this time, the primary goals concerning the patient's dysphagia were maintenance of airway integrity and provision of adequate nutrition and hydration.

The acute hospital course was complicated by recurrent pneumonitis with methicillin-resistant *Staphylococcus aureus,* which required antibiotic treatment. The patient was placed on a ventilator, from which he was fully weaned approximately 1 week before his admission to a medical rehabilitation facility.

Rehabilitation Phase

Initial status. Upon his admission to the National Rehabilitation Hospital, the patient presented with bilateral upper and lower extremity paresis. Bilateral rhonchi were present. A cranial nerve examination, performed by the attending neurologist, revealed limited extraocular movements with conjugate gaze paresis to the right; reduced touch and pinprick sensation on the right side of the face and left side of the body; right peripheral facial weakness; and inability to protrude the tongue. A feeding gastrostomy and plugged tracheostomy tube were in place. The patient demonstrated no spontaneous swallow reflex and was unable to swallow his secretions. Mandibular movements were noted to be limited. Speech production was severely dysarthric and characterized by imprecise oral articulation, a wet and harsh vocal quality, and hypernasality. Cognitive and language abilities were intact.

Stimulation and compensation. Dysphagia goals during the rehabilitation phase first focused on establishing the requisite physiologic support and protective mechanisms for the oral preparatory, oral, and pharyngeal phases of swallowing. Subsequently, goals involved developing the ability to safely consume small amounts of modified texture substances by mouth.

A program of oromotor exercises was implemented, and icing of the right facial musculature was also employed. A functionally significant improvement in lingual and mandibular range of motion was achieved over the 2-month course of the patient's inpatient rehabilitation program although the right facial musculature remained flaccid. Thermal stimulation to the anterior faucial arches was provided during three sessions each day. The consistency of subsequent swallow elicitation was noted to improve steadily, and laryngeal excursion on the swallow was increased.

Once the patient was able to swallow his secretions consistently, an initial videofluoroscopic modified barium swallow study was conducted using small amounts of pureed foods. A severe oropharyngeal dysphagia was confirmed. The characteristics included an extremely limited ability to independently propel the bolus from the mouth to the pharynx, reduced pharyngeal peristalsis with pooling in the valleculae and pyriform sinuses (greater on the right side than the left), diminished pharyngeal sensation, reduced laryngeal elevation during the swallow, and small amounts of aspiration occurring before, during, and after the swallow. Elicitation of a cough reflex following laryngeal penetration was highly inconsistent. Trial compensatory techniques, including supraglottic swallow, head turn to the right, neck flexion, and the Mendelsohn maneuver, were attempted. None was successful in reducing pharyngeal pooling or preventing small amounts of aspiration.

Oral and pharyngeal stimulation programs were continued, and therapeutic feeding of small amounts of pureed substances was initiated. These substances were dyed with food coloring, and tracheal suctioning was performed after each therapy session in an effort to check for aspirated material. The patient's oral motility continued to improve, and a more consistent cough reflex appeared to offer increased airway protection. Before the patient's discharge to home, a second modified barium study was performed. An improved oral transit time with pureed, limited mechanical soft, and thick-liquid items was evident. The initiation of the swallow reflex and protection of the airway were also improved, with trace aspiration occurring with only one bolus.

The patient's tracheostomy tube was removed, and he was discharged to his home. Ninety-five percent of the patient's nutrition continued to be provided via a gastrostomy tube, although he was taking small amounts of pureed and selected mechanical soft foods by mouth. Before discharge, S.F.'s spouse had been instructed in thermal stimulation techniques, and this procedure was continued at home.

Continued Care Phase

During the continued care phase the dysphagia therapy goals included increasing the amount and variety of the patient's oral intake while also increasing his independence in self-monitoring and in decision making about the oral feeding process.

An oral exercise program and therapeutic feeding continued to be provided through a home care speech-language pathologist. S.F.'s wife was trained to monitor the patient's lung sounds for signs of potential pulmonary complications, and the patient was also regularly monitored by a home health professional and his attending physician. His lungs remained clear. The patient and his spouse gradually expanded the menu of mechanical soft food items that he could tolerate, and his oral intake increased. While the couple initially sought approval of the speech and language pathologist for even the slightest modification in dietary selection or preparation, they gradually became more comfortable in making these decisions on their own.

Several subsequent videofluoroscopic modified barium swallow studies were conducted, and each revealed little change in physiologic functioning from that evident in the initial study. When the patient demonstrated the ability to successfully maintain his weight and hydration on a pureed, mechanical soft, and thick-liquid diet without the benefit of gastrostomy supplements, his gastrostomy tube was removed. As he and his spouse adjusted to his residual swallowing disability, their attention was gradually refocused to other aspects of their lives, and the residual dysphagia resulted in little or no functional or social handicap.

As the preceding case report illustrates, the management of dysphagia must be addressed throughout all phases of recovery from stroke. During the acute phase of recovery the emphasis is placed on protecting the airway and maintaining adequate alimentation and hydration. Efforts during the rehabilitation phase often focus on the use of stimulation and compensatory approaches designed to reduce the swallowing impairment or to minimize the functional disability resulting from that impairment. The continuing care phase involves generalization of rehabilitation techniques to the patient's own living environment. During this phase the patient and his or her family members assume greater responsibility for the integration and adaptation of recommended procedures to suit their individual needs and priorities.

Continued advancements in dysphagia assessment and treatment techniques promise to make the rehabilitation of swallowing disorders one of the most satisfying challenges faced by the stroke rehabilitation team. Dysphagia rehabilitation offers a significant opportunity to enhance the quality of a stroke survivor's life throughout all phases of recovery.

ENHANCING MOTOR FUNCTION
Nature of the Problem

The characteristic hemiplegia arising from stroke is its most prominent feature. The contralateral nature of the impairment has aided in the localization of the site of neural injuries. The pattern of impairment (of the leg versus the arm) is a reflection of the area of relative vascular insufficiency. Moreover, such impairment is not static. During the acute phase, assessment of the degree of impairment and its evolution over time foreshadows the concept that the organism is somehow responding to the existence of injury. However, the focus during the acute phase is on the degree of disruption from the normal range of activity and its prognostic implications. Preparation is also made to prevent secondary impairments, particularly in the upper extremity.

During the rehabilitation phase there is a major shift in emphasis toward assessment procedures and the conceptual framework that underlies them. Rather than a focus on impairment, there is a recognition that one must deal with the functional consequences of the sensorimotor control impairments. The problems faced are those of mobility and manipulation, and the effects are widespread, affecting more than merely the leg or hand. The entire motor system is involved. Balance in both sitting and standing is a prerequisite to use of the limbs. However, ultimately the goal is not merely to be able to use the limbs but to use the limbs to achieve the overall goals of the person in the setting in which that person seeks to act.

Moreover, the goal is to regain the ability to act via the sensorimotor control system despite the existence of neural injury and subsequent impairment. Therefore the focus of rehabilitation shifts from the degree and type of impairment to the degree and type of residual function currently available for integration into the required motor actions. Furthermore, the conditions under which one may bring about such integration must be defined. At this phase the patient learns new patterns of actions to achieve mobility, using residual motor patterns, assistive devices, and other persons to provide power and strength. The goals are to maximize the integration of existing motor patterns and to maximize function despite the continued neural injury. The patient must capitalize on what function remains and learn new ways of accomplishing life goals.

Recovery of motor function can and does occur despite the continued existence of neural injury. Thus the goal is to enhance the useful return of such function by various techniques, and this section describes methods for doing so. Successive sections of this chapter describe the training procedures by which a person with stroke may once again carry out life activities via alternative techniques, even with continued manipulation and mobility impairments. Each of the next sections describes more specific assessment and treatment techniques, including the use of assistive devices.

The ultimate goal of this phase of rehabilitation is for the patient to use the motor control system to carry out needs — to achieve mobility and self-feeding and dressing — to support "motivated behavior." The scope of the work done during this rehabilitation phase is with the upper level behaviors described in Table 10-9.[127] Levels 1 and 2 are subbehavioral outcomes involving the motor unit and the coordination of motor units composing a muscle. The lowest behavioral level is that of the muscle groups for which the patient may focus on actual muscle coordination and strength. This lowest level was the focus of the neurologic assessment during the early poststroke phase and may be an ongoing focus in this phase. For example, one may seek to increase the strength of particular muscle groups, treated as a component that supports the coordinated act of standing. The coordinated action of the muscle groups in the act of standing is generated at the level of the "organ." The coordination of the legs, trunk, and entire motor system to produce forward locomotion is an example of an outcome at this level of the "organ system."

In transection experiments on animals the various levels of the nervous system relate roughly to the levels of coordination described in Table 10-9. Loss of the forebrain entails loss of analytic and planning functions and thus limits the

TABLE 10-9 Behavioral Units of Motor Action

LEVEL	UNIT	MOTOR ACTION
6	Organism	Complex sets of actions to carry out such activities as eating and dressing, including action systems such as both locomotion and orienting in space
5	Organ system	Coordination of trunk, arms, and legs to produce locomotion
4	Organ	Coordination of the stepping of a single leg
3	Muscle groups	Coordination of antagonistic muscles on either side of joint
2	Muscle	Coordination of motor units, such as smaller motor neurons recruited early "size principle"
1	Motor unit	Individual motor neuron and the muscle fibers it innervates

degree to which motivated behavior is carried out effectively. The intact diencephalon supports motivated behavior so that actions such as walking and grooming are made to serve the animal's requirements, although this is done without focusing on the planned goal. With transection at the midbrain level, actions such as walking take place but not in such a way as to serve fundamental requirements.[127]

A comparable analysis of the levels of organization in the nervous system derives from the phylogenetic levels of the archicortex (reptilian portions), paleocortex (early mammalian portions), and neocortex (later mammalian portions) of the brain. The archi (reptilian) portion is the central core containing the autonomic nervous and reticular systems and the archicerebellovesicular system. The paleocortex constitutes the protective systems, incorporating the basal ganglia. The neocortex system represents the more discriminating localization of sensation and the exploratory components of the cortex.

Fundamental to our understanding of the nervous system has been the principle of vertically distributed functional systems.[128,129] Since the nineteenth century, the principle has been that functions are rerepresented at different levels of the nervous system. Progressively higher levels in the nervous system correspond to increasingly refined control with greater adaptive capacity. Higher levels inhibit the lower levels in the process of development. Lower levels function in a more automated fashion than higher levels. Thus damage at the higher level releases the lower levels to function, although in a less differentiated fashion. The type of motor recovery that occurs in the presence of neural injury is supported by this notion of vertical organization with the pyramidal or corticospinal tract reflecting the neocerebral, or highest level of, organization. The actions controlled by this level are those most affected by injury.

For example, distal weakness (particularly of the hand) is most likely to persist after stroke because of the relatively large component dealing with the hand in the corticospinal tract. The predilection for the recovery of strength in the flexors of the upper extremity also reflects the lesser contribution of the pyramidal tract to control of these "antigravity" muscles in the upper extremity. A major clinical implication is the high frequency of recovery of the ability to stand (and possibly walk) in those with even severe damage to the motor cortex and lateral corticospinal tract. This is based on the relatively larger contribution by the subcortical extrapyramidal motor system to the antigravity extensor muscles of the lower extremity.[148] A greater degree of functional recovery of the leg versus the arm and of the antigravity musculature in the leg results. It is postulated that the reticulospinal and rubrospinal motor tracts participate in the process of recovery despite the continued injury of the corticospinal tracts.

The level of the nervous system at which the injury has occurred determines the initial degree of disorganization and the degree of reorganization that may take place. Of equal importance is the degree to which the neural injury interferes with the transverse distribution of function. The differential effects on proximal versus more distal actions in both the arm and leg reflect the relative contribution of the components of the corticospinal tract in the control of more lateralized actions distal from the midline. The earlier return of axial and proximal limb activities reflects the relatively greater bilateral contribution to the innervation of these more midline structures. As a further example, in the context of injury affecting the facial musculature, the maintenance of the bilaterally innervated action is illustrated in the bilaterally innervated intact "emotional" smile, as distinct from the unilateral loss of the voluntary smile contralateral to the injury.[148]

The contribution of the ipsilateral portion of the brain to recovery has been confirmed by positron emission tomography (PET) scans.[120] The study group consisted of those who had substantially recovered from brachial monoparesis with a single, generally subcortical lesion demonstrated on CT or magnetic resonance imaging (MRI). PET scans were done with the subject at rest, during movement of the fingers of the previously paralyzed hand, and during movement of the fingers of the normal unaffected hand. An increase in regional blood flow was noted in both the cerebral cortex and cerebellum. In the normal fingers the increment with movement from the resting state was significantly noted only in the contralateral sensorimotor cortex and ipsilateral cerebellar hemisphere. In the recovered fingers a significant increment occurred with movement not only at the contralateral sensorimotor cortex but also at the ipsilateral cortex. For example, when the recovered fingers were moved, the ipsilateral cortical activity increase was approximately three times greater than the activity seen in the ipsilateral cortex of the normal fingers. Similarly, both the ipsilateral cerebellar hemisphere and the contralateral cerebellar hemisphere contributed to the activity of the recovered fingers.

Other studies of persons who recovered motor function in the hand measured the subjects' regional blood flow with radioactive xenon gas while the person carried out a motor task.[117] The blood flow of those with a cerebral cortex lesion and adjacent white matter involvement and those with a deep lesion sparing the cortex were studied separately. While a motor task was performed with the affected hand, regional blood flow increased not only in the contralateral primary sensorimotor area but also in the parietal regions of both hemispheres. This increase in the ipsilateral side was thought to result because substantial components of the corticospinal pyramidal tract originate from the inferior parietal region, which contributes to the uncrossed anterolateral corticospinal tract. Thus the motor recovery in those with cortical lesions required a more highly distributed contribution from both hemispheres than those who had primary subcortical lesions. Recovery in those with cortical lesions could not be attributed merely to subcortical structures.

Crucial to the development of motor recovery is the awareness of the bilateral nature of these underlying systems.[143] Only with the neocerebral system can they influence the contralateral side (with the ipsilateral neocerebellar systems). Thus laterality is an attribute of only a portion of the total action of the motor system. Even within the most recently developed corticospinal system, there is a large degree of interaction with connecting linkages. This bilaterality enables one to determine the relation of one's body to space and time. The special senses of the visual, audio, and vestibular systems enable one to orient oneself in three-dimensional space and time with bilateral receptors, pathways, and commissural fiber systems. This same bilaterality extends to the general sensorimotor system; one examines a new object bimanually to determine such characteristics as shape, weight, and temperature. Although these two hemispheres are specialized, they also share information even at the level of the neocortex.

Brain injury affects the three-dimensional nature of the neurologic systems, with the phylogenetically newer elements being more severely involved. Such involvement may be attributed to the higher metabolic demands and less well-established vascular system of the newer sections. However, the effects both are bilateral and affect the lower centers and are affected by the disruption of the connections from the lower centers and the "uninvolved" side.[136]

The following summary eloquently describes these effects[143]:

> Not only are the subcortical regulatory mechanisms released from cortical inhibition, but these lower centers lose some or most of their ability to regulate and establish the necessary foundation upon which the higher centers are dependent for normal function. Concurrently, the bilateral three dimensional nature of the system is interrupted. The involved area loses the ability to receive normal input, via commissural fibers from the non-involved side, as the

non-involved side is deprived of normal input from the contralateral areas affected by the lesion. The remaining subcortical, and especially the neo-cortical centers, once so dependent upon lower areas for normal function and vice versa, have to expend excess energies, not only in interpreting a multitude of aberrant signals, but just as important, a deficit of signals upon which they were once totally dependent.

The other principle useful to keep in mind is that of the crucial nature of midline stability. Midline stability, coupled with mobility, is the foundation on which both proximal and distal movement patterns develop. This is ultimately a feedback loop, since feedback of sensory stimuli from the periphery enters into the midline stability structures, reinforcing midline stability and mobility patterns.[143] In the presence of brain injury this entire loop can be affected by problems in either the midline control system or the periphery providing the appropriate input.

The adaptive mechanism in dealing with this state is to inhibit mobility in order to gain stability. Therefore it is necessary to reestablish head and neck control along with bilateral midline trunk control to develop proximal limb-girdle stability. The upright position requires the patient to regain sufficient balance, strength, and coordinated control of the body axis and proximal limb girdle. These phylogenetically older systems are endowed with a greater number of polysensory synaptic connections, feedback circuits, and commissural fibers. Also they are more bilaterally organized.

When higher functions are damaged as the result of brain injury, the older, once used, alternative pathways remain. If tapped or strengthened, these older pathways may provide viable "alternative potentials." These older circuits can be used and strengthened to regain some functional improvement.

Assessment of Plasticity

A basic principle is that the nervous system is plastic; it changes from moment to moment. *Plasticity* is the term given to the adaptive capacities of the central nervous system to modify its own structural organization and functioning. It is an adaptive response to a functional demand. It requires feedback on whether or not environmental demands are being met.[112] Acceptance of this notion requires a change in the perception of the brain as a malleable rather than a fixed organ. Although individual cells do not regenerate, the cell processes, axons, and dendrites are responsive to functional demand. A large component of the process of maturation is due to an increase in those cell processes and in glial cells. Such reorganization is not precluded by old age.[113]

That reorganization occurs has been demonstrated in primates. Somatosensory cortical maps in adult primates are dynamically maintained and can be relatively rapidly remodeled by use.[132] For example, in following an injury to the peripheral nerve, the portions of the cortex that deal with the representation of the nerve's input are seen to be rearranged. If the median nerve is crushed but not cut, the cortical map reorganizes with inputs from other surrounding nerves occupying the normal zone of representation. After subsequent regeneration of the peripheral nerve, there is a reemergence of normal-appearing (although not identical to preinjury) somatotropic organization. The converse has also been found. After small cortical lesions, neurons within the neighborhood of the lesion gain new receptive fields. Most of the skin surface represented in the small infarcted zone comes to be represented topographically in the surrounding uninjured cortical region.

The assessment of the degree of functional reorganization that occurs also can be measured by clinical neurophysiologic techniques. The use of such techniques includes both sensory and motor potentials, which serve as prognosticators of future recovery and as measures of the degree to which recovery has occurred.[141] In one study, motor-evoked potentials (MEPs) were elicited by electrical stimulation over the cortex and cervical spine and measured from the contralateral thenar eminence. Central motor conduction time (CMCT) was determined by the difference between the latencies of the spinally and cortically evoked responses. Somatosensory-evoked responses (SEPs) were collected in the usual manner. A correlation was also made between the findings and the degree of functional disability. "Complete" recovery was defined as an absence of functional disability. Persons were fully independent in daily living. "Partial" recovery indicated some improvement since the initial assessment at 8 days after the onset, although the patient was not fully independent.

In the study those subjects with cortical and subcortical involvement (based on CT or MRI findings) were separated. Cortical MEPs were present in 9:10 patients who made a functional recovery and absent in 8:9 who made no recovery or died. Cortical SEPs had a similar distribution. MEPs had a slightly better predictive value when related to the degree of functional recovery. Delayed CMCT was found only in those with subcortical lesions. After cortical infarction, it is suggested that the response from motor cortex stimulation is an all-or-none phenomenon that depends on the availability of corticospinal tract and cortical interneurons to propagate the stimulus. Thus the MEP is present or absent. On the whole, MEP was a more reliable prognosticator than SEP, given its more direct measurement of the motor system.

Another study used the motor central conduction time (CCT) difference between cervical and cortical stimulation recorded from biceps and abductor pollicus brevis muscles.[125] A comparison was made with the Motor Function Index described earlier in this book.[124] The initial study occurred within 72 hours of the onset of stroke, with a follow-up examination generally conducted within 60 days. Data were analyzed differently from the previous study and were examined primarily for the relationship between the initial CCT and the change in motor function. No distinction was made between cortical and subcortical lesions in the data analysis. One group, identified as having an initially prolonged

CCT and disturbances in motor function, exhibited significant improvement in motor function and CCT on follow-up. The presence of a normal CCT with motor impairment of a lesser degree was not found to be predictive, but the data may reflect a ceiling effect. Those with an absent CCT tended to have severe motor impairment initially and very little clinical improvement. The presence of a delayed CCT (although present) identified the group most likely to improve. The use of magnetic stimulation of the motor cortex offers an alternative method to determine the reorganization of motor pathways.[122] These methods offer not only techniques for prognosis but noninvasive techniques for evaluating the underlying effectiveness of training methods.

In addition to these laboratory measures, a search has been made for clinical measures to assess the degree of motor recovery that could help both with prognosis and with measuring the effect of therapeutic techniques. There are, however, serious limitations in relating clinical measures of improvements in motor impairment to function. In one such study, scores on the Brunnstrom classification described in an earlier section of this book were used to measure "motor impairment" and compared with eventual "motor performance" on self-care and ambulation items derived from the Barthel Index.[144] Improvement in motor impairment occurred in only one third of the patients studied. Despite a limited degree of improvement in impairment, lower and upper extremity performance improved to a greater degree, with particular improvement in lower extremity function as measured by ambulation. The correlation between improvement in motor impairment in the upper extremity and improvement in function in dressing and feeding was somewhat greater than that found in the lower extremity. Measures of neurologic recovery and functional recovery are not necessarily coincidental. At the very least the use of the Brunnstrom motor impairment scale does not adequately represent such improvement.

The Motor Assessment Scale (MAS)[118,145] reflects an attempt to develop a measure of motor recovery more related to functional tasks, instead of the patterns of movement used as a basis for the Fugl-Meyer Assessment (FMA) and the Brunnstrom classification.[126] There is evidence of a fairly strong correlation between the two measures with advantage to MAS on the basis of ease of administration and scoring. The upper box on p. 340 lists the functions assessed. Scoring criteria range from zero to six. The lower box on p. 340 describes the format for scoring these items, with the most reliable item given as an example.[118]

An important principle has been to develop methods for selective assessment of motor action in relation to the ability to carry out functional tasks. The Upper Extremity Function Test (UEFT) is another attempt to sample motor actions as part of a total activity rather than as discrete movements.[119] Nearly every activity brings into action the entire upper extremity and trunk. Thus the activities listed in the box on p. 341 cannot be divorced from the context of the task used and are not specific to any one task. For example, supination and

---

Motor Assessment Scale

1. Supine to side-lying positions
2. Supine position to sitting on edge of bed
3. Balance in sitting
4. Sitting to standing
5. Walking
6. Upper arm function
7. Hand movements
8. Advanced hand activities

Balanced Sitting

1. Patient sits only with support. (The therapist should assist patient in sitting.)
2. Patient sits unsupported for 10 seconds (without holding on and with knees and feet together; feet can be supported on floor).
3. Patient sits unsupported with weight well forward and evenly distributed. (Weight should be well forward at the hips, with the head and thoracic spine extended, and weight evenly distributed on both sides.)
4. Patient sits unsupported, turns head and trunk to look behind. (Feet should be supported and together on the floor. Do not allow the legs to abduct or the feet to move. Rest hands on thighs, and do not allow hands to move onto platform.)
5. Patient sits unsupported, reaches forward to touch the floor, and returns to starting position. (Feet should be supported on the floor. Do not allow the patient to hold on. Do not allow the legs and feet to move: support the affected arm if necessary. The hand must touch the floor at least 10 cm [4 in] in front of the feet.)
6. Patient sits on a stool unsupported, reaches sideways to touch the floor, and returns to starting position. (Feet should be supported on floor. Do not allow the patient to hold on. Do not allow the legs and feet to move: support the affected arm if necessary. Patient must reach sideways, not forward.)

---

pronation are assessed by a set of tasks. These include pouring water from a pitcher to a glass, then pouring water first from a glass to another glass (pronation), then back to the first glass (supination). For each item, zero to three points may be given. Note that the total score of the upper extremity function test derives equally from actions reflecting stabilization by more proximal elements of the arm and those reflecting finger movement.

Functions Sampled on the Upper Extremity Function Test

1. Grasp
2. Grip
3. Lateral prehension
4. Pinch
5. Placing
6. Arm supination and pronation
7. Shoulder abduction
8. Shoulder flexion

From Carroll D: *J Clin Dis* 18:479, 1965.

A number of other tests in this same model have been developed particularly for use in the upper extremity.[131,149] Assessing motor actions in relation to function is an integral part of planning the training program used to develop compensatory strategies for carrying out ADLs. The format for such assessments is described in a later section of this chapter.

Treatment Procedures

Treatment designed to aid in the reorganization of the system for sensorimotor control is illustrated by the techniques used in the primate studies described previously.[132] Remodeling of the somatosensory cortical maps occurred with use. The alterations in central maps were affected by differences in input conditions and were not merely the result of the injury condition. Normal monkeys were trained to carry out a task requiring continuous digital contact with a disk to obtain a food reward. The monkey's dedicated attention was necessary to regulate the force so that the pellet of food was provided. Several months of differential stimulation on the tips of one or two digits occurred during this time. There was a subsequent dramatic increase in the activity of the cortical area devoted to the stimulated skin surfaces as compared with the activity state before the use of this training procedure.

The effects of training on the reorganization of functioning underlie the entire field of rehabilitation. It is necessary to go beyond the assessment of the degree of impairment and the resultant disability to a training model that incorporates feedback from the therapist to improve results. More explicit training in sensory substitution is exemplified by electromyography (EMG) sensory feedback or EMG biofeedback to substitute for absent or altered proprioception. An external feedback loop serves as a temporary substitute for the lost internal feedback loops of proprioception, enabling the sensorimotor interaction of voluntary patterned movements.

For example, in persons with hemiplegia, postural sway is increased and often displaced laterally over the nonaffected leg. Asymmetry in lower extremity weight bearing occurs during standing. An important component of this problem is decreased sensory information from the affected side. In one study, data about the degree of deviation were obtained from the use of a pressure plate and applied to the process of training stance stability.[146] Information about the degree of lateral displacement of sway and total sway area was used. A control group was trained by ordinary physical therapy procedures using tactile, verbal, and visual cues provided by the therapist but without the direct visual feedback of results. Significant differences in lateral sway were seen between the two groups. Moreover, a large majority of the control group receiving ordinary physical therapy showed increased loading of the unaffected leg, with only 25% showing the desired increased loading on the affected leg. In contrast, 100% of the explicit direct feedback group showed the desired goal of increased loading of the affected leg. Increased lateral displacement and decreased total sway area were found in the control group. This finding suggests that, in the absence of objective data on stance symmetry, the therapists were actually helping patients to reduce body sway. This achievement may have been accomplished at the cost of increased weight-bearing asymmetry, an effort contrary to the important goal of increased weight bearing on the affected leg.

The use of biofeedback has been applied to a number of situations. Several studies have involved training of the upper extremity function in persons who remained impaired at least 6 months after stroke.[130,151] The Inglis study employed a cross-over design with two groups, wherein the second group received delayed treatment.[131] Significant improvement in all aspects of shoulder function occurred in the context of combined EMG and physical therapy. Improvement was also found in the discreteness with which movements occurred, as measured by change in the Brunnstrom stage of recovery. However, changes in functional activity were not reported in conjunction with the improvement in motor function.

The problem of hand movements was addressed in a study by Wolf and identified as particularly important for changes in function.[150] No concurrent physical therapy was provided to a control group consisting of subjects who had experienced stroke at least 12 months earlier. Improvement was significantly greater in the control of shoulder abduction; in reduced activity in the biceps, enabling more control of the triceps; in an increased range of motion of the wrist, with reduced hyperactivity within wrist and finger flexors; and in more relaxed thenar muscles. The functional tasks that showed improvement depended on improved stability from the shoulder. One such task was the ability to stack checkers. Within the treated group, those who accomplished this task were compared with those who did not to determine a better selection process for training. Those who were more successful in achieving some functional effect were found to have a more active range of motion and greater ability to reduce activity after contraction ("less spasticity"). Particularly relevant was the ability to carry out finger extension.

Still another study assessed the functional effects of muscle retraining in the lower extremities.[150] At least 12 months after stroke, patients were divided into those receiving EMG treatment alone and three control groups consisting of those receiving no treatment, those receiving "general relaxation" treatment, and those receiving upper extremity biofeedback training only. No other form of neuroeducational procedures were used. Treatment was carried out three times per week for approximately 20 weeks. The small sample size (n = 6) and marked intragroup variability made the statistical analysis of changes at the knee and hip difficult. However, ankle dorsiflexion was enhanced significantly, as was knee flexion, with the latter related to a coincident reduction of antagonists, an event compatible with the training protocol used. Significant functional changes were seen, reflected in the number of patients requiring less cumbersome assistive devices as a result of improved ankle stabilization and control. An important suggestion from this study was to focus on increasing the output from weakened musculature rather than attempting to reduce the activity of hypertonic muscles.

One recent study is representative of the extension of these theories to more difficult cases in which communication was also impaired.[114] Sensory feedback was provided by EMG to reflect muscle activity. Increases in motor performance in the affected right arm were achieved in persons with chronic (15 to 62 months) left cerebral lesions and associated communication problems. At the start of each session a goal was agreed on and results for that session were graphed (results were defined as the percentage accomplished in relation to the desired goal, whether it be active range of motion, number of repetitions, or EMG values). Retraining addressed the several different sets of problems illustrated in this variegated population, including suppression of spasticity or facilitation of contractions, depending on the state of the limb. Once the motor behavior was established, the EMG sensory feedback was gradually reduced and substituted with the patient's own sensory inputs such as sight, touch, and proprioception. Home training was eventually carried out independent of the therapists. As a result of these training procedures, spastic patients were able to apply their volitional synergistic movements toward self-care tasks and thus increased their functional level to a "gross assistance" level. Those who were flaccid showed a decrease in shoulder subluxation.

Various combinations of biofeedback have been carried out. One study, for example, used functional electrical stimulation (FES) to increase the control of the anterior tibialis muscle in ankle dorsiflexion during swing and the gastrocnemius muscle in stance with or without associated biofeedback training.[123] Still another group was trained with feedback of EMG signals to either carry out ankle dorsiflexion or relaxation of the gastrocnemius muscle. A fourth control group was treated by usual techniques. A number of indices were used to measure changes in gait pattern and changes in the affected leg as compared with the unaffected leg. The greatest gains were found in an improved speed of ambulation and shortening of gait cycle time. The combination of FES and biofeedback was associated with the greatest improvements and was more beneficial than either alone. The control group showed negative changes, with slowing of gait attributed to an increased concentration on flexing the knee and ankle.

More recently a study sought to improve the arm and hand function of persons 6 months or more after the onset of stroke.[138] EMG, induced by voluntary contraction (EMG-stim), was used. The six enrolled patients scored significantly better on the FMA than the group receiving no treatment with a lesser degree of improvement (although still significantly better than the control group) seen in grip strength. Particularly noteworthy was the contribution made by the subject to the self-stimulation paradigm. It was further suggested that the contribution of electrical stimulation to the results may reflect a basic characteristic of upper motor neuron disease. FES selectively activates type II motor units, the motor units that atrophy in persons with chronic stroke.

The most thoroughgoing application of EMG as a source of external feedback for training has been the work of Basmajian and associates.[115] Using a control group, the initial work with EMG biofeedback on "early mild" involvement of the arm suggested improved results. The comparison in the more recent study was with more classical Bobath techniques.[116,135] There has been continuing controversy concerning the effectiveness of the Bobath techniques despite the strong commitment of their adherents.[129] This study therefore sought to compare the effectiveness of an integrated EMG biofeedback method plus physical therapy with a traditional Bobath neurodevelopmental approach. The population studied had impaired motor function of the upper limb but some ability to extend the wrist and fingers and had experienced stroke less than a year earlier. The group was further stratified by the time since the stroke—for instance, if the time since the stroke was less than 4 months, the designation was "mild" motor involvement, and if greater than 4 months, the designation was "severe" motor involvement). Criteria were derived from the Upper Extremity Function test described earlier.[119] Two therapists carried out the varied treatment of a total of 29 patients, with 18 in the early severe group and 11 in the late mild group. The same test was used before and after treatment. Significant differences occurred over time in both groups. There were, however, equivalent changes between pretreatment and posttreatment increments in both groups.

It appears that, in skillful hands, changes in upper extremity function can be achieved by either of these approaches. The method of selecting which approach is preferable for which patients remains unclear. The costs in time and the level of personnel training required may be important variables in the selection of one or another method in any setting.[125] The use of EMG as a method for providing external sensory feedback to enhance motor recovery has had a limited effect on function, although a considerable effect on specific selected muscle actions has been seen even in the presence of aphasia. These effects occur in both upper and lower extremity retraining, with more direct evidence of functional effects occurring in the use of the lower extremity in gait. The intragroup variability in all studies of retraining makes the proper selection of patients and the proper selection of muscle actions the major determinants.

The use of neurodevelopmental techniques has been widespread. The focus of treatment has been to limit the effects either of abnormal unbalanced activity in the antigravity muscles or of loss of muscle tone. The treatment involves following the developmental sequence of motor control of the infant, and methods vary in terms of their active use or minimization of the reflex mechanisms.[140]

Kottke described the techniques of neuromuscular therapy to accomplish either activity in nonresponsive muscles or inhibition of excessive tone.[137] Local facilitation could be achieved by stretching the muscle through its range of motion or tapping the tendon. Manual vibration at the range of 200 cps produces facilitation. Facilitation can also be brought about by brushing or stroking, applying cold or heat, and pulling hair or slapping the skin. Inhibition of the spastic antagonist can help unblock the unresponsive muscle. For example, cooling of the skin over the antagonist muscle with ice or a procaine nerve block are among the techniques used.

Synergy patterns that actively use reflex patterns can be called into play in the treatment model. For example, flexing the hemiplegic arm above the shoulder level initiates a reflex in the upper extremity extensors and facilitates extension of the wrist and fingers. When weight bearing causes extension of the fingers and flexion of the wrist, synergistic distal stimulation facilitates contraction of the triceps and positive support of the upper extremity reaction. In the lower extremity, stretching the long toe plantar flexors causes a reflex contraction of the extensors of the hip and knee. This action (alternating with the Marie-Foix reflex, facilitating flexion of the ankle, knee, and hip by stretching the toe dorsiflexors) serves to reciprocate flexion and extension.[137]

Facilitation from the tonic neck reflexes influences the proximal muscles of the upper extremities. Turning the face to the paretic side is part of a more total effort to activate a paretic triceps muscle. Similarly, turning the head to the uninvolved side can aid in inducing flexion and abduction of the affected shoulder. Extension of the neck facilitates extension of the upper extremities and flexion of the lower extremities, whereas the opposite occurs with flexion of the neck. The general reflex tone is also influenced by the body's position in relation to gravity. For example, when the patient is lying supine, increased extensor tone exists in the lower extremities and increased flexor tone is noted in the upper extremities. This is increased even more if the patient is sitting in bed or on a chair. Therefore it may interfere with the extension of the hand when placed on the table or reaching for the rim of the wheelchair. If flexion in the lower extremities or extension in the upper extremities is to be trained, it is better for the patient to be lying prone or on his or her side. If one were to follow the treatment model to reduce the imbalance in motor control, one would strive to use these same reflexes but now to counteract the existing pattern. Positioning techniques to normalize the effects of reflex imbalance are described in greater detail in the sections of this chapter that follow.

The evaluation of these and other techniques in enhancing motor recovery remains controversial. In studies, the relatively small numbers of patients, the difficulty in identifying salient features other than time since onset, and the inadequacy of clinical measures generally used for selection make group analysis problematic. Even more questionable is the effect of specified modes of therapy on groups in which intragroup individual variation may be both considerable and unspecified. More rational methods for delineating the characteristics of motor and sensory impairment are needed. Basic to the entire process of assessing functional poststroke recovery is the critique of Wagenaar,[147] who makes a strong case for the use of controlled single-case experimental designs rather than the group statistical analysis currently in vogue.

In the absence of satisfactory recovery of motor control, the need exists for a selection of and training in appropriate compensatory strategies to overcome the patient's resultant functional disabilities. That is the subject of the sections that follow.

TRAINING IN ACTIVITIES OF DAILY LIVING

Christine Bird and Rebecca C. Mahoney

Nature of the Problem

Impairment of the sensorimotor system can limit the daily activities of a person who has sustained a stroke. The aim of the rehabilitation process is to identify these impairments and address the impact of their functional consequences or disabilities on the individual's life. Once the disabilities have been identified, the rehabilitation team, which includes the patient and caregiver, must design a treatment program based on mutually agreed on goals. The outcome sought by this program is to alleviate the disabilities through retraining of functional skills, with compensatory techniques and equipment as needed.

As the rehabilitation phase continues, so must the treatments initiated during the acute phase to prevent secondary impairments. One aspect of the rehabilitation phase is for the patient, caregiver, or both to become independent in the use of these procedures. The other aspect is for the patient, caregiver, or both to perform the identified ADLs successfully.

ADLs are defined as tasks that enable an individual to function at home, at work, and within the community. Traditionally they were viewed solely as self-care activities such as eating, dressing, and personal hygiene. However, to fit the full definition, a broader view must be taken and must include activities that allow a person to perform tasks related to work and leisure. Innate to this concept is the ability of an individual to interact with other people and objects found within the environment. Which ADLs an individual performs depends largely on the roles that person has acquired.

Roles, according to Heard, are behaviors indicating a specific position that one occupies in society.[160] The roles that a patient accepts reflect that individual's values and are often influenced by cultural and religious beliefs. As the expectations of a role change over time, so do the activities that facilitate successful role completion. For example, the activities needed to fulfill the role of mother are different for a 32-year-old stroke patient with three young children than for a 72-year-old woman with adult offspring. The nature and type of activities selected to complete the role vary from patient to patient.

As previously defined, roles can be drawn from the general areas of self-care, work, and leisure. Patients must define on their own the activities needed to achieve independence within these three areas. Within the area of work, patients may include such activities as typing, volunteering at a local organization, homemaking, or taking care of children or aging parents. Valued leisure activities include gardening, the ability to play with grandchildren, family camping trips, or visiting with family and friends. Even within the area of self-care, some patients may value the application of makeup, regular hair cuts, or polished nails over other aspects of grooming. The accomplishment of these activities may lead to the fulfillment of one of the patient's identified roles. The specific activities that bring about role obtainment vary from patient to patient and must be reflected within the rehabilitation goals.

The successful completion of ADLs makes several demands on the patient. The performance of ADLs requires that the patient is mobile within his or her environment (whether that is a bed, a house, or the community). Successful ADL performance also requires that a patient communicate his or her needs and thoughts to others. Finally, the ability to perform ADLs involves interacting with the nonhuman environment. Depending on the activity, patients need to use such items as eating utensils, soap, golf clubs, wheelchairs, or computers. Daily living skills are performed on a regular basis and are often not thought of until the ability to complete them is interrupted.

The onset of a stroke can have a devastating impact on a person's ability to perform ADLs. Hemiplegia forces the individual to learn one-handed techniques to perform activities such as dressing. However, that is not the extent of the deficits; if it were, the patient's length of hospitalization would be much shorter. Often after a stroke the patient experiences decreased trunk control, making it difficult to maintain both the static and dynamic balance needed to perform any activity. The loss of tactile sensation and proprioceptive and kinesthetic awareness and an altered body image impair the patient's mobility and ability to engage in meaningful activities. Visuoperceptual deficits, such as diplopia, hemianopsia, and neglect, have an impact on all aspects of ADLs from finding food on a plate to navigating a wheelchair to reading a simple paragraph. Communication deficits also affect the patient's ability to perform ADLs. An individual experiencing receptive aphasia has difficulty understanding directions, which may impede the speed of learning new compensatory methods. A patient with expressive aphasia encounters frustration in communicating his or her needs or feelings.

In addition, individuals who have sustained a stroke often experience cognitive deficits. Patients who demonstrate poor insight into their own abilities are often not motivated to work on ADL skills. Decreased attention can influence safety issues and affect the patient's ability to learn new techniques. The patient's success in performing varying tasks is impaired by the degree of cognitive deficits. The extent of cognitive deficits can cause an individual to experience difficulty in sequencing steps in dressing, balancing a checkbook, or preparing a balanced meal. These sensorimotor, perceptual, communication, and cognitive deficits are common in individuals who have had a stroke. How function has been affected depends on the degree of impairment.

The person who has suffered a loss of functioning through the effects of a stroke often experiences decreased self-esteem, a sense of dependency, or a feeling of being "childlike."[166] This was evident in a 72-year-old patient who was experiencing visuoperceptual deficits and who was placed on pureed foods because of swallowing problems. After several attempts to bring a tablespoon of food to his mouth, he exclaimed, "I feel like a baby. I can't even feed myself." This loss of function may bring on depression or create anxiety about whether the caregiver can provide the level of assistance needed for the patient to return home.

Multiple studies have been conducted to establish the critical factors influencing functional outcomes within the stroke population. Lincoln et al. cited several studies that indicate a variety of critical predictive factors.[164] These include perceptual problems, incontinence, decreased balance, cognitive deficits, lack of motivation, and decreased arm function. Gordon et al. states that single, specific indicators are difficult to determine, given the variables involved within this population.[158] Most studies[159] state that other contributing factors determine positive outcomes, including active family involvement, sound financial resources, a higher cognitive status on the part of the patient and an ability to make needed personal adjustments on the part of both the patient and the family. Achieving positive outcomes is the goal of the rehabilitation team. The means for doing so is the subject of this section.

Assessment

The first step to achieving the goal of performing ADLs is made by the team's assessment of the patient's level of functioning. A thorough assessment is obtained by gathering information through evaluation and by organizing that information to develop a specific treatment plan, tailor made for each patient. The assessment should reflect the total picture of that patient. It serves as a baseline of that individual's performance, reflecting strengths, deficits, and areas where change can realistically occur.[161] Patient and family participation with the development of the plan is vital. Starting on the day of admission, information is gathered to contribute to the assessment. This information is collected in both formal and informal sessions. The formal collection of information is achieved through a review of the medical record and the patient's performance on evaluations and within a "structured" interview with the patient and family. Important information is also obtained through informal exchange with or observations of the patient outside of therapy sessions. Observing how the patient and family interact, their interactions with others, and how and where they spend free time may provide information on or clarification of the patient's roles and values.

The focus of the assessment is the patient's ability to perform ADLs relevant to his or her roles. Therefore it is vital that the patient and family be part of this evaluation. This interaction with the patient and family is an exchange of information. It is important to learn the patient's various roles and the level of premorbid participation in those roles. The patient and family also need to convey which roles and activities they want to resume. The clinician needs to gather information regarding the patient's support system and expected discharge location and the patient and family's understanding of the patient's present level of functioning and how that relates to his or her future status and demands.

The patient and family are assisted in their understanding by receiving information or education on stroke recovery. The family should immediately start training on techniques to assist the patient therapeutically. This exchange provides the clinician with an opportunity to establish rapport with both the patient and family. Learning what motivates the patient and how to create an atmosphere of open communication is vital for the therapeutic relationship. The following case example illustrates this point.

CASE REPORT

J.D., a patient who had experienced a left CVA, presented with expressive aphasia with right hemiplegia, motor planning difficulties, and depression. The initial evaluation identified self-feeding as a problem. J.D. was placed in a feeding group to work on this skill. He often refused to eat and showed minimal progress in this area. Through further questioning of family, it was discovered that the patient's normal routine was to eat alone in the kitchen and that he had always been uncomfortable dining in a group. On eating alone in his hospital room, J.D. became independent in self-feeding without equipment.

Activities of daily living performance. The achievement of an accurate assessment relies on a detailed evaluation of the patient's current ADL status. Table 10-10 outlines the general ADL tasks evaluated within the stroke population. It may be inappropriate to evaluate all of these ADL tasks within the first week or even to evaluate some of them at all for several reasons. As mentioned before, the clinician needs to know which ADL tasks were incorporated into the patient's prior roles and which are included in the patient's present goals. If a patient never participated in meal preparation before the stroke, an evaluation of that task may be inappropriate. The clinician must also be aware of cultural issues. In some societies, older adults are cared for by a younger generation and are not expected to participate in certain activities.

The clinician proceeds to evaluate the level of functioning within ADLs, relating them to that patient's own goals. Optimally, the evaluation of ADL tasks should be performed in an environment and during time at which the patient is accustomed to performing such tasks. Objects that are familiar to the patient should be used. The clinician needs to observe the patient's performance, allowing for idiosyncratic methods of completion.

The clinician must decide which ADL task should be evaluated and when during the hospitalization the evaluation should occur. These ADL tasks can be tested in a continuum, reflecting the complexity of skills required to complete them successfully. The clinician must determine where on the continuum the patient's skill level falls. It may be inappropriate to perform an evaluation on checkbook management with a patient who has moderate cognitive impairments or to evaluate ambulation on an uneven surface with an individual who ambulates on level surfaces with moderate assistance. Yet evaluating simple monetary transactions or the ability of the individual to climb stairs similar to those they will encounter at home may be appropriate. Delaying an evaluation (e.g., of driving) because of the high demands inherent in that activity may be appropriate to allow time for the patient to reach his or her optimal level of functioning. The discharge location also has an impact on whether an evaluation is appropriate. For example, it is probably not necessary to evaluate meal preparation skills with an individual who is going to live in a long-term care facility.

Activity analysis. According to Abreu, the completion of any ADL task involves movement of the body toward a purpose or goal. The successful

TABLE 10-10　Activities of Daily Living

TYPE	ACTIVITY
Self-management	Feeding
	Dressing
	Grooming and hygiene
Mobility	Bed
	Transfers to and from bed, toilet, tub, and car
	Wheelchair mobility
	Ambulation on all surfaces and stairs
	Community mobility, using public transportation and driving
Home management	Meal preparation
	Home care
	Shopping
	Financial management
	Functional communication
Work and leisure	Work skills
	Volunteer, church, or community activities
	Hobbies

completion of an ADL task involves the integration of internal and external sensory input processed to elicit an appropriate response.[152] One tool used by occupational therapists for the evaluation and training in performance of ADLs is activity analysis. In activity analysis, activities are broken down into steps. These steps are further analyzed to determine the inherent characteristics within the specific step. As the occupational therapist observes a patient completing an ADL, the therapist is able to determine the altered or absent characteristic that impedes successful completion. Table 10-11 illustrates an abridged activity analysis describing the simple task of eating soup.

As illustrated through the activity analysis, different tasks have inherent characteristics or components that the therapist must monitor during the evaluation. Observing patients participating in ADL tasks does not always provide the clinician with the needed objective data. Further detailed evaluations are often required to determine the precise area and degree of impairment. Many appropriate evaluation tools are available to measure these components; only a few are highlighted in the descriptions that follow.

Sensorimotor components. Possibly the most obvious impairment is the loss of movement or the limited active range of movement (AROM) involved in

TABLE 10-11   Activity Analysis: Eating Soup

STEP	CHARACTERISTICS
1. Locate spoon on table	Motor: oculomotor to scan for spoon
	Senses: vision
	Perception: visual scanning, figure ground, form constancy, identification of spoon
	Cognition: visual attention, memory, initiation
2. Pick spoon up from table	Motor: shoulder flexion, elbow extension, forearm pronation, digit extension and flexion, ulnar deviation
	Senses: vision, tactile
	Perception: motor planning, spatial relations, figure ground, distance perception
	Cognition: visual attention, sequencing
3. Ladle soup with spoon	Motor: oculomotor, shoulder horizontal adduction, elbow flexion, radial deviation
	Senses: vision, tactile
	Perception: identification of bowl, motor planning, depth perception, spatial relations, figure ground, distance perception
	Cognition: visual attention, sequencing
4. Bring spoon to mouth	Motor: shoulder external rotation, horizontal abduction, elbow flexion, wrist flexion
	Senses: vision, tactile
	Perception: motor planning, body schema, spatial relations
	Cognition: visual attention, sequencing

hemiplegia. Limitations in AROM in the extremities and trunk can have an impact on the patient's ability to complete almost any activity. Often, limitations are present within the geriatric population before the stroke but have a greater impact on the completion of ADLs after the onset of hemiplegia. An individual may not need full AROM to be functional. As a result of AROM limitations, patients have difficulties with such activities as donning shoes or pulling a shirt over the head and bathing the back. A detailed evaluation of active and passive range of motion for the extremities and trunk provides the clinician with information on specific limitations. This and other information also assists the clinician in determining the need for assistive devices to compensate for a decreased range of motion.

Fine and gross coordination and bilateral and unilateral upper extremity use can be observed in a patient's ability to manipulate clothing or grooming items or to use a computer. Several tools are used to obtain data on coordination.[172] The Minnesota Rate of Manipulation involves bilateral and unilateral manipulation of disk patterns. The Jebson-Taylor Hand Function Test evaluates seven unilateral activities, such as writing, simulated feeding, and picking up large heavy objects, to evaluate coordination. The Purdue Pegboard evaluates both gross movement of the upper extremity and the finger dexterity needed to assemble pins, washers, and collars in a pegboard.

The measurement of muscle strength on the hemiplegic side may not be accurate as the result of tonal influences. Another factor to take into consideration is that abnormal tone may be induced in the hemiplegic extremity during manual muscle testing of the nonaffected extremity. Observations during the patient's performance of ADLs can often provide the clinician with information on the patient's functional strength.

The patient's level of overall endurance and his or her ability to participate in the rehabilitation program is influenced by several factors. The patient's premorbid activity level, coupled with deconditioning bought on by hospitalization, influences the patient's ability to perform various ADLs. Low endurance is evident in the patient who requires several rests during a low-demand task such as bathing. For another patient, activities of higher demand such as wheelchair mobility, meal preparation, or simulated work may reveal decreased endurance.

Flaccidity and spasticity are the two key motor components seen in the patient with hemiplegia. These components not only affect the extremities but are also evident in the trunk musculature, resulting in difficulty in maintaining trunk control. A patient may not be able to initiate or sustain weight shifting or weight bearing on his or her affected side. This often causes the patient to become static and thus limits the ability to reach for items or initiate correct gait patterns. A decrease in motor planning in a patient's extremities also affects the patient's ability to perform functional activities. Impaired integration of proprioception and kinesthetic information influences the patient's ability to move the extremities during tasks. During the evaluation of motor control the therapist notes not only the quality of the movement patterns but also ways in which the patient compensates with his or her nonaffected side or abnormal movement patterns that interfere with function. The patient's sense of positioning can be evaluated with the patient imitating positions of the affected arm as positioned by the therapist. Abnormal muscle tone can be determined by the degree of resistance a limb has to movement. An extremity with normal tone adjusts to changes in movement and is able to maintain a position. A flaccid extremity is heavy and reveals no ability to adjust to changes or to maintain positioning. Resistance is usually felt when a spastic extremity is moved, and the patient may not be able to maintain a position without substitution.

Interaction with the human and nonhuman environment engages the senses to varying degrees. Observing how a patient reacts to a stimulus, such as another person, a piece of furniture, or an eating utensil, can cue the clinician to possible sensory deficits. Limited vision or hearing may lead to diminished interactions or may elicit behavior perceived as inappropriate. The occupational or speech therapy departments may request the patient to perform a visual screen to assess acuity (both near and far), ocular range of motion, saccadic movement, scanning, and peripheral vision. The speech therapist may initiate a hearing screen. Depending on the results of the screen, a detailed evaluation may be requested.

Cognition. The level of cognitive demands varies greatly, depending on the complexity of the task being evaluated. Key components of cognition include orientation, attention, concentration, memory, organization, problem solving, and abstract reasoning. Deficits of cognition can be recognized during ADL performance — for instance, by the impulsivity of a patient attempting a transfer before locking the brakes or moving the footrests of the wheelchair or by the decreased attention when a person forgets to bathe several body parts. These demands are different from the integration of cognitive skills needed to plan and prepare a full meal, organize a checkbook, or prepare a legal brief as part of a work evaluation. Safety awareness and judgment are often assessed during the performance of ADLs to assist in determining the ability of the patient to be alone after discharge. The number of evaluations standardized to measure functional cognitive abilities is limited. Many of the current cognitive assessments are linked closely to visuoperceptual performance. Occupational therapists often select portions of various evaluations to put together a tool that elicits the various components of cognition, then relate the influence of these deficits on the patient's ability to perform the appropriate functional tasks. The following are examples of available standardized evaluations. The Bay Area Functional Performance Evaluation (BAFPE) is designed for the psychiatric population but can be used to evaluate the neurologic patient. It assesses the ability to perform selected daily living tasks and social interaction skills. The Rivermead Behavior Memory test scores immediate and distant recall through everyday functional tasks.

Perception. The performance of ADLs also provides the clinician with information on perceptual deficits. Visuoperceptual deficits commonly seen include figure ground (finding a sock on an unmade bed), form constancy (difficulty distinguishing close, similarly shaped objects (mistaking a water pitcher for a urinal), spatial relationship (attempting transfers from an inappropriate distance), and depth perception (misjudging the height of stairs). The Motor Free Visual Perceptual Test (MVPT) provides a profile of visuoperceptual abilities, the presence of unilateral visual neglect, and the speed of visuoperceptual processing. The Minnesota Spatial Relations Test (MSRT) measures speed and accuracy in discrimination and in placing three-dimensional geometric shapes.

The presence of apraxia causes the patient to experience difficulty executing the movement pattern needed to accomplish an activity while demonstrating intact sensory motor components. A patient may be able to identify that he has a toothbrush in his hand yet cannot initiate the brushing movement, or he may attempt to brush his hair with it.

Disturbances in body schema can also be present after a stroke. The patient may not be able to distinguish right from left, locate body parts, or understand the spatial relationship between these parts. Difficulty with any of these components can have an impact on that individual's completion of daily living skills.

Within the course of the patient's rehabilitation stay, clinicians may need to evaluate the following areas and how they influence ADL performance.

Home evaluation. The home evaluation focuses on the accessibility of the home and its adaptability to the patient's level of mobility. The evaluation also assesses the impact of the home environment on the patient's ability to perform ADL tasks. This evaluation is accomplished by either a questionnaire or a home visit. It is optimal for the patient to participate in the actual visit, although that is not always an option. The clinician evaluates the accessibility of the entrance and rooms and access to environmental devices such as light switches, phones, and cooking appliances and assists in determining emergency routes. Recommendations vary, often depending on the resources available and the level of functioning when discharge occurs. Recommendations may include ramps, permanent modifications of a kitchen or bathroom, or simply rearranging furniture or rugs.

Equipment assessment. An equipment evaluation requires the integration of five key areas. The clinician reviews (1) the anticipated level of functioning of the patient at time of discharge; (2) the cognitive status of that individual; (3) the discharge location; (4) the amount of assistance available at the discharge location; and (5) the interest of the patient toward equipment use.[165] The balance of these areas is reflected in recommendations for wheelchairs, bathroom equipment, or assistance and adaptive devices.

Driving assessment. A driving evaluation may be performed during the rehabilitation stay or on an outpatient basis. Information is collected on the patient's medical history and driving history. Present data on sensorimotor functioning, cognition, and visuoperceptual motor skills are collected. A detailed evaluation should include the patient's performance on a driving simulator or in an actual road test.

Work evaluation. Work-related evaluations may be required to assess a patient's ability to perform his or her job or the ability of the workplace to accommodate the patient's level of mobility. The assessment may require an on-site visit. Vocational rehabilitation counselors and occupational therapists often coevaluate the patient's ability to perform the same or similar work activities.

After each member of the rehabilitation team has completed an evaluation, this information must be shared to complete the assessment picture. The team may use one of the many tools (FIM, Barthel Index, or Katz Index) to organize the evaluation information and project the overall picture of that patient's present and projected level of functioning.[168] These tools also assist the team in determining the patient's interdisciplinary team goals for the rehabilitation stay.

Goal Setting and Treatment Planning

The success of treatment planning for the stroke patient depends on an integrated and consistent interdisciplinary team effort in collaboration with the patient. Patient and caregiver goals, values, and cultural background should be the driving force behind the treatment plan. The importance of these factors was studied by Chiou.[156] Through her survey of 26 patients and their therapists, she found that stroke patients and their home therapists had differing views on the importance and value of different ADL tasks. She suggested that, if additional time were spent with each patient determining goals based on individual values, the rehabilitation program might be more efficient and patient gains made in rehabilitation would more likely be maintained. Solicitation of patient goals should be the first step in the treatment planning process for all disciplines. The physician, in particular, should become familiar with all aspects of the patient's individual needs for effective team facilitation. Each discipline brings a unique perspective to the plan based on his or her expertise. For example, the psychologist may identify that depression is affecting the patient's interest in ADL independence and, through counseling and other interventions, may gain a more accurate picture of the patient's ADL goals. The physical therapist's knowledge of the patient's potential for functional ambulation and the social worker's information on the home environment assists the team in determining if the patient's goal for independent bathing and toileting is realistic or if adaptations and equipment are necessary.

Next, these patient concerns and goals are brought to the initial team conference at which the interdisciplinary plan is formulated. As previously described, the interdisciplinary treatment plan includes the identification of high-priority problem areas, interdisciplinary goals, and a plan of action for goal achievement. ADL goals are usually measured in terms of the amount of assistance, supervision, or equipment required to complete the task. The FIM rating scale (see box on p. 357) was the basis for the treatment plan in the following case example. The occupational therapist is the primary clinician

Functional Independence Measure (FIM): Description of Levels of Function and Their Scores

INDEPENDENT

Another person is not required for the activity (no helper).

7. Complete independence — All of the tasks described as making up the activity are typically performed safely; without modification, assistive devices, or aids; and within a reasonable time.

6. Modified independence — The activity involves any one or more of the following: an assistive device is required, more than a reasonable time is needed, or there are safety (risk) considerations.

DEPENDENT

Another person is required for either supervision or physical assistance for the activity to be performed, or it is not performed (requires helper).

Modified Dependence — The patient expends half (50%) or more of the effort. The levels of assistance required are the following:

5. Supervision or setup — The patient requires no more help than standby assistance, cueing, or coaxing, without physical contact; or the helper sets up needed items or applies orthoses.

4. Minimal contact assistance — With physical contact, the patient requires no more help than touching and expends 75% or more of the effort.

3. Moderate assistance — The patient requires more help than touching or expends half (50%) or more (up to 75%) of the effort.

Complete Dependence — The patient expends *less* than 50% of the effort. Maximal or total assistance is required, or the activity is not performed. The levels of assistance required are the following:

2. Maximal assistance — The patient expends less than 50% of the effort, but at least 25%.

1. Total assistance — The patient expends less than 25% of the effort.

From the Research Foundation, State University of New York: *Guide to the uniform data sheet for medical rehabilitation,* Buffalo, 1990, State University of New York Press.

responsible for implementing the ADL treatment plan, but effective and efficient goal achievement depends on coordination between all disciplines. The physical therapist may suggest gait-training strategies to be implemented by the occupational therapist and nurses during the daily self-care and toileting routine. The speech and language pathologist and psychologist work with the occupational therapist in implementing organizational and problem-solving strategies during meal preparation.

The following case study illustrates this process.

CASE REPORT

C.M. is a 62-year-old female who sustained a right CVA with resultant left hemiparesis (greater in her arm than her leg) and significant visuospatial deficits. She lives with her husband, who was also disabled by a prior CVA. He cared for himself independently but could offer no physical assistance to his wife. Their home is in a rural area miles from retail and public services.

At the initial team meeting and through their assessments, the interdisciplinary team identified C.M.'s primary concerns as independence in mobility and self-care, in view of her husband's limitations, and returning to driving.

Based on these concerns, the priority problem areas identified were ambulation, self-care, community mobility, and visuospatial skills.

Long-term goals were determined as follows:

1. Independent ambulation with assistive device during self-care and home management activities.
2. Supervision with community mobility with equipment and adaptive techniques as needed.
3. Close supervision with meal preparation and home care.

The short-term interdisciplinary goals and plan were determined as follows:

1. The patient will ambulate with close supervision during the self-care routine. (The physical therapist will instruct the nursing staff and occupational therapist on ambulation techniques to be integrated during the self-care routine.)
2. The patient will attend to her affected side and verbalize safety check items during transfers and ambulation with a 75% consistency. (The speech and language pathologist and occupational therapist will instruct the physical therapist and nursing staff on cognitive strategies for safety and left-side awareness to be used in self-care, toileting, gait training, and home management.)
3. The patient will require minimal assistance with simple meal preparation. (The speech-language pathologist and occupational therapist will cotreat with the patient to determine effective cognitive strategies. The occupational therapist will provide training with equipment and compensatory techniques.)

At the interim team meeting the short-term goals were reviewed. The first and third goals were met. The team reported that C.M. was 50% consistent with the second goal.

The following 2-week plan was determined:

Goal #1, upgraded: The patient will ambulate independently during the self-care routine and between therapies. (Continue with previous plan.)

Goal #2 will continue to be addressed.

Goal #3, upgraded: The patient will require supervision with meal preparation. (Continue with the previous plan.)

Goal #4, added: The patient will understand the equipment and training needs for a return to driving and community mobility. (Occupational therapist will conduct a driving evaluation. The patient will participate in an interdisciplinary community skills group. Therapeutic recreation and social work activities will assist patient to identify community resources.)

C.M. was successful in meeting her long-term goals for mobility, self-care, and home management. She continued to require assistance with driving as the result of visuospatial deficits, but she continued to be involved in driver training as an outpatient.

Treatment Approaches

The interdisciplinary plan provides a framework for selecting treatment interventions for ADLs in the stroke patient. The following four categories of ADL treatment approaches are most frequently used by the occupational therapist.

Retraining of performance skills. In applying a treatment approach of retraining, the therapist provides intervention to reorganize or improve the area of performance deficit, such as motor control, sensory awareness, cognition, or perception.[172] This approach is the first priority for most therapists because, if it is successful, it reduces the need for awkward compensations or expensive equipment. For example, during lower extremity dressing, the clinician can facilitate the patient's normal motor control skills using the Bobath approach. Through handling techniques and tone inhibition techniques, the following motor skills could be facilitated: inclining the trunk forward to reach the feet, manipulating clothing with the upper extremities, moving from a sitting to a standing position by moving the trunk and pelvis forward over the feet, obtaining symmetrical weight bearing through both lower extremities, performing spinal extension to stand erect, and maintaining balance while managing clothing while standing. In addition, systematic verbal cues and repetition may improve the patient's ability to select and position clothing for dressing and sequence the task efficiently. By addressing these component skills in the context of dressing, the patient can accomplish dressing in a normal manner and learn skills that can be applied to other ADLs.

Compensatory strategies. Although the retraining of performance skills is the preferred treatment approach, many stroke patients cannot achieve full independence through this method.[172] Compensatory strategies circumvent problem areas or substitute for missing performance skill areas. In other words, the therapist assists the patient to learn a new way of accomplishing the task.[166] For example, many stroke patients do not recover full function in the affected extremity, which makes putting on a shirt difficult. A one-handed technique can be taught for independence in this task. Many patients with right-sided CVA demonstrate left-sided inattention, which prevents them from seeing all of their food during a meal. The clinician may teach the patient or family to place the plate to the right of center or to rotate the plate during the meal to ensure adequate nutrition. By using compensatory strategies the patient can achieve a higher level of independence despite severe residual deficits and thus can rely less on caregivers.

Compensatory techniques are new, unfamiliar strategies and thus depend on the patient's learning ability. Some patients with cognitive and perceptual processing deficits may have difficulty learning and retaining these techniques from day to day. Learning may or may not transfer to other ADL tasks so that each particular activity may need to be practiced until learned. The learning styles of patients with right- and left-sided CVAs are often different. Thus teaching methods may need to be adapted to meet individual patient needs.[157]

This section provides an overview of some of the most common compensatory techniques in the literature, but it is important to remember that the most effective strategies often result from trial and error in the patient and therapist problem-solving process. Patient suggestions and feedback on which strategies work should always be encouraged. It is also the role of the interdisciplinary team to teach patients to be independent problem solvers so that they are prepared to meet unexpected ADL challenges after discharge.[172]

For example, a patient with a left-sided CVA demonstrated difficulty in donning slacks over her foot and ankle, and traditional methods of crossing her leg or using a stool were ineffective because her lower extremity was too heavy to be maintained in those positions. After several sessions of experimenting with her occupational therapist, the patient found that she could accomplish the task by lifting her ankle with her other leg.

Adaptive equipment. Adaptive equipment also substitutes for impaired sensorimotor and mobility skills and allows the patient to become more self-sufficient with ADL activities. Adaptive equipment includes commercially available devices, such as a tub bench, or devices fabricated by the occupational therapist, such as Velcro clothing fasteners. The patient, caregiver, or both must be trained in the use and upkeep of all devices, and thus their new learning capacity is a consideration when choosing equipment.

Remarkably few studies that investigate the use and effectiveness of adaptive equipment with the CVA patient are available. A review of studies of the general physically disabled population, however, yields some useful data. Bynum and Rogers studied equipment use by patients receiving home occupational therapy services; 52% were CVA patients.[154] They found that the overall usage rate of prescribed devices was 82% and that the use of bedside commodes and tub seats was most common. It was suggested that the high level of use of these devices may occur because bathing and toileting are basic functions that must be accomplished with or without devices. The study also noted that, even when the patient needed assistance to use a device, it was still of value in promoting independence and relieving the caregiver's burden.[167]

Several studies have begun to investigate patterns of equipment use or abandonment. In 1992 Rogers and Holm provided an extensive review of the available literature in this area.[167] In general, patients who can accomplish a task without equipment (even if the task is more difficult) often choose not to use the device.[169] Improvement or deterioration of functional capacity was found to be a common reason for changes in the use of adaptive equipment in several studies.[154,169] Other factors described as influencing the use of equipment included the patient's preference for caregiver assistance or concern about inconveniencing others[169] and compatibility (or incompatibility) with the home environment[154,169] and life-style.

A 1990 study by Batavia et al. surveyed assistive device users with a variety of physical and sensory disabilities.[153] Device characteristics that were important to users included effectiveness, ease of use and maintenance, expense, reliability, durability, safety, comfort, and attractiveness.

The results of these studies suggest that more research is needed on adaptive equipment usage specific to the stroke patient. The studies demonstrate the complexity of factors that need to be considered in equipment prescription and training. Consideration of the patient goals, values, home environment, and support systems is part of the process.

Environmental adaptation. Environmental adaptations may involve architectural changes to allow wheelchair access (e.g., widened doorways), reorganization of work areas so that ADL tasks can be accomplished efficiently (e.g., organizing the most commonly used cooking utensils in one location), or structuring both the environment and the daily routine to maximize cognitive processing. The hospital is a structured and supportive setting in which to relearn ADL skills, but it does not fully prepare the patient for return to the community. Occupational therapists and other health professionals need to be proactive in assisting the patient to anticipate the challenges of the transition to home. Thus it is important to practice all ADLs in an environment closely resembling the patient's home setting. Some rehabilitation facilities have training apartments in which the patient and family can practice ADL skills in a real-life setting with distant monitoring by health professionals.

Treatment Applications

It is important to note that these four treatment approaches are most often integrated to meet the patient's individual goals and needs. For example, short lengths of stay for stroke patients may dictate that therapists work on retraining and compensatory strategies simultaneously to achieve maximal patient independence in a short time.[252] The following examples illustrate the applications of these four treatment approaches to specific ADLs.

Feeding. The occupational therapist works closely with the speech and language pathologist, dietitian, and nursing staff to address sensorimotor and cognitive issues that affect the patient's feeding, swallowing, and nutrition.

Although often referred to in the literature as a unilateral task, incorporation of both upper extremities during feeding is important for full independence. The affected upper extremity should be supported in a weight-bearing position on the dining table with the scapula protracted and good glenohumeral alignment. This position promotes trunk symmetry, normal shoulder girdle alignment, and visual awareness of the extremity. When reaching for utensils, the patient shifts his body weight over the affected extremity, which facilitates muscle contraction around the shoulder girdle. If the patient has active movement of the affected upper extremity, hand-to-mouth patterns can be graded to facilitate active control of the biceps and triceps muscles and the forearm.

Compensatory strategies and adaptive equipment are most often used for cutting foods and stabilizing a plate during scooping. A rocker knife uses a rocker action so that the patient can cut and stabilize food using one hand. A rubber placemat can be used to prevent slippage of the plate or bowl during eating. For the patient who has sufficient control in the affected upper extremity for self-feeding, utensils with built-up handles may assist a weak grasp.

Left-sided inattention, a common problem area for the patient with a right-sided CVA, can significantly limit self-feeding independence. In the most severe cases the patient may acknowledge food and utensils only on the right side of the plate and table. Tracing around the edge of the lapboard or table with the patient's hand may assist the patient in visually locating items on the left. Anchoring is a technique in which a bright-colored line or novel object is placed on the left side to visually draw the patient's gaze. The patient is trained first to look for the anchor and then to look for other items in his visual field. If these strategies are unsuccessful, the patient can be taught to turn the plate to locate all items, or the plate can be placed to the right side (although this is least preferred because it does not facilitate awareness of affected side).

CASE REPORT

R.M., a patient with a right-sided CVA and significant left-sided inattention, was unable to acknowledge food items to the left of midline. During meals, his plate was initially placed at midline and a bright pink cup was used for beverages. R.M. was cued to look for the cup to bring his gaze to midline. With repetition he became more proficient at using this strategy and his plate was gradually positioned farther toward the left side. By talking through the strategy at each meal, the patient also learned to cue himself to look for the cup. R.M. continued to use these techniques with his family after discharge.

Other cognitive problems that interfere with safe and independent feeding include distractibility, impulsivity and a fast rate of intake, and apraxia. Most cognitive problems show improvement with repetition, consistent verbal cueing or demonstration, and a quiet environment. With practice, patients can often be trained to self-cue to reduce the effects of cognitive difficulties.

Dressing. Dressing should be practiced in a wheelchair or sturdy straight-backed chair to encourage active trunk control, weight shifts, and efficient upper extremity reaching patterns. Other motor control components that can be facilitated during dressing were previously described in the section on retraining of performance skills.

Several variations of one-handed dressing techniques have been reported in the literature. The general technique is to insert the affected extremity into the sleeve or pants leg first, followed by insertion of the unaffected side. The technique is reversed for removing clothes. Reaching the lower leg and feet for donning pants, socks, and shoes is often difficult for the patient with poor trunk control or joint limitations. Crossing the affected lower extremity over the unaffected leg or using a small stool to prop up the leg are two strategies to solve this problem. Long-handled dressing sticks, sock donners, and shoe horns are also sometimes recommended, but they are difficult to learn to use and can be awkward to use with one hand.

One-handed shoe-tying techniques, Velcro closures, and elastic shoelaces are all effective adaptations for independent shoe tying. Certain types of clothing are easier to don and doff, such as slip-on shoes, pull-over shirts, and slacks with elastic waists. Some patients would rather alter their clothing style than use unfamiliar adaptive devices. Donning and doffing braces, slings, and splints should also be considered part of the dressing process.

Dressing apraxia, a disorder of body scheme, is a phenomenon characterized by orientation mistakes such as donning clothes upside down, backward, or on the wrong body part.[170] Use of labels or color codes may assist the patient in orienting the garment correctly.

Grooming and hygiene. During grooming activities the sink provides a stable surface for upper extremity weight bearing. Incorporating the affected side in this manner improves shoulder girdle stability, body awareness, and the potential for functional upper extremity use. As recovery progresses, the affected upper extremity can be incorporated as a stabilizer (e.g., holding a toothpaste tube or shampoo bottle for opening). For the patient with proximal upper extremity active movement but limited hand and wrist control, a wash mitt with a pocket for soap allows the patient to use the affected arm effectively for bathing and to develop graded motor control. During the setup for grooming and hygiene activities, reaching patterns and active weight shifting in standing or sitting can be facilitated.

Most grooming activities can be accomplished with minimal adaptation or compensation. An electric razor is a safer and more easily managed alternative for the patient with hemiplegia. Suction cups or rubber mats can help stabilize grooming items. One-handed denture brushes, nail clippers, and files are also available. The most common difficulties with bathing for the patient with hemiplegia include bathing the unaffected arm, back, and lower leg; transferring into and out of the tub; and maintaining balance while sitting or standing. To bathe the unaffected arm, the patient is instructed to place the soaped washcloth in his lap, then move the arm over the stationary washcloth. A long-handled sponge is useful for reaching the feet and back.

Many stroke patients find it difficult to stand safely in the shower or to transfer to the bottom of the tub. As stated previously, most studies on adaptive equipment usage indicate that bath seats or benches are among the most commonly recommended devices. Fig. 10-5 shows a selection of commonly available models. Transfer tub benches are most appropriate for patients who require significant physical assistance for transfers or those who can only perform squat pivot or sliding board transfers. Transfer tub benches are the most expensive and least portable type of bathing equipment. For patients who can accomplish stand pivot transfers, a variety of economical seats that fit inside the tub or shower stall are available. The patient can either step over the tub side, which requires an ability to fully support the body's weight on one lower extremity, or back up to the tub rim, sit back onto the seat, and swing the legs into the tub. Grab bars can be installed in the tub wall or attached to the tub rim to provide stability with transfers or standing.

Toilet safety rails, grab bars, and raised toilet seats are also effective in increasing independence with transfers and standing during toileting. Toilet safety rails are usually preferred for their portability, simple installation, and cosmesis. A three-in-one commode combines the convenience of the safety rails and raised toilet seat and can be used in the existing bathroom or bedside. The other frequently encountered difficulty with toileting is clothing management. The previously described lower extremity dressing techniques should be applied during toileting. Often the biggest roadblock to bathing and toileting independence is the bathroom itself. Most bathroom doors are 22 inches wide, which will not accommodate even the narrowest wheelchair. The patient must make a decision to rely on the additional assistance of family to get into the bathroom, to use basin or sink bathing to meet hygiene needs, or to make architectural adaptations such as widened doorways. Bedside commodes are often necessary when bathroom accessibility is not feasible. The interdisciplinary team can work closely with the patient and family in choosing the most practical option and securing resources. The bathroom is also the most frequent site of falls or other accidents. Patient and caregivers must be trained to identify potential hazards, to keep floor surfaces dry, and to ensure that transfers and ambulation are accomplished in a safe manner.

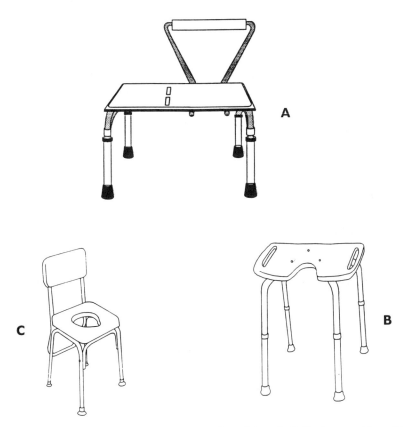

Fig. 10-5   Various forms of equipment. **A,** Transfer tub bench. **B,** Bath seat with padded seat and back. **C,** Bath seat without back. (From *Independence in the bathroom,* May 1992, National Rehabilitation Hospital, Rehabilitation Engineering Department.)

Home management. Patients with hemiplegia face numerous challenges (both physically and cognitively) in accomplishing home management. Patients must be able to maneuver in small spaces and transport items while managing wheelchair or walking aides. Reaching items from high and low cabinets and managing the bilateral demands of tasks may also prove difficult. In addition, home management activities may require a high degree of cognitive demands such as reading comprehension, organizational skills, and problem solving. Coordinating the varied skills of the interdisciplinary team is the most effective approach for maximizing independence in this area. For example, during meal preparation the physical therapist can facilitate the patient's gait training, standing balance, and trunk control; the speech and language pathologist can suggest methods to assist in the comprehension of recipes or verbal instructions; and the occupational therapist can integrate these strategies with adaptive techniques and equipment.

Work simplification is the technique of adapting a home performance task and the environment to facilitate the most efficient expenditure of energy.[172] These strategies are effective for the stroke patient with low endurance who wants to remain active. General principles of work simplification include planning and prioritizing daily activities, eliminating nonessential tasks, organizing storage areas and work space, alternating sitting with standing, and using correct equipment and body mechanics. Specific techniques are available for meal preparation, home care, yard care, and community tasks. The following are examples of common compensatory strategies, work simplification techniques, and adaptive equipment available for home management activities.

Meal preparation. The recent surge in the development of electronic convenience appliances has made cooking easier for both the disabled and the nondisabled population. Use of a microwave oven can be safer, more efficient, and more easily adaptable for the one-handed person and wheelchair user. Electric mixers are an effective one-handed alternative to the traditional eggbeater. Food processors reduce preparation time and eliminate the need for adaptive cutting devices.

Other bilateral meal preparation tasks that may require adaptations include opening boxes, carrying items, stabilizing bowls, and slicing items. By holding boxes between the knees while sitting or by stabilizing the box in a partly open drawer, the patient can use the unaffected upper extremity to open the container. As previously described, rubber placemats effectively stabilize bowls while stirring. A cutting board with three spikes holds vegetables or fruits still during cutting. A wheeled cart or walker basket can assist the homemaker with transporting items to the table. Patients are also taught to slide items along the countertop to avoid lifting while working in the kitchen. Patients with organizing and sequencing difficulties may benefit from the use of simple checklists or from the strategy of gathering all needed items and arranging them in sequence on the work area before beginning a task. The therapist may also assist the patient to select simple, familiar recipes or ready-made convenience foods to reduce the complexity or number of steps the task involves.

Home care. Long-handled, free-standing dust pans, reachers, and self-wringing sponge mops ease the difficulties of floor care for the stroke patient. All of these devices can be handled from either a standing or wheelchair level. To conserve energy, bed making can be accomplished by completing each corner before moving on to the next one. Using this method, the patient only has to walk around the bed once. Laundry, ironing, and dishwashing can usually be accomplished without compensation or equipment if the patient has sufficient motor and cognitive abilities.

Other activities of daily living. Other ADLs that should not be overlooked when developing a comprehensive interdisciplinary plan include functional communication, such as telephone use; financial management; and environmental controls, such as the ability to call for assistance. Compensatory strategies and adaptive devices are available to provide independence and safety for the stroke patient for whom these tasks are a concern. Community integration, driving, and work and leisure roles are discussed in other sections of this book.

The ultimate outcome of treatment planning in the rehabilitation setting is for the stroke patient to achieve the highest level of independence and life satisfaction in ADLs. By taking the time to understand each patient's goals, life-style, and values and to integrate the unique skills of each interdisciplinary team member, these outcomes can be achieved.

TRAINING IN MOBILITY

Richard S. Materson and Mark N. Ozer

Nature of the Problem

Mobility and regaining ambulation are the major goals of most persons with stroke. Mobility is the problem that most interferes with independent living in community settings and that largely determines the length of in-hospital rehabilitation. During the acute phase a primary aim of the assessment of the sensorimotor system was to determine the prognosis so that the proper rehabilitation program could be selected. The degree and type of impairment and the rate of recovery were assessed. However, the assessment of impairments must ultimately relate to function, rather than serve primarily to localize the lesion. For example, rather than using the finding of hemiparesis to aid in localizing the lesion, in the rehabilitation phase the finding is used to determine the relative distribution of strength between the patient's arm and leg and between the proximal and distal aspects of the affected lower limb, which has implications for the patient's ability to stand and ambulate. In addition, during the acute phase the major treatment goal of the rehabilitation program was to initiate procedures to prevent secondary impairments caused by abnormal posture of the limbs. These efforts must continue; however, during the rehabilitation phase the major treatment goal must be to alleviate the disabilities such as mobility problems, despite the continued impairment in motor control.

During the rehabilitation phase the assessment of the degree and type of impairment must shift to an assessment of the disabilities—that is, the functional consequences of those impairments in the person's life. The assessment must relate to the idiosyncratic needs and goals of the person with stroke and the physical and interpersonal environment in which he or she lives. For example, it is necessary to explore the availability of caregivers and the physical accessibility of the home in terms of bathing facilities, toilets, and stairways. A particular set of impairments affecting the sensorimotor system may have quite different consequences given these several other variables.

The determination of disabilities also requires several changes in perspective during the examination of the patient's nervous system. Rather than focusing primarily on the loss of function, one must now assess the conditions under which function can occur. For example, it has been helpful to define the functional status in terms of the degree of support necessary so that the person can carry out activities such as transferring from a bed to a chair. Patients' needs range from a major degree of physical assistance, including lifting, to merely physical guidance or supervision to prevent falls. Moreover, rather than focusing merely on the status of the remaining function, one must consider the process by which one can enhance function. The assessment must reflect the dynamic quality of the nervous system as an adaptive system attempting to maintain function in response to the effects of the impairments. Enhancing such adaptation by training in the use of compensatory strategies is the activity of the rehabilitation phase. The patient must also learn alternative ways to achieve mobility, including how to use adaptive devices such as wheelchairs and other assistive devices such as braces.

Injury affecting the upper motor neuron (pyramidal tract) has traditionally been considered to have both "positive" and "negative" features. The positive features include abnormal posture, exaggeration of proprioceptive reflexes, production of spasticity, and exaggeration of some cutaneous reflexes of the limbs, producing flexion withdrawal spasms and the Babinski response. It has been helpful to consider these phenomena as resulting not only from the release of previously inhibitory suprasegmental controls but also from changes in spinal circuits to compensate for the removal of descending circuits. It may be possible to use these phenomena in a controlled fashion to turn them to the patient's advantage rather than attempting to abolish them.[184,204]

The negative features are weakness and loss of dexterity. The greatest deficit is in the muscles acting as prime movers rather than stabilizers. In the lower extremities, upper motor neuron weakness is greater with flexion than with extension at the hip, knee, and ankle. Although there may be sufficient spinal circuitry to generate the cyclic activation of flexor and extensor muscle groups, the initiation of locomotion also requires a willful activation of muscles that may be absent.

Assessment

During the acute phase the assessment of the sensorimotor system sampled motor strength and coordination and the degree of range of motion at the various joints. The outcome of motor assessment in upper motor neuron lesions varies with bodily position and the degree of weight loading and thus must be viewed in the context of these variables. Thus during the rehabilitation phase the proper assessment of motor function must focus even more on the actual performance. Particular emphasis must be placed on motor planning, endurance, and the ability to maintain actions in the context of changing conditions. The problems of mobility in the person with stroke are those of maintaining posture over time and space. Weight bearing provides the major problem but also a major opportunity; in the context of weight bearing the previously well-developed postural patterns and reflexes can be brought into play to provide at least a partial solution to these problems.

Ambulation represents one important measure of motor function. The relation of the degree of impairment to the level of ambulation is variable. In one study of persons with unilateral lower extremity paresis, the degree of impairment was assessed at the start of rehabilitation using the Brunnstrom scale.[183,210] Although those who showed an improved degree of impairment also showed improved function, an even larger number of subjects had improved ambulation without concomitant evidence of an improvement in the degree of impairment in the lower extremity. It is clear that change in degree of impairment (at least when measured by the Brunnstrom scale) does not necessarily predict the degree of functional recovery. Lower extremity function can occur even when only a minor degree of motor ability is retained. More precise measures of those aspects that contribute to ambulation and other measures of motor function must be designed.

The traditional measures of upper motor neuron impairment involve both passive and active motion. The hyperreflexia found on examination with a reflex hammer is due to a loss of regulation of the deep tendon reflex with an elevated response to a given stimulus. Still another passive test employed by the clinician involves manipulating a portion of the limb at a joint. Increased resistance to passive stretch, or hypertonia, is another hallmark of an upper motor neuron lesion. Hypertonia has the quality of an initial high resistance with a sudden drop in resistance—hence the term *clasp knife*. The excitation of this resistance increases with the velocity with which stretch is applied. The term *spasticity* is applied to this phenomenon.[184]

In the assessment of voluntary control of movement, the finding of paresis or plegia reflects the strength of movement. Classically, with motor impairment caused by stroke, hemiparesis and the loss of strength are determined by a finding of asymmetry between the two halves of the body. The manual muscle test is used to assess the strength of specific muscles against gravity and varying resistance. A more complex, goal-directed motor activity that is organized from memory is the ability to perform a familiar gesture, such as waving good-bye. Difficulty in carrying out such purposeful actions may not be attributable to weakness or disturbance in comprehension. This phenomenon of apraxia reflects a problem in motor planning, generally found in those patients with left-sided lesions.

These findings that traditionally defined motor impairment have limited applicability to the problems of mobility in persons with stroke. The hyperreflexia and hypertonia found on passive movement are not causes of the problems found in voluntary movement. In persons with spasticity there is a dissociation between the hyperreflexia in passive movement and the coactivation that occurs in antagonist muscles in attempted voluntary movement.[223] For example, a drug that reduces the response to passive stretching of the quadriceps muscle does not affect the degree of cocontraction in alternating flexion and extension of the knee. It is the latter phenomenon that compromises the effective coordination of muscle action.

In one experimental context, persons with spasticity carried out alternating flexion and extension of the elbow. The increased time required to perform these movements indicated difficulty in reversing the direction of movement. In normal subjects flexor activity ceased before the peak of flexion was reached. In the paretic limb the EMG activity of the biceps muscle persisted throughout flexion and even during extension. There was also limited and prolonged recruitment of agonist contraction. Thus the motor disorder is one of the selection of muscles to be activated and inhibited and is not a simple consequence of the elevated stretch reflex.[217]

Still another format for studying the character of a dysfunction requires sudden flexion of the elbow.[193] In normal subjects there is a triphasic pattern to this movement. First the biceps muscle (as agonist) is activated, then the triceps muscle (as antagonist) is activated, and finally, the agonist biceps muscle is again activated. The timing of the first two components remains fixed even if the load one is working against is suddenly increased. The change that occurs is in the second burst of activity of the agonist. The preprogrammed quality of this sequence is further exemplified by its persistence in a person who lacked all peripheral feedback as the result of a degenerative condition of the peripheral nerves. In the presence of injury to the motor control system the motor deficit was linked to an inability to respond to requirements for change in motor activity and to maintain the proper timing of components. This was particularly noted in persons with cerebellar deficits in which the initial agonist burst or the first two phases may be prolonged.

Reaction time (RT) is still another measure of an abnormality in motor control.[223] In one study of patients with residual hemiparesis associated with upper motor neuron lesions following stroke, EMG records were obtained to identify the time of onset of muscle activity. The time from onset of muscle activity (as measured by EMG) to overt movement was greater on the affected side. However, there was no difference between the patient's two arms in the premotor time between a reaction signal and the EMG onset. Thus the slow onset of movement is attributable, not to a planning problem in the selection of the proper muscle, but to a difficulty in recruiting sufficient motor units to effect movement. Damage to the motor cortex, corticospinal pathways, or both is evident both in the agonist-antagonist relations and in the recruitment of activity.

Proprioceptive disturbance can also be associated with problems in motor control. In the absence of feedback about the position of a limb in space or the lack of a sense of movement, it becomes necessary for the patient to depend on visual input. Such processing can be slow, compounding any difficulties introduced by the slowing of motor output.

Therefore the traditional measures of muscle strength must be modified in light of the character of the motor control dysfunction.[213] The manual muscle test is less appropriate in the case of upper motor neuron lesions than in the assessment of disabilities of more peripheral origins, such as nerve injuries, muscle disease, and anterior horn disease. Manual muscle strength testing depends on the patient's ability to activate selectively the particular muscle being tested while simultaneously relaxing the antagonists. The assumption is that such active muscle actions are indifferent to the rate with which they occur and are unaffected by the posture of the limb or body. None of these conditions necessarily exists in the person who is paralyzed by a lesion in the brain. In one study the effect of posture on the actions of selected muscles in persons with stroke was illustrated by the response to rapid stretching of the soleus muscles.[213] On the average the sitting position doubled the intensity of response found when the patient was supine. Standing further increased the response. These differences were most evident for those who displayed minimum spasticity when supine. Hence, to identify the mechanisms responsible for deviations in gait, the muscles must be tested with the patient standing and walking. Similarly, hand and arm problems must be evaluated with the patient both sitting and standing. The supine posture displays only the patient's minimal state.

Habitual control is the subconscious mode of action used to accomplish the routine tasks that constitute day-to-day activities. The precision in timing and muscle action of a habitual performance ultimately reflects the quality of the underlying selective control. Muscle control of the ankle during walking is one example. With each step a precise reciprocal exchange occurs between the dorsiflexor and plantar flexor muscles. Each muscle also appropriately varies the intensity of action necessary while avoiding excess effort. Similarly, after heel strike, the soleus and gastrocnemius muscles become active only when their force is necessary to restrain the forward motion of the tibia over the stationary flat foot. Their intensity of action increases progressively as the forward alignment of the body magnifies the requirement to maintain a stable ankle.

The loss of selective control of those muscles and the corresponding inaccuracy of habitual performance are characteristic of hemiplegia. Often the loss is incomplete. The person may retain the ability to carry out a selective action of one segment but may be slow or limited in range. In particular, when attempting to measure strength against resistance during a manual muscle test, the selective action is replaced by a mass limb action. Similarly, the greater

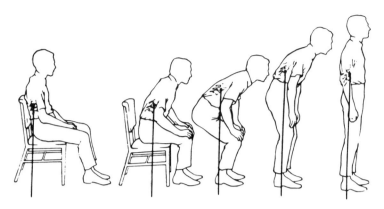

Fig. 10-6   When sitting, patient has support from seat and back of chair, as well as from area under feet. To stand, patient must bring trunk weight forward and keep it balanced over feet while he assumes erect posture. (From Perry J: *Clin Orthop* 63:32, 1969.)

demand of having to perform a complete task, such as walking, may overwhelm the limited degree of normal function, and abnormal motion patterns then dominate. These abnormal patterns also represent the unrestrained action of modes of neurologic control released from normal modulation by the injury.

The focus on ambulation as an end goal must not obscure the patient's need to perform sitting-to-standing activities.[214] These are not only prerequisite to ambulation but are a major contribution to early independence when the patient uses a wheelchair as a primary mode of mobility. Transferring from a bed to a chair and from a chair to a toilet is essential. To stand, the patient must maintain his or her balance while transferring from a broad area of support to a limited (2-foot) area (Fig. 10-6). The stage at which the patient begins to rise from a chair is particularly crucial because the trunk must be brought forward sharply to accommodate for the pelvis being so far back. Added to the demand of balance on a smaller area of support is the task of lifting the body's weight. Armrests on the chair or other types of support can enable the patient to use the upper extremity to help both with lifting and balancing.

Clarifying the usual procedure in sitting-to-standing actions for elderly persons can aid in the remediation of those with strokes, who frequently are elderly.[207] In one study a group of elderly women was asked to rise from a chair without using their arms to push off. Once the sit-to-stand motion was begun, they were free to use their arms. Three phases were identified. Phase I involves a weight shift with trunk flexion; phase II begins with a knee extension and leads to a full trunk extension during phase III. The muscles activated during these phases are successively the spinal erectors muscles, the knee extenders (vastus medialis and rectus femoris) muscles, and the gluteus maximus and biceps femoris muscles. The rectus abdominis muscle appeared to act in phase III to a variable extent. See Fig. 10-7 for a composite of these activities from kinematic data.

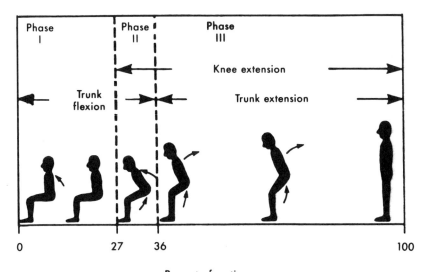

Fig. 10-7 Three phases of sit-to-stand motion defined from kinematic data. (From Millington PJ, Myklebust BM, Shambes GM: *Arch Phys Med Rehabil* 73:609, 1992.)

The requirements of the second transitional phase are particularly complex. A transition occurs between the forward and upward motions. There is concentric activity of the quadriceps muscle at the knee with eccentric activity of the biceps femoris muscle at the knee and gluteus maximus muscle at the hip. Thus cocontraction is necessary, dissimilar to the flexion of the first phase and the extension of the last phase. The peak muscle activity also occurs during this phase, despite its short duration. Weakness of the quadriceps muscle and erector muscles of the spine, in particular, contributes to difficulties during this crucial phase.

Balance is a major component of standing, even before it becomes necessary in ambulation. A measurement of sitting balance is easily made and has been useful in predicting functional outcome. In one study it was found to be highly correlated with functional status on the Barthel Index.[218] Persons able to sit unsupported for at least 15 seconds and to right themselves when nudged in several directions had significantly better Barthel Index scores than those who required some assistance in righting themselves. The relationship between sitting balance and many of the ADL tasks on the Barthel Index is not surprising; progress in achieving sitting balance during rehabilitation predicted an improvement in Barthel Index scores.

In another study a measurement of postural adjustment with induced sway in persons with hemiplegia identified several different patterns. Synchronous coactivation occurred in the several muscles involved.[174] In addition, unlike in normal subjects, there was considerable intrasubject variability in the character of these patterns. Different muscles were involved from trial to trial. The person with hemiplegia was unable to select and modulate centrally programmed adjustments and movement patterns. There was a loss of integration of the various sensory systems, such as visual, vestibular, and somatosensory, limiting the ability of the existing spinal motor programs to function effectively. This abnormality in the maintenance of stance can also be related to similar difficulties in locomotion.

An assessment of balance can include the patient's ability to maintain an equilibrium when sitting on the floor with the hands resting lightly on the legs; while sitting, the response of the patient to a quick and unexpected disturbance of the trunk is noted.[199] If the patient is able to stand with no greater than minimal physical assistance, lower extremity balance is measured by the patient's reaction to slowly applying pressure to the pelvis and observing for normal ankle response. Stepping responses were assessed by providing manual support and shifting the patient's body weight in various directions while attempting to elicit a stepping response. The relationship of balance measures to ambulation was highly predictive, accounting for 62% of the variance. In turn, the degree of motor control (determined by the degree of selective control) and proprioception were highly correlated with the degree of balance.

In one study the significance of sensory input in the management of balance in persons with hemiparesis of varying duration was measured. Subjects were able to stand on a firm surface with their eyes closed.[189] Proprioceptive input was inhibited with the use of a foam surface for standing. A reduction in the duration of stance occurred with the loss of proprioceptive feedback and, to an even greater degree, with the loss of vision. These findings suggest that, in patients with hemiparesis, difficulty exists in integrating somatosensory input and that an even greater than normal dependence is placed on visual clues for maintaining balance.

Analysis of gait. With its low energy cost, normal gait is a complex integrated activity. It involves all joint motions and muscular activity available in the lower extremities, pelvis, and trunk. With each step, three fundamental tasks are performed.[199,214] "Forward progression" consists of reaching forward with one foot while standing on the other; "single-limb balance" makes it possible to stand alternately on one foot while swinging the other; and balance, which was previously discussed, makes it possible to remain upright.

A primary requirement of ambulation is that of single-limb balance. Single-limb balance is a more advanced skill than is required for simple standing. When lifting one leg, the shift in body weight causes the body to fall to the unsupported side unless there is a counterbalancing force. Normally the trunk is shifted laterally to align the center of gravity more nearly over the supporting foot. The hip adductor muscles contract to stabilize the pelvis.

Forward progression is a generic term encompassing both the stance, or weight-bearing period, and the swing phase of ambulation. The stance period begins with heel strike. Weight acceptance is the first requirement. Several simultaneous actions are required to absorb the shock of ground contact, to make the extremity capable of supporting weight, and to preserve as much momentum as possible. Timely restraint by the ankle dorsiflexors prevents the foot from slapping the ground. The knee is passively flexed by the momentum that carries the tibia forward. Extremity stability must be maintained with the use of hip, knee, and ankle extension. Forward propulsion of the body has generally been attributed to the "push off" at the completion of stance. However, a recent study found that the swinging leg provided the major forward impetus.

Normal locomotion has been studied with surface EMG (Fig. 10-8).[191] The muscle groups sampled included the tibialis anterior, lateral head of the gastrocnemius (triceps surae), medial hamstring and quadriceps muscles. Two peaks of activity occurred with the tibialis anterior muscle: the highest occurred during the transition between the deceleration period of the swing phase and the onset of heel contact, and the second and far smaller peak occurred at the beginning of acceleration in the swing phase. The triceps surae muscle had a single peak of activity, recorded during the "push off." The medial hamstring muscles showed their greatest activity during the deceleration period of the swing phase, extending into heel contact. The quadriceps muscle showed an activity peak during the transition from the swing to the stance phase. More complete studies, which include the hip muscle groups, emphasize the contribution during stance of stabilization by the hip abductor, quadriceps, and hamstring muscles.[202] Of particular significance is the moving action of the hip abductors and calf muscles during the transition from the stance to the swing phase. The mean stance phase time was 60%, and the swing phase time was 40%.

Surface EMG has provided measures of gait patterns in patients with hemiplegia.[212] In general, the affected limb had a mean stance phase of 67% of the gait cycle with a swing phase of 33%. The unaffected limb showed a stance phase of 80% and a swing phase of 20%. The asymmetric hemiplegic gait is a product of the altered function of both the affected and the unaffected side. The shorter stance phase and longer swing phase on the affected side and the shortened swing phase on the unaffected side illustrate the unwilling dependence on the paretic leg as a stable weight-bearing support.

Gait disturbances found in persons with hemiparesis are a shortened length of stride and a reduced speed. Note that pathologic gait patterns, regardless of the type of sensorimotor disturbance, show a number of common features: they all exhibit a shortened length of step, a prolonged contact phase of heel and toe, and an increase in the support period to stride. These are compensatory strategies present in normal persons whenever their stability is

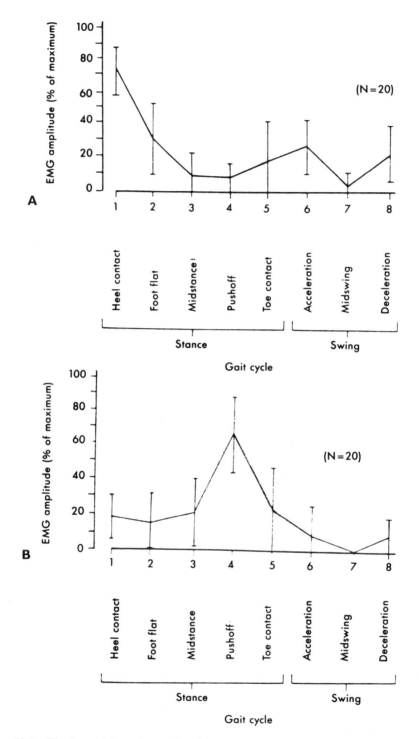

Fig. 10-8 Phasic activity of muscles in normal gait cycle. **A,** Tibialis anterior. **B,** Gastrocnemius.

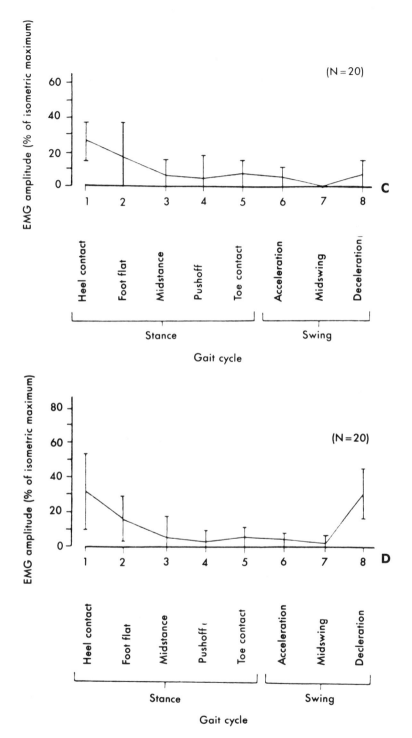

Fig. 10-8, cont'd   **C,** Vastus lateralis. **D,** Medial hamstring. (From Dubo HIC et al: *Arch Phys Med Rehabil* 57:415, 1976.)

threatened, such as in expectation of walking on slippery ground.[187] For the person with hemiparesis, the concern is the source of instability and the availability of particular compensatory strategies. Frequently in patients with hemiparesis, the knee hyperextension is increased in the stance phase and erroneous weight acceptance with the forward-reaching foot occurs, mainly with the foot flat at the start of stance.

Mass limb control is initiated when the person with hemiplegia wishes to perform an act. The actions are stereotyped because the participating muscles and the strength of their responses are the same regardless of demand. Some patients can initiate motion only when actually performing a task such as standing or walking. These locomotor patterns can indicate the muscles contributing to ambulation.[213] In the extensor synergy pattern, when one extends the knee to achieve stance, hip extension and ankle plantar flexion also occur. Similarly, when the hip is flexed, the knee also flexes and the ankle dorsiflexes. One can substitute such total actions for walking. This pattern, however, is inefficient and permits only a small step forward. With flexion synergy the limb is advanced, but as the knee extends to provide support, the hip simultaneously extends with retraction of the limb back to the body line. There is a limited amount of forward progression, arising mainly from body weight considerations.

Step length is improved with a somewhat greater selectivity of motor action. With selective control, initially available at the hip, one can maintain flexion at the hip even when the knee is extended. The forward limb posture gained by flexion is retained. However, ankle control may remain tied to the actions of the knee. Furthermore, although selective action may be present at times on command, one may revert to a locomotor pattern action when walking and when more motor units need to be recruited for any reason.

Studies of persons displaying these locomotor patterns suggest that the extensor phase (stance) is predominantly the result of the action of the gluteus maximus, gluteus medius, soleus, and vastus lateralis muscles.[213] The flexor phase (swing) requires both hip and knee flexion, and function is less consistently available with the iliacus muscle, the major primary muscle. During this phase, major deterrents to adequate knee flexion occur as the result of the frequent concomitant activity by the vastus intermedius muscle and the unavailability of the hamstring muscles because of their basic affinity with the stance phase. Moreover, patients with hemiplegia lack the ability to modify the action. Muscle timing and force are determined by the strength and completeness of patterns and not by the need to respond to changing conditions.

In general, Knuttson considered several mechanisms to be at work in the control of human locomotion.[202] Central generation of locomotor control is one. This mechanism is evident when, in stepping, the initiation of muscle activity in the calf occurs far ahead of that expected in response to the stretch. Another mechanism contributing to locomotion is feedback from the periphery, arising from the response to stretch in the hip abductors, hip adductors, hamstring, and calf muscles. A stretch of the hip abductor muscles is produced by a rapid lateral shift of the body and a medial tilt of the hip during early stance. In later stance the hip adductor muscles are stretched when the body advances ahead of the supporting foot, and the contralateral hip rotates forward. Hamstring muscles are stretched by the passive forward thrust of the pendant lower leg at the end of the swing. Calf muscles are stretched by the forward momentum that pivots the body over the fixed foot in early stance. It is also likely that reflex control modulation occurs at different parts of the cycle by preprogrammed instructions. For example, part of the activation of these muscles is prepatory to an expected strain, such as the tibialis anterior muscle being activated before weight acceptance on the heel.

A number of variables measuring motor strength, balance, and the degree of symmetry in weight bearing can be related to the quality of gait (including the degree of gait independence, speed, and cadence). Gait performance was related to balance, the degree of weight-bearing symmetry, and the degree of motor control. The sum of the static strength of the seven muscle groups, rather than the strength of individual muscle groups, was also correlated with gait performance.[179] Neither age nor the lesion side was related to gait performance in this study. However, other studies have suggested that gait is influenced by the side of the lesion, citing reports that patients with left-sided brain lesions achieve improved gait significantly faster than do those with right-sided lesions.[186]

Particularly relevant to the gait patterns described is the muscle strength assessment of the knee extensors. A positive and significant relationship between gait speed and muscle strength was found, as measured by peak torque on a Cybex dynamometer.[178] However, only about one third of the variance in gait speed could be explained. It should be noted that spasticity, as measured on the Cybex dynamometer, showed no such correlation.

The assessment of degree of symmetry in weight bearing is used as a measure of progress. A ratio of greater than 1 reflects greater support time on the unaffected side, which is consistent with the pattern found in persons with hemiplegia. Particularly relevant in clinical settings is the asymmetry of the single support phase of the gait cycle while the contralateral limb is in the swing phase. This single support phase is shortened on the affected side.[222] The extent of asymmetry and its location in the gait cycle are variables that affect the specific training program. Walking speed and temporal symmetry of swing phases are used to measure the degree of progress in motor recovery. Again, the significant factor is the measurement of single-limb support caused by shortening on the affected side and lengthening of the unaffected side.[181] A set of temporal distance measures provides a relatively simple semiquantative measure of outcome that is reliable between testers and related to the level of functional ambulation.[197] (See Table 10-12 for a measure of functional ambulation.)

TABLE 10-12 Functional Ambulation Classification

CATEGORY	DEFINITION
0 Nonfunctional ambulation	Patient cannot ambulate, ambulates in parallel bars only, or requires supervision or physical assistance from more than one person to ambulate safely outside of parallel bars.
1 Ambulator-dependent for physical assistance – level II	Patient requires manual contacts of no more than one person during ambulation on level surface to prevent falling. Manual contacts are continuous and necessary to support body weight and to maintain balance or assist coordination.
2 Ambulatory-dependent for physical assistance – level I	Patient requires manual contact of no more than one person during ambulation on level surfaces to prevent falling. Manual contact consists of continuous or intermittent light touch to assist balance or coordination.
3 Ambulatory-dependent for supervision	Patient can physically ambulate on level surfaces without manual contact of another person but for safety requires standby guard of no more than one person because of poor judgment, questionable cardiac status, or the need for verbal cueing to complete the task.
4 Ambulator-dependent for supervision	Patient can ambulate independently on level surfaces but requires supervision or physical assistance to negotiate any of the following: stairs, inclines, or nonlevel surfaces.
5 Ambulator-independent	Patient can ambulate independently on nonlevel and level surfaces, stairs, and inclines.

From Hodden MK et al: *Phys Ther* 64:35, 1984.

In summary, patients with hemiplegia exhibit a reduced speed in walking. An increased stance time on the unaffected side is reflected in the measured asymmetry. Gait disturbances include a reduction or loss of the range of knee flexion during swing. There is also a loss of dorsiflexion of the ankle in both swing and at initial contact. A measurement of work and power at the various joints offers the most fundamental analysis of gait.[209] A change in speed reflects the work done. "Positive" work is the shortening of muscles (concentric), whereas "negative" work is done against gravity and involves lengthening of the muscles (eccentric). Power is a function of force acting at a joint multiplied by velocity.

About 40% of the positive work of walking is done by the affected limb, suggesting the importance of addressing its actions, in addition to the availability of the unaffected side. A major contribution to the problem of gait speed is that less power is put into the affected limb during late stance and early swing. The ankle plantar flexors contribute about half the positive work, particularly at increased speeds, and thus merit particular attention. The hip contributes its greatest action at "push off" in moving through a neutral to a flexion position. The hip also contributes work with hip extensors, followed by lengthening of the knee flexors at the end of stance; although flexion does not occur, the leg must be cleared by the hip alone.

Motor function, proprioception, and sensory training must all be considered in providing effective systems for gait training.[214] The problem of single-limb balance can occur as the result of injury to the central balancing mechanisms, but it is more commonly the result of a loss of awareness on the affected side of the body. When standing, the person falls to the affected side because he or she fails to attempt to support or otherwise compensate for that side. Limb stability can often be enhanced by the use of orthotic devices. The problem of limb advancement can be met with an extensor synergy pattern for initial dorsiflexion of the ankle. One can compensate for this by using knee hyperextension or by leaning forward if there is sufficient hip extensor support. These strategies also require adequate proprioceptive feedback. Limb advancement may be improved by training the person to better use mass motor patterns. Electrodes may also be employed to trigger limb flexion for swing.

The level of outcome in ambulation can be assessed in several ways. One mode of assessment is that used by Keenan.[199] In this study, "community ambulators" were patients able to negotiate on all terrain and on stairs and curbs. "Limited community ambulators" were able to negotiate all terrain but required standby assistance for uneven surfaces and stairs. "Household ambulators" required supervision with level terrain ambulation and physical assistance of a minimal nature with stairs or curbs. "Physiologic ambulators" required assistance on level terrain. Nonambulators required the maximal assistance of more than one person.

Another, more specific format for assessing the level of transfer and ambulation is that provided by the Functional Independence Measure (FIM).[216] A seven-point scale reflects the degree of support required to carry out the activity. The upper box on p. 382 describes the range of scores for transfer; the box on pp. 382 and 383 describes the measure of locomotion via ambulation; and the box on pp. 383 and 384 describes the use of the wheelchair as the primary means of locomotion.

Treatment of Mobility Disorders

It is necessary to develop practical means of achieving a maximal functional return of mobility in the relatively short time available in current inpatient rehabilitation stays. One practical multistep comprehensive program for stroke recovery served as a protocol for the Hawaii Heart Association and

Transfers from Bed, Chair, and Wheelchair

Includes all aspects of transferring to and from a bed, chair, and wheelchair and coming to a standing position, if walking is the typical mode of locomotion.

NO HELPER

7. Complete independence: If walking, the patient approaches, sits down, and rises to a standing position from a regular chair; transfers from a bed to a chair; and performs safely.

   If in a wheelchair, the patient approaches a bed or chair, locks brakes, lifts footrests, removes armrest if necessary, performs either a standing pivot or sliding transfer, and returns to the wheelchair. Patient performs transfer safely.
6. Modified independence: Patient requires an adaptive or assistive device (including a prosthesis or orthosis) such as a sliding board, a lift, grab bars, or a special seat, chair, brace, or crutches; takes more than reasonable time or there are safety considerations.

HELPER

5. Supervision or setup: Patient requires supervision (e.g., standby assistance, cueing, or coaxing) or setup (e.g., positioning sliding board, moving footrests).
4. Minimal contact assistance: Patient performs 75% or more of transferring tasks.
3. Moderate assistance: Patient performs 50% to 74% of transferring tasks.
2. Maximal assistance: Patient performs 25% to 49% of transferring tasks.
1. Total assistance: Patient performs less than 25% of transferring tasks.

Comment: In the assessment of the bed-to-chair transfer, the patient should begin and end in the supine position.

Ambulation

Defined as the ability to walk on a level surface indoors once in a standing position (not in parallel bars) and to negotiate barriers.

NO HELPER

7. Independent: Patient can be left alone to walk a minimum of 150 feet safely, within a reasonable length of time and without assistive devices.
6. Independent with equipment: Patient walks a minimum of 150 feet but uses a brace (orthosis) or prosthesis on the leg; special adaptive shoes, cane, crutches, or walker; or takes more than a reasonable time.

Ambulation — cont'd

HELPER

5. Supervision: Verbal cueing, demonstration, "hands-off" guarding, or standby assistance may be necessary. Patient cannot be left alone to perform the activity safely but does not require physical assistance or contact to perform the activity. Patient walks at least 50 feet.
4. Minimal physical assistance: Patient performs 75% or more of the task. May require "hands-on" or contact guarding. Patient walks at least 50 feet.
3. Moderate physical assistance: Patient performs 25% to 50% of the task. Only one person is required for physical assistance. Patient walks at least 50 feet.
2. Maximum physical assistance: Patient performs 25% to 50% of the task. Only one person is required for physical assistance. Patient walks at least 50 feet.
1. Dependent: Patient requires total assistance and performs less than 25% of the task. One or more persons may be required for performance of the activity.

Wheelchair Propulsion

Defined as the physical ability to propel oneself in a wheelchair, to maneuver around barriers, and to manage wheelchair parts. Note that an electric wheelchair is regarded as a piece of adapted equipment. Propulsion indoors on level surfaces *only* is rated.

NO HELPER

7. Independent: Patient operates manual wheelchair independently and safely and, within a reasonable period of time, covers a distance of at least 150 feet; turns around; maneuvers the chair to a table, bed, or toilet; negotiates at least a 3% grade; and maneuvers on rugs and over door sills. (Equipment for manual wheelchairs includes projections, tubing, and wheelchair mitts.)
6. Independent with equipment: Patient operates electric wheelchair independently and safely and, within a reasonable period of time, covers a distance of at least 150 feet.

HELPER

5. Supervision and setup: Patient propels powered or manual wheelchair safely with verbal cueing, demonstration, "hands-off" guarding, or standby assistance for at least 50 feet.
4. Minimal physical assistance: Patient performs 75% or more of the task but may require "hands-on" or contact guarding. Patient propels wheelchair at least 50 feet.

Continued.

Wheelchair Propulsion — cont'd

3. Moderate physical assistance: Patient performs 50% to 75% of the task. Only one person is required for physical assistance. Patient propels wheelchair at least 50 feet.
2. Maximum physical assistance: Patient performs 25% to 50% of the task. Only one person is required for physical assistance. Patient propels wheelchair at least 50 feet.
1. Dependent: Patient requires total assistance. Patient performs less than 25% of the task.

---

enjoyed considerable success in increasing the percentage of persons receiving appropriate stroke rehabilitation services. The program is divided into phases (see the box on p. 385), with day variances based on different rates of stroke recovery. It is assumed that the patient is transferred to the rehabilitation facility or begins the rehabilitation program at 2 to 5 days after admission or when medical stability is reached and that the length of stay in a rehabilitation setting is 25 to 30 days. The services required will vary from patient to patient. Many of the recommendations are derived from the American Heart Association's *Strike Back at Stroke.*[221]

Identification phase. The identification phase is used by trained nursing staff to review with each nursing unit all admissions of patients who have stroke syndrome and who might benefit from the use of the rehabilitation protocol. The aim is to attract those patients who can benefit from the protocol early in the course of stroke care. During this phase of treatment, literature on strokes is provided to the patient and family. Clear plastic-covered cards are placed at the patient's bedside, emphasizing the proper resting positions. A triangular bandage is supplied to protect the hemiplegic shoulder from tug or subluxation during transfers within the hospital. Rehabilitation starts when someone thinks of it. The identification phase establishes a formal network in each institution so that stroke syndrome patients are discovered, and thus case finding and treatment are maximized.

In-bed phase. The key to the success of the program is to avoid the development of secondary impairments during the acute care phase when the patient is in bed and most vulnerable. Therefore, during the in-bed phase, proper attention is paid to bed positioning to avoid typical hemiplegic deformities caused by a combination of flaccidity and spasticity resulting from the perverse long-term effects of gravity on the bedridden patient and persistent faulty positioning. Common deformities are hip flexion, leg external rotation, foot plantar flexion, knee flexion, arm adduction and internal rotation, forearm flexion and pronation,

---

Stroke Rehabilitation Phases

1. Identification (of the stroke syndrome in patient admitted to an acute care facility): day 1
2. In-bed phase: days 1 to 3
3. Sit-up phase: days 3 to 7
4. Stand-up phase: days 5 to 15
5. Step-up phase: days 8 to 21
6. Step-out phase: days 18 to 30

---

and wrist and finger flexion with an indwelling adducted thumb. Other preventive measures were summarized in Part II but deserve reemphasis here.

The unmoving limb is also a sensory-deprived limb. Because sensory reintegration has been proved to occur with need and sensory experiences, cautious full-limb passive or active assisted range of motion is instituted, in which each joint is moved by the therapist or a trained family member or the patient is assisted in completing a self-initiated joint range of motion. Providing additional cutaneous cues (through skin stroking or thermal stimulation to activate cutaneous receptors or through deeper massage and vibration to activate primarily group IA afferent proprioceptors) facilitates the desired sensory stimulation and enhances the desired motor effect. These simple maneuvers are helpful and can be easily incorporated in the bedside visits of team members. Care must be taken to remain within a safe, pain-free range of motion to avoid inappropriate and undesired reflex activation from nociceptor stimulation (such as in overzealous shoulder abduction and external rotation in a patient who might not be able to communicate the history of a previous rotator cuff syndrome with subsequent unrestored range of motion and whose shoulder tissues can be harmed from overstretch).

The use of simple splints, trochanter rolls, footboards, and arm-positioning devices can play a role, although these devices must be constantly checked and repositioned to ensure their proper function.

Precautions must be taken on the patient's arrival at the hospital to avoid unnecessary tugs or pulls on the hemiplegic side, an incident that occurs all too often during transfers to the examining table, the laboratory, or the radiology department. It may be necessary to use armboards to stabilize an intravenous (IV) needle; yet, if the IV device is placed on the less-affected side, it may inhibit the only readily available, voluntary, functional upper extremity the patient has and may further limit sensorimotor experiences. If the IV is placed on the most affected side, that side will experience even more sensorimotor deprivation, and the lack of normal sensation may provoke the unreported extravasation of IV fluid and focal tissue damage. Therefore use of these devices should be minimized and the devices rotated regularly.

Protection of the patient's skin from the development of pressure ulcers is equally important. This is true not only because of the long and complicated healing process necessary once a pressure ulcer has occurred but also because of the adverse nociceptive stimuli, which can provoke unwanted flexor reflex enhancement and debilitating flexion contractures. Protein loss from such ulcers adds to the often present poor catabolic state, further complicating a timely recovery. When the patient is bedridden, "lying" sores predominate. These are found at bony prominences, which receive undue pressure from the mattress; they are often located at the sacral or trochanteric areas and the heel but may be found in other locations such as over the lateral malleolus, scapula, and elbow. On sitting, the patient's skin over weight-bearing points, such as over the ischial tuberosity, again is affected. Proper attention to both sitting posture and surfaces is necessary.

Although many special bed surfaces have been developed to reduce the likelihood of pressure ulcers, avoiding prolonged pressure that is greater than skin capillary pressure is clearly necessary. This requires frequent turning, leaning, and push-ups. An additional therapeutic benefit of the movement is neuromuscular stimulation and the prevention of contractures. A variety of aids—such as eggshell-crate foam, air-fluidized beds, artificial "fat" cushions, sheep skin, and water- or air-bead mattresses—are available, and one may choose the surface most likely to provide pressure reduction and good skin hygiene with adequate air circulation. Several manufacturers have developed heel boots fixed with both dorsiflexion assistance to prevent footdrop and antirotator bars to prevent external rotation at the hip and decrease trochanteric pressures. Similarly, devices are available to protect patients' elbows from pressure. Care must be taken when using such devices; they must be removed from time to time and the skin inspected. A red spot that blanches when pressed is a warning sign. A red spot that no longer blanches when pressed indicates dying skin. The first stage is treated by completely protecting the area at risk from pressure. Skin protection includes adequate red blood cell mass preservation because ischemia is the principal pathophysiologic cause; the identification and correction of anemia are critical. Adequate nutrition, including trace minerals and vitamins, is necessary. If a pressure ulcer develops, pharmaceutic debridement, surgical debridement, or both; proper wound care; and pressure relief are necessary. The protection must continue to be supervised by *all* members of the rehabilitation team, including the patient and family. Patients with either centrally or peripherally originating sensory deprivation are particularly vulnerable and often will not draw attention to areas that otherwise might be reported. Therefore patients receiving mind-altering drugs or whose injuries preclude safe self-attention need special monitoring.

The prevention of edema accumulation, venous stasis, and potential deep vein thrombosis can be assisted by fitting the patient with gradient pressure pumps or hose.[180,208] Many authors suggest the administration of low-dose heparin, except in cases of stroke caused by cerebral hemorrhage. (See Chapter 4 for fuller treatment of this issue.)

The location of the patient's bed during the in-bed phase can be of strategic importance. The patient with visual field impairment should be located so that he or she is in a position to observe important comings and goings in the room. For the most part, leaving the most functional side unencumbered by IV lines and other similar methods will enable the patient to begin early to practice control over his or her environment and will enhance independence. Room size must be adequate for the placement of a wheelchair or other ambulatory assistive devices. Hygiene aids, water pitcher and cups, and food should be located within the functional visual field and near the more functional hand. In the unusual case of preserved bimanual function, these placement suggestions still apply.

During the in-bed phase, one of the first opportunities to lessen the patient's feeling of helplessness and dependency is to encourage independent movement. Bedside rails, an overhead trapeze, knotted ropes, and the bed headboard and sheets all can be used (by pushing and pulling) to allow the unaffected upper and lower extremities to operate together when changing position in bed, rolling from side to side, and relieving pressure from bony prominences. Movement in bed patterns is covered in the American Heart Association's *Strike Back at Stroke.*[221] Some facilities have found it advantageous to mount pictorial directions at a patient's bedside to remind all professional and other visitors of the proper mechanics of in-bed movement and transfers. Often, diagnostic studies are carried out during the in-bed phase. Special precautions to avoid injuring the susceptible hemiplegic shoulder during transfers to a gurney or to and from an x-ray examination table are important (never pull on the hemiplegic arm). "Army-tuck" tight sheets should be avoided because they can add to gravitational pull and be a deforming force resulting in ankle equinus. Overuse of the bed head elevation and gatch controls on electric or manual hospital beds can lead to persistent faulty flexion positioning of the hips and knees, fostering unwanted flexion contractures. If a footboard device is used on the bed, hanging the bedding over it eliminates the equinus-enhancing tight sheet; however, it is unlikely alone to be effective in preventing footdrop deformity because the patient is infrequently properly positioned to take advantage of it. Devices such as the Stryker boot are available both to cradle the foot and ankle in the proper position and to protect the heel skin. Care must be taken to fasten the Velcro straps on these devices loosely enough to not gouge the dorsum of the foot or ankle.

Proper nutrition begins in the in-bed phase with a feeding and swallowing assessment and careful dietary planning. Patients with aspiration or inadequate nutrition are delayed in rehabilitation advancement if these areas fail to be addressed, and aspiration pneumonia is a difficult to treat and life-threatening complication. (This issue is discussed more fully earlier in the chapter.)

Similarly, communications means must be established early to effectively teach the patient the coping skills and safety checks that will be necessary for alternative locomotive choices and other rehabilitative solutions to work. It is also crucial to begin the speech and language pathology evaluation and team guidance at the in-bed phase.

Range-of-motion and strengthening exercises begin during the in-bed phase. Prevention of the atrophy of disuse is a clearly important mission because disuse muscle atrophy adds to the neurologic motor deficits impairing function. Brief maximal isometric exercises of functional upper and lower extremity muscles, including quadriceps muscle "setting," are useful if not contraindicated by cardiac failure or uncontrolled hypertension. In addition, active movement of movable body parts should be encouraged. To keep joints limber, gentle, full passive and (where possible) active assistive range of motion should be accomplished by the nursing staff, the physical and occupational therapy personnel, and physicians during rounds.[221] The American Heart Association's *Strike Back at Stroke* provides pictures and instructions that can be used at the bedside to guide visitors. Professional personnel should instruct family members in the proper techniques and the avoidance of overly aggressive range-of-motion exercises.

Bowel and bladder function monitoring and retraining (as necessary) are critical during this phase. The avoidance of bladder overdistention is important; once it occurs, the overstretched detrusor is ineffective at complete bladder emptying, especially "uphill," such as is often the case in in-bed micturition. This problem is compounded in elderly males with prostatic hypertrophy. Inadequate bladder emptying favors infection. Checks of postvoiding urinary residuals, preferably by noninvasive ultrasound techniques at the bedside, enhance the clinical observations and palpation for distended bladder. Clean intermittent catheterization protocols are called for if inadequate emptying is discovered. A Foley catheter is to be avoided if possible because of inevitable bacteriuria and frequent clinical infection.

Perineal hygiene is critical to the patient's physical and mental well-being. Ammoniacal or fecal odors are to be avoided. Control of bladder and bowel incontinence is also important because loss of control is one of the great nightmares of affected patients. The patient's voiding should be timed and recorded so that patterns are learned and adequate attention is given to intake and output, which are critical to control training. Frequent trials at voiding can often avoid diapering or condom catheters, which have very "regressive" overtones but may be temporarily necessary in cases of continued incontinence. Frequent changes and regular hygiene are mandatory if incontinence devices are used.

Bowel-training programs include an attention to adequate dietary or supplemental bulk formers and adequate hydration and the use of gentle low-irritant bowel stimulators, such as cocoa butter or glycerine suppositories, senna, mild nonirritant enemas, and (if necessary) cathartic agents. These methods must be planned around the patient's regular habitual evacuation times, and the goal is as rapid a return as possible to commode evacuation. One must observe the patient for signs of bowel impaction and related ileus, one of the most common complications on the rehabilitation unit. Most often, these complications can be handled with conservative medical means such as mechanical and pharmaceutic evacuation, transient nasogastric suction or rectal tubes, and careful attention to hydration and diet. Rarely, obstruction requires surgical treatment, including flexible colonoscopic lavage. If nasogastric suction tubes are used, IV alimentation must also be supplied until the crisis is over.

Sit-up phase. Of necessity, the patient's return to vertical tolerance must precede other mobility training. Cardiac instability, postural hypotension, truncal ataxia, and severe general weakness are most often the delaying factors and must be paid proper attention. Independently coming to a sitting position from a lying position demands the coordination of the most functional side and an ability to communicate and cognate. Again, the American Heart Association's *Strike Back at Stroke* has excellent visual and written instructions for attaining this posture.[221]

The patient's ability to maintain a safe sitting balance must be tested, first with the feet comfortably resting on the floor from a properly positioned bed height, then with the feet off the floor (first one foot, then both). Titubations of the body and head can be used both for testing and for challenging trunk balance. Attention to visual field deficits, positional agnosia, and hemineglect must be paid and coping strategies outlined. Wheelchair-posture devices, trunk-stabilizing back supports, lap belts, and H-pad types of patient restraints may all be considered as safety-enhancing devices for those patients with special needs.

Wheelchair transfers must be successfully carried out to complete the "sit-up" phase for patients who are unable to walk. In this stage the hemiplegic limb is usually in various degrees of flaccidity. Knee and ankle stability generally have not yet been achieved. Usually, if the patient was capable of walking before the stroke and less than 2 weeks has passed since the stroke, enough reserve strength exists in the unaffected hip and knee extensors to allow the patient to perform a standing pivot transfer from the bed to a wheelchair and back or from a wheelchair to a commode and back. The pivot transfer is accomplished by the helper placing his heels together with the feet angled to form a V. The patient's hemiplegic foot is placed in the V, and the helper's knees are aligned to either side of the patient's hemiplegic knee. Using good back mechanics, the helper flexes at the hip and knee, has the patient hold on at the waist with the most functional upper extremity, gently rocks the patient forward to move the center of gravity over the feet, then stands up with the pressure of the helper's knees against the patient's knee to lock it into extension. This maneuver usually does not require the helper to physically lift the patient; rather, the helper guides the patient and provides safety against collapse of the hemiplegic leg as the patient provides the power lift with his hip extensors and knee extensors. Once the patient is standing, a pivot placing the back of the patient's thighs against a well-placed locked wheelchair is accomplished, and the patient is allowed to sit down in a controlled fashion with the helper exercising a controlled hip and knee flexion and the patient using the unaffected arm and leg to control the sitting process. Quadriceps muscles and eccentric contraction of hip extensor by the patient are necessary. Patients with weakened quadriceps muscles or hip extensors, such as those who have had polio or diabetic multilumbar radiculopathy, may have additional difficulty with this transfer, and greater effort on the part of the helper will be required.

This same transfer technique can be successfully used to accomplish toilet transfers from the wheelchair. A toilet with a raised toilet seat and swing-out or removable side rails and a wheelchair with similar side rails facilitates this transfer. Once the patient is seated on the toilet, an antifall security system is necessary; if there is any question of instability or imbalance, a helper should be present. Patients at risk for falls from the commode must not be left alone. Those who are given privacy must also be given a nurse call system and instruction in its use to facilitate easy access to a helper. (The reader is reminded of the vasovagal effect as one bears down in defecation.)

Advancing to successful wheelchair transfers allows a patient to move about the hospital environment, reinforcing the concept of a return of independence. In particular, the patient can attend therapy in the therapy departments (as opposed to at the bedside) and can eat meals in the seated position and often in the dining room. Sitting tolerance is increased and wheelchair propulsion instructions are given. The latter not only facilitates independence but provides functional therapeutic exercise and inhibits some contractures and bedsores.

The wheelchair may be fitted with a lapboard so that eating and other activities can be done in the seated position and the hemiplegic arm can rest out of harm's way. A clear "see-through" lapboard is best because it allows a view of the lower extremities and the space immediately in front of the chair. A forearm and hand support in the shape of a foam triangular wedge may be used to elevate the hemiplegic hand to avoid dependent edema. Wrist and hand splints may be used (see Chapter 6). Some therapists advocate the use of a balanced forearm orthotic device for the hemiplegic side; however, I find those more acceptable for flaccid than spastic paresis. Others use an overhead sling (i.e., the Rancho Los Amigos overhead sling) mounted to the back of the chair and fixed with elastic or leather straps to a forearm trough. This supports the luxated shoulder joint and positions the shoulder in slight abduction and forward flexion, and it encourages early use of developing flexion synergies. It also relieves overwork fatigue strain on weakened trapezius, serratus anterior, and levator scapulae muscles, which often attempt to substitute scapular rotation for shoulder abduction. However, the overhead bar must be carefully positioned and can be an environmental hazard because it protrudes forward at a standing head height from the back of the wheelchair frame. A brightly colored tennis ball afixed to its tip provides visibility and increased safety. Some clinicians believe that elastic devices result in unwanted overwhelming flexor tone increases and prefer to avoid this device. I have found them to be particularly helpful with wheelchair-locomoting patients who have prolonged flaccidity and a tendency to distal dependent edema accumulation. The sling trough may also be adapted with a T bar and a variety of functional adaptations if there is adequate internal rotation of the shoulder and elbow flexion to mobilize the device.

Fitting the patient with a wheelchair is accomplished during this phase.[182,198] The "hemi" chair is an adult-sized wheelchair with a seat height of 17 ¾ inches from floor instead of the standard 19 ¾ inches. The lower seat height allows most average-height patients to reach the floor with the unaffected limb while the hemilimb rests on a swing-out removable footrest. The chair can then be propeled by a combination of the unaffected foot and hand action. The footrest on the unaffected side should be removed to facilitate this activity. Some patients prefer to propel the chair backward with a knee extension movement, but this requires looking backward. Forward progression with a knee flexion movement is harder to master, but the forward direction is safer and usually more rewarding. Care must be taken not to use thick wheelchair seat cushions, which take away the advantage of the lowered seat height and force the patient to struggle or slouch to reach the floor. An automotive safety belt is mandatory for safety for patients whose balance and control are untested or deficient. Although the lower seat facilitates independent propulsion, it also presents greater transfer demands on the patient whose knee and hip extensor strength is compromised, and its use is therefore not automatic but carefully considered on an individualized basis. Every rehabilitation team member should be familiar with the proper use of the "wheelchair tool," the special wrench for adjusting and removing footrest or legrest height and position. A tool and instructions are supplied with every wheelchair. The ill-fitted wheelchair that robs patients of full function and safety is common and may contribute to seated pressure sores.

An extended brake handle is useful for the patient to reach the brake on his or her impaired side; however, this handle protrudes and may present unnecessary safety problems if given to a patient who does not require it. Proper sizing of the chair to fit the patient (adult, narrow adult, junior, or extra wide) and proper depth of seat cushions, adjustable arm heights, and special weight frames are all available. If the patient must eat or work at a desk or table, removable, reversible "desk arms" are used. The high part of the arm is positioned forward during transfers, and the low part is forward during seated work. If institutional chairs are shared, refitting to each patient is necessary. Ill-fitting chairs are both dangerous and functionally inhibiting. An effective maintenance program is necessary for checking brake adjustments, air pressures for air-filled tires, proper lubrication, alignment, upholstery care, and cleaning. Often, chairs are supplied by a vendor as a rental or by an institution with little expertise in actual wheelchair fitting. Stroke patients deserve the attention of a trained physician and allied health expert for this important decision. In addition, wheelchair needs change as a neurologic return is experienced so that the chair appropriate to the first 15 days may not be correct later.

During this sit-up phase, some therapists advocate the use of neuro-developmental therapies to promote an early return of synergistic movements, generally following the Twitchell schema of motor recovery. The Rood facilitation techniques, the Proprioceptive Neuromuscular Stimulation of Knott and Voss, and the Brunnstrom methods are examples of facilitative strategies; the Bobath methods promulgate a reflex-inhibiting format. No one technique has proved most effective or even more effective than standard therapy techniques. Therefore therapists use those portions of each that seem most effective in a given case. The use of EMG-biofeedback–triggered functional electrical stimulation (FES) may represent the most sophisticated modern extension of these techniques, and early reports suggest that greater neurologic recovery is observed, as compared with standard formats.[203]

During this phase, speech and language pathology evaluations take place, and issues relating to effective communication for patients with aphasia, dysarthria, or other communication disorders such as dysprosody are addressed. The speech and language pathologist evaluates the patient's chewing and swallowing abilities in conjunction with the occupational therapist and nursing staff.[211] A modified barium-enhanced swallow videofluoroscopy may be added to the clinical testing regimen if aspiration is suspected. Oropharyngeal muscle control training is given as necessary, often using mechanical or thermal stimulation or inhibition techniques to facilitate training.

Occupational therapy ensures that functional adaptations are tested, fitted, and trained for, so that the in-bed or wheelchair locomotive patient can achieve the greatest functional independence possible. Reachers, elastic shoe ties, "sporks," and clothing fasteners are but a few of the myriad of effective but simple devices. More severely impaired patients can often benefit from the more sophisticated (and expensive) computer-controlled environment, robotic, and communication systems. A powered wheelchair may be appropriate in a small subset of patients whose physical condition precludes wheelchair self-propulsion and whose cognitive and judgmental status and visuoperceptual skills are intact. Daily living skills training proceeds with the use of these adaptive devices. Protective or assistive splinting is provided. Careful attention must be paid to visual field deficits and to potential perceptual motor dysfunction during these endeavors.

During this phase the assessment of patient roles in the family and community is made so that a care plan particular to the individual patient's needs is constructed with the guidance of the patient and family.

Also during this period the team teaches the patient and primary caregivers techniques for self-monitoring of blood pressure and blood glucose and hypoglycemic agents, as may be indicated in patients with hypertension and diabetes.

Stand-up phase. Walking requires that the patient first sit up, then stand up. Standing up requires adequate cognition to understand the process, motor planning skills, freedom from contractures, balance skills, and adequate strength or useful spasticity to support the hemiplegic limb. Ankle and knee control is necessary. If the patient has a flail ankle (such as is common early in rehabilitation) or inadequate dorsiflexion and inversion and eversion control, an ankle-foot orthosis should be provided as an ankle control device. The choice of devices is related to the deficits; the simplest, a posterior leaf spring orthosis or a dorsiflexion elastic strap assistive device, are useful only for minor dorsiflexion paresis in the presence of adequate mediolateral stability. When more serious mediolateral stability loss or dorsiflexion paresis is present, a polypropylene ankle-foot orthosis can be vacuum formed to a plaster positive mold of the patient's leg, ankle, and foot, or a presized orthosis can be heat molded for a semicustom fit. If these orthoses are cut narrowly at the ankle, less mediolateral control is obtained and more flexibility into dorsiflexion and plantar flexion is permitted. The wider the orthosis is cut to more fully enclose the malleoli, the more rigid is the orthosis, and additional mediolateral stability and dorsiflexion support are obtained. The latter is useful in the control of moderate amounts of spastic equinovarus deformity or severe degrees of hindfoot instability.

Lehmann describes the various options for hemiplegic gait correction using orthoses.[206] Some clinicians prefer the less cosmetic but more controlling double-upright ankle-foot orthosis. Usually combined with a stirrup attachment and a Klenzak or Becker type of ankle joint and calf band and cuff, these devices may be adjusted to allow for varying degrees of dorsiflexion or plantar flexion range of motion and dorsiflexion or plantar flexion spring assistance. Most often attached to a shoe, they also can be supplied with a sole plate that fits inside a tie shoe of adequate box height, allowing a change from one shoe to another and additional orthotic varus or valgus control by molding of the sole plate. A varus or valgus correcting T strap may be added to these braces. The ankle joint settings also have an effect on knee stability. Before the development of adequate quadriceps muscle spasticity control to ensure knee stability during the stance phase of walking, an anterior stop, limiting dorsiflexion to below 90 degrees, forces the knee into extension when weight bearing is applied to the leg. This is useful in patients with inadequate knee control in whom it is desirable to avoid a device that directly locks the knee (such as a hip-knee-ankle orthosis or long leg brace). When knee control is developed, plantar flexion or posterior stops can be used to limit footdrop, and spring dorsiflexion assistance can be provided with the anterior stop removed to allow free dorsiflexion. In cases of back knee hyperextension in which knee extensor control is adequate, an additional posterior stop limits plantar flexion to a few degrees of dorsiflexion and provides a knee flexor moment.

Hirschberg has long advocated a "stand-up–step-up" exercise regimen in which patients may be treated in groups or individually.[196] A simple stable chair or parallel bars may be used. To ensure success from the first therapy session, the height of the bed is adjusted upward or risers are placed on the chair so that, when the patient is asked to stand up, he can achieve the task easily. The helper may stand opposite the patient in a position similar to that for the standing pivot transfer conducted early in the training. The patient places the unaffected hand palm down and pushes on the parallel bar or chair back; at the same time the unaffected leg is used to accomplish the stand up. The patient is instructed to avoid gripping the bars or chair and to "push down, not pull up" on the bar. These are the same mechanics necessary for successful walker or cane use.

As the patient's capability to perform 10 self-paced stand-up movements improves, the task is increased in difficulty; the seat height is progressively lowered until standard heights are mastered. The patient's progress with this stand-up routine is easily measured for by noting the number of inches or risers lowered, the number of stand ups achieved, and the duration it took to achieve them. This exercise is most functional and easily followed with hand signals, even in aphasic patients. Effective and progressive strengthening of hip and knee extensors, hip abductors, elbow extensors, and shoulder stabilizers results. The program can be adapted to a therapeutic pool with underwater seats for patients who are too weak on the unaffected side to manage stand ups on dry land or who have arthritis complicating the stand-up task.

Once the stand up is achieved, the patient practices balance and weight shifts side to side at the parallel bars and may perform toe standing exercises to develop the triceps surae and toe plantar flexor function. A cadence of "stand up, balance, toe up, and sit down" is followed. To sit down, the unaffected hand is placed on the wheelchair armrest, the body is aligned with the back of the thighs at the front of wheelchair seat, and a controlled sit down is accomplished with a combination of arm and leg function. As voluntary control returns to the hemiplegic side, it too contributes to the stand-up–sit-down effort; however, the task can be completed with only one unaffected side.

Hirschberg has calculated the cardiac ergonomics of this exercise program.[194,195] As long as the patient selects the cadence, safe levels of energy expenditures are usually maintained.

The program lends itself to group exercise, which is valuable with the current constrained personnel resources of hospitals. As success is obtained with the stand-up program, a psychologic "high" may be experienced by the patient who was worried that the stroke would mean confinement forever to a bed or wheelchair. The exercise is enjoyable and meaningful to patients who can compare their own progress that of to others in the exercise group. Social interaction is also encouraged.

During the stand-up phase, other neuromuscular reeducation methods can continue to be used. Attention to the unstable shoulder, the defective wrist, and finger extension or a footdrop through EMG-biofeedback–triggered FES appears efficacious.[175] Claims are made that FES of the peroneal nerve, triggered by a heel switch, is associated with a continued facilitated function after the stimulation is discontinued.[201] The previously mentioned neurodevelopmental therapy schools offer differing approaches; each has its own merits and advocates. Knott and Voss use mat activity programs to develop general strength and endurance with movements taught in diagonal patterns to facilitate synergistic function.[200] Wood advocates vibratory facilitation and cutaneous cues to facilitate desired motor behavior.[224] Brunnstrom uses a series of posture and neural facilitative reflex techniques and stimulation to achieve therapeutic motor control return, whereas Bobath teaches reflex-inhibiting postures to allow for less primitive and more mature motor control functions.[183] Unfortunately, the latter is not compatible with current shortened rehabilitation hospital stays.

Once safe stand-up motion and balance is achieved, the patient advances in ADL skills training that takes advantage of verticality, including hygiene and lower extremity dressing skills. As mentioned elsewhere, the use of mandatory asymmetric tonic neck reflexes or other primitive reflexes can be helpful with facilitating flexion or extension of the desired body part.

Severe body neglect, hemisensory deficits, or both can delay success with the stand-up phase. Sitting balance must precede standing balance and must be attended to before this phase is advanced. Some patients have prolonged flaccidity and cannot achieve knee stability even with anterior stop ankle bracing. The use of the tilt table to stimulate antigravity reflexes and extensor spasticity and to regain cardiovascular dynamics in verticality is advocated for these patients. The use of elastic support hose and abdominal binders is especially important in these patients, who tend to experience the splanchnic blood pooling and gravity pooling of flaccid side lower extremity edema.

Although use of knee-ankle-foot orthoses for stroke patients is contraversial (those needing them rarely achieve functional ambulation), they may still be used for patients lacking adequate knee control. A Handy-Standee, which is a height-adjustable posterior splint attaching to the shoe and extending to the ischial tuberosity, locks the knee in extension. This orthosis does not unlock the knee when sitting and therefore is of use only in the clinic. Others advocate a knee-ankle-foot orthosis with upper and lower thigh bands and cuffs added to a ankle-foot orthosis with a hinged knee joint and ring drop locks, allowing the knee to be locked or unlocked without removing the brace. Velcro loop fasteners facilitate independence in donning and doffing. The ankle support is usually a type of Klenzak or Becker device with a stirrup attachment and, if needed, varus or valgus correcting T straps.

Use of such locked knee devices may allow standing and some limited level surface ambulation; however, these devices negatively affect most of the determinants of gait, making the limb a long leg, requiring either vaulting on the opposite side, abduction to clear the floor during the swing phase, or a therapist's assistance to flex the leg and place it because hip flextion and leg control is often inadequate. Heel and sole lifts on the opposite side can assist clearance. Resumption of verticality can stimulate the return of antigravity reflexes so that, in the author's experience, it is worthwhile to try this method before abandoning functional gait as a goal. Even with failure of these orthoses to provide gait, waiting for further neurologic return and working instead on wheelchair levels of independence is acceptable, with another trial of stand-up exercise occurring at each transfer.

Step-up phase. For locomotion to occur functionally, hip flexion must return to the hemiplegic side, allowing for forward progression of the leg and for uneven surfaces such as curbs or stairs to be mastered. The impaired side must also be capable of unilateral stance, with or without assistance, when the opposite limb is advanced. Gait characteristics of the patient with hemiplegia, as summarized by Perry, have already been described.[215]

Hirschberg advocated "step-up" exercises as a simply communicated and effective means of increasing hip flexor, hip extensor and abductor, and knee extensor strength. Using a stairway with handrails, the patient steps up with the unaffected leg while maintaining balance with the hemiplegic extremity and the opposite unaffected arm on the rail. Once the unaffected leg is in place on the step and the patient steps up, the hemiplegic leg is brought to the same step as the unaffected foot, balance is regained, the hand is advanced on the rail, and a repetition of the sequence for the next step is made. The patient descends backward, still facing the steps and with the hemiplegic leg lowered to the next lower step, and balances with the unaffected leg and the unaffected arm on the rail. The unaffected leg controls the rate of descent and is then lowered to the same step as the hemiplegic leg, while the hemiplegic leg and the unaffected arm maintain balance. The process is repeated until the ground is reached. Only later with mature gait does the patient attempt to descend stairs while facing the ground. Until good reciprocal leg function is regained, the one-step-at-a-time pattern is retained and alternate stepping is avoided.

Again, Hirschberg provided the cardiac-ergonomics of this exercise, which is compared favorably to mat or exercise equipment, which might give a similar major muscle group workout. Hand signals for "step up" are nearly universally understood. Although physical therapy gym stairs are commonly used, they are readily available elsewhere. Depending on the individual patient, step ups are done at the patient's chosen cadence, and progress is easily documented by the number of steps climbed and the time taken to climb them. The development of motor control, strength, and endurance is necessary for success at step-up activities and prepare a patient for the next "step-out" phase during which functional locomotion is taught. During the step-up phase, occupational therapists sometimes choose to use "standing boxes," in which pads are used to support the trunk, hip, and knee; during such exercises, vertically oriented activity is engaged and vertical tolerance is enhanced.

Equipment such as the Kinetron II provides isokinetic reciprocal lower extremity exercises and may be adjusted from full sitting to partial sitting to supported standing to standing positions, with varying degrees of paretic side assistance. This type of device is easier to mount and use than the typical bicycle ergometer device with its narrow and often high seat and lack of truncal or upper limb supports. The Restorator is a device fitted to a standard armchair or the wheelchair to facilitate reciprocal peddling and allows varied resistance to be provided.

Upper extremity ergometers, such as the Cybex UBE, can be adapted for the patient with hemiplegia and provide active exercise and range of motion safely if they are properly set up. The increased cardiac resistance of this type of exercise must be considered. Recent experience finds that the facilitation of motor control rather than the inhibition of antagonist muscle represents the most appropriate route to paresis correction.[192] The repetitive reciprocal motions also facilitate a wide range of sensory afferents with the positive benefits of sensory experience to facilitate neural plasticity and proprioceptive neuromuscular facilitation.

During this phase, continued training of the patient's attention to the hemiplegic side and to coping techniques for possible visual or perceptual field deficits and previously mentioned and other strategies are used. The computer can be arranged to provide interesting gamelike challenges, which can be varied in their degree of difficulty or speed and during which the patient's attention is drawn to a neglected side or a slow-responding motor activity is practiced with interesting repetition to gain coordination. These games provide their own reward system for "winners" and can be set so that most patients can enjoy a level of progressive success. This provides enhanced incentives to exercise and its own ego enhancement.

"Step-out" phase. At this stage the patient is ready to apply neurologic recovery and balance, motor control, and strength and endurance gains to the ultimate goal espoused by most stroke syndrome patients — "to walk again." A variety of techniques have been advocated for device-assisted gait training, and different therapists use different approaches. One school advocates using a standing pivot transfer to stand the patient in the corner of a room where adjacent walls can give physical and emotional support. Usually an assistive device is needed; commonly the wide "footprint" and enhanced stability of a "hemiwalker" are needed. The latter device has a central handle grip extending from the center of the front of a lightweight folding walker and rubber legs for better traction. The patient grasps the center grip handle with the unaffected hand for balance and picks up the walker to advance or move it side to side while maintaining balance with the unaffected leg, then pushing with the unaffected hand on the handle and maintaining balance with the walker and the hemiplegic leg while the unaffected leg is not weight bearing. As described earlier in the gait material, the stance phase on the hemiplegic side is shorter and stance on the unaffected side is prolonged. The swing phase on the unaffected side is speeded up, whereas the hemiplegic leg swing is foreshortened in stride length and (usually) in the adequacy of hip flexion and ankle dorsiflexion. The latter is made up for with a well-adjusted ankle-foot orthosis. Leg bracing cannot make up for a hip flexion deficiency. If adequate hip flexion cannot be facilitated, the trunk leans toward the opposite side; a heel and sole lift on the opposite side can provide better clearance for the swing phase of the hemiplegic side. To date, FES units are unsatisfactory for stimulating hip flexor function in the typical patient with hemiplegia, although experience is being gained in spinal cord–injured patients that may be useful in stroke patients with further research.

From the patient's supportive corner position and with a "gait belt" for safety, the patient practices forward and backward and side-stepping gait sequences, leaving the protection of the corner when these are mastered. While its wide footprint and consequent base of support are supportive, the walker is clumsy and remains the device of choice only for a limited number of patients who require greater degrees of support or controlled lower extremity weight bearing.

Progression is usually made to a four-legged quarter walker (a "hemi-cane") that is fitted on the unaffected side, and an alternate four-point gait is taught in which the hemicane is advanced, followed by the hemiplegic leg with balance on the unaffected leg and the cane. The unaffected leg and hemiplegic arm are next advanced while the unaffected hand pushes on the hemicane and the hemiplegic leg maintains balance. The process is then repeated. The more advanced, alternate two-point gait allows the hemicane and the hemiplegic leg to be advanced together while balancing on the unaffected leg; the hemiplegic leg and cane then maintain balance while the unaffected leg swings forward with a reciprocal movement of the hemiplegic arm. Some patients do well when walking a straight line but have trouble with turns, and these actions must be taught in sequential phases.

A Lofstrand or Everett crutch can be used when elbow extensor control on the unaffected side is a problem. Axillary crutches are generally discouraged because patients have a tendency to lean on the crutch at the axilla, endangering the posterior cord of the brachial plexus. When arm and forearm muscle is under good control on the unaffected side and the need for a wide base of support is less, a cane may suffice as the assistive device. A "pistol grip" cane is encouraged because the standard round-top cane causes greater pressure over the ulnar palm and can lead to ulnar nerve entrapments. The pistol grip deviates the weight bearing to the thumb web where it is more easily tolerated. Even so the clinician should be aware of possible carpal tunnel syndrome, which is associated with increased wrist use and weight bearing. Canes must have adequate rubber floor grips for adequate traction, and the tips must be replaced from time to time. Canes and crutches must be fitted at a proper height for the patient. Usually, handles are at the level of the greater trochanter when the device tip is a foot's width lateral to the midfoot. The elbow should be in no more than 25 degrees of flexion as the hand rests on the grip to facilitate extensor torques as the triceps muscle is stretched just past its rest length.

Some physical therapists choose to train patients in gait at the parallel bars. This can have the advantage of a stable starting area. However, if the patient gets into the habit of pulling up or gripping on the rail, this pattern will not work when advancement to a walker or cane is desired. A "hemibar" has been designed in which an oval area of bar is fixed so that pulling up on the bar is discouraged with a mild instability but pushing down is rewarded with stability. The patient is trained to walk around the oval with the unaffected hand pressing down on the railing. The device feels less confining to the patient than walking down the inside of standard parallel bars; it can also be used as a progression step after parallel bars and before a hemiwalker or cane is used.

This phase of training demands that the patient master more than short walks on level surfaces. Walking distances of at least 150 feet is usually necessary for successful functioning at home. Rougher terrains must be mastered, including walking over soil, rocks, and flagstones, depending on the patient's home environmental evaluation and the patient's individual preferences and priorities. For example, locomotion out of the house may be still accomplished with a wheelchair when long distances, rough terrain, or extended walking periods (such as in shopping) are anticipated; yet brace and cane ambulation may still be satisfactory at home.

The patient and caregivers must be instructed in the proper method of transferring from a bed to a chair, to and from a toilet, to a bath, and into a car. Each of these transfer training programs should be prioritized to fit the patient's environment and personal needs, although all will have to be mastered to regain independent community locomotion. Toilet and tub grab rails or transfer seats and other adaptive devices have been discussed (see p. 364). A home visit to check for safety factors should precede a "trial discharge" so that items such as throw rugs, slippery surfaces, electrical wires, and overly deep pile carpets can be identified and eliminated. Bathroom access and an analysis of entrance and egress points, stairs and steps, or other architectural barriers must be identified and adjusted. Thus the therapeutic evaluation of the patient's home is mandatory and cannot be replaced even by practice in the hospital's "family-living unit" if such barriers exist.

Because the patient's ability to drive is often impaired, in most areas training in the use of alternate transportation is a part of mobility training. When the patient's neurologic return is adequate enough to make driving a possibility, skills are best checked first in a driver simulator rather than on the road. Visual and perceptual deficits must be noted. Denial is a common defense mechanism used by patients who still wish to drive, making the development of effective and safe alternatives even more important.[185] In many states, the physician is responsible for providing accurate information to driver's license bureaus.

The timing of ankle-foot orthosis removal is sometimes a question. As long as there is fatigue of dorsiflexions or mediolateral ankle control, the orthosis should be worn, especially out of doors and on unlevel surfaces. First removal trials can often be done at home where short ambulatory distances are common. Many therapists discourage patients from wearing the ankle-foot orthosis correctly, feeling that practice will improve dorsiflexion strength and that brace substitution for muscle function may retard progression and promote atrophy. There is an obvious safety tradeoff if the brace is removed. Retaining it, yet seeing that adequate exercise is routinely done, can be an effective compromise.

Whether it is best for the patient to use a wheelchair or to perform slower and more energy-inefficient ambulatory activities out of the home is unclear. The facilitation of outside activity and social participation can be inhibited if most energy is used simply in "getting there." On the other hand, overuse of a wheelchair when unnecessary is often a sign of poor coping skills, and the increased sedentary level promotes muscle disuse and hip and knee flexion contractures. Patients who gain a level of ambulatory function should be observed for signs of regression once they leave institutional care, and some method of follow-up is mandatory. Ambulatory or home health care agency visits or stroke clubs, where the practitioner can observe the patient, all have their usefulness.

A commonly asked question today is whether "seat lift chairs" are medically indicated for persons with stroke. These chairs have been widely advertised by their manufacturers as valuable for such patients. While much can be said about the ease of powered lifts, there is no need for them if the home is adapted for higher seating surfaces for the patient who has inadequate hip and knee extensor strength but who can still walk once on his or her feet. Inexpensive chair, couch, or bed lifts can be easily made from cut 4 × 4 wooden boards. Furthermore, the seat lift chair encourages the use of the chair's power in lieu of human power and has the unwanted effect of decreasing that exercise and continuing rather than reducing hip and knee extensor weakness. Recent evidence suggests that neurologic recovery may continue for more than the roughly 2 months suggested by Twitchell's studies. Increased out-of-synergy motor behaviors can be prompted by repetitive exercise formats and by biofeedback-triggered FES even up to 2 years after stroke.[173,192] With Tax Equity and Fiscal Responsibility Act (TEFRA) caps forcing rehabilitation hospitals and units into ever earlier discharges, there is an increasing asynchrony between neurologic improvement status and daily living activity levels and discharge. This obligates institutions to responsibly provide postdischarge services until maximal recovery occurs.

During the step-out phase it is important to ensure that the patient's psychologic status matures as quickly as the neurologic recovery. As the discharge date approaches, many patients become anxious over the loss of the fully supportive rehabilitation environment and worry about "making it at home." Others are faced with the realization that the stroke will leave them with some degree of permanent impairment, often confirming their most dreaded premorbid fears. Depression is not uncommon and must be searched out and treated aggressively.[176] Counseling, encouragement, pharmaceutic agents, and patient coping strategy escalation are helpful. The program advocated clearly places the patient in the most controlling position possible and goes a long way to dispel fears of loss of control.

Locomotor skills are critical for success in the community at a maximal level of independence. Each community and each patient varies. If public transportation is to be used, an effective strategy must be planned for such activities as bus or rail access or car transfer training. The caregiver must be instructed in the proper care and maintenance of wheelchairs, walkers, and other ambulatory equipment, including automobile or public conveyance use. Included in this training is the proper use of a wheelchair when faced with stairs and curbs without cuts. Fortunately, the general public environment should become more universally accessible because of regulations written to implement the Americans with Disabilities Act.

When negotiating curbs and stairs, the caregiver must ensure that the patient is securely belted into the chair. The patient's feet rest on the footrest (or footrests). Using the foot bar at the back of the chair, the caregiver tilts the patient backward as the chair's large wheels come up against the curb or stair. Once the chair is comfortably balanced, the caregiver flexes at the hip and knee and rolls the wheelchair up the curb with the patient assisting by pushing on the handgrip of the wheel with the unaffected arm. When the curb has been negotiated and the caster wheels are clear, the helper uses the foot bar to slowly lower the patient back to the resting position. When stairs are encountered, a tilted back position is maintained and a rest in that position is taken at each step. Obviously the caregiver must have adequate physical and health skills to carry this out. Use of the chair in this position maximizes the leveraged use of the wheels to lift and makes the job much easier than it sounds.

Special Problems of Patients with Poor Neurologic Return

Up to this point the discussion has centered on the patient who obtains average or better amounts of return, according to the Twitchell sequence, and who does not have other major complications that slow or complicate the course of recovery, such as amputation, cardiovascular failure, diabetic instability with or without peripheral neuropathy and peripheral vascular disease, and previous stroke or other physically impairing disease. For those with multiple disabilities that produce problems, a well-thought-out restoration program must be designed to meet each patient's special needs.

A few patients are so ill that they are unable to sustain the greater than 3 hours per day of therapy necessary to qualify for most acute rehabilitation hospitals or units. In such cases a less demanding level of care is appropriate and may take place at a skilled nursing facility (especially at the so-called high-level Medicare skilled nursing facilities), at a "step-down unit" of an acute general hospital, or at home[29] with either standard services or, experimentally, more acute rehabilitation services.[177] A residential facility called an intermediate care unit and visiting nurse and therapy service may be the most appropriate level, depending on the patient's goals and tolerance. In each instance, periodic review of the patient's progress and status is important so that the goals of treatment are reinforced, patients are properly advanced when indicated, and proper modifications are made in the goals and program. Care must be taken to avoid secondary impairments such as pressure ulcers, contractures, disuse atrophy, urinary infection, or bowel impaction, which regularly accompany decline until pneumonia or sepsis takes its toll. Critical to this watchfulness is the assignment of a physician or other health professional to ensure that these responsibilities are carried out.

Common inhibitors of progress in stroke recovery are contractures, unwanted spasticity, cognitive deficits, and perceptual motor deficits or motor planning disorders.[219] Each patient requires individual assessment of the assets remaining with which to cope and to problem solve as independently as possible. Even a small step, such as a nursing home patient regaining wheelchair level skills from a bedridden state, is of major importance to the patient's quality of life. The ability to remain at home with family and friends is a cherished wish of all patients. Home health care services have expanded their care roles, and many conditions can be managed effectively at home and at considerable savings over institutional care. While cost savings is a compelling factor, substituting inappropriate lower levels of care for full rehabilitation services is a major mistake all too often repeated by primarily cost-driven managed care plans. Rehabilitation facilities of all levels have an obligation to use resources at the most appropriate level for only the time necessary to achieve the appropriate outcomes. Certainly, this will influence new health care system financing, with subsequent rewards in both quality and efficiency.

Finally, studies of postacute care must extend to the continuing care phase and measure the degree of return of maximal neurologic function, daily living and independent living skills enhancement, functional locomotor skills, caregiver burden, and (of course) cost to guide us to the most appropriate path.[188,220] Stroke patients may have frequent changes in living sites after stroke, and studies must be planned to see that services are appropriate in each environment. Planned care to prevent further stroke and medical deterioration, rather than crisis-oriented episodic care, provides the most successful path to allowing each patient to live long enough to use and enjoy the skills gained through rehabilitation. Because rehabilitation ultimately aspires to enable patients to once again express their human creativity and thus to contribute to private, family, and community life, quality of life scales, rather than mortality and morbidity tables alone, are required to measure meaningful outcomes.

Adaptable, creative rehabilitation professionals must consider not only a patient's medical impairments but his or her social, economic, and educational background, caregiver support, and environmental factors in selecting attainable goals for each individual. Although stereotypic treatment schemes have some strengths, the key to real success is individualization.

REFERENCES
Communication Disorders

1. American Heart Association: *Fact sheet on heart attack, stroke and risk factors,* Dallas, 1990, The Association.
2. American Speech-Language Hearing Association: Functional communication scales for adults project: advisory report, *ASHA* 32:12, 1990.
3. Ammirato T: Stroke clubs, *Urban Med* 4(3):7, 1989.
4. Aten J: Functional communication treatment. In Chapey R, editor: *Language intervention strategies in adult aphasia,* ed 2, Baltimore, Md, 1986, Williams & Wilkins.
5. Baron C: *Post stroke speech, language, and cognitive-communication disorders contrasted according to eleven relevant dimensions,* 1988.
6. Brown M, Gordon WA, Ditter L: Rehabilitation indicators. In Halpern AS, Fuhrer MJ, editors: *Functional assessment on rehabilitation,* ed 2, Baltimore, Md, 1984, Paul H Brooks.
7. Chapey R: *Language intervention in adult aphasia,* Baltimore, Md, 1986, Williams & Wilkins.
8. Darley FL, Aronson AE, Brown JR: *Motor speech disorders,* Philadelphia, 1975, WB Saunders.
9. Davis GA: *A survey of adult aphasia,* Englewood Cliffs, NJ, 1983, Prentice-Hall.
10. Frattali C: Functional assessment of communication: merging public policy with clinical views, *Aphasiology* 6(1):63, 1992.
11. Frattali C: Professional practices: perspectives and clinical outcomes, *ASHA* 33:12, 1991.
12. Frattali C: Measuring client satisfaction, *Quality Improv Dig,* Winter 1991, p 2.

13. Golper LA: Communication and dementia: a clinical perspective. In Shadden B, editor: *Communication behavior and aging: a sourcebook for clinicians,* Baltimore, Md, 1988, Williams & Wilkins.
14. Goodglass H, Kaplan E: *Assessment of aphasia and related disorders,* Philadelphia, 1972, Lea & Febinger.
15. Koppit AT: *Wings,* New York, 1978, Hill & Wang.
16. La Pointe L: Aphasia therapy: some principles and strategies for treatment. In Johns D, editor: *Clinical management of neurogenic disorders,* ed 2, Boston, 1985, Little, Brown.
17. La Pointe L: *Aphasia and related neurogenic language disorders,* New York, 1990, Thieme Medical Publishers.
18. Lomas J et al: The communication effectiveness index: development and psychometric evaluation of a functional communication measure for adult aphasia, *J Speech Hear Disord* 54:113, 1989.
19. Lubinski R: A model for intervention: communication skills, effectiveness, and opportunity. In Shadden B, editor: *Communication behavior and aging: a sourcebook for clinicians,* Baltimore, Md, 1988, Williams & Wilkins.
20. Metter EJ: Medical aspects of stroke rehabilitation. In Chapey R, editor: *Language intervention strategies in adult aphasia,* ed 2, Baltimore, 1986, Williams & Wilkins.
21. Myers P: Right hemisphere communicatin impairment. In Chapey R, editor: *Language: intervention strategies in adult aphasia,* ed 2, Baltimore, 1986, William & Wilkins.
22. Myes P, Mackisack L: Right hemisphere syndrome. In LaPointe L, editor: *Aphasia and related neurogenic language disorders,* New York, 1990, Thieme Medical Publishers.
23. National Institutes of Neurological Disorders and Stroke: *Stroke,* Bethesda, Md, 1989, US Department of Health and Human Services.
24. Ozer MN: *The management of persons with spinal cord injury,* New York, 1988, Demos Press.
25. Porch BE: *Porch Index of communication ability,* Palo Alto, Calif, 1967, Psychological Press.
26. Porch BE et al: Statistical prediction of change in aphasia, *J Speech Hear Res* 23:312, 1980.
27. Rao P: *Class notes on agnosia,* Baltimore, Md, 1985, Loyola College.
28. Rao P: The use of Amer-Ind Code by aphasic adults. In Chapey R, editor: *Language intervention strategies in adult aphasia,* ed 2, Baltimore, Md, 1986, Williams & Wilkins.
29. Rosenbek J, La Pointe L, Wertz RT: *Aphasia: a clinical approach,* Austin, Tex, 1989, Pro-Ed.
30. Sahs AL, Hartman EL, Aronson SM: *Stroke: cause, prevention, treatment, and rehabilitation,* London, 1979, Castle Publishers.
31. Sarno MT: The functional assessment of verbal impairment. In Grinby G, editor: *Recent advances in rehabilitation medicine,* Stockholm, 1983, Almquist & Widsell.
32. Sarno JE, Sarno MT, Levita E: The Functional Life Scale, *Arch Phys Med Rehabil* 54:214, 1973.
33. Schuell HM: *Differential diagnosis of aphasia with the Minnesota test,* Minneapolis, 1965, University of Minnesota Press.
34. Toner J, Gurland B, Leung M: Chronic mental illness and functional communication disorders in the elderly. In Cherow E, editor: *Proceedings of the Research Symposium on Communication Sciences,* Rockville, Md, 1990, American Speech-language Hearing Association.
35. Tonkovich J: Communication disorders in the elderly. In Shadden B, editor: *Communication behavior and aging: a sourcebook for clinicians,* Baltimore, Md, 1988, Williams & Wilkins.

36. Wertz RT, La Pointe LL, Rosenbek JC: *Apraxia of speech in adults,* New York, 1984, Grune & Stratton.
37. Weisenberg TH, McBride KE: *Aphasia,* New York, 1935, Commonwealth Fund.
38. Wilkerson D: Integrating program evaluation tools and methods with the clinical process. Paper presented at the Rehabilitation Medicine Continuous Interdisciplinary Quality Improvement Conference, Buffalo, July 1991.
39. World Health Organization: *International classification of impairments, disabilities, and handicaps,* Geneva, 1990, World Health Organization.
40. Ylvisaker M, Holland A: Coaching, self-coaching and rehabilitation of head injury. In Johns D, editor: *Clinical management of neurogenic communication disorders,* ed 2, Boston, 1985, Little, Brown.
41. Yorkston K, Beukelman D, Bell K: *Clinical management of dysarthric speakers,* San Diego, Calif, 1988, College-Hill Press.

Dysphagia and Its Management

42. Atkinson M et al: Dynamics of swallowing: normal pharyngeal mechanisms, *J Clin Invest* 36:581, 1957.
43. Barer DH: Lower cranial nerve motor function in unilateral vascular lesions of the cerebral hemisphere, *Br Med J* 289:1622, 1984.
44. Barer DH: The natural history and functional consequences of dysphagia after hemispheric stroke, *J Neurol Neurosurg Psychiatry* 52:236, 1989.
45. Bosma JF: Physiology of the mouth, pharynx, and esophagus. In Paparella M, Shumrich D, editors: *Otolaryngology. Vol 1. Basic sciences and related disciplines,* Philadelphia, 1973, WB Saunders.
46. Bosma JF: Deglutition: pharyngeal stage, *Physiol Rev* 37:275, 1957.
47. Buchholz D: Neurologic causes of dysphagia, *Dysphagia,* 1:152, 1987.
48. Buchholz DW, Bosma JF, Donner MW: Adaptation, compensation, and decompensation of the pharyngeal swallow, *Gastrointest Radiol* 10:235, 1985.
49. Castell DO, Wu WC, Ott DJ, editors: *Gastroesophageal reflux disease: pathogenesis, diagnosis, and therapy,* Mount Kisco, NY, 1985, Futura Publishing.
50. Castell D, Donner M: Evaluation of dysphagia: a careful history is crucial, *Dysphagia* 2:65, 1987.
51. Ciocon J: Indications for tube feedings in elderly patients, *Dysphagia* 5:1, 1990.
52. Curran J: Overview of geriatric nutrition, *Dysphagia* 5:72, 1990.
53. Curtis DJ et al: Timing in the normal pharyngeal swallow: prospective selection and evaluation of 16 normal asymptomatic patients, *Invest Radiol* 19:523, 1984.
54. Donner MW: Swallowing mechanism and neuromuscular disorder, *Semin Roentgenol* 9:273, 1974.
55. Donner M, Silbiger M: Cinefluorographic analysis of pharyngeal swallowing in neuromuscular disorders, *Am J Med Sci* 251(5):600, 1966.
56. Doty RW, Richmond WH, Storey AT: Effect of medullary lesions on coordination of deglutition, *Exper Neurol* 17:91, 1967.
57. Farber SD: *Neurorehabilitation: a multisensory approach,* Philadelphia, 1982, WB Saunders.
57a. Gauderer MWL, Ponsky JL, Izant RJ: Gastrostomy without laparotomy: a percutaneous endoscopic technique, *J Pediatr Surg* 15:872, 1980.
58. Gordon C, Hewer RL, Wade DT: Dysphagia in acute stroke, *Br Med J* 295:411, 1987.
59. Granieri E: Nutrition and the older adult, *Dysphagia* 4:196, 1990.

60. Groher ME: Bolus management and aspiration pneumonia in patients with pseudobulbar dysphagia, *Dysphagia* 1:215, 1987.

61. Groher ME: *Dysphagia: diagnosis and management,* Boston, 1984, Butterworth.

62. Groher ME, Bukatmen R: The prevalence of swallowing disorders in two teaching hospitals, *Dysphagia* 1:3, 1986.

63. Groher M: Managing dysphagia in a chronic care setting: an introduction, *Dysphagia* 5:59, 1990.

64. Heitmiller RF: Surgical solutions for esophageal dysphagia, *Dysphagia* 6:79, 1991.

65. Horner J et al: Dysphagia following brainstem stroke: clinical correlates and outcome, *Arch Neurol* 48:1170, 1991.

66. Horner J, Massey EW, Brazer SR: Aspiration in bilateral stroke patients, *Neurology* 40:1686, 1990.

67. Horner J et al: Aspiration following stroke: clinical correlates and outcome, *Neurology* 38:1359, 1988.

68. Horner J, Massey EW: Silent aspiration following stroke, *Neurology* 38:317, 1988.

69. Johnson LF, DeMeester TR: Evaluation of elevation of the head of the bed, bethanechol and antacid foam tablets on gastroesophageal reflux, *Digest Dis Sci* 26:273, 1981.

70. Jones B, Donner M: How I do it: examination of the patient with dysphagia, *Dysphagia* 4:162, 1989.

71. Jones B, Kramer S, Donner M: Dynamic imaging of the pharynx, *Gastrointest Radiol* 10:213, 1985.

72. Kennedy JG, Kent RD: Physiological substrates of normal deglutition, *Dysphagia* 3:24, 1988.

73. Kircher J: Pharyngeal and esophageal dysfunction: the diagnosis, *Minn Med* 50:921, 1967.

74. Langmore S, Schatz K, Olsen N: Fiberoptic endoscopic examination of swallowing safety: a new procedure, *Dysphagia* 2:216, 1988.

75. Lazzara G, Lazarus C, Logemann J: Impact of thermal stimulation on the triggering of the swallowing reflex, *Dysphagia* 1:73, 1986.

76. Leopold NA, Kagel MC: Swallowing, ingestion, and dysphagia: a reappraisal, *Arch Phys Med Rehabil* 64:371, 1983.

77. Linden P: Videofluoroscopy in the rehabilitation of swallowing dysfunction, *Dysphagia* 3:189, 1989.

78. Linden-Castelli P: Treatment strategies for adult neurogenic dysphagia, *Semin Speech Lang* 12(3):255, 1991.

79. Linden P, Shaughnessy A: Evaluating and treating the neurogenic dysphagic patient: an individual approach. Seminar presented at the American Speech-Language Hearing Association Convention, Washington, DC, 1985.

80. Linden P, Siebens AA: Dysphagia: predicting laryngeal penetration, *Arch Phys Med Rehabil* 64:281, 1983.

81. Linden P et al: Bolus position at swallow onset in normal adults: preliminary observations, *Dysphagia* 4:146, 1989.

82. Logemann JA, Kahrilas PJ: Relearning to swallow after stroke: application of maneuvers and indirect biofeedback—a case study, *Neurology* 40:1136, 1990.

83. Logemann JA: *Evaluation and treatment of swallowing disorders,* San Diego, 1983, College-Hill Press.

84. Logemann J: Control of the cricopharyngeal opening with the Mendelsohn maneuver. Paper presented at the annual meeting of the American Speech-Language Hearing Association, New Orleans, 1987.

85. Logemann JA et al: The benefit of head rotation on pharyngoesophageal dysphagia, *Arch Phys Med Rehabil* 70:767, 1989.
86. McConnel F et al: Evaluation of pharyngeal dysphagia with manofluorography, *Dysphagia* 2:187, 1988.
87. Meadows JC: Dysphagia in unilateral cerebral lesions, *J Neurol Neurosurg Psychiatry* 36:853, 1973.
88. Milazzo LS, Bouchard J, Lund D: The swallowing process: effects of aging and stroke, *Phys Med Rehabil* 3:489, 1989.
89. Miller AJ: Neurophysiological basis of swallowing, *Dysphagia* 1:91, 1986.
90. Miller AJ: Swallowing: neurophysiologic control of the esophageal phase, *Dysphagia* 2:72, 1987.
91. Morrell RM: The neurology of swallowing. In Groher ME, editor: *Dysphagia: diagnosis and management,* Boston, 1984, Butterworth.
92. Palmer J, DuChane A: Rehabilitation of swallowing disorders due to stroke, *Phys Med Rehabil Clin North Am* 2(3):529, 1991.
93. Pommerenke W: A study of the sensory areas eliciting the swallowing reflex, *Am J Physiol* 84:36, 1928.
94. Ramsey GH et al: Cinefluorographic analysis of the mechanism of swallowing, *Radiology* 64:498, 1955.
95. Robbins J, Levine RL: Swallowing after unilateral stroke of the cerebral cortex: preliminary experience, *Dysphagia* 3:11, 1988.
96. Selley W et al: The Exeter Dysphagia Assessment Technique, *Dysphagia* 4:227, 1990.
97. Selley WG: Swallowing difficulties in stroke patients: a new treatment, *Age Ageing* 14:361, 1985.
98. Sessle BJ: How are mastication and swallowing programmed and regulated? In Sessle BJ, Hannam AG, editors: *Mastication and swallowing,* Toronto, 1976, University of Toronto Press.
99. Shawker T, Stone M, Sonies B: Sonography of speech and swallowing. In *Ultrasound Annual,* New York, 1984, Raven Press.
100. Sheth N, Diner W: Swallowing problems in the elderly, *Dysphagia* 2:209, 1988.
101. Silbiger ML, Pikielney R, Donner MW: Neuromuscular disorders affecting the pharynx: cineradiographic analysis, *Invest Radiol* 136:592, 1967.
102. Silver K et al: Scintigraphy for the detection and quantification of subglottic aspiration: preliminary observations, *Arch Phys Med Rehabil* 72:902, 1991.
103. Sitzman J, Mueller R: Enteral and parenteral feeding in the dysphagic patient, *Dysphagia* 3:38, 1988.
104. Sonies B, Weiffenbach J, Atkinson J: Clinical examination of motor and sensory functions of the adult oral cavity, *Dysphagia* 1:178, 1987.
105. Sonies B, Baum B: Evaluation of swallowing pathophysiology, *Otolaryngol Clin North Am* (21)4:637, 1988.
106. Splaingard M et al: Aspiration in rehabilitation patients: videofluoroscopy vs bedside clinical assessment, *Arch Phys Med Rehabil* 69:637, 1988.
107. Storey AT: Interactions of alimentary and upper respiratory tract reflexes. In Sessle BJ, Hannam AG, editors: *Mastication and swallowing,* Toronto, 1976, University of Toronto Press.
108. Tobin MJ: Aspiration pneumonia. In Dantzker DR, editor: *Cardiopulmonary critical care,* New York, 1986, Grune & Stratton.

109. Tracy J et al: Preliminary observations on the effects of age on oropharyngeal deglutition, *Dysphagia* 4:90, 1989.

110. Veis SL, Logemann JA: Swallowing disorders in persons with cerebrovascular accident, *Arch Phys Med Rehabil* 66:372, 1985.

111. Wade DT, Hewer RL: Motor loss and swallowing difficulty after stroke: frequency, recovery, and prognosis, *Acta Neurol Scand* 76:50, 1987.

Enhancing Motor Function

112. Bach-y-Rita P: Brain plasticity as a basis for therapeutic procedures. In *Recovery of function: theoretical considerations for brain injury rehabilitation,* Baltimore, 1980, University Park Press.

113. Bach-y-Rita P: Brain plasticity as a basis for the development of rehabilitation procedures for hemiplegia, *Scand J Rehabil Med* 13:763, 1981.

114. Baillet R, Levy B, Blood KMT: Upper extremity sensory feedback therapy in chronic cerebrovascular accident patients with impaired expressive aphasia and auditory comprehension, *Arch Phys Med Rehabil* 67:304, 1986.

115. Basmajian JV et al: Stroke treatment: comparison of integrated behavioral physical therapy vs traditional physical therapy programs, *Arch Phys Med Rehabil* 68:267, 1987.

116. Bobath B: *Adult hemiplegia,* ed 2, London, 1978, Heinemann Medical Books.

117. Brion JP, Demeurisse G, Capon A: Evidence of cortical reorganization in hemiparetic patients, *Stroke* 20:1079, 1989.

118. Carr JH et al: Investigation of new motor assessment scale for stroke patients, *Phys Ther* 65:175, 1985.

119. Carroll D: Quantitative test of upper extremity function, *J Clin Dis* 18:479, 1965.

120. Challet F et al: The functional anatomy of motor recovery after stroke in humans: a study with positron emission tomography, *Ann Neurol* 29:63, 1991.

121. Cohen LG et al: Magnetic stimulation of the human cerebral cortex, an indicator of reorganization of motor pathways in certain pathological conditions, *J Clin Neurophysiol* 8:56, 1991.

122. Cozean CD, Pease WS, Hubbell SL: Biofeedback and functional electrical stimulation in stroke rehabilitation, *Arch Phys Med Rehabil* 69:401, 1988.

123. Demeurisse G, Demol O, Robaye E: Motor evaluation in vascular hemiplegia, *Eur Neurol* 19:382, 1980.

124. Dominkus M, Griswold W, Jelinek V: Transcranial electrical motor evoked potentials as a prognostic indicator for motor recovery in stroke patients, *J Neurol Neurosurg Psychiatry* 53:745, 1990.

125. Ernst E: A review of stroke rehabilitation and physiotherapy, *Stroke* 21:1081, 1990.

126. Fugl-Meyer A et al: Post-stroke hemiplegic patient: a method for evaluation of physical performance, *Scand J Med Rehabil* 7:13, 1975.

127. Gallistel CR: The organization of action: a new synthesis, *Behav Brain Sci* 4:609, 1981.

128. Goldberg G: *Principles of rehabilitation of the elderly stroke patient.* In Dunkle RE, Schmidley JW, editors: *Stroke in the elderly,* New York, 1987, Springer.

129. Goldberg G: Neurophysiologic models of recovery in stroke, *Phys Med Rehabil Clin North Am* 2:599, 1991.

130. Gordon EE: Towards a rational approach to motor disorder, *Arch Phys Med Rehabil* 68:265, 1987.

131. Inglis J et al: Electromyographic biofeedback and physical therapy of the hemiplegic upper limb, *Arch Phys Med Rehabil* 65:755, 1984.

132. Jebsen RH et al: An objective and standardized test of hand function, *Arch Phys Med Rehabil* 50:311, 1969.

133. Jenkins WM, Merzenich MM: Reorganization of neocortical representations after brain injury: a neurophysiological model of the bases for recovery from stroke, *Prog Brain Res* 71:249, 1987.
134. Jenkins WM, Merzenich MM, Recauzone G: Neocortical representation dynamics in adult primates: implications for neuropsychology, *Neuropsychologia* 28:573, 1990.
135. Johnstone M: *Restoration of motor function in the stroke patient,* New York, 1987, Churchill Livingstone.
136. Jones RD, Donaldson IM, Packin PJ: Impairment and recovery of ipsilateral sensory-motor function following unilateral cerebral infarction, *Brain* 112:113, 1989.
137. Kottke FJ: Neurophysiologic therapy for stroke. In Ficht S, editor: *Stroke and its rehabilitation,* Baltimore, 1975, Williams & Wilkins.
138. Kraft GH, Fitts SS, Hammond MC: Techniques to improve function of the arm and hand in chronic hemiplegia, *Arch Phys Med Rehabil* 73:220, 1992.
139. Kussofsky A, Wadon I, Nilsson B: The relationships between sensory impairment and motor recovery in patients with hemiplegia, *Scand J Rehabil Med* 14:29, 1982.
140. Lieberman JS: Hemiplegia: rehabilitation of the upper extremity. In Kaplan PE, Cerullo LJ, editors: *Stroke rehabilitation,* Boston, 1986, Butterworth.
141. Macdonnell RAL, Donnan GA, Bladin PF: A comparison of somatosensory evoked and motor evoked potentials in stroke, *Ann Neurol* 25:68, 1989.
142. McDowell F: Evaluation of and controversies in stroke rehabilitation, *J Stroke Cerebrovasc Dis* 2:61, 1992.
143. Moore J: Neuroanatomical considerations relating to recovery of function following brain injury. In Bath-y-Rita P, editor: *Recovery of function: theoretical considerations for brain injury rehabilitation,* Switzerland, 1980, Huber Bein.
144. Olsen TS: Improvement of function and motor impairment after stroke, *J Neurol Rehabil* 3:187, 1989.
145. Poole JL, Whitney SL: Motor assessment scale for stroke patients: concurrent validity and interrater reliability, *Arch Phys Med Rehabil* 69:195, 1988.
146. Shumway-Cook A et al: Postural sway biofeedback: its effect on reestablishing stance stability in hemiplegic patients, *Arch Phys Med Rehabil* 69:395, 1988.
147. Wagenaar RC: Functional recovery after stroke, *J Rehabil Sci* 4:13, 1991.
148. Waxman SG: Nonpyramidal motor systems and functional recovery after damage to the central nervous system, *J Neurol Rehabil* 2:1, 1988.
149. Wilson DJ, Baker LL, Craddock JA: Functional test for the hemiparetic upper extremity, *Am J Occup Ther* 38:159, 1984.
150. Wolf SL, Binder-MacLeod SA: Electromyographic biofeedback applications to the hemiplegic patient, *Phys Ther* 63:1393, 1983.
151. Wolf SL, Binder-MacLeod SA: Electromyographic biofeedback applications to the hemiplegic patient: changes in lower extremity neuromuscular and functional status, *Phys Ther* 63:1404, 1983.

Training in Activities of Daily Living

152. Abreu B: *Physical disabilities manual,* New York, 1981, Raven Press.
153. Batavia AJ, Hammer G: Toward the development of consumer based criteria for the evaluation of assistive devices, *J Rehabil Res Dev* 27(4):425, 1989.
154. Bynum HS, Rogers JC: The use and effectiveness of assistive devices possessed by patients seen in home care, *Occup Ther J Res* 7:181, 1987.
155. Carr EK: Assessment and treatment of feeding difficulties after stroke, *Top Geriatr Rehabil* 7(1):35, 1991.

156. Chiou I, Burnett C: A survey of stroke patients and their home therapists, *Phys Ther* 65:901, 1985.
157. Garrison S: Learning after stroke: left versus right brain injury, *Top Geriatr Rehabil* 6(3):45, 1991.
158. Gordon E et al: Neurophysiologic syndromes in stroke as a predictor of outcome, *Arch Phys Med Rehabil* 59:399, 1978.
159. Granger C, Sherwood C, Greer D: Functional status measures in a comprehensive stroke care program, *Arch Phys Med Rehabil* 58:555, 1977.
160. Heard C: Occupational role acquisition: a perspective on the chronically disabled, *Am J Occup Ther* 31:243, 1977.
161. Hopkins H, Smith H: *Willard and Spackman's occupational therapy,* Philadelphia, 1988, JB Lippincott.
162. Kelly J, Winogard C: A functional approach to stroke management in elderly patients, *J Am Geriatr Soc* 33:48, 1985.
163. Kottke F, Flehmann J: *Krusen's handbook of physical medicine and rehabilitation,* Philadelphia, 1990, WB Saunders.
164. Lincoln N et al: An investigation of factors affecting progress of patients on a stroke unit, *J Neurol Neurosurg Psychiatry* 52:493, 1989.
165. Millikan C et al: *Stroke,* Philadelphia, 1987, Lea & Febiger.
166. Pedretti L: *Occupational therapy: practice skills for physical dysfunction,* St Louis, 1985, Mosby.
167. Rogers J, Holm M: Assistive technology device use in patients with rheumatic disease: a literature review, *Am Occup Ther,* vol 13, 1992.
168. Shah S, Vanday F Cooper B: Improving the sensitivity of the Barthel index for stroke rehabilitation, *J Clin Epidemiol* 42:703, 1989.
169. Shipman I: Bath aids: their use by a multi-diagnostic group of patients, *Int Rehabil Med* 8(4):182, 1987.
170. Siev E, Freishtat B, Zoltan B: *Perceptual and cognitive dysfunction in the adult stroke patient,* Thorofare, NJ, 1986, Slack.
171. Sillman R, Wagner E, Fletcher R: The social and functional consequences of stroke for elderly patients, *Stroke* 42:200, 1987.
172. Trombly C: *Occupational therapy for physical dysfunction,* Baltimore, 1983, William & Wilkins.

Training in Mobility

173. Bach-y-rita P: Brain plasticity as a basis for the development of rehabilitation procedures for hemiplegia, *Scand J Rehab Med* 13:73, 1981.
174. Badke MB, Duncan DW: Patterns of rapid motor responses during postural adjustments when standing in health subjects and hemiplegic patients, *Phys Ther* 63:13, 1983.
175. Basmajian JV et al: EMG feedback treatment of upper limb in hemiplegic subjects, *Arch Phys Med Rehabil* 63:613, 1982.
176. Berk S, Schall R: Psychosocial factors in stroke rehabilitation: crucial factors for successful outcome, *Phys Med Rehabil Clin North Am* 2:549, 1991.
177. Bishop DS, Haselkorn JK: Factors predicting satisfactory home care after stroke, *Arch Phys Med Rehabil* 72:144, 1991.
178. Bohannon RW, Andrews AW: Correlation of knee extensor muscle torque and spasticity with gait speed in patients with stroke, *Arch Phys Med Rehabil* 71:330, 1990.
179. Bohannon RW: Gait performance of hemiparetic stroke patients: selected variables, *Arch Phys Med Rehabil* 68:777, 1987.

180. Brandstater ME, Roth EJ, Siebens HC: Literature review: venous thromboembolism in stroke, *Arch Phys Med Rehabil* 73S:379, 1992.

181. Brandstater ME et al: Hemiplegic gait: analysis of temporal variables, *Arch Phys Med Rehabil* 64:583, 1983.

182. Britell C, McFarland S: Adaptive systems and devices for the disabled. In DeLisa J, editor: *Rehabilitation medicine,* Philadelphia, 1988, JB Lippincott.

183. Brunnstrom S: *Movement therapy in hemiplegia,* New York, 1970, Harper & Row.

184. Burke D: Spasticity as an adaptation to pyramidal tract injury. In Waxman SG, editor: *Functional recovery in neurological disease,* New York, 1988, Raven Press.

185. Butter C, Kirsch N: Combined and separate effects of eye patching and visual stimulation on unilateral neglect following stroke, *Arch Phys Med Rehabil* 73:1133, 1992.

186. Cassvan A et al: Lateralization in stroke syndromes as a factor in ambulation, *Arch Phys Med Rehabil* 57:583, 1976.

187. Conrad B et al: Pathophysiological aspects of human locomotion. In Desmedt JE, editor: *Motor control mechanisms in health and disease,* New York, 1983, Raven Press.

188. Davidoff G et al: Acute stroke patients: long term effects of rehabilitation and maintenance of gains, *Arch Phys Med Rehabil* 72:869, 1991.

189. DiFabio RP, Badke MB: Stance duration under sensory conflict conditions in patients with hemiplegia, *Arch Phys Med Rehabil* 72:292, 1991.

190. Dillingham TR, Lehmann JF, Price R: Effect of lower limb on body propulsion, *Arch Phys Med Rehabil* 73:647, 1992.

191. Dubo HIC et al: Electromyographic temporal analysis of gait: normal human locomotion, *Arch Phys Med Rehabil* 57:415, 1976.

192. Hallet M: Personal communication, 1992.

193. Hallet M, Shahani BT, Young RR: EMG analysis of stereotyped voluntary movements in man, *J Neurosurg Psychiatry* 38:1163, 1975.

194. Hirschberg G: Energy cost of stair climbing in normal hemiplegic subjects, *Am J Phys Med* 44:165, 1965.

195. Hirschberg G et al: Energy cost of stand up exercises in normal and hemiplegia subjects, *Am J Phys Med* 43:43, 1964.

196. Hirschberg G, Lewis L, Thomas D: *Rehabilitation,* Philadelphia, 1964, JB Lippincott.

197. Holden MK et al: Clinical gait assessment in the neurologically impaired: reliability and meaningfulness, *Phys Ther* 64:35, 1984.

198. Jebsen RH: Essentials of wheelchair prescription, *Northwest Med* 67:755, 1968.

199. Keenan MA, Perry J, Jordan C: Factors affecting balance and ambulation following stroke, *Clin Orthop* 182:165, 1984.

200. Knott M, Voss D: *Proprioceptive neuromuscular facilitation,* ed 2, New York, 1968, Harper & Row.

201. Kljajic M et al: Quantitative gait evaluation of hemiplegic patients using electrical stimulation orthoses, *IEEE Trans Biomed Eng* 22:438, 1975.

202. Knuttson E, Richards C: Different types of disturbed motor control in gait of hemiparetic patients, *Brain* 102:405, 1979.

203. Kraft GH: New methods for the assessment and treatment of the hemiplegic arm and hand, *Phys Med Rehabil Clin North Am* 2:579, 1991.

204. Landau WM: Spasticity: the fable of a neurological demon and the emperor's new therapy, *Arch Neurol* 31:217, 1974.

205. Lane REJ: Facilitation of weight transference in the stroke patient, *Physiotherapy* 64:260, 1978.

206. Lehmann JF et al: Gait abnormalities in hemiplegia: their correction by ankle foot orthoses, *Arch Phys Med Rehabil* 68:763, 1987.
207. Millington PJ, Myklebust BM, Shambes GM: Biomechanical analysis of the sit-to-stand motion in elderly persons, *Arch Phys Med Rehabil* 73:609, 1992.
208. Oczkowski W, Ginsberg J, Shin A: Venous thromboembolism in patients undergoing rehabilitation for stroke, *Arch Phys Med Rehabil* 73:712, 1992.
209. Olney SJ et al: Work and power in gait of stroke patients, *Arch Phys Med Rehabil* 72:309, 1991.
210. Olsen TS: Improvement of function and motor impairment after stroke, *J Neurol Rehabil* 3:187, 1989.
211. Palmer J, DuChane A: Rehabilitation of swallowing disorders due to stroke, *Phys Med Clin North Am* 2:526, 1991.
212. Peat M et al: Electromyographic temporal analyses of gait: hemiplegic locomotion, *Arch Phys Med Rehabil* 57:421, 1976.
213. Perry J et al: The determinants of muscle action in the hemiparetic lower extremity (and their effect on the examination procedure), *Clin Orthop* 131:71, 1978.
214. Perry J: The mechanics of walking in hemiplegia, *Clin Orthop* 63:32, 1969.
215. Perry J: The mechanics of walking. In Perry J, Hislop H, editors: *Principles of lower extremity bracing,* New York, 1967, American Physical Therapy Association.
216. Research Foundation, State University of New York: *Uniform data system for medical rehabilitation,* Buffalo, 1987.
217. Sahrmann SA, Norton BJ: The relationship of voluntary movement to spasticity in the upper motor neuron syndrome, *Ann Neurol* 4:460, 1977.
218. Sandin KJ, Smith BS: The measure of balance in sitting in stroke rehabilitation prognosis, *Stroke* 21:82, 1990.
219. Soderback I et al: Video feedback in occupational therapy: its effect on patients with neglect syndrome, *Arch Phys Med Rehabil* 73:1140, 1992.
220. Stineman M, Granger C: Epidemiology of stroke-related disability and rehabilitation outcome, *Phys Med Rehabil North Am* 2:457, 1991.
221. *Strike back at stroke,* American Heart Association, New York.
222. Wall JC, Turnbull GI: Gait asymmetries in residual hemiplegia, *Arch Phys Med Rehabil* 67:550, 1986.
223. Wing AM: Disorders of movement. In Wing AM, Smythe MM, editors: *The psychology of human movement,* New York, 1984, Academic Press.
224. Wood E, Voss D, Bouman H, editors: An exploratory and analytical survey of therapeutic exercise: Northwestern University Special Therapeutic Exercise Project (NUSTEP), *Am J Phys Med Rehabil* 46:3, 1967.

PART IV

Continuing Care Phase

Edited by
Mark N. Ozer

NATURE OF THE PROBLEM
11 **Enhancing Quality of Life**
12 **Ensuring Continuity of Medical Care**

NATURE OF THE PROBLEM

When the person with stroke is able to live in the community, he or she enters the phase of "independent living" that extends throughout the life of the person. The principle of independent living must be clarified. It is not defined by the degree to which a person with stroke is independent of the need for extrinsic support; rather, it is the degree to which the person with stroke is able to manage his or her own life, including caregivers.

A characteristic of this continuing care phase is that changes occur. These changes can be the result of increased impairments caused by aging, comorbidity, or recurrent stroke leading to a greater use of health resources. Therefore one major goal is to reduce the likelihood of recurrent stroke and illness and the need for hospitalization by patient participation in the management of risk factors. One must also continue to alleviate disabilities in light of possible changes in the environment in which the person seeks to function. Environmental changes include those in the interpersonal support system or the physical environment. The development and use of assistive devices or new systems of care are responses to these changes in the interaction of the individual with his or her environment. The second major goal therefore is to enhance the patient's quality of life by maintaining the caregiver relationship and encouraging community integration.

During the acute phase the focus was on minimizing the degree of impairment; during the rehabilitation phase, on minimizing the degree of disability (i.e., the functional consequences of ongoing impairment). During the continuing care phase, problems are defined in the broader context of the social role of the person with stroke. The measurement of this goal includes those items that reflect the "quality of life" rather than the more narrow goals of the rehabilitation phase. Family and community life issues are far more complex, and therefore solutions to problems in these areas may require the employment of more large-scale coordinated social systems, such as laws protecting the rights of persons with handicaps. These systems include a physically accessible environment, such as community transportation, the availability of caregivers, and financial supports. The overall goal of this phase is to minimize the degree of handicap, which is defined as the social consequences of an impairment.

In the rehabilitation phase, disabilities are alleviated by the learning of compensatory strategies and the design of appropriate physical and interpersonal environments. The patient's reentry into community living is only the first step in the road to independent living; thereafter the patient must deal with an environment that is both more variegated at any one time and changing over time. The person with stroke and caregivers must learn not only a broader range of skills but techniques to respond to unforeseen situations. The relatively predictable and protected environment of the rehabilitation setting is replaced by a setting in which caretaker availability is limited, physical settings may be inaccessible, and public benefits and programs are often inadequate.

There must be ongoing development of compensatory strategies. This includes transferring strategies learned during the earlier rehabilitation phase to new and different settings. The patient, family members, or both must take a more independent role in the implementation of strategies. In addition, there is an ongoing need to review new problems and to seek new compensatory strategies in a collaborative fashion. For example, major issues about family life may surface that were less evident in earlier phases. There are also opportunities to consider new assistive devices or new opportunities for training that would enable the person to reenter vocational and other community settings. Overall, in the continuing care phase, the person with stroke, the caregivers, or both must learn to generate their own compensatory strategies to a greater degree.

To reduce the likelihood of recurrent stroke, a system must be established to provide a continuity of care. Many of the medical issues, such as the management of hypertension, hyperlipidemia, and other comorbidities and the maintenance of satisfactory levels of anticoagulation, are the concern of the primary physician, whose role is to provide ongoing medical supervision. In this phase the focus changes because the person with stroke can now monitor these areas and participate in their management to a greater degree as a result of the training during the rehabilitation phase. However, poststroke central pain is an example of a particularly serious ongoing impairment that can affect function and can become even more prominent. Spasticity and other results of the upper motor neuron syndrome can have significant and ongoing functional consequences. Finally, an important and ongoing need is that of preventing further impairment caused by a recurrence of stroke through an enhanced awareness of the early warning signs of stroke and by seeking medical help as soon as possible.

CHAPTER 11

Enhancing Quality of Life

Nature of the problem
Enhancing family life
  MAUREEN FREDA
  Nature of the problem
  Functional issues
  Psychosocial issues
  Sexuality
Enhancing community integration
  JAN C. GALVIN
  Nature of the problem
  Selecting appropriate assistive technology
  The Americans with Disabilities Act of 1990

NATURE OF THE PROBLEM

In the continuing care phase the focus is on the patient's ongoing adaptation to impairment. Adaptation is necessary for successful family life and community integration, including participation in productive vocational or avocational activities outside the home. The adaptations that were effective in the more limited setting of the rehabilitation facility may be less effective in this larger, more variegated outside setting. A new order of strategies may be required to deal with a more complex set of problems over a longer time period.

The outcome measures appropriate for discharge from the rehabilitation phase are no longer sufficient for independent family and community life. Although the earlier problems in mobility and carrying out activities of daily living (ADLs) may still remain, the requirements have increased. An additional set of outcome measures is needed and has been described as "instrumental ADL" (see the box on p. 417). "Quality of life" requires an additional set of outcomes. This set of measures encompasses the larger scope of problems faced by stroke survivors. In the Framingham study a group of stroke survivors whose strokes occurred at least 6 months earlier were compared with age-matched controls.[1] Those areas that were significantly different and of particularly high frequency when corrected for comorbidity, such as cardiovascular disease, are described in Table 11-1. There was a significantly greater degree of deficit in ADLs and mobility, as one would might expect. Nevertheless, major deficits were

Complex Performance Tasks (Instrumental Activities of Daily Living)

Meal preparation
Use of telephone
Money management
Ability to use transportation
Ability to self-administer medication
Shopping
Finding one's way
Manual activities such as use of hand tools

TABLE 11-1   Frequency of Functional Deficit in Stroke and Control Groups

	STROKE SURVIVORS (%)	MATCHED CONTROLS (%)	*P*
Decreased socialization outside home	32	19	<0.02
Limited in household tasks	28	7	<0.001
Decrease in interests and hobbies	27	12	<0.01
Decreased ability to use outside transportation	21	4	<0.001
Dependent on activities of daily living	14	1	<0.001
Dependent in mobility	9	1	<0.01

Modified from Gresham GE et al: *Arch Phys Med Rehabil* 60:487, 1979.

in socialization both inside and outside the home and the inability to use transportation.

In a separate analysis of this same sample, persons with stroke reaching a high level of performance in self-care (a score of 20 on the Kenny self-care test, which is analogous to a Barthel Index score of 80) were compared with their age-matched controls who were functioning at a similar level (similar in age and degree of independence).[3] When the degree of socialization outside and inside the home and the participation in hobbies or interests were assessed, those who had had a stroke were significantly more likely to have decreased their activities. Activities outside the home were particularly reduced. Such a decrease was found even when the degree of neurologic impairment was quite limited. Thus it appears that, even after physical restoration has been achieved, the patient's need for social and psychologic rehabilitation may persist. The explanation for this phenomenon remains unclear. The authors of the study attributed their findings to the stigma associated with a change in body image and the reduced sense of social status (relatively well-educated males were particularly affected).

A more recent study in Finland described a 4-year follow-up of persons

---

Leisure Time and Recreational Activities

Hobbies
Religious activities
Sexual function
Avocations
Work skills
Ability to use media (television, videotapes)
Life satisfaction (feeling of well-being)

---

who had been relatively young at the time of their stroke (mean age of 48 years) with a somewhat higher percentage of persons having experienced subarachnoid hemorrhage.[4] The four domains sampled were working conditions, activities at home, family relationships (including sexual patterns), and leisure activities in and out of the home (see the box above). These domains encompass both the so-called instrumental ADL activities and the social aspects sampled in the Framingham study group. Even when good recovery had been achieved in ADL skills and the patient had returned to work, the quality of life was not restored to the prestroke level. Again, the implications of this study suggest that, in addition to conventional measures of rehabilitation, more attention should be paid to the patient's subjective experience of disability and insufficiency.

It has been suggested that the rehabilitation team can aid in the rebuilding of relationships, social interaction, and a sense of personal participation — that is, the patient's "quality of life."[2] Essential to that goal is a sense of creative participation. Patients need to be encouraged to participate as creatively and as early as possible at each phase of rehabilitation. The recognition by the professional staff of the individual's personal contribution is one yardstick by which the disabled person can measure his or her participation. The earlier in the rehabilitation program that feedback is provided to the patient that he or she is a valued participant, the more responsive the patient will be to the rehabilitation program and the more likely he or she will be to achieve this sense of creativity.

Participation in the problem-solving and planning processes described throughout this text supports the development of creativity and contributes to improved results in the more conventional goals of rehabilitation. During the continuing care phase, effective planning requires an even greater degree of participation on the part of the person with stroke, the caregiver, or both. The questions to be addressed remain the same, but the degree of specificity in answering them requires an even greater contribution by the patient.

For example, problems can be defined more specifically in the context of a specific environment and degree of impairment. This is possible only when the family and patient learn to define their problems. For example, when a woman with left hemiparesis is asked, "What problems do you have?," her initial answer may be, "My left side is weak." In the context of her own living situation, however, she can be more specific: "I'm afraid I will lose my balance on my steep front steps." In another example, the concerns of a man with mild residual right-sided weakness may seem excessive to an observer. Although he was able to carry out all the usual ADLs, despite particular difficulty in the coordination of the right hand, he was dissatisfied. Only when taking into consideration the patient's specific needs did his concerns make sense: the patient was a dental technician who made crowns and other dental work and thus required an extraordinary degree of coordination. Similar to a specification of concerns, the goals of each patient will encompass far more than the limited spectrum of possible goals explored during the rehabilitation phase. Furthermore, the degree of participation in the design and implementation of compensatory strategies must also be greater to make solutions as effective as possible. The major readjustment in thinking during the continuing care phase is to accept a degree of ongoing impairment but to recognize the opportunity to continue life while making changes in the ways one goes about participating in those life activities.

The ongoing difficulty experienced by a person with residual right-sided weakness illustrates this. One year after the onset of stroke the patient was able to carry out all his activities, including a partial return to golf, which had been his major recreation. Nevertheless, he remained depressed and concerned about his progress. When asked about his concerns, he initially focused on his lack of balance in walking. When the therapist persisted, he mentioned how it interfered with his ability to swing a club and hit the golf ball. On further questioning, his concern that his fellow golfers saw him as a "cripple" surfaced. His specific goal was to improve his game. Solutions he arrived at were to use a golf course where he was not known, to play at a time when there were relatively few people around, and to work on his balance with the trainer in a health club to which he belonged. Persons with stroke must be encouraged to contribute their specific concerns, goals, and strategies to deal with the wide variety of both possible levels of impairment and the environment in which they are to operate.

The following case illustrates the need for ongoing assessment and problem solving in the context of changing conditions throughout the continuing care phase. The changing conditions reflect the opportunities available through further training and the use of equipment for a return to family and community living.

CASE REPORT

I.C., a 56-year-old white male, was a former economist who had experienced a left-sided cerebral hemorrhage caused by an arteriovenous malformation with subsequent right-sided hemiparesis and expressive aphasia. He was comatose for at least 1 month after ictus. The acute phase was further complicated by deep vein thrombosis with pulmonary embolus. A tracheostomy was initially required but had since been removed. A gastrostomy was also initially necessary but no longer needed. He had been living in a nursing home near his home in a relatively rural part of the state. No wheelchair had been fitted to his needs, but he used a wheelchair provided by the nursing home.

When admitted to a stroke rehabilitation facility 20 months after the onset, he was able to propel a wheelchair with one hand. He was independent in eating after setup. He was able to stand with the "maximal assistance" (greater than 75% assistance) of two people but required "moderate assistance" (50%) in transfers with a sliding board to level surfaces. His right upper extremity was flaccid and without movement. His right shoulder range of motion was limited in all directions. The right hand, fingers, and thumb were held in flexion but came to full extension with passive movement. The right leg showed trace action of the quadriceps muscle and marked limitation in hip flexion and extension. Heterotopic ossification was seen in the right axilla and the thigh. The patient's communication abilities were limited. He was able to understand and follow complex oral directions and to consistently indicate his agreement or disagreement with statements by nodding his head; however, he was unable to speak any word other than "wait," which he uttered in a variety of intonations and with considerable frustration at his limited repertoire. He was, however, relatively good humored about his communication difficulties.

The goal was to enable him to live at home. His wife worked full time and was unable to provide a major degree of physical assistance. A son-in-law was available to help with transfers on a daily basis, but he also worked full time. The patient's house was wheelchair accessible. The specific objective was to increase the patient's mobility, with a focus on transferring. The goal was to reduce the patient's physical assistance requirement so that transfers could be carried out by his wife. By the time of discharge 1 month later, he required only 25% to 50% assistance in dressing, which his wife was able to provide. He was able to transfer with the use of a sliding board to slightly higher surfaces independently. He was able to carry out a standing pivot transfer with less than 25% assistance, which his wife was able to give. He was provided with a reclining wheelchair (because of the heterotopic ossification) and other equipment, such as a bedside commode and a tub transfer bench. He also was provided with a double-upright Klenzak brace.

Two months later (23 months after the onset), the patient continued to require ongoing supervision at home because of communication problems. This was provided by a home health aide during the day while his wife was at work. He had begun to walk about 20 steps with a moderate level of support from the physical therapist, who was provided by the county health department and who came to his home twice weekly. Over the next several months he became able to rise from a wheelchair independently. In addition, he was able to draw pictures and use gestures and was beginning to say words when given the first sounds. He was also able to be left alone. However, the patient's wife could not lift the relatively heavy wheelchair into the trunk of a car, and the son-in-law was not always available to help. A rack was recommended for the back of the car to avoid lifting the wheelchair in and out of the trunk. During the next several months the patient began to leave the house with a lighter wheelchair donated by the local Rotary Club. He began taking his own meals, could answer the telephone and carry on a conversation, and was able to walk with a cane without an ankle-foot orthosis and to transfer independently. He was using more words spontaneously. His neurologic examination findings remained the same as at the outset of rehabilitation. His right-sided hemiparesis persisted.

This case illustrates the options for recovery and reintegration into the home and community over the months after the onset of stroke. Despite major problems in the acute phase, the patient was able to achieve noninstitutional living.

The patient's rural setting and the lack of speech therapy required the recruitment of the family members to provide ongoing treatment. In addition, the family carried out independent problem solving to find an alternative to the first wheelchair when their opportunities for community integration increased.

ENHANCING FAMILY LIFE

Maureen Freda

Nature of the Problem

Stroke affects the entire family. The stroke survivor is not alone in trying to deal with the myriad changes brought about by the stroke, nor is the stroke survivor the only person affected by this traumatic event. Watson states "that for all practical purposes the family itself is viewed as experiencing the stroke with each family member responding to the experience in a unique way."[28] Family life and family relationships can be negatively affected by the functional and physical limitations, psychosocial issues, and changes in sexuality of the stroke survivor. The continuing maintenance of the family relationship is a major factor permitting the person with stroke to live in a community setting. One major objective during the continuing care phase must be to support the caregiver relationship.

Specific physical, cognitive, or communicative deficits of the stroke survivor may cause a variety of problems or disruptions to a family unit. These problems may range from simple logistic difficulties to complex role change issues. The challenge for families and persons with stroke lies in the ability to adapt to these changes and to reintegrate them into their daily life in a meaningful way. Professional support for this process includes encouraging the effective use of all resources and a readiness to explore alternative strategies.

Functional Issues

Many survivors of stroke have residual physical and cognitive impairments. These impairments vary in severity and the degree to which functional ability is hampered. Some experts estimate that 30% to 60% of these survivors have some degree of dependence in at least one area of ADLs. In addition to these two areas of poststroke problems, many stroke survivors experience communication and visual deficits.

For some, these deficits translate into "losses," some real and others perceived. In a study examining the losses experienced by stroke survivors, Mumma identified three major categories of loss: activities, abilities and characteristics, and independence.[21] This study found that patients most often mentioned mobility, independence, physical abilities, shared activities, and communication as losses. Spouses in this study mentioned losses in independence, traveling, and social life. Mumma surmises that the difference in the responses from patients and spouses results because patients live with the actual limitations of the disability, whereas spouses focus on the consequences to themselves and their activities and life-styles.

The challenge for families and patients lies in the ability to adapt to these changes and to reintegrate into their daily life in a meaningful way. In part, this is made possible through reestablishing relationships with people in the community and the family. Beginning to take part in activities that played an important role in the patient's or family's life before the stroke is a good first step. However, many stroke survivors resist this out of the fear that they will not be able to participate in the activity to the same degree or at the same level as before. This turns out to be a two-tiered problem. On the first tier is the patient himself or herself and the need to participate in a way that gives him or her satisfaction, pleasure, and meaning. To this end, physical or environmental adaptations often need to be accomplished (e.g., installing a ramp to the bingo hall, playing as a one-handed card shuffler, and changing the location of a bridge game). On the second tier are the patient's feelings about being a burden to the family or social group now that he or she has some physical limitations. This is a more subtle problem and requires sensitivity and communication in expressing the importance of the presence and participation, at whatever level, of the stroke survivor in the specific activity or social gathering. A good understanding of the role the stroke survivor has played in the specific social setting is essential in making the transition successful.

Mobility deficits associated with stroke vary from minimal hemiparesis to dense hemiplegia. The functional limitations vary as much as the range of the deficits themselves. An inability to move independently affects such activities as toileting, dressing, safety, recreation, travel, sexual activity, and community reintegration. The lack of mobility on the part of the stroke survivor affects the entire family.

Family members are often put in the position of being the "helpers" or "transporters" for the patient. This can involve a fair amount of physical effort in assisting the patient to and from chairs, toilets, beds, and cars. In other cases in which the mobility deficit is not so severe, the impact is felt in increased time and organizational efforts — that is, the time it takes to schedule transportation to and from appointments and the extra effort and planning needed to include the stroke survivor in specific family activities is greater. This can include calling ahead to find out if the restaurant is accessible, calling to find out if the theater has a "handicapped" section, leaving the house early enough to give the extra time needed for the stroke survivor to walk the distance required, finding out which bus route has a bus with a ramp, and making arrangements with the airlines for a wheelchair and an aisle chair.

Communication is an essential part of family relationships and life in general. The ability to understand the spoken word or gesture and the ability to make one's own thoughts and desires understood by others is an integral component of meaningful interaction with others. Because of the relative importance of communication in a person's life, the loss of this ability is felt with a great deal of intensity by both the stroke survivor and his or her family. Adapting to this type of poststroke deficit can be devastating for the family and can cause much frustration and anxiety. A communication deficit is often seen as a disruption in the daily routine of the family's life; many families may have difficulty overcoming this obstacle.

When a communication deficit is present, the effects can be long lasting; disruptions are seen in the family's ability to cope and in their collective communication patterns.[10] The results of a 1984 study of spouses of persons with aphasia[29] indicated that, after the stroke, spouses were less satisfied with their marriages. Specific areas affected included emotional support, life-styles, and sexual relationships.

For the young stroke survivor the issues may differ somewhat from those of the older survivor. This group of individuals may find that, not only are their roles in the family different, but also the issues have an impact on the financial earning power of the family and the ability to care for dependents.[11] The loss of mobility or communication may leave the young stroke victim unable to return to gainful employment and thus may reduce the household income significantly. Alternatively, if the young stroke survivor had primary child care responsibilities, the need to find additional help for the children could put an added strain on the available financial resources (which have already been strained by the expense of health care for the patient). In these scenarios it is imperative that the rehabilitation process address these issues and attempt to resolve them through vocational intervention, job site analysis, home visits, community resources, child care training, and the use of adaptive equipment.

None of these problems is insurmountable. However, for most families they represent a drastic change from prestroke activities and necessities. The problem resides not so much in what is actually needed, but in the departure from comfortable routines and roles in each family.

Psychosocial Issues

There are several psychosocial issues for the stroke survivor and his or her family; depression is one of the most common and most significant. Depression can arise from the survivor's inability to deal with the new stressors, such as losses, the fear of another stroke, and a new body image. In some cases, depending on the lesion, alterations in biochemical and neurotransmitter processes might be responsible for poststroke depression.[26] Depression certainly can have a negative impact on many areas of the survivor's life. The desire to take part in family activities may be diminished, a general lassitude may be noted, interest and energy for continued outpatient therapy may be absent, withdrawal from social contacts and activities may occur, and a decrease in libido may be present.

For most stroke survivors who have residual physical limitations, the issue of a change in body image is an important one. Feelings of worthlessness, powerlessness, and being defective are common.[13] According to Carlson, certain psychosocial effects occur in a stroke survivor that are related to the alteration in physical appearance, the impairment of bodily function, and the loss of autonomy.[6] She describes these affected areas as self-concept, body image, and self-esteem.

One such case was that of the man described earlier who was concerned about his appearance when he tried to swing to hit the golf ball. He stated that he did not want to be seen playing golf in public. His gait was otherwise completely functional, and he had no need for a cane. He became tearful and had considerable difficulty with sleep and appetite. He benefited from treatment for his depression with medication. Still another man who had had a right-sided stroke and walked readily with an ankle-foot orthosis and cane was particularly depressed about his gait. His goal was to be able to "walk so that no one will hold a door open for me." Still another man refused to use a cane and insisted on walking with a limp. Although quite functional in his ambulation, he ceased attending the theater and other recreational activities that had been important to him because of the alteration in his appearance.

Farzan states that it is an erroneous assumption to relate successful physical rehabilitation to successful psychosocial rehabilitation.[11] It is the individual's uniqueness, personal values, and life experiences, coupled with the support and reactions of the significant others, that will determine the psychosocial impact of a stroke. For the men previously described, the least evidence of impairment to others was significantly disabling, although it might appear to the professional that they had achieved satisfactory ambulation.

The literature supports the concept that stroke is a traumatic event affecting the entire family.[5,8,10,11,27] Deteriorating family relationships have been reported by Magi and Schifano.[16] Watson stated that the effects on families vary from actual growth to deterioration to a mere "drifting along in a less than optimal level of function."[28] According to Farzan, "the event of stroke creates a family crisis affecting family unity and requires that change take place to bring about effective coping."[11] Although change may be necessary, it is often difficult and causes anxiety in the family.

Watson describes the several variables that can affect the family's ability to react to this devastating event in an "integrated manner,"[28] including the effect on the family of a stroke survivor with more severe impairment facing greater "adaptive challenges." Other factors include the perception of the patient and family, who may perceive the same degree of impairment quite differently. Those who remain hopeful actually do handle the situation more successfully. In addition, under the stress of a stroke the differences in a functional and dysfunctional family and their ability to cope effectively with the impact become clear.

Of particular importance is an awareness of the patient's family role. Watson cautions professionals to take an "unbiased estimate of the stroke patient's position in the family, and the meaning this has for the family."[28] A true understanding of the role the stroke survivor played within the specific family unit and the extent to which the stroke has affected the patient's ability to maintain that role is crucial in understanding the impact of the stroke on the relationships within that family. The degree to which the stroke survivor can be supported and assisted in a resumption of his or her premorbid role and the acceptance of that process by the family is a key factor. Rehabilitation professionals have a responsibility to hold the utmost respect for the values the family embraces and to facilitate the attainment of goals that will best assist the family unit in maintaining its integrity.

Because most caregivers of stroke survivors are family members, it is important to look at the effect of caregiving on the family. Many problems are associated with providing care to a stroke survivor, including depression, anxiety, loss of freedom, financial burdens, and decreased participation in social activities. These problems can affect the functioning of the family as a unit or can be more acutely experienced by the primary caregiver. Many primary caregivers are spouses. The specific effects felt by spouses are wide ranging. Social isolation, loneliness, and fatigue are caused by the limitations in freedom from providing ongoing care. Other emotions include guilt and revulsion. Particularly symptomatic are sexual relationship issues, especially impaired marital relationships and sexual avoidance.[8,9,12,13,18] Fitzgerald studied the intensity of some of these effects over time.[12] She found that problems in the emotional and physical health of the caregiver increased over time, as did the feeling of marital discord on the part of the caregiver. She also found that issues relating to a change in role and a sense of loss of freedom tended to diminish over time.

One such case was that of the wife described earlier who had been able to take her husband home from a nursing home despite the continued need for physical assistance. She was able to manage his care satisfactorily after retiring from her job, but after a year, she began to feel extreme fatigue. The son-in-law, who had been available to help with transfers on occasion, was no longer available, and the daughter, who now lived alone with her own child, was unable to help out. The wife also cared for her elderly mother, who was recovering from a mastectomy. She began to weep when describing the overwhelming burden she felt: "Sometimes my arms ache and I can't do any more. There are now three women who live in three separate houses. I can't take care of my mother and my husband both, yet when I even mention anything about the burden I feel, my husband gets very angry because he hated the nursing home and is afraid that he will need to go back there."

When she identified a specific need to have a means by which her husband could independently release his footrest, an assistive device was designed. By reaching under and releasing the footrest, he could now stand independently, thus enabling her to leave the house more freely.

Other caregivers are typically the "middle generation," children of the elderly person with stroke. One such case was that of the daughter of a woman who had experienced a stroke. The mother had been an active person in her community; the daughter had not married and was employed part time as a librarian. She took on the care of her mother because her only sister was physically ill. The mother required physical assistance for all transfers. After discharge the mother failed to make progress and required even more assistance than during the rehabilitation program. She became more dependent. The daughter felt herself increasingly unable to deal with this ongoing problem. She took a leave of absence from her job with the expectation that her mother would become more independent after several months. Subsequently the mother was enrolled in further physical therapy with the agreed upon goal of contributing to her transfer to a greater degree. With reenforcement she was able to do so. The daughter returned to work part time by hiring an aide to care for her mother 1 day a week. When it finally appeared possible that her mother could be cared for by a larger circle of caregivers, including the other sister (because less physical assistance was necessary), the daughter felt able to continue to care for her mother.

Goldstein et al. used the term *role constriction* to describe the loss of personal freedom often felt by caretakers of the chronically ill, including stroke survivors.[15] Caretakers suffering from role constriction have little relief from their caretaking responsibilities. These researchers also described a "role overload," in which caregivers are forced to take on a variety of new roles and responsibilities.

Role changes can be devastating to family relationships. Costello states that, because the role of caretaker quickly becomes the role of parent and interferes with the adult-to-adult relationship, most experts advise the couple to find an outsider to perform caretaking tasks. If this is not possible, discussion is needed to help the patient and partner make sharp distinctions in the roles they play.[7]

Change in the roles between the spouses can be a major concern affecting all aspects of family life. One such case was that of a 55-year-old man who had been a high-level manager in his work before experiencing an intracerebral hemorrhage several years before. He had residual left-sided weakness, which interfered with his gait, and major problems with pain on his left side that interfered with his gait but affected his life even more profoundly. He had been told that such pain was to be expected after a stroke, yet he felt unable to be hopeful because of the feeling of helplessness the pain caused him. It became the focus of his life. His wife was concerned about his depression and lack of initiative. What troubled her most was his abdication of his role in caring for the family finances. She had never been able to do so in the past and was particularly frustrated about being forced to do so now.

The change in role may not always be a problem. Still another case is that of a 63-year-old former engineer who had a left-sided stroke 1 year earlier with resultant right-sided weakness and major difficulties with communication. He was independent in caring for himself and was enrolled in a day care setting where he received speech therapy. His wife continued to work. She described herself as more tired than before. She had taken over the family finances in addition to caring for the house and making meals. Her husband had formerly been the cook in the family. Nevertheless, she felt that things were satisfactory on the whole. She described improvements in some aspects of their relationship. She found him "sweeter, more lovable. He is not as bossy as before and seems to be in a happier frame of mind." In this case the reversal in roles was accepted by both the husband and wife.

The major issues in family life are those relating to body image and changes in role. These are not necessarily related to the degree of actual impairment but to the effects of such impairments on the person experiencing them. One major area in which this sense of loss translates into dysfunction is that of sexuality after stroke.

Sexuality

Human sexual activity serves a complex need for personal expression and gratification with numerous psychologic, social, and esthetic implications. The term *sexuality* is a broad one that encompasses the expression of sexual drives through sexual acts in the context of the individual's identity—one's maleness or femaleness—and includes a wide range of behaviors.

The sexual systems of men and women who have survived a stroke undergo a certain degree of change, although most of these changes cannot be traced to a hormonal cause or to any specific anatomic site of brain injury. The frequency of intercourse has been reported to decrease following a stroke, as does the duration of foreplay.[23] Sjogren's work describes orgasmic dysfunction in women after stroke and a decrease in orgasmic frequency in men. In addition, a general decline in libido occurs in both men and women, and a decrease in both ejaculatory and erectile function is present in men.[20] Monga's study reports a significant drop in the satisfaction of both men and women with their poststroke sex lives.[20]

Medications can have an adverse effect on the sexual functioning of an individual with stroke. Of particular concern are antidepressant, anticholinergic, and antiadrenergic agents; these have been reported to cause both erection and ejaculatory problems.[19] Clinical depression after stroke has also been linked to the decrease in libido and impotency problems of males after stroke.[7]

Role changes may also have an effect on sexual functioning and satisfaction with sex in general. This can be particularly true with men who have become more passive or dependent following a stroke.[24] According to Sjogren, when the able-bodied partner takes on a more "custodial" or "mothering" role, it is difficult for the partner with stroke to engage in sexual feelings or actions. Sjogren and Fugl-Meyer report that the degree to which the partner with stroke must depend on his or her partner for assistance in activities of daily living is negatively predictive of the resumption of sexual intercourse.[25]

Miscommunication and lack of information can also add to the problems of resuming a satisfying sexual relationship. McCormick and his colleagues report that wives of men with stroke were afraid of "injuring" their husbands; these wives also felt that their husbands were "afraid" to take part in sexual activity.[18] For example, in counseling the patient with hypertension, it is important to emphasize that the incidence of cerebral hemorrhage is not necessarily related to strenuous activity. Furthermore, to reduce the degree of elevation in blood pressure during sex, the male with hypertension can sit on a low, wide chair with his feet on the floor and his partner on top.[15]

Residual physical, functional, and cognitive problems and limitations can also affect the sexual behavior of stroke survivors and their partners. The entire issue of impotence in the male stroke survivor must be dealt with in the same way as in other settings. Differentiation must be made between psychogenic and organic causes (nocturnal erections are present in the former).

Performance anxiety can complicate organic problems. Sexuality encompasses many alternatives other than intercourse. Various devices are available to assist in erections.[13] Other effects of stroke include deficits in mobility and communication, sensory loss, and specific cognitive-perceptual changes. The presence of these difficulties can affect the resumption of premorbid sexual activity and roles.[13,17] The specific problems of mobility, sensory loss, and communication are discussed in later examples.

Mobility deficits are a common poststroke problem that couples must overcome to resume sexual activity. Depending on the severity of the deficit, the couple may find that the specific positions that were enjoyable before the stroke now are more difficult or not attainable. The couple must take a practical approach in finding possible positions that allow for satisfaction. Side-lying positions can be an effective alternative. This may include lying on the affected side to free the functional arm and leg. The able-bodied partner can take on a more active role and assume the superior position. If tremor or ataxia is troublesome, a weight-bearing position or strapping weights to the affected extremity is helpful. The objective is for the couple to find a position that is both functional and comfortable.[13,22]

Communication deficits can be extremely difficult to work out. In some cases spouses may interpret the inability to verbally express sexual desire as absence of sexual desire. To maintain a healthy sexual relationship, the couple needs to change their focus somewhat. Touching and gestures may become a much more important part of the sexual "routine" as a means of communicating desires. The able-bodied partner needs to become familiar with the facial expressions of the stroke survivor and their meanings when initiating or engaging in sexual activity.[13,22]

Touching is an integral part of sexuality, and a sensory deficit may require that exploration of other parts of the body with intact sensation be incorporated into the sexual repertoire. Verbalizing the activity may be effective in lieu of the ability to experience it by touch. More specific suggestions to overcome sensory losses, such as those affecting vision and touch, relate to the degree to which there is inattention on the affected side. If the sensory field is impaired, it is important for the partner to approach the stroke survivor from the intact side and to use other senses that remain intact.[13,22]

The following case illustrates how dysfunctional relationships can affect and be affected throughout the period following a stroke and how the person with stroke can maintain himself with the aid of counseling.

CASE REPORT

P.D. was a male in his middle forties with a history of alcohol abuse. His live-in girlfriend also used alcohol and had custody of her small children. P.D. had severe hypertension, which he had treated only intermittently, primarily because of his concern about medication affecting his sexual performance. His subsequent hemorrhagic stroke resulted in left-sided hemiplegia along with sensory disturbance, including pain of central origin. When discharged home, he was able to walk with a slight limp; however, his left arm remained nonfunctional.

During his inpatient stay, P.D. suffered from acute anxiety and tension regarding his potential sexual functioning. He had begun to experience difficulty with erections. He was also beginning to worry about his future general functional ability. Added to this was his anxiety over the decision about his postdischarge destination. There were questions about whether he would be going to his parents' home in another state or home with his girlfriend. Eventually he went home with his girlfriend.

The first problem encountered on P.D.'s coming home was his inability to have an erection. This greatly increased his already high level of anxiety. In his mind this precluded sexual activity completely. His view of sex was dominated by the need for intercourse with an erect penis; other types of sexual activity were not acceptable to him nor, apparently, to his girlfriend.

As time passed and his hypertension medication was stabilized, P.D.'s impotence resolved. Instead of the expected reaction from the girlfriend, his sexual advances were rejected. At this point the girlfriend stated that she was "turned off" by his physical deficits. Although P.D. was able to sustain an erection and assume most of their previously enjoyed positions, that he "did not look normal" was repugnant to his girlfriend.

After his discharge P.D. was able to stop his substance abuse. This disrupted the balance of the previously existing relationship between him and his girlfriend. He expressed anxiety about her continued abuse of alcohol. As he became more functional and clear thinking, he began to recognize the dysfunctional nature of the relationship.

Because P.D. was unable to return to work, his girlfriend expected him to take primary responsibility for the housework and the care of her children whenever she wanted to go out with friends. P.D. was functionally unable to do all the housework, and this resulted in many arguments. P.D.'s perception was that his girlfriend was much too demanding and had little or no understanding of the implications of his functional losses. In addition, it made him uncomfortable to be left in charge of young children. He did not feel he had the ability to chase after children or keep them out of mischief. He also was fearful that his physical limitations would get in the way of keeping the children safe in an emergency. He became angry at the girlfriend's apparent lack of responsibility with the children and her total disregard of his feelings about the matter. The amount of time they spent arguing steadily rose; the amount of time spent together in a positive atmosphere or in a mutually enjoyable activity steadily decreased.

As a result of his stroke, the counseling he received, and his cessation of substance abuse, P.D. became more calm and settled. His former life-style no longer held any appeal for him. His priorities had shifted, his functional capabilities had changed, and the balance in his relationship had been disrupted; in general, he was ready for a different life-style. Although he was physically limited, he was emotionally a much healthier person and ready to get on with his "changed" life.

Still another case demonstrates the full range of family issues in a younger woman.

CASE REPORT

A.N. was 25 years of age and had a 6-week-old baby when she had her stroke. She had clerical skills and had been working as a secretary. Her husband of 3 years was a construction worker; they lived in a trailer. A.N. sustained a left-sided cerebral vascular accident that resulted in a right-sided hemiparesis and a mild expressive aphasia. She spent 3 weeks in an acute care hospital and an additional 4 weeks in rehabilitation. She was able to walk independently with an ankle-foot orthosis at a slow pace, and her right (dominant) arm was weak but somewhat functional.

A.N.'s biggest concern was her ability to care for her baby and to live independently with her family. During her rehabilitation stay, she became depressed and fearful about her ability to do the things that needed to be done for her baby and to run the household. She could not imagine being able to hold her baby or carry her from room to room. A.N.'s husband had made the decision not to bring the baby into the hospital at first because the mere thought of the baby seemed to greatly upset her. This caused her husband to take a much more active role in the day-to-day care of the infant. He rearranged his work schedule to be home fairly early in the day; his mother watched the baby during his work hours.

On her discharge from rehabilitation, A.N. was able to partially care for her baby and to get around the trailer independently. She was unable to return to work, however. This made a big difference in the financial status of the family; bills became past due, and the cash flow was drastically reduced. The family was forced to give up their second car, which in turn caused difficulty in running errands when the husband was at work.

Because of A.N.'s remaining limitations, her mother-in-law moved into the tiny trailer to assist with the daily activities. Not only was this logistically stressful (three adults with one bathroom, a living room, a kitchen, a small nursery, and one bedroom), but also it was confusing in terms of who was the primary woman of the household. A competition ensued between the mother-in-law and A.N. about who was the decision maker. This relationship was previously a pleasant and mutually agreeable one.

The couple's sex life, which was previously active, became virtually nonexistent. This was not caused by A.N.'s physical limitations, but rather by the increased stress within the family unit and the lack of privacy.

Although A.N. and her husband had a fairly stable marriage before her stroke, the financial stressors and change in their ability to be an independent family unit created a severe strain on their relationship. Their poststroke life was not altogether comfortable for them and was vastly different from their prestroke life and marriage.

This case describes a family that, with a strong foundation, remained close knit and has managed to deal with the disruption to previously established patterns.

CASE REPORT

T.M. was a 53-year-old male who had worked most recently as a supervisor for the computer programming department in a government agency. He was married and had 11 children, three of whom were in college and seven of whom lived at home. The children ranged in age from 9 to 26 years. The wife had worked for the past 3 years in a flower shop. One of the daughters was an occupational therapist; none of the other family members were in health care. T.M.'s hobbies included working on the cars, yardwork, and fishing with his sons. His major responsibilities at home had been managing finances, grocery shopping, and giving general advice to his children.

T.M. sustained a stroke resulting in a right-sided hemiplegia and severe expressive aphasia. After several months he was able to care for his daily needs without assistance and walked with use of an ankle-foot orthosis and straight cane. At that time he was using sick leave and therefore receiving full pay; within several months he would have to either return to work or receive disability payments, which were 50% of his salary. Because he was only 2 years from possible retirement, his supervisor was committed to trying to find some sort of job that he could do for that period of time.

The family's initial reaction to the stroke was surprise and fear of death. Once it was clear that T.M. would survive the stroke, the concern turned to what the functional outcome would be. The family asked questions such as what would he be able to do when he got out of the hospital and how would he be able to do the things he had always done. During his hospitalization the patient's family went to great lengths to create an environment of normalcy. All birthdays, the couple's anniversary, and other celebrations were held in the hospital with little concern about the surroundings. The family focused on continuing normal activities (this included a visit from the family dog). T.M.'s wife spent part of each day at the hospital, as did all his children, who lived nearby. The college-aged children visited each weekend to stay involved in the rehabilitation process.

The practical questions of figuring out T.M.'s personal financial system was important. Because his aphasia was so severe, this was a difficult task and one that could have had serious implications if not solved quickly. One of his children was an accountant, and she eventually deciphered the system, transferred it to a computer, and currently retains that responsibility for the family. The youngest child had the most noticeable reaction to his father's stroke and subsequent absence from the home. He became hyperactive and acted out frequently. Once his father came home, he spent much of his time "hanging onto Dad," as if he wanted to be sure T.M. was not going to leave again; he even "helped" with T.M.'s home therapy program. The 18-year-old son wanted to be sure that the tradition of his father baking multiple loaves of bread at Christmas was not lost. The first Christmas, T.M. stood by and "directed" his son's baking of 30-odd loaves for the neighbors and family members. This was his son's way of keeping the family tradition alive and helping T.M. accomplish meaningful tasks that were part of the family routine.

That T.M. did not return to work was seen as a positive choice by some members of the family. They related that he was much more involved in family activities and was without the stress of work and the responsibility of the financial issues of the family. To his children he appeared more humorous and enjoyed being at the center of family activity. The family was also enjoying this change. His daughter reported that his personality seemed to have taken a turn to the "lighter" side. He was able to laugh at situations more readily. His extended family even described him as "happier."

The relationship between T.M. and his wife was stable before the stroke and, if anything, grew stronger afterward. They began spending most of the day together, went to church together daily, ran errands together, attended therapy sessions together, and even found time to dance together in the living room from time to time. One of the daughters described them as "a team—very together." A partial role shift occurred between T.M. and his wife, who began to "take charge" more, but the change appeared to be mutually acceptable and worked well for the entire family. One daughter described the family as very close knit and supportive. She stated that their religious faith and their prayers played a large part in the family's adjustment to the stroke event and summed up her feelings by saying, "We were a strong family before, and it carried through to this time; if we hadn't been strong, it would have been much harder."

Stroke has been shown to affect many facets of family life. Stroke survivors must face psychosocial and adjustment problems, role changes, problems in the area of sexuality, and physical and functional residual impairments. The ability of the family to deal effectively with the trauma of a stroke depends on many factors, not the least of which is the premorbid health and "personality" of the family unit. Rehabilitation professionals have a responsibility to design interventions to assist the whole family in dealing with the effects of a stroke and to facilitate the resumption of roles for the stroke survivor so that an intact family emerges from the rehabilitation process.

ENHANCING COMMUNITY INTEGRATION

Jan C. Galvin

Nature of the Problem

The issues during the continuing care phase extend beyond the family into reestablishing one's social role in the larger community. Problems of residual impairment and resultant functional disability and their impact on the person with stroke, his or her individual goals, and the specific characteristics of the physical and interpersonal environment have been addressed throughout this text. When one seeks to address the issues of the patient's social role, the scope of the inquiry must extend into the wider social setting in which the person with stroke and the caregivers attempt to act. The term *handicap* has been widely used to describe the degree to which the person fails to function in his or her social role as a result of impairment and functional disability. The widely quoted World Health Organization (WHO) definition is that a handicap exists when individuals with disabilities are unable to fulfill one or more of the roles considered normal for their age, gender, and culture.[41] Based on this formulation the scope of rehabilitation outcomes broadens. "Quality of life" issues include the patient's degree of social, recreational, and occupational interaction.

One early effort to address quality of life issues was the Activity Pattern Indicators portion of the Rehabilitation Indicators Project at the Institute of Rehabilitation Medicine at New York University.[31] It sampled the frequency and duration of activities such as vocational tasks, household activities, recreation involvement, and travel. An example of a more recent measurement is that developed at Craig Rehabilitation Center.[40] It measures the degree to which the individual experiences handicaps in such areas as mobility, physical independence, occupational and social interaction, and economic self-sufficiency as compared with a paired able-bodied sample. Weights were assigned based on the attitudes of the general population and the experience of able-bodied persons.

For example, the box on p. 435 lists the components of the "occupational category"; the first four items are given twice the value of the last three when calculating the total degree of handicap. A score in that category is thus derived incorporating twice the sum of hours spent in the first four activities and the sum of the hours spent in the last three activities. The actual score is then related to the experience of able-bodied persons who represent the maximum score of 100. A score below that indicates an "occupational handicap." In another measurement, economic self-sufficiency is calculated by the total family household income from all sources less that used for medical care. Twice the poverty level — a figure approximating the median family income — is equivalent to a score of 100. Deviation from that level is a measure of handicap in the area of economic self-sufficiency. Such measures clarify the degree to which specific social roles are compromised. For example, when applied to a sample of persons with spinal cord injury, a correlation was found between the degree of impairment and the degree of handicap, yet considerable variability in handicap was found to exist between individuals with similar impairments. This finding supports the notion that the degree of handicap reflects the contribution of factors extrinsic to the degree of injury.

However, the WHO definition of "handicap" has been criticized by the independent living movement, which represents persons with disabilities. These critics suggest that the term *handicap* be applied to the limitation in social roles caused by the social environment.[32] Stairs that block entrances, poor access to transportation, economic disincentives, and negative public attitudes are some of the factors that can "handicap" the person with disabilities from carrying out his or her social role.

**Occupational Category: Craig Handicap Assessment
and Reporting Technique (CHART)**

1. How many hours per week do you spend working in a job for which you get paid?
2. How many hours per week do you spend in school working toward a degree or in an accredited technical training program (hours in class and studying)?
3. How many hours per week do you spend in active homemaking, including parenting, housekeeping, and food preparation?
4. How many hours per week do you spend in home maintenance activities such as yard work, house repairs, or home improvement?
5. How many hours per week do you spend in ongoing volunteer work for an organization?
6. How many hours per week do you spend in recreational activities such as sports, exercise, playing cards, or going to movies? (Please do not include time spent watching television or listening to the radio.)
7. How many hours per week do you spend in other self-improvement activities such as hobbies or leisure reading? (Please do not include time spent watching television or listening to the radio.)

This definition has been incorporated into a model that includes those factors that are external to the impairment and that tend to increase the negative impact of the impairment.[30] Thus handicapping conditions can exist within several contexts, including society (e.g., architectural barriers and government policy) and the individual's immediate environment (e.g., lack of an accessible vehicle or other useful technology). Access to resources is seen as the part of the solution to handicapping conditions. Indeed, money or other resources are the great equalizers. For example, the Activity Pattern Indicators measured a group of persons with spinal cord injuries who earned adequate incomes. Total time spent in vocational, recreational, and social activities was similar for persons with spinal cord injuries as compared with a control group of able-bodied persons. Thus the degree to which such activities were accomplished was not necessarily inherent in the impairment but in the availability of funds to help overcome the social aspects of the disabilities. For example, these funds provided the ability to purchase accessible means of transportation to enable persons to carry out vocational activities.

Technology is often the key to becoming independent. Many people tend to think technology means "high-tech" objects such as computers and robots; however, technology is everywhere everyday in everything people do. A car, an oven, and a vacuum cleaner are all pieces of technology, but one is so used to them that one does not consider them frightening or difficult to operate.

It is not uncommon for individuals who recently became disabled to be confronted with a wide range of new technology and assistive devices—from bathing and feeding equipment to wheelchairs with numerous options to sophisticated communication systems. Which devices will be integrated into their daily lives and which will be relegated to the closet are often determined by the individual's acceptance of the disability. Much of the assistive technology that an individual brings home from the hospital appears to be different and difficult to translate to home use and therefore is often abandoned. Clinicians must help individuals overcome the feeling that technology is a foreign element and explain that, if it is integrated into one's life, it can become a means of achieving the goals one sets and thus can help in developing a positive attitude toward technology.

In a review of the literature on accepting assistive technology, Phillips finds that early studies focused on the individual characteristics that influence technology use, such as acceptance of disability, personal values and life-style preferences, and attitudes toward devices.[37] Vash presents a variety of personal issues that affect device use and acceptance, such as acceptance of disability, motivation, perceived life tasks, and effort-reward balance.[39] She concludes that the acceptance of a disability and goal-directedness are related to positive attitudes toward devices. When devices enable the completion of tasks important to the user, they are more likely to be used. Similarly, Wright states that those who take a "coping" approach to disability are more likely to use assistive devices.[42] Such individuals recognize the difficulties of their disability but focus on managing them.

Technology must connote independence if it is to be accepted. Zola stressed the importance of defining "independence" in device selection.[43] Professionals tend to view independence in terms of physical functioning. On the other hand, consumers equate independence with social and psychologic freedom. Thus consumers prefer devices that facilitate the latter type of independence. Furthermore, Nevins suggests that, when "clients are subjected to massive doses of technology," they may react negatively and come to view technology as another dependency.[34]

The solution of handicaps lies in the availability of adequate financial resources and changes in the larger physical environment that permit persons with disabilities to enter the world beyond their homes. Technology of various sorts can aid in improving the interaction between the person with disabilities and a frequently inaccessible environment. Three laws that address the barriers confronting individuals with disabilities are helping to provide access to assistive technology devices and services through (1) community-based programs, (2) broader interpretations of consumer participation in vocational rehabilitation services, and (3) the removal of environmental and communication barriers for qualified individuals with disabilities in the workplace and to access of public and private goods and services. Those laws are the Technology Related Assistance to Individuals with Disabilities Act of 1988, the Reauthorized Rehabilitation Act of 1992, and the Americans with Disabilities Act of 1990. These federal laws are efforts to deal with the issue of handicaps by making changes in the wider social context.

Selecting Appropriate Assistive Technology

One of the keys to maximizing the benefits of assistive technology is the selection of appropriate devices — that is, devices that will be used successfully by the consumer.[33] Choosing the right piece of technology — whether that is a scooter to conserve energy when shopping or a microwave oven to make cooking safer and simpler — is a step-by-step process of deciding what is most appropriate for an individual. Decisions need to be based on the person's physical and cognitive characteristics, life-style, activities, goals, social supports, and such factors as the locale in which the device will be used, whether it will be used independently, whether it needs assembly and disassembly, and whether it is transportable.

The design of an appropriate system for community integration need not be complex but can be integrated into already existing systems. One man who walked with a straight cane despite continued hemiparesis was able to return to his recreational interest in sailing with no modification of his boat. The gangways had ropes onto which he could hold. However, he had problems using the gangplank. To solve this, he no longer used a gangplank; the sailboat was placed alongside the wharf so that he could be helped to step directly onto the boat. In a similar fashion, when about to take a train trip with his wife, the man was brought in his wheelchair onto the train by his son because of the relatively wide gap between the platform and the train in the station. While on the train he ambulated down the aisle and his wheelchair was stowed. On his arrival the platform and train were flush with each other. He could safely walk off the train, and the wheelchair was merely used to transport him down to a waiting automobile. This person with a stroke was able to travel and carry out recreation with little or no modification.

The process by which assistive technology is selected is crucial to its effective use; the process is one in which devices are "fitted" to the user[35,36] and in which the person is able to contribute to the maximal extent possible. If this is done properly, the device will not only be "fitting" (in a technical sense) but will be compatible to the person's life-style and thus more likely to be used. These steps have been emphasized throughout this book. The first step of problem identification requires the person with the problem to define the issues in the context of his or her individual characteristics.

CASE REPORT

J.S. experienced severe, almost athetoid spasms caused by brain injury following surgery. He also had difficulty in communication, yet he was able to perform his full-time job as a counselor for disabled students despite his problems. Although he was unable to speak, J.S. found it possible to communicate efficiently by pointing to a "communication board" on which key phrases and letters had been written.

While at work, J.S. was able to use his communication board and an "interpreter" was available to speak for him into a standard speaker phone rather than an ordinary telephone receiver. The speaker phone was helpful because it enabled him to hear the replies of the other person. He was able to write readily with use of a modified keyboard and a personal computer. Although to an outside observer he might appear to have significant communication problems, he had helped design a system that successfully solved those problems. He did not find it necessary to use a commercially available system to generate artificial speech.

Subsequently his spasms worsened, and he did identify a problem with the control of his power-driven wheelchair. He sustained a hip fracture following an inability to release his joystick and stop the chair. One option, which he accepted, was to have a pressure contact switch used in conjunction with the joystick. Sustained contact with the pressure switch was required to operate the joystick. When contact was not sustained, as in the case of a spasm, the wheelchair stopped automatically. The method suggested to meet the goal of greater safety in controlling the power-driven wheelchair was a suggestion J.S. accepted, although it added some complexity to the control system.

As a result of the hip fracture, J.S.'s skill in safe transfer from a wheelchair had been compromised. He had also become fearful of falling. The solution did not lie in the area of devices but in retraining his transfer process to ensure adequate safety. Thus, through a management system containing a variety of components, J.S. continued his ability to function in a satisfactory manner despite severe impairments.

The following case report explores the selection of a scooter based on the goals of the patient.

CASE REPORT

Since her stroke, B.V. had used a walker and now wished to participate more actively in her church. She decided to purchase her own transportation because driving would not make her feel as tired and she would not have to rely on lifts from her daughter-in-law to be more active and to achieve greater community mobility. After meeting with her physical therapist, B.V. decided a scooter would give her the added independence she desired.

Many individuals leave the hospital with a walker, which enables them to be independent and provides a form of physical activity. However, some patients, such as B.V., prefer to ride rather than walk to community activities so that they do not arrive at their destination late and so exhausted that they are too tired to participate. In B.V.'s case an alternative form of transportation, such as a scooter, was an appropriate alternative.

Scooters are used primarily by people who have poor endurance and difficulty walking as the result of disabilities such as arthritis, multiple sclerosis, muscular dystrophy, postpolio syndrome, emphysema, stroke, and cardiac conditions. Frequently these individuals are able to walk short distances but need a scooter or other mobility aid to travel intermediate distances or to conserve their energy. The mobility provided by a scooter allows many people to increase their independence both at home and in the community. Increased mobility can also help people return to work or maintain their current work responsibilities.[38]

During the selection process it was important to assess B.V.'s physical abilities and the locations where the scooter would be used. These factors would determine if a scooter was a safe and reasonable mobility aid. Because B.V. would be using the scooter to travel the few blocks from her home to the church, a rear-wheel-drive (RWD) scooter was first considered. RWD scooters are generally larger and more stable and are able to climb steeper hills, making them better suited for outdoor use (B.V. lived at the bottom of a small hill). However, because of their size, RWD scooters are more difficult to maneuver indoors. The therapist scheduled a visit to B.V.'s home and church. The senior center at B.V.'s church had previously installed a vertical platform lift to accommodate its members. The platform was measured to make sure the scooter chosen would fit safely on the lift. At the time the lift was installed, the senior center was also remodeled to make bathrooms easily accessible. The meeting room was large and free of obstacles. It was concluded that, even if an RWD scooter was selected, B.V. would be able to get around the senior center with few problems. The area where the church services was held could not easily accommodate a scooter. Because B.V. could still use her walker to get around, she decided that she would not need to use the scooter within the church itself for the weekly services. It was recommended that she get a second walker to leave at the church, as other members had, so she would not have to carry hers back and forth on the scooter. B.V.'s home was much less accessible. However, she had not planned on using the scooter there because she was comfortable walking about her home. Thus it appeared that an RWD scooter would be a good selection.

Other considerations still had to be discussed before a few models were selected for trial. To operate a scooter safely, B.V. first had to be able to get on and off the scooter. Once on the scooter, she had to maintain a comfortable and upright position while controlling the accelerator and steering mechanism with her arms. Additional factors to consider before selecting a seating system included B.V.'s physical abilities and sensation. For instance, individuals with poor sensation on their buttocks may require a special cushion to distribute pressure to prevent skin breakdown, and those prone to back pain or excessive spinal curves may require a special back support. Scooter operation requires the use of at least one arm to steer the scooter and control speed. If the scooter was used in more than one location, B.V. would have to consider how she would get the scooter from one location to the next. If the scooter needed to be transported in the back of a car, it would need to be disassembled into manageable pieces. One of the major components weighed at least 40 pounds and would be difficult for many people to load and unload into a car trunk. In addition, individuals such as B.V. who use assistive devices such as walking aids, leg braces, artificial legs, or an oxygen tank may need to consider which features and options will accommodate these devices while they are using the scooter.

B.V.'s cognitive abilities also had to be assessed before a scooter was purchased. For example, individuals who have uncorrected near or far vision or who demonstrate confusion, poor safety awareness, or other cognitive problems may not be able to operate a scooter safely.

A seat style that was comfortable, provided support, and placed B.V. in a proper position to operate the controls was selected. A seat that swiveled to the side and locked into place was chosen so that B.V. could sit on the scooter seat before she brought her feet to the base, although she would have to try the release mechanism before a final decision was made. Because B.V. would have to travel up and down the hill on her street, the different types of parking brakes were discussed. She decided that an automatic parking brake would be more convenient than a manual parking brake. B.V. chose gray foam-filled tires because they required no maintenance and they did not leave black scuff marks.

Over 50 scooter models are currently available in the United States. Selecting a scooter involved choosing a base unit, then deciding which features and options were necessary or desirable. In shopping for a scooter, B.V. found it useful to visit showrooms and to ask dealers to bring scooters to her home for a demonstration and trial use. Whenever possible, she test drove the scooter where it was to be used.

Outside of the hospital it is often difficult to find the same level of expertise for choosing an assistive technology device. More often the resources are not available for expert help. In many cases individuals are on their own. Individuals must be able to figure out (1) that they need something to help them accomplish their chosen goal; (2) what it is they want; (3) where to go for more information; (4) what resources are available; and (5) how to operate, maintain, and repair the device. That is a lot of information for one person to seek out.

Many states currently have federal grants that emphasize the development of community-based services to ensure access to and training in the use of assistive technology and to provide an appropriate level of expertise in the community to help individuals make decisions or to provide resources for further information. The Technology-Related Assistance to Individuals with Disabilities Act of 1988 required that states coordinate all assistive technology services for individuals of all ages and disabilities.

The law has also led to a complete survey on the funding available for assistive technology. The system is piecemeal at best, and individuals with disabilities have trouble finding funding for devices. Recommendations for improving the selection, application, and funding of assistive technology were provided to Congress in late 1992. A list of states with federal grants under the Technology-Related Assistance to Individuals with Disabilities Act of 1988 can be found in the Appendix. Also included is a list of other resources on assistive technology, including mail order catalogs.

Americans with Disabilities Act of 1990

When an older or disabled person's capabilities do not match the demands of the environment, the environment must be changed. Many environmental and communication barriers are slowly disappearing, largely as the result of the Americans with Disabilities Act of 1990. This law is modeled after the 1964 Civil Rights Act and represents a giant step forward in eliminating barriers to independence and productivity.

Title I of the Americans with Disabilities Act prohibits employment discrimination against "qualified individuals with disabilities." A qualified individual with a disability is defined as the following:

- An individual who has a physical or mental impairment that substantially limits one or more of his or her major life activities
- An individual who has a record of such an impairment
- An individual who is regarded as having such an impairment

Employers cannot discriminate against individuals with disabilities in any employment practices or terms, conditions, and privileges of employment. This prohibition covers all aspects of the employment process, including the application and testing stages and all other aspects of the job.

Reasonable accommodation is a critical component of the Americans with Disabilities Act. Reasonable accommodation is any change in the work environment or the way things are usually done that results in an equal employment opportunity for an individual with a disability. An employer must make reasonable accommodations for the known physical or mental impairments of a qualified applicant or employee with a disability unless the employer can prove that the accommodation would cause an undue hardship. One example of a reasonable accommodation is making existing facilities used by employees readily accessible to and usable by an individual with a disability. Others include modifying work schedules; acquiring or modifying equipment or devices; adjusting policies, practices, and procedures to accommodate an individual with a disability; and providing the employee with qualified readers or interpreters.

Accommodation need not be expensive. As the list shows, most accommodations are based on modifying policies and procedures rather than removing structural barriers. The key to successful accommodations that will allow employers to hire or retain an individual with a disability is based on the employer's attitude and willingness to work with the individual to find a reasonable accommodation. However, if an employee with a known disability is not performing well or is having difficulty performing the job, the employer should assess whether this is due to the disability. The law does not disturb the policies employers have about job performance, providing the employer does not discriminate against the individual with a disability by falsely claiming poor job performance as an excuse for not making an accommodation.

Title II of the Americans with Disabilities Act prohibits discrimination in public services, including public transportation. This means that public services, programs, and activities provided by state and local governments and Amtrak are prohibited from discriminating against individuals with disabilities. Any state or local government program, activity, or service must be accessible to a qualified individual with a disability. For example, if an individual using a wheelchair is to appear as a witness in a court case and the court hearing room is on the second floor of a building without elevators, the court should move the hearing to allow the individual to participate.

Title III of the Act prohibits discrimination in the provision of goods and services to individuals with disabilities. This means that places of business — such as hotels, restaurants, bars, theaters, cinemas, auditoriums, grocery stores, shopping centers, museums, libraries, amusement parks, and zoos — may not discriminate in the delivery of their goods and services.

Transportation is a major issue in permitting community reintegration. If a public office or program operates a fixed route system, such as the local bus service, it must purchase buses that are accessible to individuals with disabilities, including those who use wheelchairs. It is also discriminatory to fail to provide paratransit or other special transportation services within that geographic area. The design of all new transportation facilities must include accessibility, and any alterations to existing facilities must also be accessible. For rapid-rail and light-rail systems, "key" stations must be made accessible by July 1993, or within 30 years if the alterations involve extremely expensive structural changes. By July 1995, rapid-rail and light-rail systems, commuter rail service, and Amtrak must have at least one car per train that is accessible to individuals with disabilities, including wheelchair users. All new rail passenger cars purchased by Amtrak must be accessible to individuals with disabilities, with the capacity for a wheelchair user to park and remain in the wheelchair and to be able to use wheelchair-accessible restrooms on the train.

Facilities that are used every day, such as stores, libraries, or recreation centers, are also addressed in the Americans with Disabilities Act. Title III of the act specifies 12 types of entities that, regardless of size, are "public accommodations": places of lodging, exhibition or entertainment, public gathering, public display or collection, recreation, and exercise; private educational institutions; establishments' stations used for public transportation; and social service center establishments.

These businesses may not discriminate against individuals with disabilities by denying them the right to participate or by providing unequal or separate treatment. For example, a business cannot ask a person with a disability to leave because an employee or another customer is uncomfortable with that person's disability or because its insurance company conditions its coverage or rates on the absence of people with disabilities. In addition, people with disabilities cannot be limited to attending certain performances at a theater. Title III of the act also requires that businesses provide their services in the most integrated setting possible. For example, if just one room in a restaurant was accessible so that all people in wheelchairs who wanted to eat there would be placed together, the restaurant would be discriminating against those people. The entire restaurant should be accessible.

Businesses are also required to make reasonable modifications to their policies, practices, and procedures so that their services are accessible to individuals with disabilities, unless the business can demonstrate that doing so would fundamentally alter the nature of the goods or services provided. For example, a clothing store that allows only one person per dressing room must make an exception to that policy to allow the companion of a blind individual to assist that person.

A business is not allowed to apply eligibility criteria for its goods and services that might screen out individuals with disabilities unless the criteria are necessary to provide the goods and services being offered. For example, a retail store cannot accept only a driver's license as a valid form of identification for payment by check because some individuals with disabilities, such as those who have visual impairments, are unable to obtain a driver's license.

Effective communication with the public is a key mandate of the Act. Businesses are required to communicate effectively, by whatever means are appropriate, with their customers or clients who are deaf or hearing impaired or who have speech or visual impairments. The term used in the act to refer to the devices or services used as means of communicating effectively is *auxiliary aids.* This term includes sign language interpreters; written materials; assistive listening devices; telecommunication devices for the deaf (TDDs); taped, braille, or large-print materials; readers; and other communication tools.

The goal of the communication requirement is to find the effective means of communication appropriate for the particular circumstance. For example, jotting down the sale price of some items in a store for a deaf customer may be sufficient. However, if a deaf patient is in a physician's office seeking treatment for a serious illness, an interpreter may be more appropriate to ensure effective communication. A business is not required to provide any particular device or service that it can demonstrate would fundamentally alter the nature of the goods or services being provided or would result in an undue burden. Undue burden is defined as a significant difficulty or expense. What constitutes an undue burden is determined on a case-by-case basis.

Businesses are required to remove architectural barriers in existing facilities to ensure access for customers, clients, or patrons where it is "readily achievable" to do so. Readily achievable is defined as "easily accomplishable and able to be carried out without much difficulty or expense." For example, a business could realign parking spaces to provide extra accessible spaces, could widen a doorway or reconfigure display shelves to increase access, or if remodeling would cause an undue burden, could find an alternative way to deliver its goods or services.

Businesses have an ongoing obligation to provide accessible services. Just because they cannot afford to build a ramp this year does not mean that they are exempt from doing it the following year if their finances have improved.

No business may charge extra or assess a surcharge on an individual with a disability for auxiliary devices and services, barrier removal, or alternative measures taken in lieu of barrier removal.

All newly constructed facilities must be readily accessible to and usable by people with disabilities. The technical standards for accessible new construction are set out in the Americans with Disabilities Act Accessibility Guidelines (ADAAG). If a business is renovating its premises or adding a new wing, these renovations must be readily accessible to and usable by people with disabilities to the maximum extent feasible.

The following case describes the process at work when a stroke survivor wants to return to work after a stroke and how the American with Disabilities Act can help him attain his goal. This case study looks at how the patient, working with his therapists, approaches his decision making.

CASE REPORT

Before his stroke, C.B. was a professor of history at a university. His stroke resulted in a speech deficit, and he used a wheelchair for mobility. He was independent in his home with his wife's help.

Six months after his stroke, C.B. decided that he wanted to return to work. C.B. contacted university personnel, who said they would be glad to have him back but were concerned about his ability to continue his research and publish. His physician requested a speech evaluation and a worksite evaluation to address those concerns. C.B. worked with a speech-language pathologist and the worksite team to identify potential problems and solutions. C.B. determined that, to continue his research, he would need to compensate for the weakness in his hands because it affected his handling of written materials such as books; in addition, he would require some method to communicate with his colleagues across the country.

The worksite team worked with C.B. to evaluate his abilities to complete job tasks in his office and surrounding faculty areas. The university was accessible in terms of mobility. There were no steps blocking his way on campus, and there was an elevator to his third floor office. However, his office was extremely small and caused difficulties in maneuvering his wheelchair. As a result of the evaluation it was determined that, if his bookcases were moved from the floor to the wall and if the desk were moved against the same wall, there would be enough room to maneuver the wheelchair. Four desk blocks would elevate the desk height to allow C.B. to roll up to the desk without hitting his knees. The door could be equipped with offset hinges to allow a width of 32 inches, which was not perfect but wide enough for C.B. to roll his chair through. C.B. was worried about trips to the library and carrying books. The solution to this problem and his communication concern was to attach a modem to his computer, which allowed for communication with his colleagues, the downloading and uploading of files, and direct access to library files. The university provided C.B. with a graduate assistant to obtain the books he needed for research.

Under the American with Disabilities Act, C.B. was considered a qualified individual with a disability. He could carry out the essential functions of the job—research and publishing—with reasonable accommodations. Therefore the university could not refuse to allow him to return to work. The university worked with C.B., his physician and therapists, and the local vocational rehabilitation agency to ensure that funds were available to pay for the necessary assistive technology devices.

REFERENCES

Nature of the Problem

1. Gresham GE et al: Epidemiologic profile of long term stroke disability: the Framingham study, *Arch Phys Med Rehabil* 60:487, 1979.
2. Kottke FJ: Philosophic considerations of quality of life for the disabled, *Arch Phys Med Rehabil* 63:60, 1982.
3. Labi MLC, Phillips TF, Gresham GE: Psychosocial disability in physically restored long term stroke survivors, *Arch Phys Med Rehabil* 61:561, 1980.
4. Niemi ML et al: Quality of life 4 years after stroke, *Stroke* 19:1101, 1988.

Enhancing Family Life

5. Bishop DS et al: Stroke: morale, family functioning, health status, and functional capacity, *Arch Phys Med Rehabil* 67:84, 1986.
6. Carlson CE: Psychological aspects of neurological disability, *Nurs Clin North Am* 15:309, 1980.
7. Costello SP: The sexual recovery of the stroke patient, *Sexual Med Today* 5:6, 1981.
8. Ebrahim S, Nouri F: Caring for stroke patients at home, *Int Rehabil Med* 8:171, 1986.
9. Emick-Herring B: Sexual changes in patients and partners following stroke, *Rehabil Nurs* March-April:28, 1985.
10. Evans RL et al: Family intervention after stroke: does counseling or education help? *Stroke* 19:1243, 1988.
11. Farzan DT: Reintegration for stroke survivors: home and community considerations, *Nurs Clin North Am* 26:1037, 1991.
12. Fitzgerald G: Effects of caregiving on caregiver spouses of stroke victims, *Axon*, June 1989, pp 85-88.

13. Freda M, Rubinsky H: Sexual function in the stroke survivor, *Phys Med Rehabil Clin North Am* 2(3): 643, 1991.
14. Garden F, Smith B: Sexual function after cerebrovascular accident, *Curr Concepts Rehabil Med* 5:2, 1990.
15. Goldstein V, Regenery G, Wellin E: Caretaker role fatigue, *Nurs Outlook* 29(1):24, 1981.
16. Magi G, Schifano F: Psychological fitness after stroke, *J Neurol Neurosurg Psychiatry* 47:567, 1984.
17. Marron KR: Sexuality with aging, *Geriatrics* 37(9):135, 1982.
18. McCormick GP, Riffer DJ, Thompson NM: Coital positioning for stroke afflicted couples, *Rehabil Nurs* 11:17, 1986.
19. Mims FH, Awenson M: *Sexuality: a nursing perspective,* New York, 1980, McGraw-Hill.
20. Monga TN, Lawson JS, Inglis J: Sexuality dysfunction in stroke patients, *Arch Phys Med Rehabil* 67:19, 1986.
21. Mumma CM: Perceived losses following stroke, *Rehabil Nurs* 11:19, 1986.
22. Neistadt M, Freda M: *Choices: a guide to sex counseling with physically disabled adults,* Melbourne, Fla, 1987, RE Kreiger Publishing.
23. Sjögren K: Sexuality after stroke with hemiplegia. II. With special regard to partnership adjustment and to fulfillment, *Scand J Rehabil Med* 15:63, 1983.
24. Sjögren K, Damber JE, Liliquist B: Sexuality after stroke with hemiplegia. I. Aspects of sexual function, *Scand J Rehabil Med* 15:55, 1983.
25. Sjögren K, Fugl-Meyer AR: Adjustment to life after stroke with special reference to sexual intercourse and leisure, *J Psychosom Res* 26:409, 1982.
26. Stankstein SE, Robinson RG: Lateralized emotional response following stroke. In Kinsbourne M, editor: *Cerebral hemisphere function in depression,* Washington, DC, 1988, American Psychiatric Press.
27. Wade DT, Leigh-Smith J, Hewer RL: Effects of living with and looking after survivors of stroke, *Br J Med* 293:418, 1986.
28. Watson PG: Stroke in the family: theoretical consideration, *Rehabil Nurs* 11:15, 1986.
29. Williams SE, Freer CA: Aphasia: its effects on marital relationships, *Arch Phys Med Rehabil* 67:250, 1986.

Enhancing Community Integration

30. Brown M, Gordon W, Ragnarsson K: Unhandicapping the disabled: what is possible, *Arch Phys Med Rehabil* 68:206, 1987.
31. Diller L et al: *Rehabilitation indicators,* New York, 1979, Institute of Rehabilitation Medicine.
32. Finkelstein V: Attitudes and disabled people: issues for discussion, *World Rehabilitation Fund Monographs,* No. 5, 1980.
33. McFarland S: Product evaluation: issues and options. In *Provision of assistive technology: planning and implementation,* Washington, DC, 1989, Electronic Industries Foundation.
34. Nevins B: Grassroots rehabilitation technology and the delivery systems: gap in the system. In Redden MR, Stern VW, editors: *Technology for independent living. Vol 2. Issues in technology for daily living, education, and employment,* Washington, DC, 1983, American Association for the Advancement of Science.
35. Ozer M: Participatory planning process for wheelchair selection: choosing a wheelchair system, *J Rehabil Res Dev,* clin. suppl. 2, p 31, 1990.
36. Payton O, Nelson C, Ozer M: *Patient participation in program planning: a manual for therapists,* Philadelphia, 1989, FA Davis.
37. Phillips B, Zhao H: Predictors of technology abandonment, *Assistive Technology,* vol 5.1, 1993.

38. Request Rehabilitation Engineering Center on Evaluation of Assistive Technology: *Product comparison and evaluation of scooters,* Washington, DC, 1991, National Rehabilitation Hospital.
39. Vash CL: Psychological aspects of rehabilitation engineering. In Redden MR, Stern VW, editors: *Technology for independent living. Vol 2, Issues in technology for daily living, education, and employment,* Washington, DC, 1983, American Association for the Advancement of Science.
40. Whiteneck GG et al: Quantifying handicap: a new measure of long-term rehabilitation outcomes, *Arch Phys Med Rehabil* 73:519, 1992.
41. World Health Organization: *World Health Organization's international classification of impairments, disabilities and handicaps: a manual of classification relating to the consequences of disease,* Geneva, 1980, World Health Organization.
42. Wright BA: *Physical disability: a psychosocial approach,* ed 2, New York, 1983, Harper & Row.
43. Zola I: Involving consumers in the rehabilitation process: easier said than done. In Redden MR, Stern VW, editors: *Technology for independent living,* vol 1, Washington, DC, 1982, American Association for the Advancement of Science.

CHAPTER 12

Ensuring Continuity of Medical Care

Nature of the problem
Stroke prevention
   Nature of the problem
   Monitoring outcome
   Maintaining regimens
   Emergency response
Management of spasticity
   Nature of the problem
   Assessment
   Treatment
Central poststroke pain
   MARK N. OZER AND LORENZ K.Y. NG
   Nature of the problem
   Treatment

NATURE OF THE PROBLEM

One goal of the continuing care phase must be to minimize the degree of medical illness — that is, the morbidity and mortality in persons with stroke. A major source of such subsequent illness is related to stroke recurrence. Other factors contributing to morbidity are those impairments likely to be ongoing that reflect the injury to the motor and sensory systems, including spasticity and central pain as late sequelae of stroke.

The progressive nature of vascular disease in the pathogenesis of stroke has been the basis for emphasizing stepped-up training in the management of risk factors such as hyperlipidemia and hypertension during the rehabilitation phase. One of the objectives of the rehabilitation phase has been to engender a greater degree of cooperation on the part of the person with stroke, ensuring that he or she seeks a continuity of primary medical care. The surveillance responsibility during this continuing care phase is shared to a greater degree with the person with stroke. Nevertheless, several major opportunities to prevent recurrent stroke involve ongoing medical supervision. One specific outcome sought in all persons with stroke is the identification of a primary care physician (with an actual appointment made by the time of discharge). A measure of success during the continuing care phase, therefore, is the degree to which a continuity of care is achieved and maintained.

In addition to the collaboration of the patient with the monitoring process, a greater degree of participation is required to ensure adherence to treatment regimens. Frequently in the case of both hypertension and hyperlipidemia, these include drugs that both are expensive and cause inconvenient side effects. During the rehabilitation phase, efforts were devoted to knowledge of and commitment to the medication regimen, while simultaneously seeking to reduce the complexity of such regimens. In addition, efforts were made to minimize stroke recurrence by encouraging the patient to abstain from drugs such as tobacco and alcohol, change his or her diet, increase the amount of exercise, and participate in other techniques independent of the health system. A further measure of success in the continuing care phase is the degree to which the person with stroke adheres to such stroke prevention regimens.

For the future, a major effort lies in the early treatment of persons with stroke to inhibit the progression of cerebral ischemia to infarction. Ischemia is a potentially reversible altered state of the brain tissue to reduced oxygen and glucose; infarction is death of tissue. Most successes in reducing infarct size in animal models of stroke have occurred when treatment was given soon after the onset of ischemia. For success of a similar sort to occur in humans, it appears necessary to institute much earlier treatment for stroke than has been the case in the past. One of the objectives of the rehabilitation phase was to increase the awareness of the person with stroke and caregivers in the warning signs of stroke and to train them in emergency responses to these warning signs. A comparable type of emergency response on the part of professionals is available only in some settings. It is anticipated that, in the future, the use of protocols for early treatment of stroke will be more widespread.

STROKE PREVENTION
Nature of the Problem

One objective of the continuing care phase is to minimize the likelihood of recurrent stroke. One method to accomplish this is by maintaining medical supervision to support the ongoing monitoring and the use of regimens designed to control treatable risk factors. Still another objective is to minimize the degree of infarction and brain injury that occurs in the presence of subsequent ischemia by educating the patient to seek early medical care if warning signs of stroke appear.

It is important to note that, although regimens for stroke prevention frequently benefit from a degree of professional support, the desired changes in life-style are actually under the control of the patient. Activities to reduce the incidence of primary or secondary stroke involve identifying goals, measuring outcomes, and ensuring that treatment is appropriate. The relationship between

TABLE 12-1   Quality of Interaction

INTERACTION	PROFESSIONAL	PATIENT
Independent		Asks questions of self
Free choice	Asks open questions	Answers freely
Choice	Offers suggestions (at least three)	Selects
Adherence	Makes recommendation (one)	Agrees (or disagrees)
Compliance	Orders and prescribes	Complies (or does not)

the patient and the health professional and the character of the data discussed can provide support in such activities. Throughout this text, it has been emphasized that the quality of the interaction must enable the patient to participate to the greatest extent possible. Table 12-1 defines the possible levels of interaction between the patient and the professional. The common use of the term *compliance* is inappropriate for the quality of interaction actually sought. Evidence indicates that a relatively high level of agreement about problems and outcomes between the patient and the practitioner can lead to better outcomes.[8] An effective program for stroke prevention requires just such a higher level of collaboration by the person with stroke. It is necessary to maintain the highest possible level of patient participation in this ongoing effort.

Monitoring Outcome

During the rehabilitation phase the person with stroke can be familiarized with the goals in managing blood pressure, hyperlipidemia, and anticoagulation. The role of the professional is to make clear recommendations to which the patient can agree. Once the goals have been defined and agreed on, the patient can take an even greater role in the next step—measuring outcomes. During the continuing care phase the patient can self-monitor his or her blood pressure with the use of readily available instruments. Information concerning the selection of blood pressure monitors is available to consumers.[2] At this time, monitoring serum lipid levels and prothrombin time requires the use of a laboratory; however, educating the patient about the results sought can contribute to the effectiveness of treatment. When anticoagulant medication is used, the maintenance of effective stroke prevention is particularly problematic.

The following cases illustrate the crucial nature of continued monitoring of the proper level of anticoagulant medication and the advantage of educating the patient about the outcomes sought and of encouraging the patient's active participation in the monitoring process.

CASE REPORT

A.T. was a 53-year-old, right-handed scientist who had experienced sudden onset of numbness and tingling of the left arm that resolved over several days. A computed tomography (CT) head scan demonstrated a small lesion on the right side of the brain. The patient had an atrial septal defect and was administered warfarin because the brain lesion indicated the presence of emboli from the peripheral venous circulation. His prothrombin time was checked on a regular basis, but the patient was unaware of the specific range within which it was to be maintained. Since discharge he had moved to another city and had maintained monthly monitoring by a laboratory, but he had not personally been kept apprised of the prothrombin level being achieved. The degree to which the prothrombin time data was followed by the physician, who should have been monitoring the warfarin level, remains unclear.

Approximately 1 year later, A.T. noted an onset of numbness in his right hand that progressed over several hours to hemiparesis involving the entire right side and global aphasia. When admitted to an acute care setting, his prothrombin time was 20 seconds. A CT head scan revealed a medium-sized left internal capsular hemorrhage. No evidence of aneurysm or arteriovenous malformation was found on arteriography. When transferred to the rehabilitation setting several weeks later, he continued to have a major degree of weakness with persistent difficulties in expression and impairments in memory and attention.

This patient had a somewhat higher prothrombin time than that generally sought. Subsequently, he experienced a cerebral hemorrhage with major sequelae of both a cognitive and a communication nature, which could have a significant effect on the continuation of his scientific career.

The following case illustrates another common problem in managing a regimen that incorporates anticoagulant medication.

CASE REPORT

M.S., a 47-year-old, right-handed food service supervisor, had a history of chronic atrial fibrillation (AF) and valvular disease caused by rheumatic fever in childhood. She had been receiving on a consistent dose of warfarin for several years but was not aware of the goals of such treatment or the range of prothrombin time sought. She had been followed by a physician but at irregular intervals. Her prothrombin time was checked even less frequently.

M.S. experienced an acute onset of right hemiparesis and aphasia. A CT head scan yielded negative findings for hemorrhage. On admission to an acute care facility, M.S.'s prothrombin time was 13.2 seconds with the control 12.5. Echocardiographic studies showed a mild mitral regurgitation and a dilated left atrium but no evidence of thrombus. The electrocardiogram showed continued evidence of AF.

On admission to a rehabilitation program, 2 weeks after the onset she continued to have motor weakness, difficulty finding words, and impairments in cognition, such as problems with memory and problem solving. Her language difficulties extended to reading and writing. After completion of her rehabilitation program (6 weeks after the onset), she continued to have communication difficulties in oral expression, reading, and writing. However, she was mobile and could carry out daily living skills independently. Her prothrombin time was maintained at 1.5 times the control (16 to 18 seconds) on substantially higher dose of warfarin than before. She was also now familiar with the treatment goal and the range sought. Continuity of care for more frequent monitoring of her prothrombin time was instituted.

The preceding case illustrates the need for proper supervision to achieve and maintain an adequate therapeutic level of anticoagulation. Unlike the first patient, M.S.'s stroke was her first. However, in both cases the impairments from the stroke were likely to prevent a return to the level of work each had previously carried out. The problem in both these cases does not lie in the selection of the regimen or in the adherence of patients to the agreed on regimen; rather, it lies in the proper degree of supervision. The likelihood of achieving satisfactory prothrombin times in both these patients might be enhanced by the patient's knowledge of the goals and insistence that the patient participate with the physician in monitoring.

In both these cases it is unclear whether intervening variables may have affected the prothrombin time inadvertently. Neither of these patients had been familiarized with the effects of drugs or diet on the level of anticoagulation. The patient's knowledge about the potential effects of common drugs on the anticoagulant effect of a fixed dose of warfarin could have been of value. It is important that all persons be warned about potential hazards and be instructed against the use of any drug, including nonprescription products, without the advice of a physician or pharmacist. The patient's knowledge of the dietary sources of vitamin K and of drug interactions can reduce the likelihood of problems arising from either excessive or insufficient anticoagulation medication. (See Table 12-2 for the vitamin K content of foods, a list to be shared with patients receiving warfarin. The box on p. 454 lists the more common nonprescription drugs affecting action of warfarin.)

TABLE 12-2   Vitamin K Content*

FOOD	MEAN (µg)*
BEVERAGES	
Coffee—6 fl oz (180 g)	68
Tea, green—8 fl oz (240 g)	1709
FATS	
Oil, corn—3½ oz (100 g)	50
Oil, soybean—3½ oz (100 g)	500
MEAT	
Beef, ground—3½ oz (100 g)	7
Beef, ground, gamma irradiated—3½ oz (100 g)	0
Beef, liver, raw—3½ oz (100 g)	92
Liverwurst—1 oz (28 g)	34
MILK	
Cow milk, whole—1 liter	60
Human milk—1 liter	15
VEGETABLES	
Asparagus, raw—5-6 spears (100 g)	57
Broccoli, raw—1 cup (126 g)	252
Brussels sprouts, raw—3½ oz (100 g)	(800-3000)
Cabbage, raw—1 cup (124 g)	155
Cauliflower, raw—3½ oz (100 g)	3600
Green beans, raw—3½ (100 g)	290
Lettuce, raw—1 cup (74 g)	95
Peas, green, unripe—3½ oz (100 g)	300
Peas, green, boiled—½ cup (85 g)	221
Potato, raw—3½ oz (100 g)	80
Spinach, raw—3½ oz (100 g)	89 (40-3000)
Tomato, raw—1 med (148 g)	7
Turnip greens, raw—1 cup (54 g)	54
Watercress, raw—25 sprigs (25 g)	14

From Pennington JAT, Church HN: *Bowes and Church's food values of portions commonly used*, ed 15, Philadelphia, 1989, JB Lippincott.
*Numbers in parentheses are range.

Nonprescription Drugs Affecting Warfarin

Aspirin
Cold and cough medicines
Antacids
Laxatives
Medication for aches and pains
Vitamin preparations containing vitamin K or large amounts of vitamin A,
   E, or C
Diet products, such as liquid food supplements
Alcohol

Maintaining Regimens

The appropriateness of any set of recommended activities—whether the use of drugs, assistive devices, or newly learned procedures—is ultimately measured by the degree to which these activities are actually carried out independently by the patient. The degree to which adherence to any regimen can be maintained is enhanced by the patient's perceived efficacy of the activity in achieving goals.[5] The patient's knowledge of the outcomes being sought is basic to adherence to any regimen. If there is a clear indication that a result has been achieved, the next step is to establish a relationship between those outcomes and the actions that were taken. If medication has been one of the methods employed, the relationship between the medication and the results must be clearly established in the mind of both the patient and the professional. The patient must view this relationship as one that is useful to maintain.

When a positive outcome has been achieved (e.g., the patient has met the agreed on goal for blood pressure or lipid level), a method by which the relationship between the regimen and the outcome can be clarified is to explore answers to the question of "What has worked?" In the context of such success the dialog is most usefully expanded to an exploration of the methods used. In addition, the ongoing independent use of these means by the client can be enhanced to the degree that the answers come from the client rather than the professional. It is desirable to work at the level of "choice" or higher, such as is defined by the scale in Table 12-1 (see p. 450). When medication is part of the regimen, the client should be encouraged to describe the medication used in all its detail—that is, its name, frequency of dosing, and actual dose in the context of its perceived success. In such a review both an increased awareness of the means used and a renewed commitment to its use can be generated.

Still another result can be achieved by exploring questions about the actions taken. In a relatively mutualistic discourse, there is an opportunity to make modifications so that such treatments can be properly fitted to the person.[4] This process of "tailoring," itself, contributes to the result. Not only are changes made that can enhance the likelihood of efficacy, but the very process of seeking a fit can lead to enhancement. The patient being asked about the degree of fit accommodates to the treatment by virtue of being asked to modify it. For example, changes can be made in the choice of drug and its dosage and frequency on the basis of input from the client. Crucial to this entire process is the degree to which the client perceives that the changes have arisen out of mutual interaction. This ongoing process makes it more likely that adherence to a regimen will be enhanced.

However, problems with adherence to a regimen do not always lie solely with the patient. Many regimens are expensive and require strong commitment. It is important to recognize the concept of medication burden. One way to measure this burden is to multiply the number of different medications and the number of doses to be taken each day.[2] The need to fill several prescriptions and recall the various times and pills to be taken adds to the burden, as do side effects caused by polypharmacy.

Emergency Response

Ongoing studies of several new therapies in stroke suggest the need for early intervention if brain reperfusion and neuronal protection are to be successful.[7] It is likely that in the near future new methods will be forthcoming that require a far more expeditious handling of persons who appear to have had a stroke. In particular, some studies describe the use of tissue plasminogen activation.[9]

A number of recent studies explored the specific factors for delay in seeking treatment. Delays in presentation for more definitive care can be attributed to either the patient or physician (the degree of contribution varies with the character of the catchment area). In one study, education programs aimed mainly at physicians substantially increased the numbers of patients reaching an acute stroke center within 24 hours of onset.[1] The physician education program was coupled with multimedia information to the general public describing the signs and symptoms of stroke and the need for early treatment.

An awareness of the warning signs of stroke in persons who have already had a stroke is particularly important. These warning signs have been widely broadcast, but it appears that widespread publicity is only one way to bring about a more prompt response. A focused effort on those who have had a stroke would be a more useful approach. Yet, in one study of persons who had a stroke and

Recognition of Stroke Warning Signs

Includes an awareness of early warning signs of stroke and a plan for seeking help promptly.

7. No problem: Patient and family recognize all early warning signs of stroke and have independently generated a plan for dealing with such, including knowing the name and telephone number of a physician, clinic, emergency room, or other source to alert.

6. Minimal problem: Patient and family recognize early warning signs and generate a plan at the team's request for dealing with such, including knowing the name and telephone number of a physician, clinic, emergency room, or other source to alert.

5. Mild problem: Patient and family recognize all pertinent early warning signs and require suggestions by the staff to generate a plan for dealing with such, including knowing the name and telephone number of a physician, clinic, emergency room, or other source to alert.

4. Mild to moderate problem: Patient and family recognize 75% of the early warning signs of stroke and require suggestions by the staff to generate a plan to seek emergency care.

3. Moderate problem: Patient and family recognize 50% of the early warning signs of stroke and require specific recommendations to generate a plan to seek emergency care.

2. Moderately severe problem: Patient and family recognize less than 25% of the warning signs and have no plan to seek emergency care.

1. Severe problem: Patient or family recognize none of the early warning signs of stroke and will require supervision to create a plan to seek emergency care.

WARNING SIGNS

1. Numbness or weakness of your face, arm, or leg
2. Difficulty speaking or understanding
3. Difficulty swallowing
4. Sudden confusion
5. Severe headaches
6. Dizziness or loss of balance
7. Sudden blurred or decreased vision
8. Sudden change in mental ability

COMPONENTS OF PLAN

1. Actions to be taken on one's own, such as lying down
2. Name of physician, clinic, or emergency room source they might alert and telephone numbers such as 911.

were enrolled in a stroke club, only a small percentage were able to identify the warning signs and the proper response to those signs.

To remedy this problem, a program should be instituted during the rehabilitation phase to increase the awareness of this issue. The box on p. 456 lists the warning signs and a scale of the degree of awareness that can be used to measure the outcome of such an educational program.

The following case illustrates the need for a continuity of care for persons with stroke. There may be limits to what can be achieved in reducing stroke recurrence, yet the systems must be in place to ensure that these limits are reached, that strokes are prevented to the fullest extent possible, and that care is sought as early as possible.

CASE REPORT

M.B. is a retired housekeeper with a long history of non-insulin-dependent diabetes and hypertension. She had been followed by a prepaid health program for both problems while employed. She had no knowledge of her blood pressure or diabetes goals and had not been trained to monitor either one. At 59 years of age she had the first of a series of strokes. This initial stroke affected her right side, but she recovered within a few weeks and was able to return to work. Several months later she had another episode with subsequent difficulty with gait. She retired from her job as the result of disability. At this time she was approximately 60 years of age. Her husband had died the previous year. Although eligible for survivor's benefits under Social Security, she was denied Medicare coverage on the basis of her disability. Her membership in the prepaid health program expired 1 year after her retirement. She ran out of medication for blood pressure, and she could identify no physician to prescribe medication. The cost of the drugs was apparently an additional factor.

At 62 years of age, M.B. had a third stroke. Again, her right side was affected. It was at least 24 hours before she was brought to the emergency room of a local acute care hospital. A CT head scan demonstrated bilateral old infarcts involving the right central semiovale, left parietooccipital region, and right occipital lobe. Carotid Doppler ultrasonography showed a 60% to 80% stenosis of the left internal carotid artery; dipyridamole- and thallium-enhanced radiologic tests showed posterolateral left ventricular ischemia. The patient was administered acetylsalicylic acid (325 mg qd) and antihypertensive medications. At this time she first enrolled in an intensive stroke rehabilitation program.

When M.B. was discharged 6 weeks after the onset, the neurologic examination showed homonymous hemianopsia with right facial droop and marked dysarthria. She also had swallowing problems and right hemiparesis (greater in her arm than her leg) with impaired position sense on the right. She was able to propel her wheelchair on her own and required some assistance to transfer from a bed to a wheelchair, to dress, and to perform other activities of daily living (ADLs). A major effort was devoted to identifying a physician who would provide continuity of medical care and to training the patient's daughter in both blood pressure and blood sugar monitoring. The daughter (with whom the patient would live) was aware of the goals and the need to seek medical advice if the parameters established were exceeded or the warning signs of stroke occurred.

When seen 10 weeks after the onset, the patient had met with the identified primary physician and brought her record of blood pressure and blood sugar measurements to him. Her antihypertensive medication had been adjusted because she reported her blood pressure level had exceeded the recommended range. She was taking acetylsalicylic acid and the other medication prescribed. A system for a continuity of medical care had been established. She was now ambulating and meeting her daily needs without the need for physical assistance.

Eight weeks later the patient had difficulty with urinary incontinence and was found to have an elevated blood sugar level. Her daughter brought her to her primary physician who found evidence of a urinary tract infection and prescribed insulin. The plan was to readmit the patient to an acute care hospital if her blood sugar levels remained elevated. However, 48 hours later, she had a sudden onset of difficulty with the left side of her body and was promptly brought to the emergency room and admitted. Evaluations of her left side yielded improved findings over the next several days, but her dysarthria worsened and she exhibited difficulty with swallowing liquids safely.

The problems of this person cannot be solved in their entirety; both an availability of medical care and the receipt of that care by the family were achieved. Changes were made in the behavior of the patient and family, who learned to seek medical care appropriately and to monitor the patient's blood pressure and blood sugar levels; the regimen was modified on the basis of their input, and adherence was obtained to an agreed on medical regimen. The patient and family promptly responded to the existence of a problem in blood sugar levels and later signs of a possible recurrent stroke. The presence of such behaviors earlier in the course of her illness might have enabled the patient to avoid some of the more devastating effects of her multiplicity of strokes. The incidence of such tragic stories must be reduced.

In many instances the person who enters the health care system during the acute phase reenters it on a recurrent basis. Stroke is the localized evidence of a diffuse progressive vascular disease, and it must be treated in the context of its ongoing nature. In at least one third of persons with stroke, it is a recurrent stroke that brought about hospitalization, and the effects of each successive stroke were increasingly devastating. Major opportunity still exists for stroke prevention. Ongoing surveillance by both the person with stroke and the professional offers the most likely method for the cost-effective accomplishment of this goal.

MANAGEMENT OF SPASTICITY
Nature of the Problem

The deficits that primarily disable persons with spastic hemiparesis are the so-called negative symptoms, such as weakness, fatigability, lack of dexterity, and an inability to produce isolated movements. In addition to such deficits, persons with central nervous system (CNS) lesions notice the emergence of a number of "positive" symptoms, including heightening of flexor withdrawal reflexes and spasticity, which are attributed to the release of lower level reflex behaviors disconnected from the more rostral controls in the corticospinal system.[17]

The clinical criteria of "spasticity" that are evident on examination (e.g., velocity-dependent increases in resistance to passive movement and exaggerated tendon jerks at rest) are only components of the total upper motor neuron syndrome. These clinical findings dealing with abnormalities of the stretch reflex do not necessarily reflect the symptoms most frequently disabling to the person with upper motor neuron impairment. For example, flexor spasms caused by heightening of the normal flexor withdrawal reflex cause significant disability in persons with spinal cord injury.[16]

In persons with cerebral lesions the effect of an imbalance of both motor power and exaggerated tonic stretch reflexes can lead to further impairment and subsequent disability. For example, joint contractures that can limit future function are related to an imbalance in strength of the antagonistic muscle groups acting across a joint. The imbalance may be due to weakness, excessive muscle contraction, or both. Commonly, the arm is affected by the relative weakness of the elbow extensors and the excessive muscle contraction of the flexors.[19]

In addition to the effects attributed to spasticity arising from injury in the corticospinal system, concomitant lesions frequently affect the extrapyramidal system. "Rigidity" results from abnormally increased, non-velocity-dependent muscle activity. Again, the distribution of effect is unbalanced. Muscle groups such as the flexors of the upper extremity and the extensors of the lower extremity preferentially and actively contract even while "at rest." Thus the contractures are more likely to occur in the presence of these combined lesions affecting both the pyramidal and extrapyramidal motor systems.[18]

Such effects apparently also extend to changes in the mechanical property of the muscles.[10,13] However, it is unclear whether the effects of immobilization bring about changes in the character of the muscle. Lower threshold motor units develop increased fatigability, whereas fast-twitch and larger units become slower.[18]

The long-term effects of the motor neuron syndrome generally persist into the continuing care phase. Although limited functional results occur from treatment of these "positive" effects of the upper motor neuron syndrome, such treatment can be occasionally useful in increasing motor function and limiting the likelihood of contractures.

Assessment

Understanding the pathophysiologic factors that produce spastic hyperreflexia can help determine an appropriate treatment. The basic cause of the upper motor neuron syndrome is the disinhibition within the CNS of extrafusal motor efferents. Particular emphasis is placed on the effects on Ia interneurons, which mediate reciprocal inhibition within the spinal cord.

A number of different systems are considered to be affected. One is that of the presynaptic inhibition associated with γ-aminobutyric acid (GABA) release. Receptors for benzodiazepine are adjacent to this same area. Suprasegmental lesions reduce the excitation of this inhibitory activity. In addition, the normal supraspinal control of Renshaw cells, which activate a negative feedback loop during voluntary movement, is reduced in persons with hemiplegia. Failure of this aspect of the inhibitory system is thought to account for some of the clonus seen in the soleus muscle when contraction of the tibialis anterior muscle occurs.

The problems caused by spasticity are evident when the patient attempts to move. If one group of spastic muscles is contracting, difficulties arise when abnormal reflexes are induced in the stretched antagonist muscles rather than their appropriate inhibition. Reciprocal inhibition uses the Ia interneurons. For example, when a person voluntarily contracts the tibialis anterior muscle, descending pathways activate not only the α motor neurons to that muscle but also the Ia inhibitory interneurons that end in the antagonist soleus muscle motor neurons. These several systems are all affected, reducing the degree of reciprocal inhibition in persons with spasticity.

Studies involving the H reflex have been used to identify which of the several components have been affected, information that has implications for the more appropriate selection of treatment. The H reflex of Hoffmann can be observed with low-intensity stimulation of a mixed nerve. It can be applied to muscles other than the soleus muscle, although it is most commonly applied to excitation of that muscle. The H reflex has been identified as a monosynaptic reflex associated with activation of large afferent Ia fibers. As such, the ratio of response to electrical stimulation of the H reflex in the soleus muscle is related to the maximum response to stimulation of the motor action potential as a measure of the excitability of the motor neuron pool. The normal reduction of the H reflex by vibratory stimulation of the muscle is considered to be a measure of the presynaptic inhibition system. Patients with a deficient response to vibration respond preferentially to diazepam administration. A deficiency in the reciprocal inhibition by the Ia inhibitory interneurons is measured by the effect on the H reflex in the soleus when concomitant contraction of the anterior tibial muscle is present. The normal inhibition of the antagonist is particularly noticeable during voluntary contraction. Animal studies indicate that glycine serves as the neurotransmitter in this system.[12] In patients with such abnormal H reflex recovery curves, baclofen has been found to be particularly efficacious.

Motor nucleus excitability is measured by still another procedure. When a motor nerve is stimulated at supramaximal intensity, an inconsistent late response of low amplitude is elicited. First observed in the foot, it is called the F response. Reflecting the response of antidromically activated neurons, it is a supplementary index of motor neuron excitability. The F response is helpful in studies of the motor nuclei supplying muscles in which a monosynaptic reflex is unavailable.

Treatment

Medical treatment with diazepam therapy has been advocated for the treatment of spasticity, but the results have been less helpful in those with spasticity arising from cerebral lesions than in those with spinal cord lesions. The indication for the use of diazepam is the suggested effect of GABA-mediated presynaptic inhibition. Some evidence also indicates that baclofen has limited clinical effects in the person with spasticity of cerebral origin.[5] In physiologic studies these effects were noted to occur predominantly in the interneuron system rather than at the sites for presynaptic inhibition. Therefore it has been recommended that the use of baclofen is more likely to be efficacious in those with demonstrated changes in that system.

More recently, botulinus toxin has been used for the selective treatment of spasticity.[11] The toxin acts presynaptically to prevent release of acetylcholine with resultant flaccid weakness. Local injection at motor points in an uncontrolled series of patients with severe spasticity relieved spasticity involving the flexors of the arm. Botulinus toxin was helpful in increasing the range of movements, with subsequent improvement in the overall functional status and in specific activities. The required frequency of such injections has not been determined, but it is likely that the results will not be permanent.

The major approach to the treatment of contractures and associated spasticity is to prevent shortening of the muscle by early and frequent passive movement.[15] Passive stretching of the spastic muscle is presumed to lead to fatigue, thereby exposing the fibrous tissue elements to the stretching force. Stimulation of the antagonists can also lead to contralateral relaxation, permitting more complete stretching of the contracture. Serial plaster casting can maintain the joint at rest. Under these circumstances the stretch response is not elicited and the soft tissues are exposed to the correcting force. In addition, various orthotic devices may be used to maintain the joint in a neutral functional position (see Chapter 10).

A more direct means of inducing muscle activity is through functional electrical stimulation (FES) of the affected muscle. For example, a 66-year-old patient experienced left upper extremity pain and flexor spasticity several months after experiencing an intracranial hemorrhage. He was unable to use his left arm for dressing and other activities without assistance from his wife. Serial plaster casting was ineffective despite an active home program of stretching. Limited flexion and abduction of shoulder joint and extension of elbow were present, with particular limitations in finger flexion (40%). FES was applied to both agonist and antagonist muscles of the forearm, including the triceps, extensor carpi ulnaris, biceps, and flexor carpi radialis muscles, with a subsequent total excursions of the fingers. The patient's wife was instructed in a home program of FES and stretching. After several weeks the patient was observed to voluntarily fully extend the fingers of the hand. Extension at the elbow had also improved, although contractures remained. The follow-up home program was continued to maintain a degree of stretch.

In another case of difficulty in using the left arm, an 80-year-old woman complained of decreased function 12 months after the onset of a stroke involving the basal ganglion. She could not use her hand even as a stabilizer and found that this interfered significantly with her ability to dress herself. On examination it was noted that her shoulder was adducted, her left forearm held in flexion (90 degrees) at the elbow, and her left wrist and fingers held in flexion (90 degrees). Her left leg was also noted to be adducted, and she exhibited scissor gait and inversion of her foot. The patient set a goal of being able to use her hand as a stabilizer. FES was applied on several occasions to her upper extremity muscles: the extensor carpi radialis, triceps, supinator, and adductor pollicis. Only minimal effects were seen despite follow-up stretching exercises carried out by a therapist immediately following FES. However, at this time the patient was able to use her resting hand splint at night and was committed to carrying out a home program of stretching. The outcomes in this patient were less successful, reflecting a lack of intensity of follow-through stretching.

Surgery is reserved for those few persons with stroke who have reached a stable neurologic state and for whom the abnormal position significantly interferes with function. In surgery the spastic muscles are released or lengthened to allow a functional position; postoperative splinting is employed to prevent a recurrence of the deformity. Bony surgery is not recommended for the correction of spastic deformities. Joint contractures unmasked by the release of the spastic muscle can often be corrected by serial casting and stretching exercises after surgery. Surgery is performed to improve function or to aid nursing care, not to improve cosmesis. Practically speaking, this means that spastic hemiplegia in the lower limb can often be improved with safe and relatively minor surgery. Spasticity in the upper limb is not treated unless skin breakdown occurs or residual selective function is overpowered by limited spasticity.

One of the most common deformities after a stroke treated surgically is equinovarus of the involved foot. In this condition a relatively unopposed action of the plantar flexors and invertors occurs and interferes with foot clearance during the swing phase of walking. In some instances it is necessary to intervene to provide a stable platform for stance during transfers by achieving a more neutral position of the dorsiflexor ("plantigrade foot").

For example, a 46-year-old woman had a 24-month history of left-sided weakness and an area of attenuation of the parietal lobe seen on CT head scan. She was ambulatory with the use of an ankle-foot orthosis; however, she complained of difficulty in maintaining her foot in proper alignment when walking: "My foot twists in my shoe." On examination she was unable to maintain foot placement when walking but went into plantar flexion and inversion. This was not a problem when standing.

Surgical treatment requires a determination of the contribution of the soleus or gastrocnemius muscles to the equinus (plantar flexion). An EMG performed while the patient walks is recommended to make this determination.[15] Because only the gastrocneumius muscle crosses the knee, spastic equinus that occurs with extension but not with flexion is attributed to that muscle. If the position of the knee makes no difference, the soleus muscle is credited. In the most common surgery for this problem the Achilles tendon is elongated, permitting forcible dorsiflexion of the foot. Generally, varus of the forefoot is caused by overactivity of the tibialis anterior muscle, which surgery can also correct.

CENTRAL POSTSTROKE PAIN

Mark N. Ozer and Lorenz K.Y. Ng

Nature of the Problem

Central poststroke pain (CPSP) is defined as "pain associated with a lesion of the central nervous system." It is important to differentiate such pain from the neuropathic pain related to disease or injury of the peripheral nerves, wherein the pathophysiologic factors may be quite different.[23] CPSP may be present after injury to either the spinal cord or the brain. In those with brain lesions the most common cause is vascular disease. Its incidence is difficult to establish, but the severity of the problem does not lie merely in its incidence; the pain can become the major cause of disability, extending into the continuing care phase when these persons have otherwise developed compensatory strategies to alleviate other disabilities, such as those in mobility.

Since Dejerine's classic description in 1906, CPSP has been considered synonymous with lesions in the region of the thalamus. Although particularly frequent in lesions of the ventroposterior thalamus, in one large series the incidence remained less than 20%.[22] CPSP is more appropriately related to lesions anywhere along the course of the spinothalamic tract. In another group of 40 patients with CPSP and adequate lesion localization, only 25% had lesions of the thalamus.[37] In the majority of cases in still another recent study of cerebrovascular lesions and central pain, the lesions involved extrathalamic structures.[28] Of the known lesions, 38% were thalamic and the remainder occurred in the brainstem and elsewhere in the cerebrum outside the thalamus.

The clinical pathologic correlation between CPSP and lesions is incom-

TABLE 12-3   Quality of Steady Pain Reported by Patients with Central Poststroke Pain*

DESCRIPTORS	PERCENT
Burning	64.4
Cold	10.6
Numb, tingling, fuzzy, stinging, itchy	31.6
Aching, bruising, sore, throbbing, pulling, pressing, swelling, cramping, rushing, tight, grabbing, pinching, tearing	38.6

From Teijon G, Bowie J: *Pain* 36:13, 1989.
*Some patients used multiple descriptors.

plete. In one study pain was almost always unilateral, affecting the face and body in 55% of patients, the face alone in 10%, and only the body opposite to the side of the lesion in 30%. The quality of the pain was almost always steady, with an intermittent lancinating quality also present in approximately 17%. Table 12-3 lists descriptors of the quality of the steady pain. Although "burning" is the most frequent descriptor, it is important to note that a variety of descriptors may be used by an individual patient. Intensity may vary, with some persons reporting exacerbation on movement, temperature changes, emotions, or a combination of these. The quality of the pain had some correlation to the site of the lesion. In at least one study of large groups of such patients, intermittent lancinating pain tended to be associated with lesions outside the thalamus. In addition, pain was found in a higher percentage of persons with right-sided thalamic brain lesions than in those with lesions involving the left side of the thalamus.[37]

The pathophysiology of CPSP is also somewhat controversial.[37] The usual delay in onset (1 to 6 months) suggests that the causative process may take time to develop. The triggering factor appears to be a somatosensory disturbance, although sometimes this is subclinical with a particular involvement of the spinothalamic tract. The most common steady, usually burning, spontaneous pain may reflect possible denervation neuronal hypersensitivity in the CNS. One group of investigators documented that the abnormal temperature and pain sensibility were common elements in all their cases.[27] However, variability exists in the degree to which touch sensibility was affected. Thus it appears that injury to the medial lemniscal (touch) pathways is not necessary for the development of this syndrome.

The accepted model of pain transmission portrays the perception of pain as heavily affected by central modulation and controlled by supraspinal inhibition.[39] This model supports the use of various techniques for increasing central inhibition to the entry of nociceptive stimuli from the periphery. Central modulation of pain is extremely complex and involves the interaction of multiple systems: these include the monoamines norepinephrine (NE) and serotonin (5-HT), GABA, and the adrenergic systems. Endogenous opioid peptides have also been implicated in the intrinsic analgesia system at the midbrain, medullary, and spinal levels.[21] The role of opioids in pain modulation is being reevaluated in light of recent findings suggesting that opioids, when properly administered, have a useful role in the control of central and neuropathic pain.[26,33]

Treatment

The medications most commonly used to treat CPSP are antidepressant and anticonvulsant agents. In a controlled study, amitriptyline has been shown to effectively relieve the pain of CPSP.[29,30] The analgesic effect obtained with antidepressant agents is unrelated to its antidepressant effect. The analgesic effect is observed to occur with a shorter onset and at a lower dose. Amitriptyline has also been shown to potentiate the effect of morphine analgesia by a direct action on the central nervous system.[24] Anticonvulsant agents also may be effective in the treatment of central pain syndromes.[36] Phenytoin and carbamazepine probably exert their analgesic effect by inactivating sodium channels. Clonazepam and sodium valproate are thought to relieve pain through GABA-mediated inhibition.

Modulation of adrenergic systems may also be effective in the treatment of neurogenic pain. Clonidine, an α_2-adrenergic agonist, is thought to modulate 5-HT and NE release in the dorsal horn, thereby inhibiting pain transmission.[25]

Local anesthetic agents may also be tried. Intravenous lidocaine has been reported to be effective.[35] Similarly, oral mexiletine, a close structural analog of lidocaine, has been used in the treatment of thalamic pain syndrome.[20] The mechanism by which these drugs induce pain relief is unknown.

Transcutaneous electrical nerve stimulation (TENS) and percutaneous nerve stimulation have been used with some beneficial effect in nociceptive and neurogenic pain. The effects of TENS (either low or high frequency) are reported to be variable. In one study 20% of patients did achieve good and long-lasting relief. It has been suggested that the subset of persons with relatively normal touch or vibration sensibility may benefit most from such treatment.[31] The intensity of the stimulus and the frequency and waveform are also important variables that need to be considered.[34]

Despite these efforts to delineate the pathophysiology of central pain and to establish a more rational basis for the selection of treatment, only a minority of patients can be relieved of pain satisfactorily with presently available pharmacologic agents or conditioning stimulation therapies. In a recent monograph the author concluded that a majority of patients do not achieve effective relief.[32]

In most instances the treatment of chronic pain, of which CPSP is an example, requires a more total approach to the person and his and her environment.[38] Many patients believe that, if only the pain were removed, they would recover. The focus on pain relief and the use of various techniques for achieving relief support this notion. Unfortunately, in many persons the pain cannot be relieved. The pain is an impairment similar to the hemiplegia or the loss of sensation. The goal is to maintain life functions and to relieve the disabilities that have occurred as the result of these various impairments. In the case of CPSP the disabilities can be profound and can affect social and family roles and the patient's psychologic state. The goal must shift from focusing on the impairment (pain) to relieving the consequent disabilities of the pain.

The approach described here is a method by which the person and family members deal with the disabilities arising from the pain and regain their lives and the freedom to enter into their social roles despite the existence of the pain. The pain recedes into the background and ceases to be the focus of the person's life.

The following case report illustrates the application of the problem-solving and planning approach to the problem of CPSP. The process is one in which the person with pain establishes a goal relating to the disabilities. In this instance the disability was the patient's housebound situation. The goal was to "get out of the jail his house had become." The patient was able to state this more functional goal soon after the initial session; the wording is optimally that of the patient and becomes the focus rather than the pain itself. Once the overall goal has been established, the person can set short-term goals for each interim and log the times he met these goals. Eventually the patient should also be able to describe the methods used. In this case, although medication was used and appeared to the wife to be helpful, the patient consistently disagreed with her perception but agreed to continue his medication therapy.

CASE REPORT

D.C., a 54-year-old white male, had had non-insulin-dependent diabetes for the past 10 years. His hypertension was well controlled. The patient experienced a right carotid occlusion 4 years earlier. At the time a CT scan showed an infarct in the right temporal region. The patient had loss of sensation to pinprick, temporarily followed by tingling that began 10 weeks after the stroke. Pain began several weeks later. The pain was aching in quality, constant and located in the left axilla and breast. The pain sometimes intensified in this site and extended to the entire left side of the body (from the thorax to the arm to the leg). When this occurred, the patient felt nauseated. The pain changed in character, becoming more burning in quality and more intense. More severe pain began to occur as often as several times a day. The pain was precipitated by physical activity and emotional stress. The patient learned to control and eliminate anger and other stressors. However, he was limited in his ability to leave his house and occasionally could not get out of bed. When asked about any positive experiences during the recent past, he stated that he walked as much as

100 yards on one occasion to visit a neighbor and was able to converse with the neighbor for over an hour. He also was able to mow his lawn by using a riding mower. The neurologic examination demonstrated a reduction of sensation to pinprick and touch on the left side, with extinction of touch to simultaneous stimulation.

Initially the patient set several functional short-term goals; in particular, he wanted to be able to ride in a car so that he was not so uncomfortable "that I would feel I couldn't come here again." On the next visit several weeks later, he stated for the first time that his overall goal was to "get out of the house. I want to get out of the jail I have been in for the past 4 years." At that time he was able to get out of the house for several hours on rare occasions but needed about 48 hours of rest to recover sufficiently to go out again. He was able to specify his next goal for the short term: "to be able to get out of the house for at least an hour and for the subsequent pain to be below 4.5 on a scale of 1 to 10."

One month later he reported that he had made a 45-mile automobile ride that met his criteria and that he was able to go out 2 days consecutively. He set further short-term goals to get out of the house to visit his neighbor and to take an automobile trip to visit his son several hundred miles away. On a visit several weeks later, he reported that he was getting out of the house but that his subsequent pain was at an unacceptable level. The pain caused him to be nauseated and made him unable to sleep because of its severity. On subsequent visits he continued to report the times when he met his goal of leaving the house without a cost in pain of an intensity so excessive as to cause nausea.

At this time amitriptyline was prescribed to be taken at bedtime because sleeplessness was one consequence of his pain. The patient did not report improvement with up to 50 mg of amitriptyline. Although he slept better, he said he felt "drained." Next he was prescribed fluoxetine (20 mg in the AM). The following month he reported that nausea no longer was associated with pain. He described himself as doing more: He drove himself to the barbershop for the first time and went on an automobile trip.

At this time he addressed the question of "What worked?" His wife thought the medication was helpful. The patient stated, "I was looking for a miracle cure. I have learned to appreciate the strides I have made. I have been handling the pain much better." He went on to state that what had been most helpful was "becoming realistically aware that I have to learn to live with the pain and need to figure out what works so that I can manage the pain so that it does not control my life." His wife agreed that focusing on functional goals, rather than on the pain itself, was helpful.

The frequency of therapy visits was reduced. Two months later the patient reported that he had celebrated Thanksgiving and Christmas and had had lunch with his son. His wife stated that he had fewer outbursts of anger and was able to cope with his pain. In answer to a question about what worked, he stated that he had been finding "crutches." He found that it helped to sit on chairs that provided support. When riding in a car, it helped to use a pillow to support his left arm. He found himself finding ways to minimize the effects of the pain on his life. Two months later he described himself as going out each day. He went out to dinner and attended a seminar with a neighbor. At this time his goal was "to come and go when I want to."

Two months later the patient reported several breakthroughs toward his goal. He went to the library and gave his first dinner party since his stroke. He was able to parallel park when he went to the library, which necessitated turning his body. He had minimal pain, lasting 4 hours, after the dinner party. The patient stated, "What worked was that I told myself I was going to do it. I did it and it didn't hurt as much as I thought. Monitoring it helped. What also helped was my commitment to you that I was going to do it."

Six months later the patient reported that company visited him at his home at least once each Wednesday. He gave a wedding reception for his son. Driving in a car as much as 100 miles each day, he had travelled over 1200 miles to his son's wedding. At this time, he described that what worked for him was "accepting the pain better. I realize it is going to be there; that there is no magic antidote." He also commented on the process, stating that it was "setting goals and seeing progress; building on success gave me the incentive to explore further." Therapy sessions were reduced to an "as needed" basis, but the patient agreed to continue his use of fluoxetine.

Although results vary from patient to patient, the preceding approach to CPSP illustrates the overall importance of patient involvement in the planning process and a focus on the methods for solving problems.

REFERENCES

Stroke Prevention

1. Alberts MJ et al: Effects of public and professional education on reducing the delay in presentation and referral of stroke patients, *Stroke* 23:352, 1992.
2. Blackwell B: The drug regimen and treatment compliance. In Haynes RB, Taylor DW, Sackett DL, editors: *Compliance in health care,* Baltimore, 1979, Johns Hopkins University Press.
3. Blood Pressure Monitors, *Consumer Reports,* May 1992, p 295.
4. Dunbar DM, Marshall GD, Hovell MF: Behavioral strategies for improving compliance. In Haynes RB, Taylor DW, Sackett DL, editors: *Compliance in health care,* Baltimore, 1979, Johns Hopkins University Press.
5. Ozer MN: *The measurement of the efficacy of technology: a participatory process,* Washington, DC, 1987, Proceedings of 10th Annual Conference, Rehabilitation Engineering Society of North America, p 11.
6. Ozer MN: Planning with patients: a feedback loop engendering health. In Lasker GE, editor: *Applied systems and cybernetics,* vol 4, New York, 1981, Pergamon Press.
7. Sheinberg P: The biologic basis for the treatment of acute stroke, *Neurology* 41:1867, 1992.
8. Starfield B et al: The influence of patient-practitioner agreement on outcome of care, *Am J Public Health* 71:127, 1981.
9. Wardlaw JM, Warlow CP: Thrombolysis in acute ischemic stroke: does it work? *Stroke* 23:1826, 1992.

Management of Spasticity

10. Berger W, Horstmann G, Dietz V: Tension development and muscle activation in the leg during gait in spastic hemiparesis: independence of muscle hypertonia and exaggerated stretch reflexes, *J Neurol Neurosurg Psychiatry* 47:1029, 1984.
11. Das TK, Park DM: Effect of treatment with botulinum toxin on spasticity, *Postgrad Med J* 65:208, 1989.
12. Delwaide PJ: Electrophysiologic testing of spastic patients: its potential usefulness and limitations. In Delwaide PJ, Young RR, editors: *Clinical neurophysiology in spasticity,* Elsevier, 1985, Amsterdam.
13. Dietz V, Quintern J, Berger W: Electrophysiological studies of gait in spasticity and rigidity: evidence that altered mechanical properties contribute to hypertonia, *Brain* 104:431, 1981.
14. Milanov IG: Mechanisms of baclofen action on spasticity, *Acta Neurol Scand* 85:305, 1992.
15. Roper BA: The orthopedic management of the stroke patient, *Clin Orthop* 219:78, 1987.
16. Shahani BT, Young RF: Human flexor spasms. In Desmedt J, editor: *New developments in electromyography and clinical neurophysiology,* Basel, 1973, Karger.
17. Young RR: Physiologic and pharmacologic approaches to spasticity, *Neurol Clin* 5:529, 1987.
18. Young JL, Mayer RF: Physiological alterations of motor units in hemiplegia, *J Neurol Sci* 54:401, 1982.
19. Young RR, Weigner AW: Spasticity, *Clin Orthop* 219:50, 1987.

Central Poststroke Pain

20. Awerbuch G: Treatment of thalamic pain syndrome with mexiletine, *Ann Neurol* 28:233, 1990.
21. Basbaum AI, Fields HL: Endogenous pain control mechanisms: brain stem spinal pathways and endorphia circuitry, *Annu Rev Neurosci* 7:309, 1984.
22. Bogouslavsky J, Regli F, Uske R: Thalamic infarcts: clinical syndromes, etiology and prognosis, *Neurology* 38:837, 1988.
23. Bonica JJ: Semantic, epidemiologic and educational issues In Casey KL, editor: *Pain and central nervous system disease: the central pain syndromes,* New York, 1991, Raven Press.
24. Botney M, Fields HL: Amitriptyline potentiates morphine analgesia by a direct action on the central nervous system, *Ann Neurol* 13:160, 1983.
25. Glynn C, Dawson D, Sanders R: A double-blinded comparison between epidural morphine and epidural clonidine in patients with chronic cancer pain, *Pain* 34:123, 1988.
26. Hammond DL: Do opioids relieve central pain? In Casey KL, editor: *Pain and central nervous system disease: the central pain syndromes,* New York, 1991, Raven Press.
27. Leijon G, Bowie J, Johansson I: Central post-stroke pain: neurological symptoms and pain characteristics, *Pain* 36:13, 1989.
28. Leijon G, Bowie J, Johansson I: Central post-stroke pain: a study of the mechanisms through analysis of the sensory abnormalities, *Pain* 37:173, 1989.
29. Leijon G, Bowie J: Central post-stroke pain: a controlled trial of amitriptyline and carbamazepine, *Pain* 36:27, 1989.
30. Leijon G, Bowie J: Pharmacological treatment of central pain. In Casey KL, editor: *Pain and central nervous system disease: the central pain syndromes,* New York, 1991, Raven Press.
31. Leijon G, Bowie J: Central post-stroke pain: the effect of high and low frequency TENS, *Pain* 38:187, 1989.

32. Lindblom U: New direction for basic and clinical research in central pain syndromes. Casey KL, editor: *Pain and central nervous system disease: the central pain syndromes,* New York, 1991, Raven Press.

33. Melzack R, Wall PD, editors: *Textbook of pain,* New York, 1989, Churchill Livingstone.

34. Ng LKY, Liao SJ: Acupuncture: traditional and scientific prospectives. In Weiner RS, editor: *Innovations in pain management: a practical guide for clinicians,* Orlando, Fla, 1992, Paul M. Deutsch Press.

35. Peterson P et al: Chronic pain treatment with intravenous lidocaine, *Neurol Res* 8:189, 1986.

36. Swerdlow M: Anticonvulsants in the therapy of neuralgic pain, *The Pain Clinic* 1:9, 1986.

37. Tasker RR, de Carvalko G, Dostrovsky JO: History of central pain syndromes with observations concerning pathophysiology and treatment. In Casey KL, editor: *Pain and central nervous disease: the central pain syndromes,* New York, 1991, Raven Press.

38. Tunks E, Roy R, Bellissimo A: Synthesis and future directions. In Roy R, Tunks E, editors: *Chronic pain: psychosocial factors in rehabilitation,* Baltimore, 1982, Williams & Wilkins.

39. Zimmerman M: Central nervous mechanisms modulating pain related information: do they become deficient after lesions of the peripheral or central nervous system? In Casey KL, editor: *Pain and central nervous system disease: the central pain syndromes,* New York, 1991, Raven Press.

Community Resources

Organizations
Mail Order Catalogs
Technology-Related Assistance

Organizations*

The following is a list of organizations that may be of aid to persons with stroke and their caregivers.

American Association of Homes for the Aging
901 E Street, N.W., Suite 500
Washington, DC 20004
(202) 296-5960

American Association of Retired Persons
601 E. Street, N.W.
Washington, DC 20049
(202) 434-AARP
Health care information and publications such as caregiving, insurance, safety, and long-term care. Some available materials are audiotapes; videotapes in Spanish. Write for free catalog. No orders via phone.

The American Diabetes Association (ADA)
1660 Duke Street
Alexandria, VA 22314
Voluntary health organization supporting diabetes research and education. Array of services and materials for any age group. Contact local ADA in white pages or call 1(800) 232-3472.

American Foundation for the Blind
15 West 16th Street
New York, NY 10011
(800) 232-5463
(212) 620-2147 in New York

Products for people who are blind or visually impaired. Free catalog, *Products for People with vision problems.*

American Health Care Association (Nursing Homes)
1201 L Street, N.W.
Washington, DC 20005
(202) 842-4444

American Heart Association
7272 Greenville Avenue
Dallas, TX 75231
(214) 706-1220
Call for free newsletter. For information about stroke, contact your local American Heart Association.

American Occupational Therapy Association
1383 Piccard Drive
P.O. Box 1725
Rockville, MD 20849-1725
(301) 948-9626

American Physical Therapy Association
1111 North Fairfax Street
Alexandria, VA 22314
(703) 684-2782

American Printing House for the Blind, Inc.
P.O. Box 6085
Louisville, KY 40206-0085
(502) 895-2405
Produces products for the visually impaired: braille, large print, and talking books and magazines; educational and daily living aids. Free catalog and newsletter.

*This list is modified from that made available by the National Stroke Association.

American Speech-Language-Hearing Association
10801 Rockville Pike
Rockville, MD 20852
(800) 638-8255
Information on aphasia. Referral to speech-language pathologists in your area.

The Arthritis Foundation
P.O. Box 19000
Atlanta, GA 30326
(800) 283-7800
Information and referral, publications, support groups, local chapters. Guide to independent living for people with arthritis.

Bible Alliance, Inc.
P.O. Box 621
Bradenton, FL 34206
(813) 748-3031
Free service for those who cannot read conventional print because of a physical disability or visual impairment that prevents handling the printed material. The Bible on cassette, available in 33 languages, is given free of cost or obligation with proper verification of the impairment.

Children of Aging Parents
1609 Woodbourne Road
Woodbourne Office Campus
Suite 302-A
Levittown, PA 19057
(215) 945-6900

The Dole Foundation
For organizations seeking information about Dole Foundation grants, write or phone:
1819 H Street, N.W., Suite 850
Washington, DC 20006
(202) 457-0138
Publication. *Workplace Workbook: Illustrated Guide to Job Accommodations and Assistive Technology,* a book to assist employers making accommodations for workers with disabilities. Order through:

National Easter Seal Society
Publications Department
70 East Lake Street
Chicago, IL 60601
Cost: $32.00

Eastern Paralyzed Veterans Association
Barrier Free Design and Communication
75-20 Astoria Boulevard
Jackson Heights
New York, NY 11370-1178
(800) 803-0414
Free booklet on modifying existing house and new home for wheelchair accessibility.

Epilepsy Foundation of America (EFA)
4351 Garden City Drive
Landover, MD 20785
(301) 459-3700
(800) 332-1000
Information and referral. Printed materials. Physician referral legal advocacy. Free catalog.

Family Survival Project
425 Bush Street, Suite 500
San Francisco, CA 94108
(415) 434-3388
(800) 445-8106 in California only
Family support services for brain-impaired adults. Information and referral, fact sheets and printed materials available nationwide. Service program for California residents only.

Help for Incontinent People, Inc.
P.O. Box 8306
2375 E. Main Street, Suite A - 106
Spartanburg, SC 29035
(803) 579-7900
Help for Incontinent People (HIP) is a not-for-profit organization dedicated to improving the quality of people with incontinence. HIP is leading source of education, advocacy, and support to the public and to the health profession about the causes, prevention, diagnosis, treatments, and management alternatives for incontinence. Available are a quarterly newsletter (*The HIP Report*), a *Resource Guide of Continence Products and Services,* audiovisual programs, and educational leaflets.

IBM National Support Center for Persons with Disabilities
P.O. Box 2150
Atlanta, GA 30055
(800) 426-2133
(404) 238-4806 - TDD

Information on how computers can help people with vision, hearing, speech, learning, mental retardation, and mobility problems. Assistive devices, software, and services.

National Aphasia Association
Murray Hill Station
P.O. Box 1887
New York, NY 10156-0611
Information about aphasia: reading list, fact sheet, and newsletter.

National Association for Hispanic Elderly
(Formerly National Association for Spanish-Speaking Elderly)
2025 I Street, N.W., Suite 219
Washington, DC 20006
(202) 293-9329

National Association for Music Therapy
8455 Colesville Road, Suite 219
Silver Spring, MD 20910
(301) 589-3300
(301) 589-5175
Information and printed materials on the use of music therapy. Referral to music therapists in client's area.

National Association of Private Geriatric Care Managers
655 B. Alvemon Way, Suite 108
Tuscon, AZ 85711
(602) 881-8008

National Association for Sickle Cell, Inc.
3345 Wilshire Boulevard, Suite 1106
Los Angeles, CA 90010-1880
(800) 421-8453
Education material and information on sickle cell anemia. Have 65 chapters. Free newsletter.

National Council on the Aging, Inc.
409 Third Street, S.W.
Suite 100, West Wing
Washington, DC 20024
(202) 479-1200

Nation Council on Disability
800 Independence Avenue, S.W., Suite 814
Washington, DC 20591
(202) 267-3846
Federal agency developing policy for persons with disability.

National Digestive Diseases
Information Clearinghouse
Box NIDDIC
9000 Rockville Pike
Bethesda, MD 20892
(301) 468-6344
Provide information on products and services about digestive diseases and disorders.

National Easter Seal Society
70 East Lake Street
Chicago, IL 60601
(312) 726-6200
Agency dedicated to increasing the independence of adults and children with disabilities. Information and printed materials available.

National Hispanic Council on the Aging
2713 Ontario Road, N.W.
Washington, DC 20009
(202) 745-2521

National Information Center for Children and Youths with Handicaps
P.O. Box 1492
Washington, DC 20013
(703) 893-6061
(800) 999-5599

National Institute on Aging—Public Information Office
Federal Building, Room 6C12
Bethesda, MD 20892
(301) 496-1752

National Rehabilitation Association
1910 Association Drive
Reston, VA 22091-1502
(703) 715-9090

National Rehabilitation Information Center (NARIC)
8455 Colesville Road, Suite 935
Silver Spring, MD 20910-3319
(800) 34-NARIC (346-2742)
(301) 588-9284
Computer database for information on rehabilitation and health-related problems. Publications and materials available; library; mailing list rental.

National Self-Help Clearinghouse
Graduate School and University Center
of the City University of New York
25 West 43rd Street, Room 620
New York, NY 10036
(212) 642-2944

National Senior Citizens Law Center
1815 H Street, N.W., Suite 700
Washington, DC 20006
(202) 887-5280

National Stroke Association (NSA)
300 E. Hampden Avenue, Suite 240
Englewood, CO 80110-2654
1 (800) STROKES
NSA is the national voluntary health care
organization committed to stroke prevention,
treatment, rehabilitation, and support for
stroke survivors and their families. NSA
sponsors research; promotes the national
awareness of stroke warning signs and risks;
advocates reintegration of stroke survivors
into meaningful roles in society; provides
medical education to effect more rapid and
aggressive treatment; elevates awareness of
the effectiveness of rehabilitation; supports
and encourages stroke survivors and families;
and builds a national network of chapters to
expand on and concentrate national and local
resources in the fight against stroke. NSA
publishes and distributes a broad array of
information about stroke, including a newsletter for persons with stroke and their
families.

North American Riding for the
Handicapped, Inc.
P.O. Box 33150
Denver, CO 80233
(800) 369-RIDE
(303) 452-1212
Promotes the recovery of individuals with
disabilities through therapeutic horseback
riding.

Parent Care
Gerontology Center
4089 Dole
Human Development Center
University of Kansas
Lawrence, KS 66045
(913) 864-4130

Resources to assist family caregivers. Sample
copy of newsletter.

The President's Committee on Employment
of People with Disabilities
1331 F Street, N.W.
Washington, DC 20004-1107
(202) 376-6200 - Voice
(202) 376-6205 - TDD
Public and private partnership of national
and state organizations and individuals working to improve the lives of people with
disabilities. Information and referrals primarily with employment. Free monthly newsletter.

Rehabilitation Research and Training
Center for Brain Injury and Stroke
University of Washington
Department of Rehabilitation Medicine,
RJ-30
Seattle, WA 98195

The Simon Foundation for Continence
P.O. Box 835
Wilmette, IL 60091
(800) 238-4666–Patient information
(708) 864-3913–Foundation

Very Special Arts USA
Education Office
The John F. Kennedy Center for
Performing Arts
Washington, DC 20056
(800) 933-8721
(202) 7373-0645 - TDD
International opportunities in music, dance,
drama, literature, and the visual arts to
individuals with mental and physical challenges. Organizations in each state.

Visiting Nurse Associations of America
3801 E. Florida Avenue, Suite 206
Denver, CO 80210
(800) 426-2547
Information and referrals for home health
care service: speech, physical, and occupational therapies and general nursing. 426
organizations nationwide. Free brochure.

Mail Order Catalogs*

Many companies currently respond to the needs of persons with disabilities by offering mail and phone order services. For the consumer, this means greater ease, selection, and independence in shopping for often hard to find products. The following list is a sample of the many mail order catalogs available that carry products of interest to persons with disabilities. Catalogs were chosen from a wide range of companies, all of which sell directly to the consumer. For additional information about particular products from these catalogs, please contact the company directly.

Name: Ableware
Address: Maddak, Inc.
Pequannock, NJ 07440-1993
Catalog: Ableware: Independent Living from Maddak, Inc.
Specialty: Daily living aids, household
Cost: Free

Name: Access with Ease, Inc.
Address: P.O. Box 1150
Chino Valley, AZ 86323
Catalog: Access with Ease
Specialty: Daily living aids
Cost: Free

Name: AdaptAbility
Address: P.O. Box 515
Colchester, CT 06415-0515
Catalog: Adaptability
Specialty: Daily living aids
Cost: Free

*List produced by the Rehabilitation Engineering Center on the Evaluation of Assistive Technology, National Rehabilitation Hospital, Washington, DC.

Name: Aids Unlimited, Inc.
Address: Alternative Independence Devices & Services
1101 N. Calvert Street
Suite 405
Baltimore, MD 21202
Catalog: Aids Unlimited
Specialty: Daily living aids, household
Cost: Free

Name: American Foundation for the Blind
Address: Consumer Products
15 West 16th Street
New York, NY 10011
Catalog: Products for People with Vision Problems
Specialty: Household, games, visual aids
Cost: Free

Name: Ann Morris Enterprises, Inc.
Address: 26 Horseshoe Lane
Levittown, NY 11756
Catalog: Ann Morris
Specialty: Aids for the visually impaired and blind, household
Cost: Free

Name: Brookstone
Address: 5 Vose Farm Road
Peterborough, NH 03458
Catalog: Brookstone Homewares
Specialty: Daily living aids
Cost: Free

Name: Comfort Clothing
Address: Kingston, Inc.
21 Harvey Street
Kingston, Ontario K7K 5C1
Catalog: Comfort Clothing
Specialty: Women's clothing
Cost: Free

Name: Enrichments
Address: 145 Tower Drive
P.O. Box 579
Hinsdale, IL 60521
Catalog: Enrichments for Better Living
Specialty: Daily living aids, household, health
Cost: Free

Name: The Fuller Brush Company
Address: P.O. Box 1020
Rural Hall, NC 27098-1020
Catalog: Fuller Brush
Specialty: Household, daily living aids
Cost: Free

Name: Healthy Home
Address: 5844 Alessandro Avenue
Temple City, CA 91780
Catalog: Healthy Home
Specialty: Daily living aids
Cost: Free

Name: Hello Direct
Address: 140 Great Oaks Blvd.
San Jose, CA 95119
Catalog: Hello Direct
Specialty: Telephone, telecommunications
equipment, and accessories
Cost: Free

Name: Hold Everything
Address: Mail Order Department
P.O. Box 7807
San Francisco, CA 94120-7807
Catalog: Hold Everything
Specialty: Devices for storage, transport,
and holding
Cost: Free

Name: Irwin Taylor
Address: 80 Superior Road
Rochester, NY 14625
Catalog: Irwin Taylor
Specialty: Women's clothing
Cost: Free

Name: JC Penney Easy Wear Catalog
Address: Catalog Distribution Center
Atlanta, GA 30390-0370
Catalog: Ease Wear Catalog
Specialty: Clothing
Cost: $1.00

Name: LS&S Group, Inc.
Address: P.O. Box 673
Northbrook, IL 60065
Catalog: LS&S
Specialty: Household products for persons
with low vision
Cost: Free

Name: Mature Wisdom
Address: P.O. Box 28
Hanover, PA 17333-0028
Catalog: Mature Wisdom
Specialty: Daily living aids and innovative
household products
Cost: Free

Name: SelfCare Catalog
Address: P.O. Box 130
Mandeville, LA 70470-0130
Catalog: SelfCare Catalog
Specialty: Daily living aids and innovative
household products
Cost: Free

The publication *Mail Order Catalogs* is a product of the Request Program, a Rehabilitation Engineering Center at the National Rehabilitation Hospital. The focus of the Request Program is on evaluation of assistive technology. Results of the research conducted through this program are disseminated to persons with disabilities, clinicians, and third-party payors in an effort to educate these consumers to make informed, appropriate choices about assistive technology products. Implementation of the Request Program's objectives will result in the greater use of assistive technology, improved products and environments, and an increased market for products.

Mail Order Catalogs
Edited by: Brian M. Kemlage
Request Program
Rehabilitation Engineering Center
National Rehabilitation Hospital
102 Irving Street, N.W.
Washington, DC 20010-2949

Technology-Related Assistance*

The following is a listing of state programs funded under the National Institute on Disability and Rehabilitation Research (NIDRR) to provided assistive technology–service delivery to persons with disabilities. For further information, contact the program within your state. Further information is also available from the RESNA Technical Assistance Project in Washington, DC.

RESNA
Technology-Related Assistance Project
1101 Connecticut Avenue, N.W., Suite 700
Washington, DC 20036
(202) 857-1140 Voice/TDD

ALASKA
Assistive Technology Service
400 D Street, Suite 230
Anchorage, AK 99501
(907) 274-0138

ARKANSAS
Increasing Capabilities Access Network
(ICAN)
2201 Brookwood, Suite 117
Little Rock, AR 72202
(501) 666-8868

COLORADO
Colorado Assistive Technology Project
Rocky Mountain Resource and Training
Institute
6355 Ward Road, Suite 310
Arvada, CO 80004
(303) 420-2942

---

*List produced by the Rehabilitation Engineering Center on the Evaluation of Assistive Technology, National Rehabilitation Hospital, Washington, DC.

CONNECTICUT
Connecticut State
Department of Human Resources
Bureau of Rehabilitation Services
1049 Asylum Avenue
Hartford, CT 06105
(203) 566-3318

DELAWARE
Applied Science and Engineering
Laboratories
University of Delaware
A.I. duPont Institute
1600 Rockland Road
Wilmington, DE 19899
(302) 651-6834

FLORIDA
Florida Department of Labor and
Employment
Division of Vocational Rehabilitation
Bureau of Client Services
Rehabilitation Engineering Technology
1709-A Mahan Drive
Tallahassee, FL 32399-0696
(904) 488-6210

GEORGIA
Georgia Assistive Technology Program
Division of Rehabilitation Services
878 Peachtree Street, N.E., Room 702
Atlanta, GA 30309
(404) 894-7593

HAWAII
Hawaii Assistive Technology System
(HATS)
100 Bishop Street, Suite 302
Honolulu, HI 96813
(808) 521-8489

IDAHO
Idaho State Program for Technology-Related Assistance for People with Disabilities
University of Idaho
Idaho Center on Developmental Disabilities
Professional Building
129 W. Third Street
Moscow Latah, ID 83843
(208) 885-6849

ILLINOIS
Illinois Technology-Related Assistance
Project
411 East Adams
Springfield, IL 62701
(217) 785-7091

INDIANA
Accessing Technology Through Awareness
in Indiana (ATTAIN)
Department of Human Services
Office of Vocational Rehabilitation Services
Technical Assistance Unit
150 W. Market Street, P.O. Box 7083
Indianapolis, IN 46207-7083
(317) 233-3394

IOWA
Technology-Related Assistance for
Individuals with Disabilities
University of Iowa
Division of Developmental Disabilities
Iowa City, IA 52242
(319) 353-6386

KENTUCKY
The Kentucky Assistive Technology
Network (KATS)
Coordinating Center at Kentucky
Department for the Blind
427 Versailles Road
Frankfort, KY 40601
(502) 564-4665

LOUISIANA
Louisiana Assistive Technology Project
P.O. Box 3455
Baton Rouge, LA 70821-3455
(504) 342-6804 Voice/TDD

MAINE
Maine CITE
Maine CITE Coordinating Center
University of Maine at Augusta
University Heights
Augusta, ME 04330
(207) 621-3195

MARYLAND
Maryland Assistive Technology Project
Governor's Office for Handicapped
Individuals
300 W. Lexington Street
Box 10
Baltimore, MD 21201
(301) 333-3098

MASSACHUSETTS
MATP Center
Gardner 529
Children's Hospital
300 Longwood Avenue
Boston, MA 02116
(617) 735-7820 (Voice)
(617) 735-7301 (TDD)

MICHIGAN
Michigan Department of Education
Rehabilitation Services
P.O. Box 30010
Lansing, MI 48909
(517) 373-3391

MINNESOTA
A System of Technology to Receive Results
(STAR)
Governor's Advisory Council on
Technology for People with Disabilities
300 Centennial Building
685 Cedar Street
St. Paul, MN 55155
(612) 297-1554

MISSISSIPPI
Division of Rehabilitation Service
Project START (Success Through Assistive/
Rehabilitative Technology)
P.O. Box 1698
Jackson, MS 39215-1698
(601) 354-6891

MISSOURI
Missouri Assistive Technology Project
UMKC, School of Education
5100 Rockhill Road
Kansas City, MO 64110
(816) 235-5337

MONTANA
MonTech
Rural Institute on Disabilities
The University of Montana
52 Corbin Hall
Missoula, MT 59812
(406) 243-4597

NEBRASKA
Nebraska Assistive Technology Project
301 Centennial South
P.O. Box 94987
Lincoln, NE 68509
(402) 471-0735 Voice/TDD

NEVADA
Assistive Technology Services, Advocacy,
and Systems Change
Rehabilitation Division, PRPD
505 East King Street, Room 501
Carson City, NV 89701
(702) 687-4452 Voice/TDD

NEW HAMPSHIRE
New Hampshire Technology Partnership
Project
Institute on Disability
14 Ten Ferry Street
The Concord Center
Concord, NH 03301
(603) 224-0630

NEW JERSEY
New Jersey Department of Labor
Office of the Commissioner
Labor Building, CN 110
Trenton, NJ 08625
(609) 984-6550

NEW MEXICO
New Mexico Technology Related
Assistance Project (NMTAP)
State Department of Education
Division of Vocational Rehabilitation
604 W. San Mateo
Santa Fe, NM 87503
(505) 827-3533 Voice/TDD

NEW YORK
New York State Office of Advocates for
the Disabled
TRAID Project
One Empire State Plaza, Tenth Floor
Albany, NY 12223-0001
(518) 474-2825 (Voice)
(518) 473-4231 (TDD)

NORTH CAROLINA
North Carolina Assistive Technology
Project
Department of Human Resources
Division of Vocational Rehabilitation
Services
1110 Navaho Drive, Suite 101
Raleigh, NC 27609
(919) 850-2787 Voice/TDD

OHIO
Ohio Rehabilitation Services Commission
Division of Public Affairs
400 E. Campus View Boulevard
Columbus, OH 43235-4604
(614) 438-1236

OKLAHOMA
Oklahoma Dept. of Human Services
Rehabilitation Services Division
DHS, RS #24
P.O. Box 25352
Oklahoma City, OK 73125
(405) 424-4311

OREGON
Technology Access for Life Needs (TALN)
Department of Human Resources
Vocational Rehabilitation Division
2045 Silverton Road, N.E.
Salem, OR 97310
(503) 378-3830 Ext. 386

PENNSYLVANIA
Pennsylvania's Initiative on Assistive
Technology (PIAT)
Temple University
Institute on Disability/UAP
13th St. & Cecil B. Moore Avenue
Philadelphia, PA 19122
(215) 787-1356

SOUTH CAROLINA
South Carolina Assistive Technology
Program
Vocational Rehabilitation Department
P.O. Box 15
1410-C Boston Avenue
West Columbia, SC 29171-0015
(803) 822-5362 Voice/TDD

SOUTH DAKOTA
South Dakota Dept. of Human Services
Division of Rehabilitation Services
Kneip Building
700 Governors Drive
Pierre, SD 57501
(605) 773-3195

TENNESSEE
Tennessee Technology Access Project
(TTAP)
Developmental Disabilities Council
Department of Mental Health and Mental
Retardation
Doctors' Building, Suite 300
706 Church Street
Nashville, TN 37243-0675
(615)741-7441

TEXAS
The University of Texas at Austin UAP of
Texas
Department of Special Education
P.O. Box 7726
Austin, TX 78713-7726
(512) 471-7621

UTAH
Utah State Program for Technology-
Related Assistance for Individuals with
Disabilities
Utah State University
Developmental Center for Handicapped
Persons
UMC 6855
Logan, UT 84322-6800
(801) 750-1982

VERMONT
Assistive Technology Development Grant
Department of Aging and Disabilities
Agency for Human Services
103 South Main Street
Weeks Building, First Floor
Waterbury, VT 05671-2350
(802) 241-2620 Voice/TDD

VIRGINIA
Virginia Assistive Technology System
(VATS)
Department of Rehabilitative Services
Office of Planning
4901 Fitzhugh Avenue
P.O. Box 11045
Richmond, VA 23230
(804) 367-2445

WEST VIRGINIA
West Virginia Assistive Technology System
Division of Rehabilitation Services
Capital Complex
Charleston, WV 25301
(304) 766-4698

WISCONSIN
WisTech
Division of Vocational Rehabilitation
P.O. Box 7852
1 W. Wilson Street, Room 950
Madison, WI 53707
(608) 267-6720 (Voice)
(608) 266-9599 (TDD)

Index

A

Abulia, 107
ACA strokes; *see* Anterior cerebral artery strokes
Accommodation, reasonable, Americans with Disabilities Act of 1990 and, 441-442
Achromatopsia, 105
Acquired disorders of written language, 95-97
Active range of motion (AROM), activities of daily living and, 351-352
Activities of daily living (ADL)
    active range of motion and, 351-352
    activity analysis and, 350-351, 352
    adaptive equipment and, 360-361
    assessment of, 349-356
    cognition and, 354
    communication deficits and, 348
    compensatory strategies and, 359-360
    definition of, 347
    dressing and, 363
    driving assessment and, 355
    environmental adaptation and, 361
    equipment assessment and, 355
    feeding and, 361-363
    goal setting and treatment planning and, 356-359
    grooming and hygiene and, 363-364
    home care and, 366
    home evaluation and, 355
    home management and, 365-367
    instrumental, 416, 417
    meal preparation and, 366
    perception and, 354-355
    retraining of performance skills and, 359
    role changes and, 347
    sensorimotor components and, 351-354
    training in, in rehabilitation management, 346-367
    treatment applications and, 359-367
    visuoperceptual deficits and, 348
    work evaluation and, 355-356
Activity analysis, activities of daily living and, 350-351, 352
Activity Pattern Indicators portion of Rehabilitation Indicators Project, 434
Acute care phase, 12, 14, 27-142
Acute medical care setting, types of patient behavior reinforced in, 242
ADA; *see* American Diabetes Association
ADAAG; *see* Americans with Disabilities Act Accessibility Guidelines

Adaptive equipment, activities of daily living and, 360-361
Adjustment disorder, depression as, 236
ADL; *see* Activities of daily living
Adult neurogenic communication disorders following stroke, decision tree for, 285, 286-287
Age, rationing of health care on basis of, 116
Aging
  dysphagia and, 316-317
  normal, 220-225
    cognitive factors and, 222-224
    neuropsychologic aspects of, and stroke rehabilitation, 219-250
      behavioral and psychologic adjustment to stroke and, 233-245
      facilitating adaptation and new learning in, 245-250
      neurobehavioral syndromes and, 225-233
    personality factors and, 220-221
    psychosocial factors and, 221-222
Agnosia, 287, 291
  after left cerebrovascular accident, 283
  auditory, 291
  definition of, 284
  tactile, 291
  visual, 291
Agraphia, 96
  alexia with, 96
  apraxic, 96
  fluent, 97
Alcoholic Korsakoff's syndrome, procedural memory and, 247
Alexia, 95, 96
Alzheimer's disease, neurobehavioral syndromes and, 228, 232
Alzheimer's Disease and Related Disorders Association, 307
Ambulation, 379, 380, 382-383
Ambulatory cardiac rhythm monitoring in detection of arrhythmias, 80
American Association of Homes for the Aging, 471
American Association of Retired Persons, 471
American Diabetes Association (ADA), 471
American Foundation for the Blind, 471
American Health Association, 186
American Health Care Association, 471
American Heart Association, 281, 307-308, 384, 387, 388, 389, 471
American Occupational Therapy Association, 471
American Physical Therapy Association, 471
American Printing House for the Blind, Inc., 471
American Psychiatric Association, 235
American Speech-Language-Hearing Association, 307, 472
Americans with Disabilities Act Accessibility Guidelines (ADAAG), 444
Americans with Disabilities Act of 1990, 401, 437, 441-445
Amer-Ind Code, Broca's aphasia and, 302
Amitriptyline in treatment of central poststroke pain, 465
Amnesia
  abnormalities of temporooccipital lobes and, 106-107
  retrograde, 106
Amphetamines, 83, 91
Amtrak, Americans with Disabilities Act of 1990 and, 442
Amyloid angiography, 66
Analgesics, nonsteroidal, 127

Aneurysm, 78, 83
  rebleeding from, hypertension and, 84
  rupture of, 63
Angiography in evaluation of stroke patient, 80, 82
Angioma, 83
Ankle equinus, development of, 387
Ankle-foot orthosis, 395-396
  flail ankle and, 393
  hemiplegic gait correction using, 393-394
  timing of removal of, 400
Anomic aphasia, 95, 96, 285, 289
Anosognosia, 100, 229-231, 237
  attention allocation processes in, 230
  left neglect and, 230-231
Anterior cerebral artery (ACA) strokes, neurobehavioral syndromes and, 229
Antiadrenergic medications, adverse effect of, on sexuality, 428
Anticholinergic medications, 49
  adverse effect of, on sexuality, 428
  dysphagia and, 317
Anticipatory phase of dysphagia, 313-314, 325
Anticoagulant medications
  dietary sources of vitamin K and, 452, 453
  in prevention of recurrent stroke, 164, 180, 450, 451-452
  in treatment of deep vein thrombosis, 40, 42
  in treatment of occlusive thrombus, 87
  in treatment of "red" fibrin-erythrocyte thrombi, 87
Anticonvulsant agents in treatment of central poststroke pain, 465
Antidepressant medications, 128
  adverse effect of, on sexuality, 428
  dysphagia and, 317
  in treatment of central poststroke pain, 465
  in treatment of poststroke depression, 239
Antiepileptic drugs (AEDs), 50, 51-57
Antihistamines, dysphagia and, 317
Antihypertensive medications, 84, 91
  dysphagia and, 317
  in prevention of recurrent stroke, 172, 176-179
Antiplatelet medications in prevention of recurrent stroke, 164
Antispasticity pattern, 129
Anton's syndrome, 229
Anxiety disorders, normal aging and, 221-222
AOS; *see* Apraxia of speech
Aphasia, 92-95, 246, 285-290
  after left cerebrovascular accident, 283
  alexia and, 95
  anomic, 95, 96, 285, 289
  apraxia and, 97
  Broca's; *see* Broca's aphasia
  caused by left hemisphere lesions, 228
  classification system for, 285
  comprehension and, 285, 289
  conduction, 94, 96-97, 101
  definition of, 284
  expressive, 348

Aphasia—cont'd
  fluent; *see* Fluent aphasia
  global, 93, 94, 96
  jargon and, 289
  literal paraphasias and, 289
  neologistic jargon and, 289
  nonfluent, 92-94, 285
  phonemic paraphasias and, 289
  prognostic variables important to, and related neurogenic communication disorders following stroke,
     295, 297
  receptive, 348
  repetition and, 285-289
  semantic paraphasias and, 289
  syndrome approach to, 285, 288, 289
  transcortical motor, 93
  transcortical sensory, 95
  verbal paraphasias and, 289
  Wernicke's; *see* Wernicke's aphasia
Aphasia syndrome decision tree, 285, 288, 289
Apraxia
  after left cerebrovascular accident, 283
  constructional, 102-104
  difficulty in executing movement pattern and, 355
  dressing, 363
  ideational, 97
  ideomotor, 97
  limb-kinetic, 97
  of speech (AOS), 287, 290-291
    versus Broca's aphasia, 290
    definition of, 284
    versus dysarthria, 291-292
    versus Wernicke's aphasia, 290
  tests for, 97
  truncal, 97
Apraxic agraphia, 96
Archicortex, phylogenetic levels of, 334
Arm function tests, 121
"Army-tuck" tight sheets, avoidance of, 387
AROM; *see* Active range of motion
Arteries, thickening of walls of, 66
Arteriovenous malformation (AVM), 78
Arthritis Foundation, 472
Aspiration pneumonia, dysphagia and, 327
Aspirin
  in treatment of occlusive thrombus, 87
  in treatment of "white" platelet-fibrin thrombi, 87
  versus warfarin, 180
Assistive technology, appropriate, selection of, 437-441
Ataxia, 109
Atheromatous plaque, 66
Atherosclerosis, neurobehavioral syndromes and, 228
Atherothrombotic infarction, 3
Atrial fibrillation, brain embolism and, 80
Attention allocation processes in anosognosia, 230
Auditory agnosia, 291

Auxiliary aids, Americans with Disabilities Act of 1990 and, 443
AVM; *see* Arteriovenous malformation
Axillary crutches, 398-399

B
Babinski's syndrome, 229
Baby Broca's aphasia, 93-94
Baclofen
  H reflex and, 460
  in treatment of spasticity, 461
BAFPE; *see* Bay Area Functional Performance Evaluation
Balance
  in analysis of gait, 374
  assessment of, 373-374
  single-limb, 381
  sitting, 340, 373, 395
  standing, 395
Balint's syndrome, 95, 105-106
Barbiturates to reduce energy needs of brain, 88
Barthel Index, 16, 32, 122, 132, 133, 137, 204, 205, 339, 356, 373, 417
Bath, transfers from, 399
Bathing, difficulties in, 364, 365
Bathroom accessibility, 364, 399-400
Bay Area Functional Performance Evaluation (BAFPE), 354
Bed, transfers from, 211-212, 382, 399
Bedside commode, 364
Behavior, problem, in rehabilitation setting, 245
Behavioral adjustment to stroke, 233-245
Behavioral changes, abnormalities of temporooccipital lobes and, 107
Behavioral disturbances, regression as model for, 240-241
Behavioral units of motor action, 333, 334
Benzodiazepines, 91, 460
Bible Alliance, Inc., 472
Bile acid sequestrants in treatment of hyperlipidemia, 190
Biofeedback, electromyography, training in sensory substitution and, 341-345
Blacks, prevention of recurrent stroke and, 165-166
Bladder function
  disturbances in, 30
  monitoring and retraining of, during in-bed phase of stroke rehabilitation, 388
Bladder management, 43-49
Bladder outlet obstruction, 48
Blindness, cortical, 105
Blood, in cerebrospinal fluid, complications of, 83
Blood tests in evaluation of stroke, 78-79, 82
Bobath method, 344, 392
Bobath sling, 127
Body language, 101
Body schema, disturbances in, 355
Boston Diagnostic Aphasia Examination, 285
Botulinus toxin in treatment of spasticity, 461
Bowel function monitoring and retraining during in-bed phase of stroke rehabilitation, 388, 389
Bowel impaction and ileus during in-bed phase of stroke rehabilitation, 389
Bradycardia, 161-162
Brake handle, extended, for wheelchair, 391
Broca's aphasia, 93-94, 95, 96, 285

Broca's aphasia—cont'd
  Amer-Ind Code and, 302
  versus apraxia of speech, 290
  baby, 93-94
  neurobehavioral syndromes and, 228-229
Brunnstrom six-stage motor recovery scale, 117, 339, 392
Burden of care, 206

C

CAD; *see* Coronary artery disease
Calcium antagonists, 49
Calcium channel-blocking agents
  in treatment of hypercholesterolemia, 182
  in treatment of vasoconstriction, 84
Canadian Neurological Scale, 32
Cane in step-out phase of stroke rehabilitation, 399
Car, transfers from, 399
Carbamazepine, 54, 55, 56, 465
Cardiac disease, 30, 33-34
  management of
    in prevention of recurrent stroke, 166, 180-192
    in rehabilitative care phase, 157-162
Cardiac failure, mortality from, 32
Cardiac testing in evaluation of stroke patient, 80
Cardiovascular disease, 2-6, 32
Care, burden of, 206
Caregiver, role overload and, 426
Caregiver anxiety, 259, 272
Caregiver Education Program, 266, 271
Caregiver potential in psychosocial assessment for continued care planning, 259-260, 261
Caregiving, effect of, on family, 425-426
CARF; *see* Commission on Accreditation of Rehabilitation Facilities
Carotid artery disease, 33-34
Carpal tunnel syndrome, use of cane and, 399
Case fatality rate (CFR), 3, 4
Case history, dysphagia and, 319
CCT; *see* Central conduction time
CE; *see* Cerebral embolism
CEA; *see* Cost-effectiveness analysis
Central conduction time (CCT), 338-339
Central poststroke pain (CPSP)
  definition of, 463
  ensuring continuity of medical care and, 463-468
  treatment of, 465-468
Cerebral embolism (CE), 3
Cerebrospinal fluid, blood in, complications of, 83
Cerebrovascular accident (CVA); *see* Stroke
Cerebrovascular disease
  leading to stroke, 2-6
  program for rehabilitation of patients with, and associated cardiovascular disease, 158, 159
CFR; *see* Case fatality rate
Chair, transfers from, 211-212, 382, 399
Change in body image, effect of, on stroke survivor, 424
CHART; *see* Craig Handicap Assessment and Reporting Technique (CHART)
Chicago Stroke Study, 174

Chief complaint in interview, 20
Children of Aging Parents, 472
Choking episodes, 313
Cholesterol, elevated levels of, management of, in prevention of recurrent stroke, 5, 182-190
Cholestyramine in treatment of hyperlipidemia, 190
Cigarette smoking, prevention of recurrent stroke and, 5, 6, 166, 180-182
Clasp knife, 369
Clonazepam in treatment of central poststroke pain, 465
Clonidine, 91
   in treatment of central poststroke pain, 465
   in treatment of hypertension, 178
Coaching, communication disorders and, 305-307
Cocaine
   prevention of recurrent stroke and, 166
   subarachnoid hemorrhage and, 83
Cognition, activities of daily living and, 354
Cognitive communication disorders, poststroke, 295, 296
Cognitive decline, normal aging and, 224
Cognitive factors, normal aging and, 222-224
Collaboration in planning process, 22, 24, 25
Commission on Accreditation of Rehabilitation Facilities (CARF), 198, 212
Communication
   functional, 282-285
   gestures used in, 213
   during in-bed phase of stroke rehabilitation, 388
   nonlinguistic, 101
Communication assessment, functional, 283-285
Communication care plan, interdisciplinary, establishment of, 301
Communication deficit
   adverse effect of, on sexuality, 428, 429
   effect of, on family, 423
Communication disorders, 281-310
   activities of daily living and, 348
   adult neurogenic, following stroke, decision tree for, 285, 286-287
   assessment of left cerebrovascular accidents in, 283-292
   coaching and, 305-307
   comprehensive assessment and diagnostic therapy and, 295-299
   comprehensive assessment of, 297
   continuous quality improvement and, 308-310
   definition of, 282
   development of treatment plan for, 299-304
   multiple-infarct dementia and, 294-295
   nature and extent of problem in, 281-283
   neurogenic, poststroke, prognostic variables important to aphasia and, 295, 297
   patient education and, 307-308
   philosophy and implementation of treatment of, 304-310
   in rehabilitation management, 281-310
   right hemisphere; *see* Right hemisphere communication impairment
Communication Effectiveness Index, 302
Community ambulators, 381
Community integration, enhancement of, 433-445
Community reentry group in preparation of family for discharge, 267-268
Community resources for persons with stroke and their caregivers, 471-480
Comorbidity, 32-34
Compensatory strategies, 24-25, 197

Compensatory strategies—cont'd
 activities of daily living and, 359-360
 feeding and, 362
Compliance, quality of interaction between client and professional and, 450
Comprehension, aphasia and, 285, 289
Comprehensive assessment of poststroke communication disorders, 297
Comprehensive inpatient rehabilitation, 199
Comprehensive program, multistep, for stroke recovery, 381-384
Compression stockings, deep vein thrombosis and, 39
Computed tomography (CT) in evaluation of stroke, 77-78
Conduction aphasia, 94, 95, 96-97, 101
Confusional states, acute, neurobehavioral syndromes and, 232-233
Constructional apraxia, 102-104
Continuing care phase, 12, 413-470
 enhancing quality of life in, 416-447
 ensuring continuity of medical care in, 448-470
Continuous quality improvement, communication disorders and, 308-310
Coordination
 assessment of, 353
 of planning process, 25
Coronary angiography in evaluation of stroke patient, 80, 82
Coronary artery disease (CAD), 33-34
Cortical blindness, 105, 229
Cortical deafness, 95
Corticosteroids, 90, 127
Cost-effectiveness analysis (CEA), application of, to health care, 42
Courage Stroke Network, 308
CPSP; *see* Central poststroke pain
Craig Handicap Assessment and Reporting Technique (CHART), 435
Craig Rehabilitation Center, 434
Crutches, axillary, 398-399
Crystallized intelligence, normal aging and, 224
CT; *see* Computed tomography
Cultural information, assessment of, in psychosocial assessment for continued care planning, 257
Curbs, negotiating, with wheelchair, 401-402
CVA; *see* Cerebrovascular accident
Cybex UBE, 397

D

DA; *see* Dopamine agonists
Daily living skills (DLS), assessment of, 302
Daily log, communication disorders and, 308-310
Day pass assignments in preparation of family for discharge, 267
Deafness, cortical, 95
Decubitus ulcers, protection of patient's skin from, 386
Deep vein thrombosis (DVT), 30, 34-43
 in calf, 40
 identification of, 36-38
 prevention of, 38-40
 in thigh, 40
Defective visual perception, 95
Delay in seeking treatment for stroke, 455-458
Delirium, neurobehavioral syndromes and, 232-233
Dementia, 287
 definition of, 284

Dementia — cont'd
  of depression, normal aging and, 222
  multiple-infarct; *see* Multiple-infarct dementia
  preexisting, neurobehavioral syndromes and, 228
  subcortical, neurobehavioral syndromes and, 232
Dementia syndrome with marked cognitive impairment, depression and, 237
Demographic factors, stroke mechanisms and, 69-70
Denial of illness, right hemisphere neurobehavioral syndromes and, 229-231
Denial syndrome versus lability of laughter, 232
Depression
  base rate of, 238
  caregiver anxiety and, 259
  definition of, 235
  dementia of, normal aging and, 222
  dementia syndrome with marked cognitive impairment, 237
  dexamethasone suppression test and, 238
  versus emotional lability, 236-237
  versus mood disturbance, 236
  neurochemical marker of, 238
  normal aging and, 221-222
  poststroke, 235-241, 424, 428
  pseudobulbar lability of tears versus, 232
  during step-out phase of stroke rehabilitation, 401
Depressive crisis, 241
Depth perception, assessment of, 354
Desk arms for wheelchair, 391-392
Detrusor hyperreflexia, 47
Detrusor sphincter dyssynergy, 47
Devolution, prevention of recurrent stroke and, 171
Dexamethasone suppression test (DST), depression and, 238
Diabetes, 5, 6, 30, 32, 33
  management of, in rehabilitation care phase, 147-157
  neurobehavioral syndromes and, 228
  prevention of recurrent stroke and, 165
Diagnostic and Statistic Manual of Mental Disorders (DSM-III-R), 235
Diary, daily, communication disorders and, 308-310
Diaschisis, 14, 90, 226-227
Diazepam
  H reflex and, 460
  in treatment of spasticity, 461
Dicyclomine hydrochloride, 49
Diet modifications to lower blood cholesterol levels, 186, 187-188, 190, 191
Diplopia, 109
Disability
  versus impairment, 11
  World Health Organization's model of consequences of pathology and, 299, 300
Discharge
  and patient's right to self-determination, 252-253
  preparation of family for, 251-273
Disconnection syndromes, neurobehavioral syndromes and, 227
Disease versus illness, 19-20
Disuse muscle atrophy during in-bed phase of stroke rehabilitation, 388
Diuretics, dysphagia and, 317
Dizziness, 109
DLS; *see* Daily living skills

Dole Foundation, 472
Dopamine agonists (DA), 91
Dressing
  activities of daily living and, 363
  lower extremity techniques of, 364
  one-handed, 363
Dressing apraxia, 363
Driving, assessment of, 355, 400
DSM-III-R; *see* Diagnostic and Statistic Manual of Mental Disorders
DST; *see* Dexamethasone suppression test
Dual admission of older adult into hospital, 243
DVT; *see* Deep vein thrombosis
Dysarthria, 108, 287, 291-292
  after left cerebrovascular accident, 283
  versus apraxia of speech, 291-292
  classification of, 292
  definition of, 284
Dyslexia, 95
Dysphagia, 30, 109
  acute phase concerns and, 321-323
  aging and, 316-317
  anticipatory phase of, 313-314, 325
  aspiration pneumonia and, 327
  assessment of, 318-321
  case history and, 319
  characteristics of, in stroke population, 313-323
  clinical evaluation of, 318-320
  clinical manifestations of, 313-315
  clinical swallowing examination and, 320
  continuing care issues and, 329-332
  course of recovery of, 315-316
  esophageal phase of, 315, 329
  goal setting and, 323-324
  head-turning and head-tilting postural adjustments and, 327-329
  jejunostomy and, 323
  management of, 310-332
  medications and, 317
  Mendelsohn maneuver and, 327, 329
  neuropathology of, 313
  nonoral feeding alternatives and, 322-323
  oral phase of, 315, 326
  oral preparatory phase of, 314-315, 325-326
  oral prosthesis and, 327
  palatal training appliance and, 327
  percutaneous endoscopic gastrostomy and, 322-323
  pharyngeal phase of, 315, 316, 317, 326-329
  physical examination and, 319-320
  pocketing of residual food substances and, 325-326
  in rehabilitation phase, 323-329
  screening for, 318
  specialized diagnostic procedures and, 320-321
  supraglottic swallow and, 327
  surgical gastrostomy and, 322-323
  texture modification and, 322
  therapy techniques and, 324-329

Dysphagia — cont'd
  tracheostomy tubes and, 318
  videofluoroscopy and, 321
Dyspraxia, orofacial, 97
Dysprosody, 93, 94, 100-101, 392
Dyssynergy, true, 48

E

Easter Seal Society, 307-308
Eastern Paralyzed Veterans Association, 472
Echocardiography in evaluation of stroke patient, 80
EFA; *see* Epilepsy Foundation of America
Elastic shoelaces, 363
Electrical stimulation, functional, 343-344
Electromyography (EMG) biofeedback, training in sensory substitution and, 341-345
Electromyography (EMG) sensory feedback, 341-345
Elementary dysfunctions, 107-109
Embolism, 71, 75-77
  cerebral, 3
  definition of, 65-66
  paradoxic, 66
  pulmonary, 32, 34-43
Embolus, 66, 67
EMG biofeedback; *see* Electromyography biofeedback
EMG sensory feedback; *see* Electromyography sensory feedback
EMG-biofeedback–triggered functional electrical stimulation, 392, 395, 401
EMG-stim, 344
Emotional lability versus depression, 236-237
Emotional smile versus voluntary smile, 335
Empowerment, patient's, principle of, 26
Endogenous opioid peptides, central modulation of pain and, 465
Environmental adaptation, activities of daily living and, 361
Environmental impact statement, communication disorders and, 301
Environmental resources, assessment of, in psychosocial assessment for continued care planning, 258-
    259, 261
Ephedrine in treatment of low blood pressure, 88
Epilepsy Foundation of America (EFA), 472
Epinephrine, 156
Equinovarus of involved foot after stroke treated surgically, 462-463
Equipment, assessment of, activities of daily living and, 355
Ergometer, upper extremity, 397
Erikson's theory of human development, normal aging and, 220-221
Esophageal phase
  of dysphagia, 315, 329
  of swallowing, 311, 312, 313
Ethnic differences, prevention of recurrent stroke and, 165-166
Euphoria, organic, versus lability of laughter, 232
Everett crutch, 398-399
Evolving lesions, neurobehavioral syndromes and, 226-227
Excitotoxic injury, 89
Exercise
  program of, for patients with cardiac disease and brain injury, 151-152
  range-of-motion; *see* Range-of-motion exercises
  relationship between metabolic response and, diabetes and, 153-157
  stand-up–step-up, during stand-up phase of stroke rehabilitation, 394-395

Exeter Dysphagia Assessment Technique, 320-321
Expert Panel of the National Cholesterol Education Program, 184
Expressive aphasia, 348
Extinction, 99
Extralinguistic communication deficits, right hemisphere communication impairment and, 292-293

F

F response, 461
Facial weakness, 109
Fair assist, definition of, 123
Family
    active participation of, in continued care planning process, 253-254
    definition of, 252
    effect of communication deficit on, 423
    effect of poststroke depression on, 424
    effect of role changes on, 427
    emotional unit of, information about, in psychosocial assessment for continued care planning, 259, 261
    health and nutrition education for, in preparation for discharge, 267
    participation of, in planning patient care, 209
    preparation of, for discharge, 251-273
    programmatic interventions to prepare, for discharge, 266-271
Family conference in preparation for discharge, 268
Family counseling in preparation of family for discharge, 270-271
Family life, enhancement of, 421-433
    functional issues in, 422-424
    psychosocial issues in, 424-427
    sexuality in, 427-433
Family support groups for preparation of families for discharge, 267
Family Survival Project, 472
Family training for preparation discharge, 267
Family-oriented interdisciplinary goals, 269
Feeding
    activities of daily living and, 361-363
    assessment of, during in-bed phase of stroke rehabilitation, 387-388
    nonoral alternatives to, dysphagia and, 322-323
FES; *see* Functional electrical stimulation
Fibromuscular dysplasia, 66
Figure ground, assessment of, 354
FIM; *see* Functional Independence Measure
Flaccidity, 353
Flail ankle, ankle-foot orthosis and, 393
Flavoxate hydrochloride, 49
Flexion contractures, development of, 387
Fluent agraphia, 97
Fluent aphasia, 92-94, 285, 289
Fluid intelligence, normal aging and, 224
FMA; *see* Fugl-Meyer Assessment
Focal brain ischemia, 27, 65-66
Footboard device, prevention of equinus development and, 387
"Footprint," standing pivot transfer and, 398
Form constancy, assessment of, 354
Forward progression in analysis of gait, 374, 375
Framingham Heart Disease Epidemiology Study, 3, 166, 167, 173, 180, 181, 196

Frontal lobe, neglect and, 99
Frontal lobe lesions, 107
Frontal lobe syndrome, normal aging and, 223-224
FSR; *see* Functional Status Report
Fugl-Meyer Assessment (FMA), 91, 118, 125, 339
Functional Assessment Measures, 261
Functional communication, 282-285
Functional electrical stimulation (FES), 343-344, 392, 395, 401, 461-462
Functional Independence Measure (FIM), 204-206, 207, 261, 356, 357, 381
Functional Life Scale, 302
Functional range of motion, 123, 124
Functional Status Report (FSR), 261-264

G

GABA; *see* Gamma-aminobutyric acid
Gait
    disturbances of, in persons with hemiplegia, 375-378
    quality of, 379
Gait belt, standing pivot transfer and, 398
Gamma-aminobutyric acid (GABA), 91
    central modulation of pain and, 465
    spastic hemiplegia and, 460
Gastrostomy, percutaneous endoscopic, dysphagia and, 322-323
General deficits, 246
Gerstmann's syndrome, 96, 105
Gestures used in communication, 213
Global aphasia, 93, 94, 96
Global brain hypoperfusion, 67
Global ischemia, 85
Goal setting, coaching and, 305
Good assist, definition of, 123
Grab bars, 364, 399
Gradient pressure pumps, prevention of edema accumulation and, 387
Grooming, activities of daily living and, 363-364
Gross assist, definition of, 123

H

H reflex of Hoffmann, spastic hemiplegia and, 460
Habitual control in assessment of motor control, 371-372
Haloperidol, 91
Hand movements, improvement in, 342-343
Hand splints, 130
Handicap, 16
    definition of, 304, 433-434
    enhancement of functional capacity and, 304
    occupational, 434
    provision of assistive devices and, 304
    reduction of demands of environment and, 304
    World Health Organization's model of consequences of pathology and, 299, 300
Handy-Standee, 395
Harris hemisling, 127
Hawaii Heart Association, 381
HDL; *see* High-density lipoproteins
Headache at onset of stroke, 73

Head-turning and head-tilting postural adjustments, dysphagia and, 327-329
Healing relationship, aim of, 25-26
Health care, rationing of, on basis of age, 116
Heel boots, prevention of footdrop and, 386
Help for Incontinent People (HIP), 472
Hematoma, 64-65, 71, 84-85
   pontine, enlarging, 65
   surgical drainage of, 85
"Hemi" chair, 391
Hemianopia, 105, 108
Hemibar in step-out phase of stroke rehabilitation, 399
Hemicane in step-out phase of stroke rehabilitation, 398
Hemiinattention, 98, 230-231, 362
Hemiparesis, 11, 107-108, 459-463
Hemiwalker, 398, 399
Hemodilution, hypervolemic, in treatment of vasoconstriction, 84
Hemorrhage, 81
   intracerebral, 3, 11, 31, 34, 63-65, 71, 73, 74, 81, 84-85
   versus ischemia, 63, 81
   mortality from, 31-32
   subarachnoid, 3, 11, 34, 63, 71, 73, 81, 83-84
   supratentorial, 31
Heparin
   low-dose
      deep vein thrombosis and, 39, 40
      prevention of edema accumulation and, 387
   low-molecular-weight, in treatment of occlusive thrombus, 87
Heparinoid in treatment of occlusive thrombus, 87
High-density lipoproteins (HDL), management of, in prevention of recurrent stroke, 182-190
HIP; *see* Help for Incontinent People
Hispanics, prevention of recurrent stroke and, 165-166
Home care, activities of daily living and, 366
Home evaluation, activities of daily living and, 355
Home management, activities of daily living and, 365-367
Household ambulators, 381
Hygiene, activities of daily living and, 363-364
Hypercholesterolemia, 92, 182-190
Hyperlipidemia, treatment of, in prevention of recurrent stroke, 166, 182-192
Hyperreflexia in assessment of motor control, 369, 370
Hypertension, 4-5, 6, 92
   intracerebral hemorrhage and, 11, 63
   management of, in prevention of recurrent stroke, 165, 172-179
   neurobehavioral syndromes and, 227-228
   rebleeding from aneurysms and, 84
   sexuality and, 428
Hypertensive arteriopathy, 66
Hypertonia in assessment of motor control, 369, 370
Hypervolemic hemodilution in treatment of vasoconstriction, 84
Hypoglycemia, 153, 156
Hypoperfusion
   global brain, 67
   systemic, 65-66
Hypotension, diffuse vascular ischemia caused by, 27
Hypothermia to reduce energy needs of brain, 88

I

IBM National Support Center for Persons with Disabilities, 472-473
ICH; *see* Intracerebral hemorrhage
Idazoxan, 91
Ideational apraxia, 97
Ideomotor apraxia, 97
Illness versus disease, 19-20
Imipramine, 49
Impairment, 14
   versus disability, 11
   effects of, in terms of patient's needs, 20-21
   World Health Organization's model of consequences of pathology and, 299, 300
Impotence, sexuality and, 428
Inattention, left-sided, 362
In-bed phase of stroke rehabilitation, 384-389
Inconstancy, principle of, neurobehavioral syndromes and, 226-227
Incontinence, 30, 43-44, 45, 48-49
   during in-bed phase of stroke rehabilitation, 388
   interdisciplinary goals for, 213
Independent living (IL), 16, 198
Infarct, presence of, ischemia and, 78
Informal team interventions in preparation of family for discharge, 271-273
Information gathering process to define problem, 24, 25
Ingestion and swallowing, models of, 311
Instrumental activities of daily living, 416, 417
Insulin-dependent diabetes, exercise and, 153-154
Intelligence, normal aging and, 224
Intensive inpatient rehabilitation, definition of, 146
Interactional information, assessment of, in psychosocial assessment for continued care planning, 257, 261
Interdisciplinary communication care plan, establishment of, 301-304
Interdisciplinary goals, 213-219, 268-270
Interdisciplinary plans, 214, 219
Interdisciplinary team
   formulation of interdisciplinary plans by, 212-219
   versus multidisciplinary team, 251-252
   outcome measures in, 200-212
   in psychosocial assessment for continued care planning, 261-264
   in rehabilitation management, 198-219
Intervention, Lubinski's model of, 299, 300
Interview, 19-20
Intracerebral hemorrhage (ICH), 3, 11, 31, 34, 63-65, 71, 73, 74, 81, 84-85
Intravenous (IV) needle, placement of, 385-386
Ischemia, 65-66, 81, 85-92
   definition of, 87-88
   diffuse vascular, caused by hypotension, 27
   focal brain, 27, 65-66
   global, 85
   versus hemorrhage, 63, 81
   presence of infarct and, 78
   systemic hypoperfusion causing, 66-67
Ischemic lesion, localization of, to anterior or posterior circulation, 82
Ischemic penumbra, 89
IV needle; *see* Intravenous needle

J

Jargon, aphasia and, 94, 289
Jebson-Taylor Hand Function Test, 353
Jejunostomy, dysphagia and, 323
Judgment, affect, memory, cognition, and orientation (JAMCO), multiple-infarct dementia and, 294

K

Katz Index, 356
Kenney scale, 137
Kenny self-care test, 417
Kinetron II, 397
Knee-ankle-foot orthosis, 395-396
Korsakoff's syndrome, alcoholic, procedural memory and, 247

L

Labetalol in treatment of hypertension, 88
Lability
    emotional, versus depression, 236-237
    of laughter, versus organic euphoria, 232
    pseudobulbar, of tears versus depression, 232
Language
    assessment of, during sit-up phase of stroke rehabilitation, 392
    body, 101
    normal aging and, 223
    written, acquired disorders of, 95-97
Language communication disorders, poststroke, 295, 296
Lapboard, wheelchair fitted with, 390-391
Laughter, lability of, versus organic euphoria, 232
LDL; *see* Low-density lipoproteins
Learning
    new, in rehabilitation setting, 245-250
    normal aging and, 223-224
Left cerebral hemispheric deficits, 92-98
Left cerebrovascular accidents, assessment of, in communication disorders, 283-292
Left hemiinattention in anosognosia, 230-231
Left hemisphere, neurobehavioral syndromes and, 228-229
Left neglect in anosognosia, 230-231
Left-sided inattention, 98, 230-231, 362
Lehigh Valley study, 180
Lesion, localization of, 73-77
Lesion momentum, neurobehavioral syndromes and, 226-227
Lidocaine, intravenous, in treatment of central poststroke pain, 465
Limb apraxia, 97
Limb-kinetic apraxia, 97
Limited community ambulators, 381
Linguistic communication deficits, right hemisphere communication impairment and, 292-293
Literal paraphasia, aphasia and, 289
Localization of lesion, 73-77
Locked knee devices, 395-396
Locomotion, normal, muscle groups involved in, 375, 376-377, 378-379
Lofstrand crutch, 398-399
Long-term memory, normal aging and, 223
Losses experienced by stroke survivors, 422
Low-density lipoproteins (LDL), management of, in prevention of recurrent stroke, 182-190

Lower extremities, muscle retraining in, functional effects of, 343
Lower extremity dressing techniques, 364
Lubinski's model of intervention, 299, 300
Lumbar puncture, 81, 83-84

M

Magnetic resonance angiography (MRA) in evaluation of stroke, 79-80, 82
Magnetic resonance imaging (MRI) in evaluation of stroke, 77-78
Mail order catalogs for persons with stroke and their caregivers, 475-476
Maladaptive responses, definition of, 236
Mania, 235
Manual muscle strength testing in assessment of motor control, 371
MAS; *see* Motor Assessment Scale
MCA strokes; *see* Middle cerebral artery strokes
McMaster Family Assessment Device, 255
Meal preparation, activities of daily living and, 366
Meals on Wheels, 219
Medical care, ensuring continuity of, 448-470
    central poststroke pain and, 463-468
    management of spasticity and, 459-463
    stroke prevention and, 449-458
Medical management plan, 30-60
    bladder management in, 43-49
    comorbidity and, 32-34
    deep vein thrombosis and pulmonary embolism and, 34-43
    management of seizures in, 50-60
    in rehabilitation care phase, 146-163
        cardiac disease management in, 157-162
        diabetes management in, 147-157
Medication maintenance skills, 208-209
Medications
    adverse effect of, on sexuality, 428
    dysphagia and, 317
Memory
    normal aging and, 223-224
    procedural, 247
Mendelsohn maneuver, dysphagia and, 327, 329
Metabolic equivalents of task (METs), 148, 149-154
Methylphenidate, 91
METs; *see* Metabolic equivalents of task
Mexiletine, oral, in treatment of thalamic pain syndrome, 465
Micturition, 46, 47
Middle cerebral artery (MCA) strokes, neurobehavioral syndromes and, 229
Midline stability, principle of, 337
Minnesota Rate of Manipulation, 353
Minnesota Spatial Relations Test (MRST), 354-355
Miscommunication, adverse effect of, on sexuality, 428
Mobility
    analysis of gait in, 374-381
    assessment of, 368-381
    training in, in rehabilitation management, 367-403
Mobility disorders
    adverse effect of, on sexuality, 429
    identification phase of, 384
    patients with poor neurologic return and, 402-403

Mobility disorders—cont'd
    treatment of, 381-402
Mood disorders following stroke, 215, 235-240
Motor action, behavioral units of, 333, 334
Motor Assessment Scale (MAS), 339, 340
Motor Free Visual Perceptual Test (MVPT), 354
Motor function, enhancement of, 332-346
    assessment of plasticity in, 337-341
    in rehabilitation management, 332-346
    treatment procedures in, 341-346
Motor Function Index, 338
Motor impairment, stages of, 119
Motor impersistence, 102
MRA; *see* Magnetic resonance angiography
MRST; *see* Minnesota Spatial Relations Test
Multidisciplinary team versus interdisciplinary team, 251-252
Multiple-infarct dementia, 294-295
    in communication disorders, 294-295
    deficits in judgment, affect, memory, cognition, and orientation and, 294
Multistep comprehensive program for stroke recovery, 381-384
Muscle retraining in lower extremities, functional effects of, 343
Musculotropic relaxants, 49
MVPT; *see* Motor Free Visual Perceptual Test
Myocardial disease, management of, in prevention of recurrent stroke, 166, 180-192
Myocytolysis, 34

N

NARIC; *see* National Rehabilitation Information Center
National Aphasia Association, 307, 308, 473
National Association for Hispanic Elderly, 473
National Association for Music Therapy, 473
National Association for Sickle Cell, Inc., 473
National Association of Private Geriatric Care Managers, 473
National Council on Disability, 473
National Council on the Aging, Inc., 473
National Digestive Diseases, 473
National Easter Seal Society, 473
National Hispanic Council on the Aging, 473
National Information Center for Children and Youths with Handicaps, 473
National Institute of Neurological Disorders and Stroke, 281
National Institute on Aging, 473
National Rehabilitation Association, 473
National Rehabilitation Hospital, 261-264, 266, 295
National Rehabilitation Hospital Stroke Recovery Program, 206
National Rehabilitation Information Center (NARIC), 473
National Self-Help Clearinghouse, 474
National Senior Citizens Law Center, 474
National Stroke Association (NSA), 307, 474
National Survey of Stroke, 2-3
Natural Family Systems Theory, 259
NE; *see* Norepinephrine
Neglect, 98-100
Neocortex, phylogenetic levels of, 334
Neologisms, aphasia and, 94, 289

Nervous system
    assessment of, 368
    levels of organization in, 334
Neurobehavioral syndromes, 225-233
    acute confusional states and, 232-233
    concurrent diseases and, 227-228
    left hemisphere, 228-229
    lesion characteristics and, 226-227
    rehabilitation strategies for, 245-247
    right hemisphere, 229-231
    subcortical vascular disease and, 231-232
Neurogenic communication disorders following stroke
    decision tree for, 285, 286-287
    prognostic variables important to aphasia and, 295, 297
Neuroimaging in evaluation of stroke, 77-78, 81
Neurologic assessment of acute stroke, 63-82
    for hemorrhagic lesion, 81-82
    identifying stroke mechanism in, 68-73
    laboratory evaluation in, 77-80
    localizing lesion in, 73-77
    review of various stroke mechanisms in, 63-67
Neurologic impairment, patterns of, 92-109
Neurologic management plan, 61-113
    neurologic assessment of acute stroke in, 63-82
    patterns of neurologic impairment in, 92-109
Neurologic signs
    development of, in stroke, 71
    fluctuation of, 71-72
    gradual progression of, 72
Neuromuscular therapy, 345
Neuropsychologic aspects of normal aging and stroke rehabilitation, 219-250
Neurotransmitters, ischemia and, 89
New learning
    normal aging and, 223-224
    in rehabilitation setting, 245-250
Nicotinic acid in treatment of hyperlipidemia, 190
Nonambulators, 381
Nonfluent aphasia, 92-94, 285
Nonhemorrhagic stroke, mortality from, 31-32
Nonlinguistic communication, 101
Nonlinguistic communication deficits, right hemisphere communication impairment and, 292-293
Nonneurologic symptoms of stroke, 72-73
Non-insulin-dependent diabetes, exercise and, 154
Nonoral feeding alternatives, dysphagia and, 322-323
Nonpyramidal hemimotor syndromes, 108
Nonsteroidal analgesics, 127
Norepinephrine (NE)
    central modulation of pain and, 465
    in treatment of hypertension, 178
Norepinephrine (NE) system agonists, 91
North American Riding for the Handicapped, Inc., 474
NSA; *see* National Stroke Association
Nutrition
    during in-bed phase of stroke rehabilitation, 387-388

Nutrition — cont'd
in management of hyperlipidemia, 186, 187-188, 190, 191
Nutrition maintenance knowledge, 208

O

Occupational handicap, 434, 435
One-handed dressing techniques, 363
Operational deficits, 245-246
Ophthalmoplegia, 109
Opioid peptides, endogenous, central modulation of pain and, 465
Oral phase
of dysphagia, 315, 326
of swallowing, 311
Oral preparatory phase
of dysphagia, 313-314, 325-326
of swallowing, 311
Oral prosthesis, dysphagia and, 327
Organic causes of impotence, sexuality and, 428
Organic euphoria versus lability of laughter, 232
Organizations for persons with stroke and their caregivers, 471-474
Orientation seminars for preparation of families for discharge, 266
Orofacial dyspraxia, 97
Orthosis
ankle-foot; *see* Ankle-foot orthosis
hemiplegic gait correction using, 393-394
knee-ankle-foot, 395-396
limb stability and, 381
wrist-hand, 130
Oscillopsia, 109
Outcome, Wilkerson's model of, 299, 300
Oxybutynin chloride, 49
Oxygen free radicals, 89

P

Pain, central poststroke; *see* Central poststroke pain
Palatal training appliance, dysphagia and, 327
Paleocortex, phylogenetic levels of, 334
Palinopsia, 105
Papez circuit, 104, 106
Paradoxic embolism, 66
Parallel bars in step-out phase of stroke rehabilitation, 399
Paranoia, normal aging and, 222
Paraphasias, aphasia and, 94, 289
Parent Care, 474
Paresis, 107-108, 369
Parietal lobe, neglect and, 99
Paroxysmal atrial fibrillation, 43
Partial seizures, 51
Passive assist, definition of, 123
Pathology, World Health Organization's model of, 299, 300
Patient
active participation of, in continued care planning process, 253-254
activity of, at onset of ischemic symptoms, 70-71
behavior of, in acute medical care setting versus rehabilitation environment, 242
degrees of participation of, in planning process, 23

Patient—cont'd
    effects of impairment in terms of needs of, 20-21
    empowerment of, principle of, 26
    goals for participation of, in planning care, 209, 210
    health and nutrition education for, in preparation for discharge, 267
    with poor neurologic return, special problems of, 402-403
    right of, to self-determination, discharge and, 252-253
Patient education, communication disorders and, 307-308
Pattern matching in locating cause of stroke, 75
Patterned motion, 117
PCA strokes; *see* Posterior cerebral artery strokes
PE; *see* Pulmonary embolism
PEG; *see* Percutaneous endoscopic gastrostomy
Perceived Exertion Scale, 151
Perception, activities of daily living and, 354-355
Percutaneous endoscopic gastrostomy (PEG), dysphagia and, 322-323
Percutaneous nerve stimulation for nociceptive and neurogenic pain, 465
Performance anxiety, adverse effect of, on sexuality, 428
Performance skills, retraining of, activities of daily living and, 359
Perineal hygiene during in-bed phase of stroke rehabilitation, 388
Personal information, assessment of, in psychosocial assessment for continued care planning, 258, 261
Personality changes, frontal lobe lesions and, 107
Personality factors, normal aging and, 220-221
PET scans; *see* Positron emission tomography scans
Pharyngeal phase
    of dysphagia, 315, 316, 317, 326
    of swallowing, 311, 312
Phenobarbital, 54, 55, 91
Phenothiazines, dysphagia and, 317
Phenoxybenzamine, 91
Phenytoin, 53, 54, 55, 56, 91, 465
Phonemic paraphasia, aphasia and, 289
Phylogenetic levels of archicortex, paleocortex, and neocortex, 334
Physical examination, dysphagia and, 319-320
Physiologic ambulators, 381
Pistol grip cane, 399
Pivot transfer
    standing, in step-out phase of stroke rehabilitation, 397-398
    wheelchair transfer and, 389
Plantigrade foot, 462-463
Plaque, atheromatous, 66
Plasticity, assessment of, in enhancement of motor function, 337-341
Plegia, 369
Pneumonia
    aspiration, dysphagia and, 327
    mortality from, 32
PNF techniques; *see* Proprioceptive neuromuscular facilitation techniques
Pocketing of residual food substances, dysphagia and, 325-326
Pontine hematoma, enlarging, 65
Porch Index of communicative abilities, 285
Positron emission tomography (PET) scans, contribution of ipsilateral portion of brain to recovery
    and, 335
Posterior cerebral artery (PCA) strokes, neurobehavioral syndromes and, 229
Poststroke pain, central; *see* Central poststroke pain
Powered wheelchair, 392

Pragmatics, 292
Prazosin, 91
President's Committee on Employment of People with Disabilities, 474
Primary memory, normal aging and, 223
Primidone, 55
Problem behaviors in rehabilitation setting, 245
Problem solving and practical reasoning, coaching and, 305
Procedural memory, 247
Professionals in rehabilitation environment, 242
Propantheline bromide, 49
Proprioceptive disturbance in assessment of motor control, 371
Proprioceptive neuromuscular facilitation (PNF) techniques, dysphagia and, 325
Proprioceptive Neuromuscular Stimulation of Knott and Voss, 392
Prosopagnosia, 105
Pseudobulbar lability of tears versus depression, 232
Pseudobulbar states, neurobehavioral syndromes and, 232
Pseudodyssynergia, 48
Psychogenic causes of impotence, sexuality and, 428
Psychologic adjustment to stroke, 233-245
Psychosocial assessment for continued care planning, 255, 257-261
Psychosocial factors, normal aging and, 221-222
Pulmonary embolism (PE), 32, 34-43
Purdue Pegboard, 353
Pure alexia, 96
Pure word blindness, 96
Pure word deafness, 95

Q
Quadrantanopsia, 104-105
Qualified individuals with disabilities, Americans with Disabilities Act of 1990 and, 441-445
Quality of life, 16
    enhancement of, 416-447
    enhancement of community integration and, 433-445
    enhancement of family life and, 421-433

R
Radioiodine-labeled fibrinogen uptake test (RFUT), 38
Raised toilet seats, 364
Rancho Los Amigos overhead sling, 390-391
Range-of-motion (ROM) exercises, 123, 124
    functional, 123, 124
    during in-bed phase of stroke rehabilitation, 388
Rationing of health care on basis of age, 116
Reaction time (RT) in assessment of motor control, 370
Rear-wheel-drive (RWD) scooter, 439-440
Reasonable accommodation, Americans with Disabilities Act of 1990 and, 441-442
Reauthorized Rehabilitation Act of 1992, 437
Recent memory, normal aging and, 223
Receptive aphasia, 348
Recombinant tissue plasminogen activator (rTPA) in treatment of vasoconstriction, 84
Recurrent stroke; *see* Stroke, recurrent
Red thrombus, 66
Reflex sympathetic dystrophy (RSD), 125-126
Regression as model for behavioral disturbances, 240-241

Rehabilitation care phase, 114-142, 143-412
  activities of daily living in, 114
  alleviating specific disabilities in, 279-412
  communication disorders in, 281-310
  disorders of sensorimotor control in, 116-131
  dysphagia in, 310-332
  efficacy of, 131-140
  enhancing motor function in, 332-346
  in-bed phase of, 384-389
  intensive patient, definition of, 146
  interdisciplinary team in, 198-219
  medical management in, 146-163
  neuropsychologic aspects of normal aging and, 219-250
  phases of, 12, 385
  preparing family for discharge in, 251-273
  prevention of recurrent stroke in, 164-194
  principles of rehabilitation management in, 195-278
  sit-up phase of, 389-393
  stages of, 12
  stand-up phase of, 393-396
  step-out phase of, 397-402
  step-up phase of, 396-397
  training in activities of daily living in, 346-367
  training in mobility in, 367-403
Rehabilitation environment, 241-242, 245-250
Rehabilitation Indicators Project, Activity Pattern Indicators portion of, 302, 434
Rehabilitation Institute of Chicago Functional Assessment Scale (RIC-FAS), 206-208, 261
Rehabilitation Research and Training, 474
Rehabilitation strategies for neurobehavioral syndromes, 245-247
Remote memory, normal aging and, 223
Renshaw cells, supraspinal control of, spastic hemiplegia and, 460
Repetition, aphasia and, 285-289
Residual food substances, pocketing of, dysphagia and, 327
Resolving lesions, neurobehavioral syndromes and, 226-227
Resting hand splint, 130
Restorator, 397
Retrograde amnesia, 106
RFUT; *see* Radioiodine-labeled fibrinogen uptake test
RHCI; *see* Right hemisphere communication impairment
RIC-FAS; *see* Rehabilitation Institute of Chicago Functional Assessment Scale
Right cerebral hemisphere abnormalities, 98-104
Right hemisphere, neurobehavioral syndromes and, denial of illness and, 229-231
Right hemisphere communication impairment (RHCI), 287, 292-294
  in communication disorders, 292-294
  definition of, 284
Rigidity, 459
Rivermead Behavior Memory test, 354
Rivermead Stroke Assessment, 118
Rocker knife, 362
Role changes, 347
  adverse effect of, on sexuality, 428
  effect of, on family, 427
  between spouses, 427
Role overload, caregivers and, 426

Role release, 262
Role restriction, caregivers and, 426
ROM exercises; *see* Range-of-motion exercises
Rood facilitation techniques, 392
Rostral brainstem reticular activating system, neglect and, 99
RSD; *see* Reflex sympathetic dystrophy
RT; *see* Reaction time
rtPA; *see* Recombinant tissue plasminogen activator
Rubber placemat, 362
Rupture of aneurysm, 63
RWD scooter; *see* Rear-wheel-drive scooter

S

Safety belt for wheelchair, 391
SAH; *see* Subarachnoid hemorrhage
SC group; *see* Stepped-care group
Scooter, rear-wheel-drive, 439-440
Seat cushions, wheelchair, 391
Seat lift chairs, 400-401
Secondary memory, normal aging and, 223
Seizures, 30
    management of, 50-60
    at onset of stroke, 50, 73
    partial, 51
    temporal relation of stroke and, 50-51
Self-awareness, coaching and, 305
Self-determination, patient's right to, discharge and, 252-253
Self-efficacy, 248-250
Self-esteem in adjustment to stroke, 233-235
Self-instruction, coaching and, 305
Self-monitoring, coaching and, 305
Self-motivation, coaching and, 305
Semantic paraphasia, aphasia and, 289
Seminars, orientation, for preparation of families for discharge, 266
Sensorimotor components, activities of daily living and, 351-354
Sensorimotor control, disorders of, 116-131
Sensorimotor system, examination of, 115
Sensory deprivation of unmoving limb, 385
Sensory memory, normal aging and, 223
Sensory symptoms, 108
Sentinel bleeds, 70
SEPs; *see* Somatosensory-evoked responses
Serial lesion effect, neurobehavioral syndromes and, 226-227
Serotonin, central modulation of pain and, 465
Sexuality
    in adjustment to stroke, 233-235
    in enhancement of family life, 427-433
Shoulder-hand syndrome (SHS), 125, 126, 127
Sick sinus syndrome, brain embolism and, 80
Silfverskiold test, 463
Simon Foundation for Continence, 474
Single-limb balance, 374, 381
Sinistrals, 98
Site visit by team, communication disorders and, 301
Sitting balance, 340, 373, 395

Sitting-to-standing activities, performance of, 372-373
Situational information, assessment of, in psychosocial assessment for continued care planning, 257, 261
Sit-up phase of stroke rehabilitation, 389-393
Smile, emotional, versus voluntary smile, 335
Social activities in preparation of family for discharge, 268
Sodium valproate, 54, 56, 465
Somatosensory-evoked responses (SEPs), 124
Spastic hemiparesis, management of, 459-463
Spasticity, 353, 369
    assessment of, 460-461
    management of, ensuring continuity of medical care and, 459-463
Spatial neglect, unilateral, 99
Spatial relationship, assessment of, 354
Speech, assessment of, during sit-up phase of stroke rehabilitation, 392
Speech communication disorders, poststroke, 295, 296
Spinal taps, 31
Spouses, role changes between, 427
Stairs
    Functional Independence Measure for, 207
    negotiating, with wheelchair, 401-402
Standing balance, 395
Standing pivot transfer in step-out phase of stroke rehabilitation, 397-398
Stand-up phase of stroke rehabilitation, 393-396
Stand-up–step-up exercise regimen during stand-up phase of stroke rehabilitation, 394-395
Status epilepticus, 55-57
Step-out phase of stroke rehabilitation, 397-402
Stepped-care (SC) group in treatment of hypertension, 174-175, 179
Step-up exercises in step-up phase of stroke rehabilitation, 396-397
Step-up phase of stroke rehabilitation, 396-397
Stockings, compression, deep vein thrombosis and, 39
Strike Back at Stroke, 384, 387, 388, 389
Stroke
    behavioral and psychologic adjustment to, 233-245
    definition of, 63
    differential diagnosis of, 63, 64
    distribution of symptoms in body and, 74-75
    fluctuation of neurologic signs in, 71-72
    gradual progression of neurologic signs in, 72
    headache at onset of, 73
    incidence of, 7, 8
    morbidity from, 5-6
    mortality from, 2-3, 5-6
    natural history of, 11-18
    patient's activity at onset of ischemic symptoms and, 70-71
    principles of management of, 1-26
    recurrent, 2-3, 32
        prevention of, 23, 24, 28, 164-194
            emergency response in, 455-458
            ensuring continuity of medical care and, 449-458
            maintaining regimens in, 454-455
            management of cardiac factors in, 180-192
            management of hypertension in, 172-179
            monitoring outcome in, 450-454
            treatment of hyperlipidemia in, 182-190

Stroke — cont'd
 seizures at onset of, 50
 temporal relation of seizure and, 50-51
 time of onset of ischemic symptoms and, 70-71
 "walking through" course of, 71-72
 warning signs of, 70, 208, 455-457
Stroke Club, 307-308
Stroke Data Bank, 11, 33, 165
Stroke mechanism
 identification of, 68-73
 medical factors and, 68-69
 risk factors and, 68-69
Stroke recovery, multistep comprehensive program for, 381-384
Stroke Recovery Program, 261-264, 266
Stroke rehabilitation; *see* Rehabilitation care phase
Stryker boot, prevention of footdrop and, 387
"Stunned" brain, 78
Subarachnoid hemorrhage (SAH), 3, 11, 34, 63, 71, 73, 81, 83-84
Subcortical vascular disease, neurobehavioral syndromes and, 231-232
Subluxation, 126-127
Suicide, normal aging and, 221-222
Supraglottic swallow, dysphagia and, 327
Supratentorial hemorrhage, 31
Surgical gastrostomy, dysphagia and, 322-323
Swallowing
 assessment of, during in-bed phase of stroke rehabilitation, 387-388
 esophageal phase of, 311, 312, 313
 impairment in; *see* Dysphagia
 models of, 311
 neural control and regulation of, 312-313
 normal, 311-313
 oral phase of, 311
 oral preparatory phase of, 311
 pharyngeal phase of, 311, 312
 supraglottic, dysphagia and, 327
Sympathomimetic agents in treatment of low blood pressure, 88
Syndrome approach to aphasia, 285, 288, 289
Systemic hypoperfusion, 65-66
Systolic Hypertension in Elderly study, 174

T

Tactile agnosia, 291
Tax Equity and Fiscal Responsibility Act (TEFRA), 401
TCD ultrasonography; *see* Transcranial Doppler ultrasonography
Tears, pseudobulbar lability of, versus depression, 232
Technology, appropriate assistive, selection of, 437-441
Technology related assistance for persons with stroke and their caregivers, 477-480
Technology Related Assistance to Individuals with Disabilities Act of 1988, 437, 440, 441
TED hose, deep vein thrombosis and, 39
TEFRA; *see* Tax Equity and Fiscal Responsibility Act
Temporooccipital lobes, abnormalities of, 104-107
TENS; *see* Transcutaneous nerve stimulation
Tertiary memory, normal aging and, 223
Texture modification, dysphagia and, 322
Thalamic pain syndrome, oral mexiletine in treatment of, 465

Three-hour rule, rehabilitation goal and, 301
Thromboembolic ischemic strokes, treatment of, 86-87
Thrombolytic agents in treatment of vasoconstriction, 84
Thrombosis, 74
  deep vein; *see* Deep vein thrombosis
  definition of, 65-66
Thrombus, 66
  red, 66
  white, 66, 87
TIAs; *see* Transient ischemic attacks
Ticlopidine in treatment of "white" platelet-fibrin thrombi, 87
Tilt table, 395
Tissue plasminogen activation, 455
Toilet, transfers from, 390, 399
Toileting independence, 364
Tone of motor control, 122
Tracheostomy tubes, dysphagia and, 318
Transcortical motor aphasia, 93
Transcortical sensory aphasia, 95
Transcranial Doppler (TCD) ultrasonography in evaluation of stroke patient, 79
Transcutaneous nerve stimulation (TENS) for nociceptive and neurogenic pain, 465
Transesophageal echocardiography in evaluation of stroke patient, 80
Transfer training programs, 211, 213, 382, 399
Transfer tub benches, 364, 365
Transient ischemic attacks (TIAs), 3, 34, 70, 71
Transportation, Americans with Disabilities Act of 1990 and, 442
Transtentorial herniation, 31, 35
Tricyclic antidepressants, 49
Truncal apraxia, 97
Twitchell schema of motor recovery, 392, 402

U
UEFT; *see* Upper Extremity Function Test
Ultrasound tests, noninvasive, in evaluation of stroke patient, 79
Undue burden, Americans with Disabilities Act of 1990 and, 443
Unilateral spatial neglect, 99
Upper extremity, impairment in, assessment of, 118-125
Upper extremity ergometer, 397
Upper Extremity Function Test (UEFT), 339, 341, 344
Upper motor neuron impairment, assessment of, 369-371
Urgency, 43-44, 48-49
Utensils with built-up handles, 362

V
Valproic acid, 55
Vasoconstriction, 66
Vasodilation, 66, 73
Velcro closures, 363
Verbal paraphasia, aphasia and, 289
Versaframes, 364
Vertically distributed functional systems, principle of, 334
Very Special Arts USA, 474
Videofluoroscopy, dysphagia and, 321
Visiting Nurse Associations of America, 474
Visual agnosia, 291

Visual field loss, bilateral, abnormalities of temporooccipital lobes and, 105
Visual symptoms, abnormalities of temporooccipital lobes and, 104-106
Visuoperceptual deficits, activities of daily living and, 348, 354-355
Vitamin K, dietary sources of, anticoagulation medication and, 452, 453
Voiding, neurologic pathways involved in, 46, 47
Voluntary control of movement, assessment of, 369
Voluntary smile versus emotional smile, 335
Vomiting at onset of stroke, 73

W

WAIS; *see* Wechsler Adult Intelligence Scale
WAIS-R; *see* Wechsler Adult Intelligence Scale-Revised
Walker, four-legged quarter, 398
Warfarin
  versus aspirin, 180
  effects of common drugs on anticoagulant effect of, 452, 454
  in treatment of cardiovascular disease in prevention of recurrent stroke, 180
  in treatment of occlusive thrombus, 87
Warning signs of stroke, 70, 208, 455-457
Wechsler Adult Intelligence Scale (WAIS), 224
Wechsler Adult Intelligence Scale-Revised (WAIS-R), 224
Wernicke's aphasia, 94, 95, 96-97, 285, 289, 290
Western Aphasia Battery, 298
Wheelchair, 16
  fitted with lapboard, 390-391
  fitting patient with, 391-392
  negotiating curbs and stairs with, 401-402
  powered, 392
  transfers from, 382, 389-390
  use of, outside of home, 399, 400, 401
Wheelchair propulsion, 383-384
Wheelchair tool, 391
White thrombus, 66, 87
Whites, prevention of recurrent stroke and, 165-166
WHO; *see* World Health Organization
Wilkerson's model of outcome, 299, 300
Wings, 281
Word blindness, pure, 96
Work evaluation, activities of daily living and, 355-356
Work simplification, activities of daily living and, 366
World Health Organization (WHO) model of consequences of pathology, 299, 300
Wrist-hand orthosis, 130